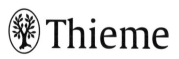

Endonasal Endoscopic Surgery of Skull Base Tumors: An Interdisciplinary Approach

Wolfgang Draf[†], MD, PhD
Formerly Professor and Director
Department of Otolaryngology–Head and Neck Surgery
Klinikum Fulda
Fulda, Germany
International Neuroscience Institute
Hannover, Germany

Ricardo L. Carrau, MD
Professor and Director
Comprehensive Skull Base Surgery Program
Department of Otolaryngology–Head and Neck Surgery
James Cancer Center and Solove Research Institute
Wexner Medical Center at The Ohio State University
Columbus, Ohio, USA

Ulrike Bockmühl, MD, PhD
Professor and Director
Department of Otolaryngology–Head and Neck Surgery
Klinikum Kassel
Kassel, Germany

Amin B. Kassam, MD
Vice President
Neurosciences System Clinical Program
Aurora Neuroscience Innovation Institute
Medical Director, Neurosurgery
Aurora St. Luke's Medical Center
Milwaukee, Wisconsin

Peter Vajkoczy, MD, PhD
Professor and Director
Department of Neurosurgery
Charité University Medicine
Berlin, Germany

498 illustrations

Thieme
Stuttgart • New York • Delhi • Rio de Janeiro

Library of Congress Cataloging-in-Publication Data
Endonasal endoscopic surgery of skull base tumors :
an interdisciplinary approach / [edited by] Wolfgang Draf,
Ricardo L. Carrau, Ulrike Bockm|hl, Amin B. Kassam,
Peter Vajkoczy.
  p. ; cm.
 Includes bibliographical references and index.
   ISBN 978-3-13-154671-5 (hardback) –
ISBN 978-3-13-154811-5 (eISBN)
   I. Draf, Wolfgang, 1940- , editor. II. Carrau, Ricardo
L., editor. III. Bockm|hl, Ulrike, editor. IV. Kassam, Amin B.,
editor. V. Vajkoczy, Bockm|Peter,
editor.
   [DNLM: 1. Skull Base Neoplasms–surgery. 2. Endoscopy–
methods. WE 707]
   RD529
   617.5'14–dc23
                                                    2015006970

© 2015 by Georg Thieme Verlag KG

Thieme Publishers Stuttgart
Rüdigerstrasse 14, 70469 Stuttgart, Germany
+49 [0]711 8931 421, customerservice@thieme.de

Thieme Publishers New York
333 Seventh Avenue, New York, NY 10001 USA
+1 800 782 3488, customerservice@thieme.com

Thieme Publishers Delhi
A-12, Second Floor, Sector -2, NOIDA -201301
Uttar Pradesh, India
+91 120 45 566 00, customerservice@thieme.in

Thieme Publishers Rio, Thieme Publicações Ltda.
Argentina Building 16th floor, Ala A, 228 Praia do Botafogo
Rio de Janeiro 22250-040 Brazil
+55 21 3736-3631

Cover design: Thieme Publishing Group
Typesetting by Thomson Digital, India

Printed in Germany by Aprinta   5 4 3 2 1

ISBN 978-3-13-154671-5

Also available as an e-book:
eISBN 978-3-13-154811-5

Important note: Medicine is an ever-changing science undergoing continual development. Research and clinical experience are continually expanding our knowledge, in particular our knowledge of proper treatment and drug therapy. Insofar as this book mentions any dosage or application, readers may rest assured that the authors, editors, and publishers have made every effort to ensure that such references are in accordance with **the state of knowledge at the time of production of the book.**

Nevertheless, this does not involve, imply, or express any guarantee or responsibility on the part of the publishers in respect to any dosage instructions and forms of applications stated in the book. **Every user is requested to examine carefully** the manufacturers' leaflets accompanying each drug and to check, if necessary in consultation with a physician or specialist, whether the dosage schedules mentioned therein or the contraindications stated by the manufacturers differ from the statements made in the present book. Such examination is particularly important with drugs that are either rarely used or have been newly released on the market. Every dosage schedule or every form of application used is entirely at the user's own risk and responsibility. The authors and publishers request every user to report to the publishers any discrepancies or inaccuracies noticed. If errors in this work are found after publication, errata will be posted at www.thieme.com on the product description page.

Some of the product names, patents, and registered designs referred to in this book are in fact registered trademarks or proprietary names even though specific reference to this fact is not always made in the text. Therefore, the appearance of a name without designation as proprietary is not to be construed as a representation by the publisher that it is in the public domain.

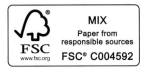

In Memoriam

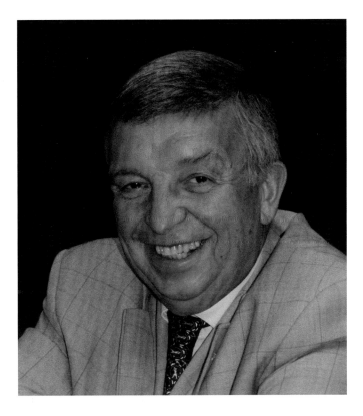

We dedicate this book to Professor Wolfgang Draf (1940–2011).

As the main surgical teacher of Ulrike Bockmühl, and as a close friend of Ricardo Carrau, Amin Kassam, and Peter Vajkoczy, he was the initiator and father of this book. But, unfortunately, he departed from us before we could finish it.

Wolfgang was an eclectic clinician and surgeon with interest in all the subspecialties of our discipline (otology, facial plastic surgery, head and neck oncology, rhinology, and skull base surgery). However, his heart would beat faster for rhinology and skull base surgery. His innovative and revolutionary contributions will mark forever the history of these two fields and his name will be passed on to future generations. He was among the first otolaryngologists to study and expand the indications of endoscopy as a diagnostic tool in paranasal sinus diseases. Additionally, he enthusiastically pioneered the use of the operative microscope in the field of sinonasal and skull base surgery for transnasal as well as external procedures. In the tireless effort of refining endonasal approaches to the sinuses, he realized that the microscope had limitations that could be overcome by the combined use of a microscope and endoscope, for which he coined the term "microendoscopic approach."

Among Wolfgang's numerous scientific contributions, the systematization of endonasal approaches to the frontal sinus, known as Draf type I to III drainages, which stands as a milestone in the history of modern rhinosurgery, deserves a special mention. His interest for frontal sinus surgery was a guiding theme in his professional life. He continued to refine his philosophy of management, remaining open to cooperation with other surgeons. He was also a pioneer in understanding the potential role of microendoscopic techniques in the transnasal resection of benign and malignant tumors. He strongly believed in the power of cooperation between different disciplines; therefore, he promoted the creation of multidisciplinary teams to take profit from the professional and surgical expertise of specialists in different areas.

Wolfgang authored many papers, books, and book chapters, as well as hundreds of invited lectures at meetings and courses worldwide and his contributions to the scientific sessions were marked by clarity, intuition, and balance. He was always open to new ideas ("never be dogmatic" was one of his preferred mottos) and he infected people with his unequaled humanity and enthusiasm. We will always miss his invaluable teachings, his sharp and balanced comments, and his witty and friendly company.

In commemoration of this honorable personality we completed this book.

The Editors

Contents

Foreword

Some years ago, I received a letter from Professor Draf inviting me to write a foreword for this book. I felt honored for such proposal, coming from such a renowned teacher. I consider myself privileged to have lived these years inside a true evolutionary process, i.e. the endoscopic endonasal approach to skull base tumors. There are no secrets to explain the success of these techniques; one must only consider four major explanations:

The first is the widespread recruitment and active involvement of young surgeons. Their energy and enthusiasm have turned a mere "attempt to change" into a continuous and high pace development.

The second is the commitment to surgical competency rather than to titles, ranks, or interspecialty turf battles, academic or not.

The third is the partnership and exchange of ideas and concerns with pharmaceutical companies and instrument manufacturers. Day after day this relationship has helped satisfy the surgeon's quest for performance improvement.

The fourth and last reason, but by no means the least important, is the cooperation among different specialists. I cannot imagine the progress of our school in Naples without giving proper credit to the professionals of contiguous disciplines, which have contributed significantly to improve our outcomes. One should consider and ponder that we would have never understood the relevant anatomy without the contributions of Manfred Tschabitscher and his peers; that we could not be abreast of evolving diagnostic and therapeutic possibilities of contemporary neuroradiology without close contact with colleagues that deal and develop these techniques, namely neuroradiologists, interventional radiologists, and endovascular neurosurgeons; that we have a better understanding of the relationships of a surgical corridor and its target with the surrounding vasculature and neural structures due to Amin Kassam's obsession with acquiring a thorough anatomical knowledge and following meticulous pre- and intraoperative preparation; that we could not have understood the design of a transnasal approach or learn to respect nasal function without the tremendous experience and didactic perspectives of otolaryngologists such as Paolo Castelnuovo and other distinguished endoscopic surgeons; that we could not achieve an intraoperative

systemic balance of the patients without the help of our operating room partners, the neuroanesthesiologists; that we depend on the collaboration with the pathologists to gain insight into our surgical specimens; and, that many times we owe our successes and ability to overcome the pitfalls of our surgeries to the interspecialty cooperation with endocrinologists.

Professor Draf has passed away, but his lessons stay; his legacy is immense and displays his extraordinary ability to share knowledge, his enthusiastic support for the scientific community and his will to participate in the process, his joy of learning, and the realization that one learns from teaching. Many times, hearing his name still sounds like music to me, like the music he loved.

The kind invitation from Professor Draf was repeated by Ulrike Bockmühl on the occasion of the 5th World Congress for Endoscopic Surgery of the Brain, Skull Base and Spine, held in Vienna in 2012, under the superb leadership of Professor Stammberger, and has been ultimately renewed by Ricardo Carrau. Ric represents the link between the otolaryngology and neurosurgical worlds, a master role model and a pioneer, a man and a "pro" per vocation, with an extraordinary sense of proportion, talented in adjusting everyday's balance, trying to find always the right distance; he figures as a paramount figure in the development and progress of skull base surgery.

This surgical opera collects the contributions from many big actors. In this current and wonderful season, it comprises the bright movement of humans and ideas around the world; thus promoting crossfertilization among different specialties and in turn impacting all of us, from the individual to entire populations. I have experienced this change; I have crossed paths and connected with extraordinary men and women and with unique people that have changed my life. Ed Laws has offered his special values of science and humanism, and Dr A. Michael Apuzzo his sharp and broad mind. I owe many others, from around the world, who by visiting my service have exposed my residents, coworkers, professional partners, and myself to multiple and new stimuli; thus creating a virtuous mechanism, a method to move frontiers forward under the realities of a team approach.

I feel proud, as a neurosurgeon, to have the task of writing this foreword. In the endonasal team approach to the skull base many figures are complementary; however, I found myself thrown into the "parterre de roi" while still considering myself as just a soldier. As a soldier, I am proclaiming the multidisciplinary teams' knowledge, competence, and respect for each other. All those who contribute to the progress are welcome, whether the contribution is strictly technological, surgical, biological, molecular, or other. Our common goal is to create a better future for the patients, and for the young generations of surgeons and physicians, those with the will to grow professionally and to better understand the disease processes. Together with constant improvement of our knowledge, techniques, and technologies we must be ready to accept novel forms of medicine, surgery, and engineering, targeted deeper toward the submolecular structures.

Nonetheless, one of the most significant innovations by those who have contributed to this book is the acceptance of the work and interventions by other specialists without feeling threatened or bothered in any way. On the contrary, they are and feel rather lucky to be able to grow and to exchange knowledge and know-how, and to live in the middle and be the caretakers of this evolution involving diseases and techniques, and impacting generations of patients and surgeons.

Paolo Cappabianca

Preface

"In times of change learners inherit the earth; while the learned find themselves beautifully equipped to deal with a world that no longer exists."

—Eric Hoffer

During the past 20 years neurosurgery and otolaryngology–head and neck surgery have evolved exponentially, bringing no less of a dramatic transformation to the treatment of skull base pathologies. In turn, the cross-pollination of multiple specialties with interest in the skull base has amplified the effect and spread of many alternative paradigms; thus, breeding a transmutation in both neurosurgery and otolaryngology–head and neck surgery. We have witnessed the introduction of subcranial approaches and pedicled flaps, and the evolution toward novel minimal access approaches such as endonasal endoscopic approaches and mini craniotomies. In conjunction with advancements in the fields of diagnostic and interventional radiology, radiation, and medical oncology, as well as technological innovations, we have improved our surgical armamentarium; henceforth, we have improved the surgical outcomes and quality of life of our patients.

The magnitude and speed of change are astounding; therefore, presenting a great challenge in keeping abreast of this ever-expanding and exciting bounty of information. Further progress can be expected as a result of ongoing experience and contemporary training by leading centers. This never-ending effort toward perfecting our care provides momentum and guidance in the search for new ideas. We remain both learned and enthusiastic learners and look forward to being humbled by new and advanced techniques that will turn our previous attempts into seemingly primitive tools.

Even in this era of digital information we rely on traditional time-proven methods to continue our medical education. A book still provides an experience and service that is different to that acquired online or with other digital media. However, books focused on the skull base are, by the very rare nature of the specialty, sparse; and that is especially true if we address those dealing with endoscopic endonasal techniques. These circumstances triggered the inception of our journey to edit a multidisciplinary book revolving around current endoscopic endonasal skull base surgery.

We have made a concerted effort to address the fundamentals of skull base anatomy and pathology that in conjunction with current diagnostic and interventional imaging techniques will serve to provide the reader with a deep understanding of these topics. Novel endoscopic endonasal surgeries are just a complement of pre-existent techniques and part of the continuous evolution of the specialty. As they mature, they will become the foundation of newer ones. Therefore, we offer a chapter where skull base pathologies are addressed from a 360° panoramic view, putting the endonasal approaches into the context of a complete skull base practice. A discussion of the general principles and management of the sinonasal corridor, addressing various perioperative concerns, follows this pivotal overview. At the core, various skull base surgery groups have favored us by presenting their experience, philosophy of treatment, technique, results, and clinical pearls. We are grateful for the altruistic spirit of all our contributors and feel extremely lucky that we were able to attract some of the most experienced skull base surgery groups from Europe and North America. Oskar Hirsch and Walter Dandy would be spellbound by the evolution of endonasal skull base surgery and the ensuing exchange of ideas more than 100 years after their independent introduction of transsphenoidal pituitary surgery.

We offer this comprehensive book on the management of skull base pathologies with the hope that it will serve as a study guide and reference work for "learners" in both neurosurgery and head and neck surgery. Notwithstanding, reader beware that although all the information offered was current at the time of writing, we do not claim to provide eternal certainties. Being "learned" is but a flitting moment.

The Editors

Acknowledgments

Although it is not possible to list all the formidable individuals who contributed to this project, we would like to express our gratitude to everyone involved in the creation of this book. Special recognition must be given to those who made this book possible:

Many thanks go to all the authors for dedicating their time, and for enriching this book with wonderful manuscripts and suggestions.

Without the constant dedication, insistence, direction, and organization of Stephan Konnry of Thieme Publishers, this project would have never become a reality.

We would like to also thank Sibylle Toenjes, MD, and Nidhi Chopra for elegant implementation of the manuscripts.

Contributors

Isam Alobid, MD, PhD
Department of Otorhinolaryngology, Rhinology Unit
Hospital Clinic de Barcelona
Faculty of Medicine
Universitat de Barcelona
Barcelona, Spain

Paolo Battaglia, MD
Otorhinolaryngologist
Division of Otorhinolaryngology,
   Ospedale di Circolo Fondazione Macchi
Department of Biotechnology and Life Sciences,
   University of Insubria
Varese, Italy

Manuel Bernal-Sprekelsen, MD, PhD
Professor and Director
Servicio de ORL
Hospital Clinic Universitat de Barcelona
Barcelona, Spain

Ulrike Bockmühl, MD, PhD
Professor and Director
Department of Otolaryngology–Head and
   Neck Surgery
Klinikum Kassel
Kassel, Germany

Ricardo L. Carrau, MD
Professor and Director
Comprehensive Skull Base Surgery Program
Department of Otolaryngology–Head and
   Neck Surgery
James Cancer Center and Solove Research Institute
Wexner Medical Center at The Ohio State University
Columbus, Ohio

Paolo Castelnuovo, MD, FRCS(Ed)
Professor and Chairman
Division of Otorhinolaryngology, Ospedale di Circolo
   Fondazione Macchi
Department of Biotechnology and Life Sciences,
   University of Insubria
Varese, Italy

Iacopo Dallan, MD
First ENT Unit
Azienda Ospedaliero-Universitaria Pisana
Pisa, Italy

Wolfgang Deinsberger, MD, PhD
Professor and Director
Department of Neurosurgery
Kassel Hospital
Kassel, Germany

Wolfgang Draf[†], MD, PhD
Formerly Professor and Director
Department of Otolaryngology–Head
   and Neck Surgery
Klinikum Fulda
Fulda, Germany
International Neuroscience Institute
Hannover, Germany

Joaquim Enseñat, MD, PhD
Division of Neurosurgery
Hospital Clinic de Barcelona
Faculty of Medicine
Universitat de Barcelona
Barcelona, Spain

Davide Farina, MD
Radiologist
Department of Radiology
Spedali Civili of Brescia
Brescia, Italy

Juan C. Fernandez-Miranda, MD
Assistant Professor
Department of Neurological Surgery
University of Pittsburgh Medical Center
Pittsburgh, Pennsylvania

Leo F. S. Ditzel Filho, MD
Clinical Instructor
Department of Neurological Surgery
Wexner Medical Center
The Ohio State University
Columbus, Ohio

Giorgio Frank, MD
Center of Surgery for Pituitary Tumors and Endoscopic
   Skull Base Surgery
Neurosurgical Department
Bellaria Hospital
Bologna, Italy

Dietmar Frey, MD, PhD
Attending Physician
Department of Neurosurgery
Charité University Medicine
Berlin, Germany

Marco Faustini Fustini, MD
Consultant Endocrinologist
Department of Neurosurgery
IRCCS Istituto delle Scienze Neurologiche
Ospedale Bellaria
Bologna, Italy

Stefania Gallo, MD
Otorhinolaryngologist
Division of Otorhinolaryngology, Ospedale di Circolo
    Fondazione Macchi
Department of Biotechnology and Life Sciences,
    University of Insubria
Varese, Italy

Fred Gentili, MD, MSc, FRCSC
Professor and Director of the Skull Base Centre
Deputy Chief of the Division of Neurosurgery
University of Toronto
Toronto, Canada

Erich Hofmann, MD, PhD
Professor and Director
Department of Diagnostic and Interventional
    Neuroradiology
Fulda Hospital
Fulda, Germany

Apostolos Karligkiotis, MD
Otorhinolaryngologist
Division of Otorhinolaryngology, Ospedale di Circolo
    Fondazione Macchi
Department of Biotechnology and Life Sciences,
    University of Insubria
Varese, Italy

Pornthep Kasemsiri, MD
Lecturer
Department Otorhinolaryngology
Khon Kaen University
Khon Kaen, Thailand

Amin B. Kassam, MD
Vice President
Neurosciences System Clinical Program
Aurora Neuroscience Innovation Institute
Medical Director, Neurosurgery
Aurora St. Luke's Medical Center
Milwaukee, Wisconsin

Daniel F. Kelly, MD
Director
Brain Tumor Center & Pituitary Disorders Program
John Wayne Cancer Institute
Providence Saint John's Health Center
Santa Monica, California

Danielle de Lara, MD
Department of Neurological Surgery
Wexner Medical Center
The Ohio State University
Columbus, Ohio

Davide Lombardi, MD
Otorhinolaryngologist
Department of Otorhinolaryngology
University of Brescia
Brescia, Italy

Diego Mazzatenta, MD
Department of Neurosurgery
IRCCS Istituto delle Scienze Neurologiche
Ospedale Bellaria
Bologna, Italy

Nancy McLaughlin, MD, PhD, FRCSC
Assistant Clinical Professor
Department of Neurosurgery
University of California
Los Angeles, California

Philip Michael, FRCS(ORL-HNS), MA(ODE)
Consultant
Department Rhinology
The Royal Victorian Eye and Ear Hospital
Honorary Senior Clinical Fellow
University of Melbourne
Melbourne, Australia

Amir Minovi, MD, PhD, MHA
Department of Otorhinolaryngology,
    Head and Neck Surgery
Ruhr University of Bochum
St. Elisabeth Hospital
Bochum, Germany

Piero Nicolai, MD
Professor and Chairman
Department of Otorhinolaryngology,
    Head and Neck Surgery
University of Brescia
Brescia, Italy

Matteo de Notaris, MD, PhD
Department of Neuroscience
Division of Neurosurgery
G. Rummo Hospital
Benevento, Italy

Eng H. Ooi, MBBS, PhD, FRACS
Head of Otolaryngology Head and Neck Surgery
Department of Surgery
Flinders Medical Centre
Flinders University
Adelaide, Australia

Bradley A. Otto, MD
Assistant Professor
Department of Neurological Surgery
Wexner Medical Center
The Ohio State University
Columbus, Ohio

Ernesto Pasquini, MD
Chief of ENT Unit Metropolitan Area
Azienda Unità Sanitaria Locale di Bologna
Bologna, Italy

Carlos Diogenes Pinheiro-Neto, MD, PhD
Assistant Professor
Co-Director, Cranial Base Surgery Program
Department of Otolaryngology
Albany Medical College
Albany, New York

Andrea Pistochini, MD
Otorhinolaryngologist
Division of Otorhinolaryngology, Ospedale di Circolo
    Fondazione Macchi
Department of Biotechnology and Life Sciences,
    University of Insubria
Varese, Italy

Andreas Prescher, MD, PhD
Professor
Department of Pathology
Institute for Molecular and Cellular Anatomy
University Hospital of the RWTH Aachen
Aachen, Germany

Daniel M. Prevedello, MD
Associate Professor
Department of Neurological Surgery
Wexner Medical Center
The Ohio State University
Columbus, Ohio

Federica Sberze, MD
Otorhinolaryngologist
Division of Otorhinolaryngology, Ospedale di Circolo
    Fondazione Macchi
Department of Biotechnology and Life Sciences,
    University of Insubria
Varese, Italy

Alberto Schreiber, MD
Otorhinolaryngologist
Department of Otorhinolaryngology,
    Head and Neck Surgery
Spedali Civili of Brescia
Brescia, Italy

Bernhard Schuknecht, MD, PhD
Professor
Diagnostic and Interventional Neuroradiology
Neuroradiology, Head and Neck Radiology
Medical Radiological Institute
Zurich, Switzerland

Vittorio Sciarretta, MD
Department of Otolaryngology
University of Bologna
Bologna, Italy

Ralf Siekmann, MD, PhD
Chief Physician Neuroradiology
Center for Radiology
Institute of Neuroradiology
Klinikum Kassel
Kassel, Germany

Domenico Solari, MD
Division of Neurosurgery
Universita' degli Studi di Napoli Federico II
Naples, Italy

Manfred Tschabitscher, MD
Professor
Department of Clinical and Experimental Sciences
Brescia University
Brescia, Italy

Mario Turri-Zanoni, MD
Otorhinolaryngologist
Division of Otorhinolaryngology, Ospedale di Circolo
    Fondazione Macchi
Department of Biotechnology and Life Sciences,
    University of Insubria
Varese, Italy

Peter Vajkoczy, MD, PhD
Professor and Director
Department of Neurosurgery
Charité University Medicine
Berlin, Germany

Andrea Bolzoni Villaret, MD
Otorhinolaryngologist
Department of Otorhinolaryngology,
    Head and Neck Surgery
Spedali Civili of Brescia
Brescia, Italy

Gerhard Franz Walter, MD, PhD
Professor and Dean
PhD-Program Clinical Neurosciences
International Neuroscience Institute Hannover
Hannover, Germany

Ian J. Witterick, MD, MSc, FRCSC
Professor and Chair
Department of Otolaryngology,
    Head and Neck Surgery
University of Toronto
Toronto, Canada

Matteo Zoli, MD
Center of Surgery for Pituitary Tumors and Endoscopic
    Skull Base Surgery
Neurosurgical Department
Bellaria Hospital
Bologna, Italy

Chapter 1

History of Endonasal Tumor Surgery

1 History of Endonasal Tumor Surgery

Wolfgang Draf[†], Philip Michael, Amir Minovi

1.1 Introduction

Endonasal tumor surgery developed from the interactions of the field of rhinology and the field of skull base surgery. Rhinology initially arose as a specialty centered on the management of infectious diseases of the nose and paranasal sinuses. Skull base surgery arose from the combined efforts of otolaryngologists–head and neck surgeons, craniofacial surgeons, and neurosurgeons devoted to the treatment of congenital, traumatic, neoplastic, and other various pathologies affecting this complex area. Importantly, skull base surgeons established the principles of management and surgery of the neurovascular anatomy that are critical to achieve optimal outcomes. Major advances in rhinology such as the introduction of microscopic and endoscopic visualization tools and techniques, and developments in radiology including computer-assisted tomography, magnetic resonance imaging, and interventional radiology, facilitated the benefits of endonasal tumor surgery. More recently these developments have been complemented through the use of powered instrumentation and intraoperative image guidance that have helped to optimize the results of endonasal surgery.

In this chapter, we hope to provide a brief summary highlighting major contributions from related specialties and significant developments that have led to improvements in endonasal skull base surgery (▶ Fig. 1.1) and have allowed it to become a fascinating and rapidly evolving concept.

1.2 The Origins of Sinus Surgery

Egyptian papyrus writings discuss rhinological techniques that were used by Egyptian surgeons to remove brain tissue transnasally as part of the mummification procedure.[1,2] In the second decade AD, Galen of Pergamum presented detailed anatomical studies of the nose describing the lamina papyracea and nasolacrimal duct.[3] It was later, during the Renaissance period, when Leonardo da Vinci (1452–1519) described different paranasal sinuses, including the maxillary sinus, and produced illustrations of the nasal conchae and the paranasal sinuses drawn from observations of anatomical specimens. Subsequently, Andreas Vesalius (1514–1564) differentiated between maxillary, frontal, and sphenoid sinuses, and Giovanni Filippo Ingrassia (1510–1580) delineated the anterior ethmoid cells. Furthermore, Nathaniel Highmore (1651) provided a detailed description

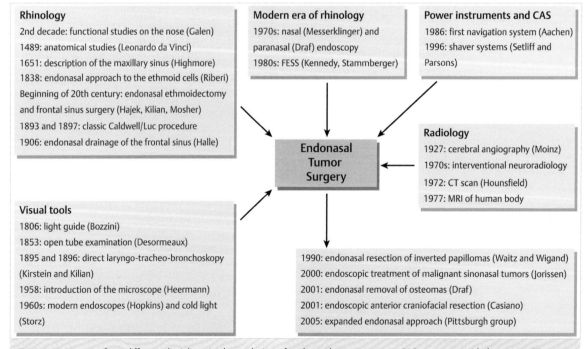

Fig. 1.1 Major steps from different disciplines in the evolution of endonasal tumor surgery. CAS, computer-aided surgery; CT, computed tomography; FESS, functional endoscopic sinus surgery; MRI, magnetic resonance imaging.

of the maxillary sinus, which subsequently conveyed his name: "Highmore's antrum."[4]

In 1660, C. V. Schneider (Wittenberg, Germany) concluded that the nasal mucus is not produced by the brain, but rather by the mucosa lining the paranasal sinuses.[5] Consequently, multiple approaches to the maxillary sinus were described to access these secretions. Molinetti (1675) published the description of an approach to the anterior maxillary sinus wall via an incision in the cheek[6] and Cowper and Drake reported the treatment of maxillary sinus suppuration through an opening of the alveolus.[3] Subsequently, Jourdain (1761) and Hartmann (1883) opened and irrigated the maxillary sinus through its natural ostium in the middle nasal meatus while Lichtwitz (1890, Bordeaux) performed the first irrigation of the maxillary sinus via puncture of the inferior meatus. Lamorier (1743) and Desault (1789) mentioned the canine fossa approach, which was also practiced by Küster (Marburg, Germany) a century later. However, unlike Lamorier, who suggested an opening through the tuber maxillae, Küster used a more anterior approach through the canine fossa utilizing a local cheek flap to line the opening creating a fistula, which was then used for further irrigation. Thereafter, Caldwell (1893) and Luc (1897) independently described a more radical surgery that included opening the anterior maxillary sinus wall in combination with an inferior meatal antrostomy. This classic Caldwell–Luc procedure remained the gold standard option in the treatment of maxillary sinusitis for many decades.

In 1905 Denker proposed enlarging the maxillary sinus approach by resecting the piriform crest. Of interest, Denker recommended the preservation of healthy mucosa as much as the procedure allowed. Although the pathophysiology of mucosa regeneration was not fully understood, a functional surgical strategy was advocated.[3]

Riberi (1838) first described an endonasal approach to the ethmoid cells in a case involving the management of the frontal sinus by resecting the lamina papyracea using a chisel. Subsequently, the endonasal ethmoidectomy technique was further refined by Gruenwald (1893), Hajek (1899), Killian (1900), and Uffenorde (1907).

In English publications, Mosher was regarded as the founder of endonasal ethmoid sinus surgery, describing a more detailed and structured surgical technique.[3] In 1912, Mosher suggested that the natural "ostium" of the frontal sinus could be reached more easily through an endonasal approach. At the beginning of this new period in rhinology, few surgeons were able to perform a successful ethmoidectomy and simple drainage of the frontal sinus, but Halle successfully performed endonasal drainage of the frontal sinus in 1906. In this pre-antibiotic and pre-endoscopic era, endonasal surgery of the paranasal sinuses was a life-threatening procedure with a high incidence of catastrophic complications including meningitis, brain abscesses, and encephalitis. Consequently, despite some early successes of endonasal surgery, Mosher declared that intranasal ethmoidectomy had been "proven to be one of the easiest ways to kill a patient." Furthermore, anesthesia techniques were inadequate to provide a bloodless operative field.[3] It was for these reasons that for many decades most rhinologists advocated an external approach to paranasal sinus surgery. From 1920 to almost 1980, endonasal surgery was generally abandoned worldwide and remained relegated to a handful of centers.

1.3 Development of Visual Tools in Sinus Surgery

Endonasal sinus surgery was revolutionized and entered a new era with the introduction of the operating microscope and subsequently the rod-lens endoscope. In the middle of the 20th century, Heermann (1958) introduced the microscope in endonasal sinus surgery.[7] A decade before, the microscope was mainly used to aid surgery of the middle ear, as it provided excellent visualization of the surgical field. This development, together with the introduction of the self-retracting speculum, facilitated bimanual surgical techniques, which enabled the surgeon to apply suction with one hand and dissect in a relatively bloodless surgical field with the other hand.

However, it was the advent of rod-lens endoscopes that renewed interest in endonasal surgery. The roots of endoscopy can be traced to the 18th century, starting with the development of visual tools for examination of organs that were deeply located. Philipp Bozzini is regarded as one of the founding fathers of endoscopy. His "Lichtleiter" (light guide) consisted of a housing in which a candle was placed.[8] In 1853, for the examination of the genitourinary passages Antonin Jean Desormeaux[9] described an open tube, which contained condenser lenses to gain a higher light intensity. Subsequently this open tube endoscopy technique was used for direct laryngo-tracheo-bronchoscopy, first described by Kirstein in 1895 and then by Killian in 1896.[10]

In 1877, Max Nitze achieved another breakthrough when he developed the first cystoscope.[11] Following Edison's invention of the filament globe in 1879, Nitze and his team were able to miniaturize it to a size that was small enough to fit into the tip of a cystoscope. However, Nitze's lens system had many limitations including poor image quality and rigidity.

To overcome these deficiencies, Harold Horace Hopkins (▶ Fig. 1.1), a British physicist, began to use glass fibers for image transmission[12]; these transported the optical image with lower degradation of quality over a greater distance, thus revolutionizing endoscopic technology.[13] However, Hopkins' innovation was ignored by industry and he was unable to continue his research. Despite this obstacle, in 1960, J. G. Gow, a British urologist, encouraged Hopkins to develop a cystoscope with improved image quality. Hopkins replaced the previous lens and air-interspace optical relays with glass rods. This development led to improved light transmission, which resulted in brighter and more detailed images. Furthermore, the viewing angle could be increased giving the examiner significantly better orientation. Using this technology, Hopkins was able to construct telescopes measuring 2 to 3 mm in diameter, which also revolutionized pediatric endoscopy. In early 1960s, Hopkins' endoscopic system was mostly ignored until Karl Storz, the head of Karl Storz Company, recognized the high potential of Hopkins' telescopes. In 1964 a very fruitful collaboration between Hopkins and Storz began. The value of these telescopes was further increased with the development of "cold light," provided by an external halogen light that transported the light through the entire length of the telescope.[13]

1.4 Diagnostic and Radiological Tools

Modern endonasal skull base surgery could not have been initiated without the parallel development of novel diagnostic tools including computed tomography (CT), magnetic resonance imaging (MRI), and angiography. In 1972, Godfrey N. Hounsfield, developed the CT scan in the UK, heralding a new era in diagnostic imaging.[14] Improvements in resolution of newer and faster CT scanners made this imaging technique increasingly popular and economical. At the beginning of the 1980s, W. Draf suggested the use of routine preoperative CT scans prior to embarking upon endoscopic sinus surgery.[15] This concept, which was initially heavily mistrusted and declined, is nowadays regarded as a matter of course. Development of a systematic preoperative CT evaluation for the treatment of chronic sinusitis ensued shortly afterwards.[16] Furthermore, CT was also advocated for the preoperative evaluation and treatment planning of sinonasal tumors.[17] Parallel to the development of CT, the diagnostic use of MRI started in the 1970s.[18] The first publication of MRI of the human body appeared in 1977. Subsequently, in the mid-1980s, the first reports of MRI of sinonasal tumors were published,[19,20] and in the following two decades MRI rapidly became the routine method of preoperative imaging of sinonasal tumors in addition to CT scans.[21]

Developments in angiography and interventional techniques, including embolization, greatly facilitated the endonasal management of highly vascularized tumors such as angiofibromas. In 1927, Egas Moniz, a neurologist from Portugal, reported opacification of the carotid artery by using a contrast medium; a technique that he called cerebral angiography.[22] Another major development was that of Seldinger, a Swedish radiologist, who introduced the percutaneous technique for cardiac catheterization in 1953. Further advances established interventional

neuroradiology as a subspecialty of radiology and led to the development of endovascular neurosurgery. Consequently, the application of interventional neuroradiology and endovascular neurosurgery embolization of highly vascularized tumors has significantly broadened the options of endonasal tumor surgery.[23]

1.5 Powered Instrumentation and Navigation in Sinus Surgery

Orthopedic surgeons used soft-tissue shavers or microdebriders during knee arthroscopy for many years before they were introduced into endonasal surgery. Dr J. C. Urban held the patent for the original instrument that was named as a "vacuum rotatory dissector." In 1996, Setliff and Parsons introduced the use of soft-tissue shavers in endoscopic sinus surgery.[24] They rapidly became one of the most commonly used powered instruments in endonasal surgery. Additionally, bone-cutting drills have been especially beneficial in endonasal skull base surgery when there is a need for extended removal of the underlying bony structures.[25]

Image-guidance systems were first used in the field of neurosurgery[26] but were subsequently found to be beneficial in endoscopic sinus surgery. In 1985, RWTH Aachen University, Aachen, Germany, designed a prototype specific for rhinology. Schloendorff proposed the term "computer-aided surgery" (CAS), which was introduced in 1986.[26] Introduction of the first CAS system in otorhinolaryngology provided real-time information regarding the location of surgical instruments. Thus, CAS aided the localization of tumors and allowed radiological confirmation of nearby hazardous areas such as the orbit and brain. CAS systems are continuously being improved by the incorporation of new technologies such as real-time updated perioperative CT[27] and they are now regarded as useful tools during endonasal tumor surgery.[28] However, it has been highlighted that CAS systems should remain an adjunct to surgical procedures rather than a replacement for surgical technique and experience.[29]

1.6 Functional Endonasal Sinus Surgery

In the period from the 1950s to the 1970s, the development of new optical aids including the operating microscope and rod-lens endoscopes revolutionized the surgical management of rhinosinusitis. Improvements in the understanding of the pathophysiology of paranasal sinus inflammatory disease played an important role in the rebirth of endonasal sinus surgery.

Endoscopes with a smaller diameter, higher illumination, and improved resolution motivated surgeons such as Messerklinger to switch from a microscope to the endoscope for functional studies of nasal and paranasal sinus mucosa (function).[30] On the basis of Messerklinger's studies regarding the pathogenesis of chronic rhinosinusitis, his student Heinz Stammberger introduced a conservative method of sinus surgery. David Kennedy, in the United States, adopted this technique and their combined efforts propelled functional endoscopic sinus surgery to a global scale.[31,32] They declared that the main goal of this surgery was to "maintain mucociliary function where possible."[33]

Complementing the findings of Messerklinger, who investigated the anatomy and pathophysiology of the nose and its relationship to chronic sinusitis, Wolfgang Draf examined the different sinuses systematically and directly,[34] becoming the first person to perform endoscopy of the frontal and the sphenoid sinus. His primary goal was to formulate more robust indications for sinus surgery, thereby avoiding unnecessary radical procedures; especially taking into consideration that imaging techniques at that time were limited and offered only plain radiograms and only occasionally conventional tomography. Subsequently, and emulating Messerklinger, Draf began to utilize endonasal techniques to manage inflammatory sinonasal disorders using the operating microscope in combination with rigid endoscopy and powered instrumentation. Between 1980 and 1984, the Fulda School developed a system of endonasal drainage procedures directed at the frontal and sphenoid sinuses.[35]

1.7 The Development of Endonasal Oncologic and Skull Base Surgery

After the new era of endonasal sinus surgery was established, a few surgeons adopted an exclusively endonasal approach for the removal of benign tumors. In 1990, Waitz and Wigand were the first to present such an exclusive endonasal endoscopic approach for the resection of inverted papillomas in a large series of patients.[36] Later, others reported the endonasal resection of other benign tumors such as osteomas.[37] The increased recognition of endonasal tumor surgery did not come without controversy, debate, and mistrust. Many surgeons argued that a purely endonasal approach may compromise the ability to remove tumor in its entirety resulting in potentially higher recurrence rates.[38] Others advocated that a complete, en bloc tumor resection was essential. Nevertheless, further developments of endonasal surgery over the last two decades have led to the wide acceptance of the concept that the endonasal approach for benign tumors is adequate in most cases.

Several authors have reported large series highlighting the possibilities, and also the limitations, of endonasal tumor surgery.[21,39] In particular, endoscopes afford an improved assessment of deeper structures and provide the capability to "look around the corner." Subsequent to the acceptance of the endonasal technique for the excision of benign lesions, a few authors presented their experience with endonasal resection of malignant tumors.[40] Casiano described endoscopic anterior craniofacial resection for the management of esthesioneuroblastoma[41] and the Fulda group reported a large series of selected malignant tumors managed through an endonasal approach.[25]

Several authors have demonstrated that in selected cases endonasal tumor surgery using en bloc or piecemeal resection and controlled by intraoperative histologic analysis (i.e., frozen sections)[42,43,44] produces equal or superior results in comparison with the traditional external procedures such as lateral rhinotomy, midfacial degloving, and subcranial operations. However, this does not mean that traditional surgical techniques are obsolete, as surgeons advocate their use in patients with large tumors.

Whereas the initial developments in nasal endoscopy were directed at the nose and paranasal sinuses, the advent of the aforementioned technological advancements in imaging coupled with procedure-specific surgical instrumentation has broadened the anatomical access afforded via the transnasal route. Interdisciplinary groups of endoscopic skull base surgery have been based upon the earlier initiatives of Sethi et al (1995) in Singapore[45] and Jho et al (1997) in Pittsburgh[46] with the endonasal approach to pituitary surgery now being commonplace. Subsequently, through the use of thorough surgical planning and training, the Pittsburgh group further developed the so-called expanded endonasal approaches. These approaches enable access to the entire ventral skull base with a minimally invasive approach associated with oncological outcomes that are comparable with conventional techniques.[47]

The first Interdisciplinary Congress of Endoscopic Surgery of the Skull Base, Brain and Spine took place in Pittsburgh in 2005 as a result of the efforts of Ricardo Carrau (otolaryngologist–head and neck surgeon), Amin Kassam (neurosurgeon), and Carl Snyderman (otolaryngologist–head and neck surgeon). This meeting brought together the Pittsburgh group with many other pioneers of endonasal endoscopic surgery from already advanced interdisciplinary groups from all over the world, for example: Paolo Castelnuovo (otolaryngologist–head and neck surgeon) from Varese, Italy, and Piero Nicolai (otolaryngologist–head and neck surgeon) from Brescia, Italy, and their neurosurgical partner Davide Locatelli (neurosurgeon); Wolfgang Draf and his neurosurgeon Robert Behr, Fulda, Germany; Georgio Frank (neurosurgeon) and Ernesto Pasquini (otolaryngologist–head and neck surgeon), Bologna, Italy; Paolo Cappabianca (neurosurgeon), Naples, Italy; Alexandre Felippu, Aldo Stamm, and Velutini (otolaryngologists and neurosurgeon from São Paulo, Brazil); Heinz Stammberger (otolaryngologist–head and neck surgeon) and Michael Mokry (neurosurgeon) from Graz, Austria; Vijay Anand (otolaryngologist) and Theodore Schwartz (neurosurgeon) from New York, United States; Alfredo Herrera (otolaryngologist–head and neck surgeon), Bogota, Colombia; and many others. It was a highly stimulating event and it was decided to continue this exchange in different cities around the world.

1.8 Conclusions

As described above, the evolution of endonasal tumor surgery was achieved through a variety of new inventions and contributions from related specialties. In particular, close interdisciplinary collaboration(s) between otolaryngologists–head and neck surgeons, neurosurgeons, and neuroradiologists during the last four decades has significantly contributed to the progress in this field.

More recent developments in techniques and equipment have increased the breadth of anatomical access afforded by minimally invasive, endonasal routes to areas previously restricted to conventional, external, neurosurgical approaches. Consequently, endonasal tumor surgery remains a fascinating field and further advancement of its techniques with fewer complications, together with a higher quality of life, is expected.

References

[1] Nogueira JF, Hermann DR, Américo RdosR, Barauna Filho IS, Stamm AE, Pignatari SS. A brief history of otorhinolaryngology: otology, laryngology and rhinology. Braz J Otorhinolaryngol 2007; 73: 693–703

[2] Stammberger H. History of rhinology: anatomy of the paranasal sinuses. Rhinology 1989; 27: 197–210

[3] Draf W. Surgical treatment of the inflammatory diseases of the paranasal sinuses. Indication, surgical technique, risks, mismanagement and complications, revision surgery [in German]. Arch Otorhinolaryngol 1982; 235: 133–305

[4] Highmore N. Corporis Humani Disquisitio Anatomica. S Broun, Hagae Comitis; 1651

[5] Feldmann H. The maxillary sinus and its illness in the history of rhinology. Images from the history of otorhinolaryngology, highlighted by instruments from the collection of the German Medical History Museum in Ingolstadt [in German]. Laryngorhinootologie 1998; 77: 587–595

[6] Lund V. The evolution of surgery on the maxillary sinus for chronic rhinosinusitis. Laryngoscope 2002; 112: 415–419

[7] Heermann H. Endonasal surgery with utilization of the binocular microscope [in German]. Arch Ohren Nasen Kehlkopfheilkd 1958; 171: 295–297

[8] Bozzini PH. Light guide, an invention for illustrative internal parts and diseases [in German]. J Prak Heilk 1806; 24: 107

[9] Berci G, Forde KA. History of endoscopy: what lessons have we learned from the past? Surg Endosc 2000; 14: 5–15

[10] Killian G. About direct bronchoscopy [in German]. Munch Med Wochenschr 1898; 27: 845

[11] Nitze M. Observation and examination method for urinary bladder urethra and rectum [in German]. Vienna Med Wochenschr 1879; 24: 651

[12] Hopkins HH, Kapany NS. A flexible fiberscope. Nature 1954; 173: 39

[13] Grunert P, Gaab MR, Hellwig D, Oertel JM. German neuroendoscopy above the skull base. Neurosurg Focus 2009; 27: E7

[14] Ambrose J, Hounsfield G. Computerized transverse axial tomography. Br J Radiol 1973; 46: 148–149

[15] Draf W. Micro-endoscopic sinus surgery. In: Advanced course of endonasal sinus surgery. Fulda, Germany; 1981

[16] Zinreich SJ, Kennedy DW, Rosenbaum AE, Gayler BW, Kumar AJ, Stammberger H. Paranasal sinuses: CT imaging requirements for endoscopic surgery. Radiology 1987; 163: 769–775

[17] Maroldi R, Ravanelli M, Borghesi A, Farina D. Paranasal sinus imaging. Eur J Radiol 2008; 66: 372–386

[18] Lauterbur PC. Image formation by induced local interactions: examples of employing nuclear magnetic resonance. Nature 1973; 242: 190–191

[19] Schroth G, Gawehn J, Marquardt B, Schabet M. MR imaging of esthesioneuroblastoma. J Comput Assist Tomogr 1986; 10: 316–319

[20] Som PM, Shapiro MD, Biller HF, Sasaki C, Lawson W. Sinonasal tumors and inflammatory tissues: differentiation with MR imaging. Radiology 1988; 167: 803–808

[21] Minovi A, Kollert M, Draf W, Bockmühl U. Inverted papilloma: feasibility of endonasal surgery and long-term results of 87 cases. Rhinology 2006; 44: 205–210

[22] Leeds NE, Kieffer SA. Evolution of diagnostic neuroradiology from 1904 to 1999. Radiology 2000; 217: 309–318

[23] Valavanis A, Christoforidis G. Applications of interventional neuroradiology in the head and neck. Semin Roentgenol 2000; 35: 72–83

[24] Setliff RC, Parsons DS. The "Hummer": new instrumentation for functional endoscopic sinus surgery. Am J Rhinol 1994; 8: 275–278

[25] Bockmühl U, Minovi A, Kratzsch B, Hendus J, Draf W. Endonasal micro-endoscopic tumor surgery: state of the art [in German] Laryngorhinootologie 2005; 84: 884–891

[26] Klimek L, Mösges R, Schlöndorff G, Mann W. Development of computer-aided surgery for otorhinolaryngology. Comput Aided Surg 1998; 3: 194–201

[27] Woodworth BA, Chiu AG, Cohen NA, Kennedy DW, O'Malley BW, Palmer JN. Real-time computed tomography image update for endoscopic skull base surgery. J Laryngol Otol 2008; 122: 361–365

[28] Doshi J, Youngs R. Navigational systems in rhinology: should we all be using them? J Laryngol Otol 2007; 121: 818–821

[29] Fried MP, Parikh SR, Sadoughi B. Image-guidance for endoscopic sinus surgery. Laryngoscope 2008; 118: 1287–1292

[30] Messerklinger W. Endoscopy of the nose. Baltimore: Urban and Schwarzenberg; 1978

[31] Kennedy DW, Zinreich SJ, Rosenbaum AE, Johns ME. Functional endoscopic sinus surgery. Theory and diagnostic evaluation. Arch Otolaryngol 1985; 111: 576–582

[32] Stammberger H. Endoscopic endonasal surgery—concepts in treatment of recurring rhinosinusitis. Part I. Anatomic and pathophysiologic considerations. Otolaryngol Head Neck Surg 1986; 94: 143–147

[33] Kennedy DW. Sinus surgery: a century of controversy. Laryngoscope 1997; 107: 1–5

[34] Draf W. Die Endoskopie der Nasennebenhöhlen. [English edition 1983: Endoscopy of the paranasal sinuses]. Berlin Heidelberg New York: Springer; 1978

[35] Draf W. Endonasal micro-endoscopic frontal sinus surgery: the Fulda concept. Oper Tech Otolaryngol Head Neck Surg 1991; 2: 234–240

[36] Waitz G, Wigand ME. Endoscopic, endonasal removal of inverted papillomas of the nose and paranasal sinuses [in German] HNO 1990; 38: 242–246

[37] Schick B, Steigerwald C, el Rahman el Tahan A, Draf W. The role of endonasal surgery in the management of frontoethmoidal osteomas. Rhinology 2001; 39: 66–70

[38] Phillips PP, Gustafson RO, Facer GW. The clinical behavior of inverting papilloma of the nose and paranasal sinuses: report of 112 cases and review of the literature. Laryngoscope 1990; 100: 463–469

[39] Lawson W, Patel ZM. The evolution of management for inverted papilloma: an analysis of 200 cases. Otolaryngol Head Neck Surg 2009; 140: 330–335

[40] Goffart Y, Jorissen M, Daele J et al. Minimally invasive endoscopic management of malignant sinonasal tumours. Acta Otorhinolaryngol Belg 2000; 54: 221–232

[41] Casiano RR, Numa WA, Falquez AM. Endoscopic resection of esthesio-neuroblastoma. Am J Rhinol 2001; 15: 271–279

[42] Hatano A, Aoki K, Iino T, Seino Y, Kato T, Moriyama H. Endoscopic endonasal surgery in the management of selected malignant naso-ethmoidal tumors. Auris Nasus Larynx 2010; 37: 334–339

[43] Podboj J, Smid L. Endoscopic surgery with curative intent for malignant tumors of the nose and paranasal sinuses. Eur J Surg Oncol 2007; 33: 1081–1086

[44] Lund V, Howard DJ, Wei WI. Endoscopic resection of malignant tumors of the nose and sinuses. Am J Rhinol 2007; 21: 89–94

[45] Sethi DS, Pillay PK. Endoscopic management of lesions of the sella turcica. J Laryngol Otol 1995; 109: 956–962

[46] Jho HD, Carrau RL. Endoscopic endonasal transsphenoidal surgery: experience with 50 patients. J Neurosurg 1997; 87: 44–51

[47] Snyderman CH, Pant H, Carrau RL, Prevedello D, Gardner P. Kassam AB. What are the limits of endoscopic sinus surgery?: the expanded endonasal approach to the skull base. Keio J Med 2009; 58: 152–160

Chapter 2

Anatomy of Anterior, Central, and Posterior Skull Base

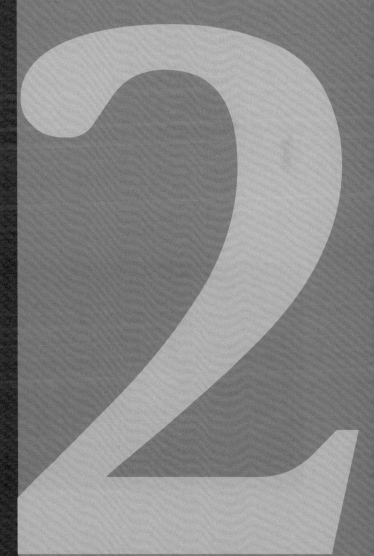

2 Anatomy of Anterior, Central, and Posterior Skull Base

2.1 The Osseous Anatomy of the Skull Base and Related Regions

Andreas Prescher

2.1.1 Introduction and General Aspects

The human skull base is a very complicated anatomical structure, which has intensive topographical relations to important neurovascular structures and sense organs. Therefore, the skull base demands a specialized and very detailed anatomical knowledge to achieve a successful surgery. Furthermore, the skull base involves different medical disciplines such as neurosurgery, ear, nose, and throat surgery, maxillofacial surgery, ophthalmology, neuropathology, and neuroradiology. Anatomy, embryology, and developmental sciences, as well as comparative anatomy, are also involved. In particular, the radiological and neuroradiological exploration of the skull base demands a very distinct knowledge of the topography, the variations, the abnormalities, and the pathology. Because of this exhaustive complexity of the structure "skull base" the International Skull Base Study Group was founded in 1979 in Montpellier by Hermann Dietz, Wolfgang Draf, Claude Gros, Jan Helms, Pierre Rabischong, Madjid Samii, and Kurt Schürmann.

In presenting an anatomical survey of the anatomy of the human skull base, the first step is to consider the osseous structures, which are fundamental. In the second step the muscles, vessels, and nerves are important and must be added to the osseous structures. In the last step the surgical and endoscopic anatomy will complete the whole survey and present the essential landmarks, the topography, and practical important facts. The overview of skull base anatomy in this book follows this concept. The important developmental history (ontogeny as well as phylogeny) of the skull base, which is the key to the different variations and malformations, is not addressed in this section, and only some hints to essential abnormalities are given. On the other hand, the paranasal sinuses are described in detail, because their conditions are relevant for the anatomy of endoscopic approaches.

The human skull base is a terracelike base plate for the cerebrum, cerebellum, and brain stem, and it can be divided into the anterior, middle, and posterior cranial fossa (▶ Fig. 2.1). In each fossa typical parts of the central nervous system are localized. In addition, each fossa can be subdivided for systematic description into two lateral parts and a medial one. The anterior cranial fossa consists of three osseous components: the frontal bone, the ethmoidal bone, and the sphenoid bone. Dorsally the anterior fossa is bordered by the margins of the lesser sphenoid wings, which are medially ending as anterior clinoid processes and the anterior margin of the prechiasmatic sulcus. The medial cranial fossa has only two components: the sphenoid bone and the temporal bones. This important fossa is bordered dorsally by the superior angle of the petrous pyramid in its lateral parts, whereas the dorsum sellae constitutes the dorsal border of the medial part. The posterior fossa is composed of the temporal bones and the occipital bone, with its basilar part, its lateral parts, and the inferior part of the squama ossis occipitalis.

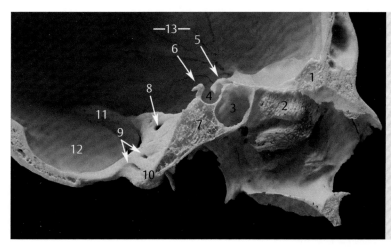

Fig. 2.1 Median sagittal section of the skull base presenting the terracelike architecture with the anterior, middle, and posterior cranial fossa.
1, Crista galli; 2, concha nasalis superior; 3, sphenoid sinus; 4, sella turcica; 5, processus clinoideus anterior; 6, dorsum sellae with processus clinoideus posterior; 7, clivus; 8, porus acusticus internus; 9, bipartite canalis hypoglossi; 10, condylus occipitalis; 11, sulcus sinus transversi and sigmoidei; 12, fossa cerebellaris; 13, sulci arteriosi of the middle meningeal artery.

2.1.2 Anterior Cranial Fossa

Medial Area

In the medial part, the olfactory fossa is visible; this consists of the fragile lamina cribrosa and the crista galli as midline structures. The height of the crista galli decreases from anterior to posterior. Different morphologic types of the crista galli, as well as of the cribriform plate, have been described.[1] In front of the crista galli the foramen cecum can be seen, which is normally obliterated in the adult. Posteriorly this foramen is bordered by the alar processes of the ethmoid, and anteriorly it is formed by the frontal bone. During development, an extension of the superior sagittal sinus passes through the foramen cecum and joins the venous system of the nasal cavity. Only in rare cases do this duct and its venous connection persist into adulthood. In contrast to this widely accepted concept, other authors[2] state that only connective tissue can be found within the foramen cecum, even in young children or fetuses. In front of the foramen cecum the crista frontalis is localized as an osseous ridge, which is often divided by the sulcus for the superior sagittal sinus. Both structures, the crista galli and the crista frontalis, are important for the insertion of the falx cerebri.

The cribriform plate presents a lot of little foramina olfactoria: 43 on the right side and 44 on the left side.[1] Furthermore, it is important that the foramina olfactoria often present larger foramina, often adjacent to the crista galli. At the bottom of these larger foramina, smaller foramina can be recognized. Therefore Sieglbauer[3] described the lamina cribrosa as a multilayered sieve. In the anterior part a distinct foramen for the passage of the anterior ethmoidal artery, accompanied by the anterior ethmoidal nerve and vein, can be described: the foramen cribro-ethmoidale.

The lateral border of the olfactory groove is formed by the thin lamella lateralis (see next). This lamella lateralis usually presents also a small foramen or cleft in its anterior or medial part, where the orbitocranial canal, containing the anterior ethmoidal artery, vein, and nerve, enters the endocranium. In the posterolateral corner of the olfactory fossa, between the cribriform plate, the sphenoid bone, and the pars orbitalis ossis frontalis, the posterior ethmoidal artery usually enters the endocranial cavity, accompanied by some little nerves and veins (▶ Fig. 2.2). This small entrance is often covered by a little osseous lamella, so that it can be difficult to recognize. Posteriorly, a variable osseous ridge borders the olfactory fossa from the planum sphenoidale, which ends at the anterior margin of the prechiasmatic sulcus. This slight osseous margin is known as limbus sphenoidalis.

Lateral Area

The lateral parts of the anterior cranial fossa are formed by the partes orbitales ossis frontalis, which often show irregular prominences, the juga cerebralia, as well as depressions, the impressiones digitatae. It is important that the lateral parts are not horizontally oriented, but present a typical declination from lateral to medial. Moreover, two characteristic depressions must be described: the fovea endofrontalis lateralis and medialis. These two foveae are separated by the slight eminentia endofrontalis (▶ Fig. 2.2 and see also ▶ Fig. 2.16). In the posterior lateral part, the frontosphenoidal suture can be recognized, whereas in the medial part the variable sphenoethmoidal suture appears, especially in younger skulls.

Important Variations and Pathologies of the Anterior Cranial Fossa

1. In elderly people the pars orbitalis ossis frontalis often can be markedly thinned, and also with the formation of dehiscences.
2. In some patients, mostly females (90% female and 10% male[4]), a condition called the hyperostosis frontalis interna affects the frontal bone as well as the anterior cranial fossa (▶ Fig. 2.3). This pathology is characterized by smooth, white-colored osseous excrescences of the inner surface of the frontal bone, in many cases including the major wing of the sphenoid bone and the temporal bone. The affected structures are also greatly thickened, but the outer surface is always

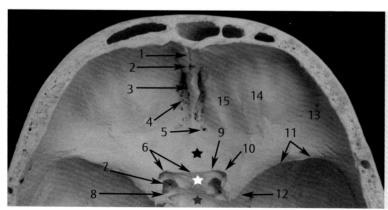

Fig. 2.2 Anterior cranial fossa. 1, Crista frontalis; 2, foramen caecum; 3, crista galli; 4, lamina cribrosa; 5, osseous corner, where the canalis orbitoethmoideus enters the endocranium; 6, limbus sphenoidalis; 7, foramen caroticoclinoideum (Henle); 8, processus clinoideus medius; 9, sulcus prechiasmaticus; 10, canalis opticus; 11, ala minor ossis sphenoidalis; 12, processus clinoideus anterior; 13, fovea endofrontalis lateralis; 14, eminentia endofrontalis; 15, fovea endofrontalis medialis. *Black star,* planum sphenoidale; *white star,* sulcus prechiasmatis; *red star,* sella turcica.

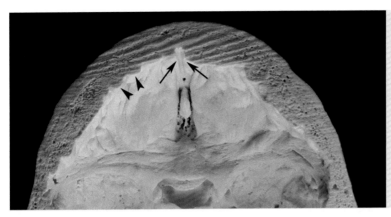

Fig. 2.3 Hyperostosis frontalis interna. Typical thickening of the frontal bone and anterior cranial fossa. Note the characteristic smooth osseous excrescences (*arrowheads*) and the pronounced sulcus for the superior sagittal sinus (*arrows*).

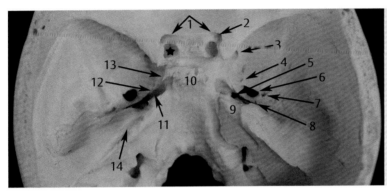

Fig. 2.4 Middle cranial fossa. 1, Limbus sphenoidalis; 2, canalis opticus; 3, canalis rotundus; 4, foramen vesalianum; 5, foramen lacerum; 6, foramen ovale; 7, foramen spinosum; 8, fissura sphenopetrosa; 9, incisura trigeminalis; 10, dorsum sellae; 11, sulcus caroticus; 12, lingula sphenoidalis; 13, processus clinoideus posterior; 14, sulcus sinus petrosi superioris. *Star*, foramen caroticoclinoideum (Henle).

unaffected and smooth. Frequently the region of the superior sagittal sinus and the adjacent areas also remain unaffected, so that the condition is divided in the midline. The dura mater adheres strongly at the osseous excrescences and cannot be separated from the underlying bone. The hyperostosis frontalis interna is often part of a triad, including hirsutism and obesity. This triad is known as Morgagni syndrome. It is questionable whether this syndrome has any clinical significance beyond contributing to the differential diagnosis. For surgery it can be important because of the exhaustive thickening of the bone and the extremely fixed dura mater.

3. At the margin of the ethmoidal incisure, where the chondrially developed ethmoidal complex fits to the frontal bone, typical clefts can persist. These osseous clefts are positioned within the frontoethmoidal sutures or the directly neighboring osseous areas. These defects are responsible for the formation of celes in this region.[5]

2.1.3 Middle Cranial Fossa

Medial Area

The medial part of the middle cranial fossa (▶ Fig. 2.4) is dominated by the corpus ossis sphenoidalis and its typical

surface structures. Anteriorly there is the prechiasmatic sulcus, which continues to the optic canal, positioned just anteromedial to the root of the anterior clinoid process. In 1 to 2% of individuals the optic canal presents a small inferior portion, separated by a complete or incomplete osseous bar termed the ophthalmic canal (foramen clinoideo-ophthalmicum), containing the ophthalmic artery.

The anterior clinoid processes, which are pneumatized in some cases, are important for fixing the anterior petroclinoid fold of the tentorium cerebelli. Furthermore, the anterior clinoid process is an important anatomical landmark for the internal carotid artery (ICA), which lies directly medial to the process. Just behind the prechiasmatic sulcus, the variable tuberculum sellae (s. eminentia olivaris) can be recognized. Behind this landmark the sella turcica is visible. The anterior edges of the sella can be bordered by variable small osseous protuberances known as the medial clinoid processes. The floor of the sella turcica presents in its center a small depression, called the fossa hypophyseos, which contains the hypophysis cerebri. The dorsum sellae borders the sella against the posterior cranial fossa. According to the shape of the dorsum sellae, four types can be distinguished[6]: forklike (10.4% of individuals), transitional form (37.5%), wall-like (45.8%), and sticklike (6.2%). In addition, the dorsum often presents as a filigree and fragile osseous structure with a cranially thickened margin. Laterally this margin forms the posterior clinoid processes, which also present in different shapes.[7] At the posterior clinoid process, the posterior petroclinoid fold of the tentorium cerebelli is fixed.

Somewhat lower to the posterior clinoid process at the lateral margin of the dorsum sellae the small inconstant processus clinoideus posterior inferius can be seen; this is the origin of a small ligament, termed the superior sphenopetrosal ligament of Gruber. The ligament inserts at the superior petrous crest, so that the foramen sphenopetrosum fibrosum is formed.[8] In some cases the Gruber ligament ossifies, so that a foramen sphenopetrosum osseum anomalum (Gruber) results. The abducens nerve passes through the foramen sphenopetrosum (fibrosum or osseum) and is fixed at the superior margin of the petrous pyramid. In this narrow area, the nerve can be compressed or stretched, especially during traumatic events. In literature, this special passage for the abducens nerve is also known as the Dorello canal. But it must be mentioned that the concept of Dorello canal is no longer convincing.[9,10]

Lateral Area

The lateral parts of the middle cranial fossa (▶ Fig. 2.5) comprise the ala major of the sphenoid bone and the facies anterior of the petrous pyramid. In addition, there is a semilunar line of different entrances and egressions in this fossa. The contents of these osseous canals and foramina are summarized in ▶ Table 2.1.

Anteriorly we can see the superior orbital fissure between the greater and lesser wing of the sphenoid bone. This fissure is hidden under the lesser wing. Then we can see the foramen rotundum, better termed as canalis rotundus,[11] because it is not a simple foramen, but a short canal with a length of approximately 2 mm.[12]

Table 2.1 Contents of the osseous canals and foramina of the middle cranial fossa

Opening	Content
Canalis opticus	Nervus opticus Arteria ophthalmica
Fissura orbitalis superior	
Intraconal	Nervus oculomotorius Nervus nasociliaris Nervus abducens
Extracoronal	Nervus trochlearis Nervus frontalis Nervus lacrimalis Vena ophthalmica superior Ramus recurrens (arteria ophthalmica) [Ramus anastomoticus cum arteria lacrimalis?]
Canalis rotundus	Nervus maxillaris Arteria canalis rotundum Plexus venosus canalis rotundum
Foramen ovale	Nervus mandibularis Plexus venosus foraminis ovalis [Arteria pterygomeningea]
Foramen spinosum	Arteria meningea media Ramus meningeus recurrens (nervus mandibularis)
Fissura sphenopetrosa	Lateral: nervus petrosus (superficialis) minor Medial: nervus petrosus (superficialis) major
Foramen innominatum (Arnold)	Nervus petrosus (superficialis) minor

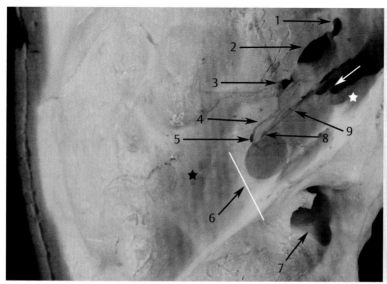

Fig. 2.5 Facies anterior of the petrous pyramid.
1, Foramen vesalianum; **2**, foramen ovale; **3**, foramen spinosum; **4**, sulcus n. petrosi (superficialis) minoris; **5**, apertura superior canalis n. petrosi (superficialis) minoris; **6**, eminentia arcuata (marked by white solid line, which is rectangularly oriented to the superior margin of the petrous pyramid); **7**, margo terminalis sigmoidea; **8**, hiatus canalis facialis; **9**, sulcus n. petrosi (superficialis) majoris. *Black star*, tegmen tympani; *white star*, impressio trigeminalis; *white arrow*, apertura interna canalis carotici; *red area*, planum meatale.

The canalis rotundus lies at the medial end of the superior orbital fissure and is separated from it by a small osseous bridge. The canalis rotundus develops as a part of the superior orbital fissure and separates secondarily. Only in rare cases does this continuity persist (foramen orbitorotundum), so that the maxillary nerve passes through the medial inferior end of the superior orbital fissure. Furthermore, the canalis rotundus is intimately related to the lateral wall of the sphenoid sinus. The next large foramen of the middle cranial fossa is the foramen ovale, positioned somewhat more laterally, which can be incompletely bordered at its dorsomedial margin.

Dorsolateral to the oval foramen the foramen spinosum (canalis spinosus) becomes obvious. In some patients this small foramen is incomplete at its dorsomedial side, so that only a spinal notch results. Rarely a fusion with the oval foramen takes place. From the foramen spinosum, osseous sulci containing the medial meningeal artery and vein run laterally. In some patients these sulci are closed or incompletely bridged by osseous material, so that canals are formed. Frequently (~42%) in the area between the canalis rotundus and the foramen ovale an accessory variable opening becomes visible.[13] This structure is termed the emissary sphenoidal foramen of Vesalius (foramen Vesalii or Vesalianum). It contains an emissary vein that connects the pterygoid plexus with the cavernous sinus. This venous route can be important for the spread of inflammation.

Dorsally the middle cranial fossa is bordered by the facies anterior of the petrous pyramid (▶ Fig. 2.5). Near the pyramidal apex we can see the trigeminal impression, containing the triangular part of the trigeminal ganglion of Gasser. The trigeminal nerve often produces a slight incisura trigeminalis at the superior crest of the petrous pyramid. According to this topographical relation the fifth nerve can be affected by pathologies of the petrous apex.

Laterally the eminentia arcuata of Henle can be seen as a longitudinal eminence, oriented nearly vertically to the superior margin of the petrous pyramid. If these typical features (longitudinal structure and vertical orientation to the pyramid) are taken into account, the arcuate eminence can be distinguished from the irregular osseous eminences in this region. The arcuate eminence is related to the superior (anterior) semicircular canal and can be used as landmark for the localization of the internal acoustic meatus while performing the transtemporal approach through the middle cranial fossa. Recent investigations show that the arcuate eminence is a reliable landmark in only 37% of patients.[14]

Lateral to the eminence, a thin osseous plate can be seen, termed the tegmen tympani, which is the roof of the tympanic cavity as well as of the antrum mastoideum. The roof above the antrum is also termed as tegmen antri.

The anterior area of the petrous pyramid contains two small osseous sulci, running from a lateral superior to a medial inferior direction. The medial rim, usually better expressed, starts at the hiatus canalis facialis (Fallopii) (s. hiatus canalis n. petrosi majoris) and runs toward the medial part of the fissura sphenopetrosa (▶ Fig. 2.5). This sulcus contains the (superficial) greater petrosal nerve, which penetrates the fibrobasal cartilage. Traction of this nerve must be avoided, for example during the dural reflexion performed by a middle cranial fossa approach toward the meatus acusticus internus, because traction may cause a lesion of the facial nerve. Laterally in the parallel sulcus the (superficial) lesser petrosal nerve is embedded. This small nerve enters the middle cranial fossa at the hiatus canalis n. petrosi minoris at the anterior facies of the pyramid, and runs toward the sphenopetrous fissure. In some cases a separate foramen for this nerve is expressed: the innominate foramen of Arnold. Both nerves are accompanied by small arteries branching from the middle meningeal artery: the (superficial) greater petrosal nerve is accompanied by the superficial petrosal artery, the (superficial) lesser petrosal nerve by the superior tympanic artery. Both small vessels are important, because they contribute in a variable manner to the vascularization of the facial nerve within its canal. Therefore these vessels should be preserved during surgical procedures in this region.

The osseous field determined by the arcuate eminence and the hiatus canalis facialis was termed planum meatale by Fisch (▶ Fig. 2.5). This planum meatale is important for the topographical orientation performing the subtemporal middle fossa approach toward the internal acoustic meatus. In the elderly, cribriform dehiscences are seen often in the tegmen tympani and the tegmen antri. Joseph Hyrtl, the famous anatomist from Vienna, assumed that these osseous changes were due to high pressure in the tympanic cavity produced by indecently loud and forceful sneezing. This kind of sneezing does not occur today, but the frequency of dehiscences is the same as in Hyrtl's day. Therefore Hyrtl's hypothesis cannot be verified. The dehiscences develop as atrophic osseous changes, due to the continuous pulsation of the brain. Similar changes can be observed in the region where the temporal lobe is adjacent to the greater wing of the sphenoid bone. The dehiscences of the tegmen tympani may be important for the spread of inflammation from the middle ear toward the endocranium. But it must be stated that small veins connecting the tympanic cavity with the endocranium are more important for these pathological conditions than the dehiscences.[15]

The carotid canal opens at the apex of the petrous pyramid with its superior aperture. This aperture, also termed the foramen lacerum anterius internum,[16] is a very variable opening in the upper frontal part of the carotid canal. Frequently the aperture reaches far laterally, so that the ICA is positioned directly under the dura mater of the middle cranial fossa. After entering the endocranium the artery lies directly above the foramen lacerum, which is closed by the thick and resistant fibrobasal cartilage. Above this cartilage the artery bends upwards and has an intimate position to the lateral wall of the sphenoid body. This osseous wall is often slightly depressed, so that a sulcus caroticus appears. In such cases the ICA protrudes slightly into the sphenoid sinus. A various osseous spur, the lingula sphenoidalis, fixes the ICA to the lateral wall of the sphenoid body. Five different types of the lingula sphenoidalis are distinguished.[17]

Important Variations

Foramen Meningo-orbitale

In 21% of individuals,[13] an accessory small foramen meningo-orbitale occurs at the lateral end of the superior orbital fissure. This foramen contains the small meningo-orbital artery, which anastomoses the lacrimal artery with the middle meningeal artery. In some cases the middle meningeal artery is completely branching from the lacrimal artery, so that no foramen spinosum exists.

Foramen Caroticoclinoideum (Henle)

In some cases the middle clinoid process fuses with the anterior clinoid process (▶ Fig. 2.2 and ▶ Fig. 2.4), so that an accessory foramen for the ICA results. This structure is termed the foramen caroticoclinoideum (Henle) and appears with a frequency about 7.7%.[18] The condition can be identified in X-ray films as well as in computed tomography (CT) scans.

Taenia Interclinoidea

The fusion between the anterior and posterior clinoid processes is known as the taenia interclinoidea and occurs in 5.9% of individuals.[19] The different forms of osseous connections between the clinoid processes are also known as "sella bridging" or "ponticuli sellae." A great deal of literature has been published concerning the question of whether "sella bridging" accompanies hormonal and nervous ailment. This question has not yet been answered clearly.

Trigeminal Bridge

A variable osseous or calcified bridging over the trigeminal incisure at the superior margin of the petrous pyramid is termed the trigeminal bridge. This bridge can be explained phylogenetically, but is of no clinical importance.

Ductus Craniopharyngeus Persistens (Landzert)

Rarely in adulthood can a small duct be present in the floor of the sella turcica, which opens into the epipharynx. This duct, the ductus craniopharyngeus persistens, is an embryologic remnant from the Rathke pouch, which is important for the development of the adenohypophysis. A complete canal can be observed in 0.3 to 0.52% of individuals, whereas an incomplete form occurs somewhat more frequently.[20]

Canalis Craniopharyngeus Lateral (Sternberg) (Sternberg Canal)

During development of the sphenoid bone an incomplete fusion between the greater wing and the presphenoid/basisphenoid leads to the lateral craniopharyngeal canal. This canal was originally described by Sternberg in 1888.[21] Sternberg[21] observed this canal regularly in children at the age of 3 to 4 years, but in only about 4% of adults. Therefore this canal must be seen as an embryologic remnant. The Sternberg canal may cause an intrasphenoidal meningocele.[22]

Aplasia of Foramen Spinosum

If the foramen spinosum is missing, two varieties can be assumed. First, the medial meningeal artery can be perfused completely by a persistent stapedial artery, which is usually combined with the absence of the foramen spinosum (see below). In the second case the medial meningeal artery branches from the lacrimal artery of the orbit and enters the endocranial cavity through a large meningo-orbital foramen. In such cases the foramen is also missing.

2.1.4 Posterior Cranial Fossa

The large and deep posterior cranial fossa (▶ Fig. 2.6) is bordered mainly by the temporal and occipital bone as well as by the dorsum sellae at the anterior end of the clivus. The posterior fossa can also be subdivided into a medial and two lateral parts.

Medial Area

The central part is formed by the clivus of Blumenbach, which starts just behind the dorsum sellae. In youth, we can recognize the large synchondrosis sphenooccipitalis directly behind the dorsum sellae. This synchondrosis acts as an important growth area for the skull base and ossifies between 16 and 20 years. If this fissure has been synostosized, the occipital bone is fixed firmly to the sphenoid bone. This unit is often called the os basilare. Virchow[23] termed this central part of the skull base the os tribasilare. The third part of this structure is the presphenoid component of the sphenoid bone, which contacts the basisphenoid in the synchondrosis intersphenoidalis. The clivus, which often presents a slender concavity on its endocranial surface, ends at the foramen magnum as its anterior margin. Laterally this mighty foramen is bordered by the lateral parts of the occipital bone, which mainly form the occipital condyles.

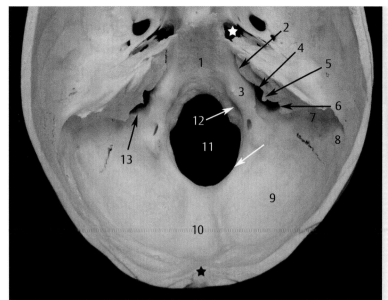

Fig. 2.6 Posterior cranial fossa.
1, Clivus; 2, synchondrosis petrooccipitalis and sulcus sinus petrosi inferioris; 3, tuberculum jugulare; 4, foramen jugulare: pars nervosa; 5, processus intrajugularis; 6, foramen jugulare: pars venosa; 7, sulcus sinus sigmoidei; 8, sulcus sinus transversi; 9, fossa cerebellaris; 10, trigonum vermianum; 11, foramen occipitale magnum; 12, canalis n. hypoglossi; 13, margo sigmoidea terminalis. *White star,* foramen lacerum; *black star,* protuberantia occipitalis interna.

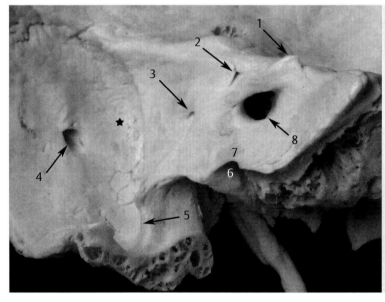

Fig. 2.7 Facies posterior of the petrous pyramid.
1, Exostosis supra meatum; 2, hiatus subarcuatus; 3, apertura externa canaliculi vestibuli; 4, emissarium mastoideum; 5, margo sigmoidea terminalis; 6, apertura externa canaliculi cochleae; 7, janua arcuata; 8, porus and meatus acusticus internus. *Star,* sulcus sinus sigmoidei.

The basis of the occipital condyle is traversed by the canalis hypoglossi, which can be subdivided into two canals (canalis hypoglossi bipartitus) in about 56.2% of individuals.[24] The hypoglossal canal contains the hypoglossal nerve as well as a mighty venous plexus. On the endocranial surface the entrance of the canalis hypoglossi is marked by the tuberculum jugulare, which is positioned somewhat anteriorly to the canal. The medial part of the posterior margin of the foramen magnum rarely presents an osseous process, called the Kerckring process.[25] Newborns frequently have a small notch in this region, the incisura occipitalis posterior, which can persist to adulthood. Dorsally the medial region is formed by the squama ossis occipitalis with the protuberantia occipitalis interna and the crista occipitalis. The crista occipitalis can be divided so that an oval fossa, the trigonum vermianum, results, which contains the vermis of the cerebellum.

Lateral Area

The lateral part is bordered by the posterior facies of the temporal pyramid (▶ Fig. 2.7). This posterior area shows essential anatomical structures. As a major structure the somewhat medially positioned porus acusticus internus, leading into the meatus acusticus internus, can be

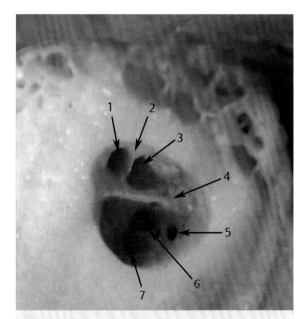

Fig. 2.8 Fundus meatus acustici interni (right side).
1, Area n. facialis; **2**, crista verticalis (Bill's bar); **3**, area vestibularis superior; **4**, crista transversa s. falciformis; **5**, foramen singulare; **6**, area vestibularis inferior; **7** area cochleae with tractus spiralis foraminosus and with foramen centrale cochleae.

separates a superior half from an inferior one. The superior region is further subdivided by a smaller, dorsally inclined crest, the crista verticalis (or Bill's bar according to William House). Bill's bar separates topographically the facial nerve from the n. utriculoampullaris (s. vestibularis superior) and therefore represents an important landmark. The different areas of the fundus meatus acustici interni contain the openings for the different nerval structures. These functionally important nerves are summarized in ► Table 2.2. It is topographically important that only the delicate osseous plate of the fundus forms the medial wall of the labyrinth. An injury of this plate may lead to a serious cerebrospinal liquor fistula.

Superior and somewhat lateral to the internal acoustic porus, the hiatus subarcuatus can be recognized. Here the thin subarcuate artery is running into the subarcuate s. petromastoid canal. Moreover, between the internal acoustic porus and the anterior edge of the sigmoid sinus sulcus a flat tray can be observed, which contains the apertura externa canaliculi (s. aquaeductus) vestibuli. Normally this opening is hidden under a small osseous edge. Under this structure the endolymphatic duct forms the endolymphatic sac. The pars rugosa of the endolymphatic sac, important for the resorption of the endolymphatic fluid, is normally positioned in the osseous canal, whereas the capillary cleft of the pars intraduralis lies between the dural sheets. The endolymphatic sac lies within the Trautmann triangle, which is bordered laterally by the sigmoid sinus, cranially by the superior petrous sinus, and medially by the jugular bulb.

At the medial inferior border of the pyramid the sulcus sinus petrosi inferioris is located. Just behind this the jugular incision can be seen. Furthermore, a variable osseous spur, the intrajugular process, must be mentioned, which subdivides the jugular foramen.

Vertically under the internal acoustic porus a smooth osseous bridge, the janua arcuata, is visible. This bridge lies above the apertura externa canaliculi cochleae like a

recognized. The porus is bordered by a lateral osseous lip and a medial, smooth rounded margin. Just above the porus an exostosis supra meatum is often expressed. It is topographically important that the internal acoustic meatus is lying under the floor of the medial cranial fossa. Therefore the meatus can be reached surgically by drilling the planum meatale (transtemporal or subtemporal approach through the middle cranial fossa).

The meatus acusticus internus ends with the fundus meatus acustici interni, which is subdivided by osseous crests (► Fig. 2.8). The crista transversa (s. falciformis)

Table 2.2 Structures of the fundus meatus acustici interni

Opening	Nerve	Function
Area nervi facialis, synonym: introitus canalis facialis	Nervus intermediofacialis	Motoric: mimic muscles, musculus stapedius, and some suprahyoidal muscles. Sensitive: auditory canal, ear concha. Sensory: anterior two-thirds of the tongue. Parasympathetic: Gll, lacrimalis, submandibularis and sublingualis
Area vestibularis superior, synonym: area utriculoampullaris	Nervus utriculoampullaris	Equilibrium
Area vestibularis Inferior, synonym: area saccularis	Nervus saccularis	Equilibrium
Area cochleae with tractus spiralis foraminosus	Pars cochlearis Nervus vestibulocochlearis	Auditory
Foramen singulare	Nervus ampullaris posterior	Equilibrium

roof. In adulthood this aperture is usually closed by a meshwork of arachnoidal fibers and proliferations.

Laterally the large sulcus sinus sigmoidei can be seen, which terminates at the margo sigmoidea terminalis. After passing this osseous ridge the sinus passes over into the internal jugular vein. The emissarium mastoideum, very variable in size and position, opens into the sigmoid sinus. The distal part of the sigmoid sinus and the jugular bulb present different and important variations: the anterior position of the sigmoid sinus must be mentioned as well as the medial or lateral high-positioned bulbus. The anterior position of the sigmoid sinus is characterized by an intimate relation of the sinus to the external acoustic meatus.

In cases of an anterior position of the sigmoid sinus the approach towards the antrum, the tympanic cavity or the labyrinth can be difficult. A medially positioned high bulb projects just laterally of the internal acoustic porus, whereas a lateral high-positioned jugular bulb projects into the tympanic cavity. This projection may cause osseous dehiscences in the floor of the tympanic cavity, so that the wall of the jugular bulb is lying directly at the mucous membrane of the tympanic cavity.[26] In such cases a paracentesis must be performed very carefully in order not to lacerate the jugular bulb. In addition, pathological conditions, for example inflammations, easily can involve the venous structures and cause a thrombosis of the jugular vein.

Important Variations of the Posterior Cranial Fossa

Basilar Canals

In some cases a canalis basilaris (medianus) can be present in the basal part of the occipital bone. Usually this canal contains a vein or venous plexus, which can be seen as former basivertebral veins of the vertebral material, which was incorporated into the skull base. In adults, the frequency of a persistent canalis basilaris is 7.86%.[27] Different entities (canalis basilaris medianus superior, canalis basilaris inferior 1, canalis basilaris medianus bifurcatus, and canalis basilaris inferior 2) are summarized by Lang.[12]

Basilar Transverse Fissure (Sauser Fissure)

The extraordinarily rare basilar transverse fissure is a unilaterally or bilaterally incomplete or complete cleft or groove in the pars basilaris ossis occipitalis at the level of the pharyngeal tubercle. For the various types of segmentation of the basioccipital bone see Le Double.[28] Confusion with the synchondrosis sphenooccipitalis belonging to normal anatomy in children and juveniles should be avoided.

Platybasia and Basilar Impression

For these typical pathologies, which are not synonymous, see Klaus[29] and Graf von Keyserlingk and Prescher.[30]

2.1.5 Paranasal Sinuses

The Ethmoid Sinus

The ethmoid sinus represents the most complicated part of the paranasal sinus system, so that it is also called the ethmoidal labyrinth. This is composed of several minor pneumatic cells located bilaterally beside the upper part of the nasal cavity. These ethmoidal cells are separated from the orbit by the very thin lamina orbitalis ossis ethmoidalis, also termed the lamina papyracea. This very thin structure is stabilized by the walls of the ethmoidal cells (▶ Fig. 2.9). Cranially the ethmoid labyrinth reaches the anterior cranial fossa beside the olfactory groove and forms part of the so-called rhinobase, a term introduced by Wullstein and Wullstein in 1970.[31] Dorsally the ethmoid complex is bordered by the sphenoid sinus, and caudally it reaches the maxillary sinus and the nasal cavity. Anteriorly it is confined by the frontal and nasal bones.

For the description of the ethmoidal complex, the fixing line of the middle turbinate, called "basal lamella of the middle turbinate," is essential (▶ Fig. 2.10). This "basal lamella" can be divided into three parts: the first part is oriented vertically, the medial part frontally, and the posterior part horizontally. These three parts present a constant attachment at the osseous structures of the lateral wall of the nasal cavity. The vertical part is fixed at the

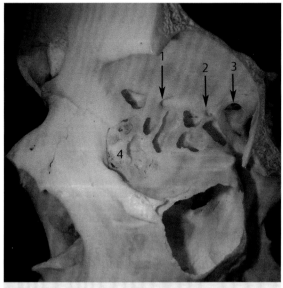

Fig. 2.9 Medial wall of the orbit with cellulae ethmoidales. **1**, Foramen ethmoidale anterius; **2**, foramen ethmoidale posterius; **3**, canalis opticus; **4**, os lacrimale and fossa sacci lacrimalis.

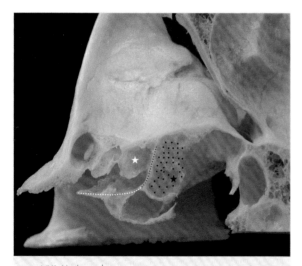

Fig. 2.10 Horizontal section of the ethmoid, showing the basal lamina and its different parts. *Dotted line*, basal lamella of the middle turbinate; *white dotted line*, anterior, vertically oriented part; *red dotted line*, medial, frontally oriented part; *scattered black points*, posterior, horizontal part, forming the roof of the middle nasal meatus; *white star*, anterior ethmoid; *black star*, posterior ethmoid.

lateral edge of the lamina cribrosa; it is often termed the "lamina conchalis."[32,33] The medial part is fixed at the lamina orbitalis and the posterior part also at the lamina orbitalis and additionally at the medial wall of the maxillary sinus. This complicated fixing line provides a three-dimensional stabilization and therefore contributes essentially to the stability of the middle turbinate. Furthermore, this constant osseous attachment of the middle turbinate is used for the division of the ethmoidal complex (▶ Fig. 2.10): in front of the line the anterior ethmoidal cells are located, whereas behind this line the posterior ethmoidal cells are found. The openings of the

anterior cells are located in front of and beneath the basal lamella, whereas the posterior ethmoidal cells open behind and above the basal lamella. A classification that describes middle ethmoidal cells is not supported by topographical or developmental arguments.[34] In addition, the middle turbinate can be pneumatized, and contain a large cavity. This condition is termed concha bullosa and appears in approximately 8% of individuals.[35]

For the endoscopic orientation at the lateral wall of the nasal cavity two osseous structures of the ethmoidal complex are very important: the prominent ethmoidal bulla and the uncinate process (▶ Fig. 2.11). The sickle-shaped uncinate process was first described by Johann Friedrich Blumenbach in 1790.[36] This structure represents a thin brittle osseous lamella, which is sagittally oriented and dorsally has quite a concave margin and an anterior convex one. Dorsally and inferiorly the uncinate process is attached to the perpendicular lamina of the palatine bone and at the ethmoidal process of the inferior turbinate. Cranially the uncinate process may be fixed at different structures, so that systematically three different topographical situations can be classified (▶ Fig. 2.12):

- Type A: the uncinate process inserts at the lamina papyracea.
- Type B1: the uncinate process inserts at the skull base.
- Type B2: the insertion is at the middle turbinate.

These conditions are important for the opening of the frontal sinus. In the type A situation the sinus opens into the middle nasal meatus, whereas in the type B1 or B2 situation it opens into the ethmoidal infundibulum. It is important to mention that at the anterior margin osseous dehiscences may occur, which are termed anterior nasal fontanelles (Zuckerkandl fontanelles) (▶ Fig. 2.11). Posterior nasal fontanelles are located in the region of the dorsal end of the uncinate process, where it is fixed at the perpendicular lamina of the palatine bone. Regularly

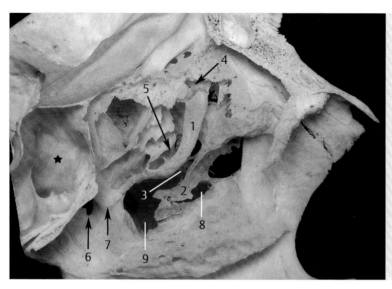

Fig. 2.11 Ethmoid complex at the lateral wall of the nasal cavity after removing the middle turbinate.
1, Bulla ethmoidalis; 2, processus uncinatus; 3, infundibulum ethmoidale; 4, recessus suprabullaris; 5, recessus retrobullaris; 6, foramen sphenopalatinum; 7 crista ethmoidalis; 8, anterior fontanelle (of Zuckerkandl); 9, posterior fontanelle (of Giraldes). *Star*, sinus sphenoidalis

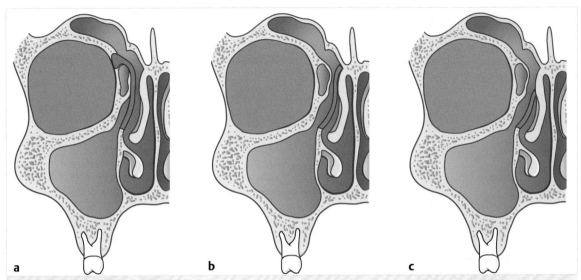

Fig. 2.12 a–c Different types of uncinate process. Type A: the uncinate process (red) is inserted at the lamina papyracea; therefore the frontal sinus opens into the middle nasal meatus (**a**). Type B1: the uncinate process (red) is inserted at the lateral border of the cribriform plate. The frontal sinus opens in the ethmoidal infundibulum. A terminal recess occurs (**b**). Type B2: the uncinate process (red) is inserted at the basal lamella of the middle turbinate. The frontal sinus also opens into the ethmoidal infundibulum and a terminal recess is present (**c**).

the osseous nasal fontanelles are enclosed by the mucous membrane, but accessory openings of the maxillary sinus may occur in about 10% of these positions,[37] which lead directly to the lumen of the maxillary sinus. In some cases the uncinate process is bent into the nasal cavity and often reaches the lateral surface of the medial turbinate. This anatomical variation can be seen as an atavism and was called "doubled medial turbinate" by Kaufmann in 1890.[38] In rare cases the uncinate process can be pneumatized or it can deviate laterally into the maxillary sinus.

The term ethmoidal bulla was introduced by Zuckerkandl in 1893,[39] although this structure was well known before. Samuel Thomas Sömmering described this structure as "Pars turgida ossis ethmoidalis" and Zoja called it "Eminentia fossae nasalis" in 1870. The ethmoid bulla is the largest and most constant anterior ethmoidal cell, positioned with a broad base on the lamina papyracea. In 30% of individuals the ethmoidal bulla lacks pneumatization, so that an osseous torus is formed.[32,33] This variation should be termed the "Torus ethmoidalis." The topographical relations to the neighboring structures are important. If the ethmoidal bulla reaches the skull base, the bulla forms the posterior border of the frontal recess. If it does not reach the skull base, an accessory recess is formed above the ethmoidal bulla, and this is termed as suprabullar recess (▶ Fig. 2.11). If the dorsal border of the ethmoidal bulla does not reach the middle turbinate a retrobullar recessus will be established. Grünwald (1925)[35] termed the irregular spaces of the suprabullar and the infrabullar recesses together as "lateral sinus."

Between the ethmoidal bulla and the uncinate process the semilunar hiatus is located. This structure shows a sagittally oriented cleft, which represents the entrance into the ethmoidal infundibulum. The ethmoidal infundibulum, the term was introduced by Boyer in 1805 but termed primarily the recessus frontalis, forms an atrium of the maxillary sinus. The frontal sinus can open into the ethmoidal infundibulum, usually in the region between the medial and posterior third.

If an exhaustive pneumatization takes place, some accessory cells or cell groups may occur within the ethmoidal labyrinth. The lacrimal cells are located within the lacrimal bone. The sphenoethmoidal cells of Onodi-Grünwald are in intimate position to the optic canal (▶ Fig. 2.13) and, in rare cases, the entire optic canal can be surrounded by these pneumatic cells. If a close relationship between the optic nerve and a sphenoethmoidal cell is present, the optic nerve can bulge into the pneumatic space. This bulging structure is termed the optic nerve tubercle. Onodi-Grünwald cells occur in approximately 11.4% of individuals.[32,33] These cells are very important because of the very close relationship between the cells and the content of the optic canal. As a consequence of this topography the optic nerve can be easily damaged during surgical procedures in the posterior ethmoidal labyrinth. Otherwise inflammations of the cells can spread easily into the optic canal, especially if there are dehiscences in the osseous wall of the optic canal. In the region of the agger nasi pneumatizations can occur often, called agger cells. These cells are present in approximately 89% of individuals, and can therefore be

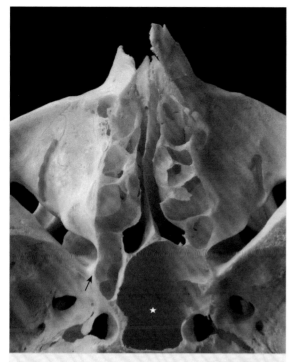

Fig. 2.13 Horizontal section of the ethmoid. Onodi–Grünwald cell (red star) beside the sphenoid sinus (white star). *Arrow*, floor of the optic canal.

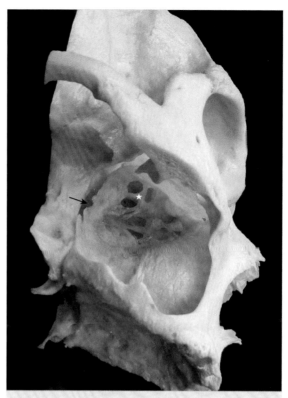

Fig. 2.14 Maxillary sinus, opened laterally. *Star*, infraorbital cells (v. Haller); *arrow*, fissura pterygomaxillaris, which is the entrance into the pterygopalatine fossa.

considered to be anatomically normal.[40] They are in direct contact with the laterally positioned nasolacrimal duct. This topography should be kept in mind during operations. On the other hand a dacryocystorhinostomy can be easily performed at this site. In the medial infraorbital region, accessory pneumatizations may also occur (▶ Fig. 2.14). These cells are called "infraorbital ethmoidal cells (v. Haller cells)," first described by Albrecht von Haller in 1743. The infraorbital ethmoidal cells may originate from the anterior or from the posterior ethmoid. These pneumatic cells are important for the orientation during operation. Performing a transmaxillary approach to the ethmoidal labyrinth, the v. Haller cells can be used. If they are not established, a false route can be taken and the orbita can be damaged. In some cases the infraorbital cells include the infraorbital nerve, which can also be a dangerous topographical situation. Large infraorbital cells narrow the ethmoidal infundibulum and can therefore be responsible for the pathology of the maxillary sinus. The frontal cells or bullae frontales occur in about 20% of individuals (see ▶ Fig. 2.17). These cells are typical anterior ethmoidal cells that bulge into the floor of the frontal sinus and distort the frontal infundibulum of Killian, so that there is a considerable narrowing of the outlet structure of the frontal sinus. Nowadays it is important to differentiate the frontal cells (bullae frontales) from cells of the Kuhn type. The posterior wall of the bullae frontales is formed by the wall of the cranial vault, whereas the

Kuhn type III or IV cells have an individually separated border.

The ethmoidal labyrinth is crossed by two important arteries, accompanied by small veins and nerves: the anterior ethmoidal artery and the posterior ethmoidal artery. Both arteries arise from the ophthalmic artery and belong therefore to the area supplied by the ICA. At the medial border of the orbit, regularly at the superior margin of the lamina papyracea (synonym: lamina orbitalis ossis ethmoidalis), two foramina can be found: the anterior ethmoidal foramen and the posterior ethmoidal foramen (▶ Fig. 2.9). Both foramina can be doubled and show a large range of variations.[41] The anterior foramen leads into the orbitocranial canal and the posterior one into the orbitoethmoidal canal. The orbitocranial canal normally lies in the gusset between the first orbital ethmoidal cell and the frontal sinus.[42] Often this canal is not a complete osseous canal, but shows dehiscences in its walls, so that the vessels are lying directly under the mucous lining of the ethmoidal cells. Its internal opening into the endocranium is located just above the lamina cribrosa of the olfactory groove within the anterior half of the lateral lamella. In this region, often still in the orbitoethmoidal canal, the anterior ethmoidal artery splits off the anterior meningeal artery, which fans out anteriorly embedded in

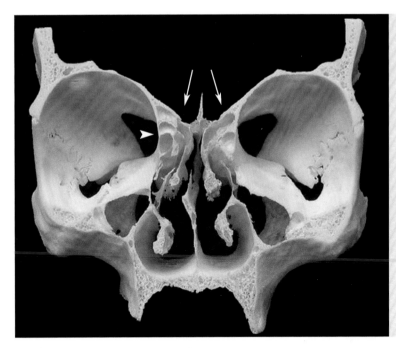

Fig. 2.15 Keros type I. The arrows point toward the flat lateral wall of the olfactory fossa. The arrowhead marks the very thin lamina papyracea, stabilized by the osseous septs of the ethmoidal cells.

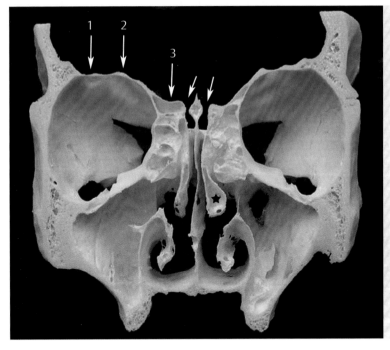

Fig. 2.16 Keros type III, so-called dangerous ethmoid. The arrows point toward the high lateral lamellas. Deep in the olfactory groove the horizontal plate of cribriform can also easily be recognized.
1, Fovea endofrontalis lateralis; **2**, eminentia endofrontalis; **3**, fovea endofrontalis medialis. *Star*, concha bullosa.

slight osseous sulci. The posterior ethmoidal artery supplies the dura mater of the planum sphenoidale, the posterior ethmoidal labyrinth, some posterior parts of the nasal cavity, and the posterior septum. The ethmoidal arteries are of great surgical importance because they run obliquely through the ethmoidal labyrinth, where they can be easily damaged. If a transection occurs, the artery may retract into the orbit, producing a retrobulbar hematoma, which threatens the optic nerve. In addition to these anatomical details of the ethmoidal labyrinth, three general ethmoidal types were defined by Keros in 1965[43] according to the expression of the olfactory groove:

- Keros type I (► Fig. 2.15) describes a flat olfactory fossa (1–3 mm).
- Keros type II describes a deeper olfactory fossa (4–7 mm).
- Keros type III (► Fig. 2.16) describes a deep olfactory fossa (8–16 mm) with a high lamella lateralis. Type 3 is also termed the deep standing ethmoid.

Type I and especially type III present potential dangers for the endonasal surgeon.

The Frontal Sinus

The frontal sinus is a bilaterally expressed pneumatization within the squama of the frontal bone, which presents a lot of anatomical variations. Hypoplasias and aplasias can be observed, with racial differences. For example, 52% of Eskimos do not present a frontal sinus. If the frontal sinus is largely pneumatized, it will extend into the orbital roof, so that a double-layered structure results. In rare cases, the septum of the frontal sinus lies in the median sagittal plane; often it is bent asymmetrically to one side. Frequently, small incomplete accessory septal ridges can be seen, which are called "septula"[44] (▶ Fig. 2.17). The left sinus is usually larger than the right one.[45] If the frontal sinus extends largely to the dorsal region, it will reach the olfactory groove. The anterior borders of this groove will then form a prominent ridge projecting into the frontal sinus. These ridges consist of a fragile thin osseous substance and are termed "crista olfactoria." This typical situation, which results from the excessive pneumatization, was termed "dangerous frontal bone" by Boenninghaus (1913).[46] During surgical procedures the crista olfactoria can be easily damaged, and an opening of the endocranium will result. In cases of a dangerous frontal bone the crista galli is also often

pneumatized and contains a pneumatic cell, termed the recessus cristae galli or recessus of Palfyn. In these cases the pneumatization originates from the frontal sinus. Additionally, it must be mentioned, that pneumatization of the crista galli can also be established from the bullae ethmoidales. It is important that cases of a pneumatized crista galli must not be combined with an asymmetrically expressed interfrontal septum.[47]

An important structure of the frontal sinus is the funnel-shaped outlet structure, called the frontal sinus infundibulum,[48] which opens into the frontal recess. According to the developmental history of this region the frontal recess must be seen as an anterior ethmoidal cell. This cell was responsible for the pneumatization of the frontal bone and therefore for the development of the frontal sinus.[48] The frontal recess can be seen as the cranially directed continuation of the ethmoidal infundibulum and presents typical anatomical boundaries: it lies dorsal of the agger nasi and ventral to the ethmoidal bulla. The lateral border is the lamina papyracea and the medial border is formed by the lateral lamella of the middle turbinate. Two main situations must be differentiated: if the outlet duct is longer than 3 mm it is described as a nasofrontal duct (77.3% of individuals); if the duct is shorter, the term frontal ostium (22.7%) is preferred.[32,33] Unfortunately there are many different definitions used to describe structures in this region, and these cannot be discussed in detail in this overview. However, it must be mentioned that the term "nasofrontal duct" is not a synonym for the frontal recess.[34] A simple connection between the frontal sinus and the nose can be found in only one-third of patients.[49] In the other cases the drainage route is divided during the passage of the ethmoidal cell system and therefore complicated topographical situations occur. It must be mentioned that aberrant olfactory fibers may occur in the region of the frontal recess anterior and lateral to the middle turbinate.[47] This is a dangerous variation, because the damage of these fibers opens the lymphatic vaginas and produces a continuation with the subarachnoidal space, so that meningitis may develop.

The Maxillary Sinus

The maxillary sinus, also termed the Highmore cave according to the classical description of the English practitioner Nathanael Highmore in 1651,[50] presents the largest pneumatic cave of the skull. Furthermore, the morphology is quite constant and presents only few anatomical variations. The first, not published, description was made by Leonardo da Vinci. The maxillary sinus lies within the body of the maxillary bone beneath the orbita. According to this typical topography the floor of the orbita is simultaneously the roof of the maxillary sinus. For traumatology it is very important that the orbital floor has no support or strengthening (▶ Fig. 2.18). These anatomical facts explain a typical injury that was first

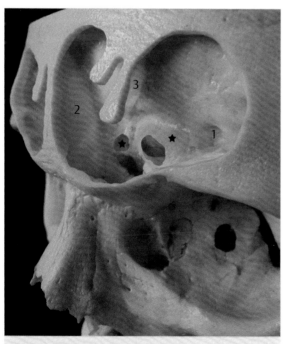

Fig. 2.17 Frontal sinus with bullae frontales.
1, Recessus supraorbitalis; **2**, septum interfrontale; **3**, septula. *Stars*, bullae frontales.

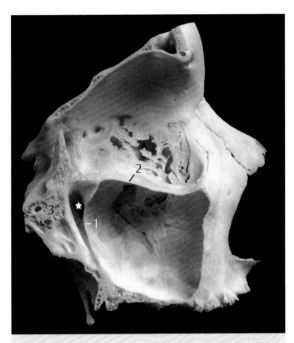

Fig. 2.18 Maxillary sinus.
1, Tuber maxillae; 2, orbital floor; 3, processus pterygoideus. *Star*, foramen sphenopalatinum in the depth of the pterygo-palatine fossa.

described in 1889 by Lang[51] as traumatic enophthalmos, and is known as "blow-out fracture" today. This injury is characterized by a bursting out of the orbital floor into the maxillary sinus and this bursting out is often accompanied by a herniation of adipose tissue as well as the inferior rectus muscle, which explains diplopia. Two hypotheses have been established for explaining the development of a blow-out fracture. The first is also called the hydraulic pressure hypothesis. According to this the force is transmitted to the orbital content, which is more or less incompressible, and therefore the force is transmitted to the osseous boundaries of the orbit. The weakest point will break out, and this is the orbital floor. The second hypothesis is known as the buckling force hypothesis. According to this explanation, the force is transmitted to the osseous orbital frame, which is elastically deformed. As a result of the suddenly increasing pressure within the orbital compartment, the orbital floor is crinkled and broken out into the maxillary sinus.

The dorsal wall of the maxillary sinus is next to the infratemporal fossa on the lateral side and the pterygopalatine fossa on the medial side (▶ Fig. 2.18). This typical relationship is important for the transmaxillary approach to the sphenopalatine artery and also to the pterygopalatine ganglion. Dependent on the grade of pneumatization, accessory recesses of the maxillary sinus can be described. The alveolar recess is especially important because in cases of excessive pneumatization the apices of the roots of the teeth can project into the maxillary

sinus and cause a maxilloantral fistula during extraction. Furthermore, the structures for the dental roots and the dental plexuses of nerves and vessels, lie directly beneath the mucosal lining of the maxillary sinus, so that these structures can be easily damaged.[52] Septations are also not rare events. Often irregular septa can be observed in the region of the alveolar recess separating the molar from the premolar region. These septa are called Underwood septa.[53] Rarely, horizontally or sagittally extending septa are observed as well as complete vertical septa, separating an anterior from a posterior maxillary sinus. Within the roof of the maxillary sinus the infraorbital nerve and the infraorbital artery are located. These structures often are protruding into the infraorbital recess, so that they run in an osseous trabecular structure.

The Sphenoid Sinus

The sphenoid sinus is a structure presenting a large amount of variations, which are due to different grades of pneumatization. Three types of sphenoid sinus can be differentiated[54]: the conchal type, the presellar type, and the sellar type. In approximately 1.5% of individuals a complete aplasia of the sphenoid sinus can be observed.[35] The bilaterally expressed sphenoid sinuses are separated from each other by a septum sinuum sphenoidalium. This septum is rarely a symmetrical structure; in most cases it is asymmetrically bent to the right or the left side. In some cases the septum inserts in the region of the carotid canal. This is a dangerous situation for the surgeon because careless manipulation at the septum may lead to carotid injury. Besides the main intersinus septum, incomplete additional septa often occur, which may complicate the architecture of the sphenoid sinus remarkably. Horizontal septa do not occur in the sphenoid sinus. Sometime posterior ethmoidal cells are misinterpreted in this sense. If a large amount of pneumatization has taken place, several additional recesses may occur. In such cases it is important that essential neighboring structures can bulge into the sphenoid sinus (▶ Fig. 2.19).

The ICA forms the prominentia arteriae carotidis and the optic nerve forms the prominentia nervi optici, both on the lateral side. Just above the floor, the maxillary nerve can also produce a slight prominence. In older patients with rarefying osseous processes dehiscences may occur in the region of these prominences, so that these important structures are not covered by bone, but lie directly beneath the mucosa. Therefore it is essential to open the sphenoid sinus in the middle part of its anterior wall, to avoid the dangerous lateral structures. The posterior end of the middle turbinate marks the level of the perforation in order to avoid laceration of the posterior septal branches (nasopalatine ramus) of the sphenopalatine artery. It should further be kept in mind that in rare cases an aneurysm of the ICA may bulge into the sphenoid sinus.[55] In other also rare cases, the so-called "kissing carotids" may protrude into the sella turcica

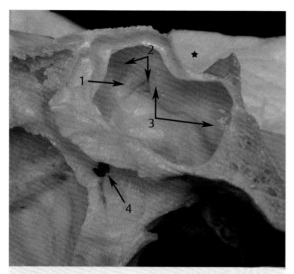

Fig 2.19 Sphenoid sinus.
1, Prominentia nervi optici; 2, recessus lateralis superior;
3, prominentia arteriae carotidis; 4, foramen sphenopalatinum.
Star, sella turcica.

Table 2.3 Content of the three entrances and egressions of the pterygoid fossa

Entrances	Egressions
Fissura sphenomaxillaris: arteria maxillaris	Foramen sphenopalatinum: Arteriae nasales posteriores (3–4) Rami nasales posteriores superiores laterales (~10) Rami nasales posteriores superiores mediales
Canalis rotundus: Nervus maxillaris Arteria canalis rotundum Plexus venosus canalis rotundum	Canalis pterygopalatinus: Nervi palatini Arteria palatina descendens
Canalis pterygoideus: Nervus canalis pterygoidei	Fissura orbitalis inferior: Nervus/arteria infraorbitalis Nervus zygomaticus Rami orbitales (2–3)

reaching the midline.[56] In these pathological cases osseous dehiscences are often present, so that the arterial structures lie directly under the mucosal lining of the sphenoid sinus.

In the floor of the sphenoid sinus the nerve of the pterygoid canal (Vidian nerve) runs toward the pterygoid fossa. If there is a large amount of pneumatization of the sphenoid sinus the superior osseous wall of the pterygoid canal can be absorbed, so that the nerve is in direct contact with the mucosal membrane of the sphenoid sinus. Furthermore, the nerve can protrude into the sphenoid sinus and is then running in an osseous ridge.

The sphenoid sinus opens with a round or elliptic aperture into the sphenoethmoidal recess behind the superior turbinate. This recess is present in the described typical anatomy of only 48.3% of individuals.[57] This recess can be an important source of bleeding because a small arterial ramus can be present in this region. This artery arises constantly from the nasopalatine ramus (posterior septal branches) of the sphenopalatine artery, runs upwards toward the sphenoethmoidal recess, and lies in the lateral part of this location.[58]

2.1.6 Pterygopalatine Fossa (s. Sphenomaxillary Fossa)

The pterygopalatine fossa is a small hidden space with a triangular shape (▶ Fig. 2.18). Topographically it lies beneath the apex of the orbit. It is bounded above by the body of the sphenoid bone, anteriorly by the tuber maxillae, posteriorly by the anterior surface of the pterygoid

process, and medially by the lamina perpendicularis ossis palatini with the sphenoidal and orbital process. The lateral border is the plane of the sphenomaxillary fissure. It is essential, that the pterygoid fossa possesses three entrances and three egressions (▶ Table 2.3). At the dorsal wall the foramen rotundum and the pterygoid canal can be seen (▶ Fig. 2.20). It is important that the aperture of the pterygoid canal lies somewhat caudally and medially to the foramen rotundum (▶ Fig. 2.20). At the medial wall there is the great foramen sphenopalatinum, which can be subdivided in some cases.[59] Caudally the pterygopalatine fossa narrows and runs into the pterygopalatine canal (▶ Fig. 2.20). The caudal orifices of this canal are the foramina palatina minora and the foramen palatinum major. Furthermore, the pterygopalatine fossa communicates with the orbita via the inferior orbital fissure.

Canalis Caroticus

The canalis caroticus begins at the outer surface of the skull base with the foramen caroticum externum just anteromedial to the jugular foramen. Its dorsal wall forms the anterior wall of the tympanic cavity, termed the paries caroticus. In some cases dehiscences may occur in this wall. After a short ascending part there should be a nearly rectangular bend in the anteromedial direction. Then the canal runs horizontally to the apex of the petrous bone, where it ends with the foramen caroticum internum. In some cases the floor of the carotid canal is lacking, so that a carotid sulcus occurs. The superior aperture presents variable osseous structures. In this region the osseous covering of the canal can be very thin or even lacking. In such cases the carotid artery lies directly beneath the dura mater of the middle cranial fossa. In the dorsal wall of the carotid canal there should be two small osseous canals, termed canaliculi caroticotympanici.

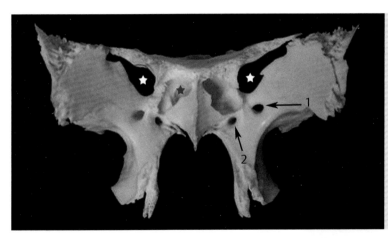

Fig. 2.20 Anterior facies of the processus pterygoideus.
1, Canalis rotundus; **2**, canalis pterygoideus. *White star*, fissura orbitalis superior between the lesser and greater wing of the sphenoid bone; *red star*, sphenoid sinus.

These canals contain sympathetic nerve fibers arising from the carotid plexus and the small caroticotympanic artery. All these structures terminate in the tympanic cavity.

Two essential vascular varieties must be mentioned: the intratympanic course of the ICA[60] and the persistent stapedial artery.[61] In cases of an intratympanic course of the carotid artery the ascending part of the artery is aplastic, and the distal part is reached by collateral arteries. This atypical communication uses the ascending pharyngeal artery, the inferior tympanic artery, and the caroticotympanic artery, which communicates with the distal part of the ICA. In normal cases these vessels are small structures. Increased blood flow enlarges these vessels to the diameter of the ICA; therefore it seems as if the carotid artery passes through the tympanic cavity. For the differential diagnosis it is important that the ascending part of the carotid canal is missing.[62] In such cases the ICA is positioned laterally to the line of Lapayowker in the A-P radiogram. In normal cases the artery would be positioned medially. The line of Lapayowker is defined as a vertically positioned tangent at the lateral part of the vestibulum. In patients with an intratympanic ICA, a high-positioned jugular bulb, aneurysm, and glomus tumor must be ruled out.

The entity of the persistent stapedial artery was first described in Vienna by Joseph Hyrtl in 1836. The stapedial artery should be seen as an embryologic communication between the ICA and the middle meningeal artery. During normal development this communicating vessel disappears. If this stapedial artery persists, an atypical vessel is formed, which enters the foramen inferius a. stapediae, positioned laterally to the jugular fossa, and then runs into the tympanic cavity. It passes between the crura of the stapes and leaves the tympanic cavity by passing the foramen superius a. stapediae, which opens into the middle cranial fossa. The middle meningeal artery is perfused by the persisting stapedial artery. Therefore the middle meningeal artery is not a branch of the maxillary artery and the foramen spinosum is typically lacking in

such cases. Furthermore, it is important that the persisting stapedial artery can be positioned into the facial canal, which will be enlarged importantly in such cases.[61,62]

Jugular Foramen

The jugular foramen is an important opening of the posterior cranial fossa, positioned just behind the inferior aperture of the carotid canal. The jugular foramen lies between the petrous portion of the temporal bone and the lateral part of the occipital bone. It is subdivided by irregular intrajugular processes (processus intrajugularis partis petrosae and processus intrajugularis ossis occipitalis) into two parts. The anteromedial part is termed the pars nervosa, whereas the posterolateral part forms the pars vasculosa (s. venosa) (► Fig. 2.6). The pars nervosa contains the inferior petrosal sinus, the glossopharyngeal, vagus, and accessory nerves. In the pars vasculosa the internal jugular vein with its bulb and some meningeal branches from the pharyngeal ascending and occipital artery are positioned. Above the jugular foramen the internal acoustic meatus is located. Generally the jugular foramen is larger on the right than on the left side.[63] The entrance into the canaliculus mastoideus is located at the lateral wall of the jugular foramen, whereas the apertura externa aquaeductus cochleae can be seen just before the processus intrajugularis of the petrosal bone in the lateral wall. A few essential variations may occur: in some cases cranial nerve IX runs in a separate osseous canal, the canalis n. glossopharyngei. A canalis sinus petrosi inferioris can also be present.[64] Different forms of bridging can subdivide the jugular foramen in completely or incompletely separated parts.[20] In some cases dehiscences in the roof, which is also the floor of the tympanic cavity, may be present.[26] In addition, it should be mentioned that the osseous wall between the jugular foramen and the carotid canal presents at its inferior surface the small fossula petrosa. In this fossula the orifice of the tympanic canal can be seen, and this leads to the tympanic nerve of

Jacobson, branching from the glossopharyngeal nerve, toward the tympanic cavity.

2.1.7 Craniocervical Junction

Normal Anatomy

The development of the craniocervical junction is complicated, because embryologic material of the spine is incorporated into the skull base.[25] In normal anatomy the craniocervical junction includes the osseous structures surrounding the foramen magnum, the atlas, and the axis. The ringlike atlas articulates with the occipital condyles forming the atlanto-occipital articulations. These articulations are crucial for nodding of the head. The atlas constitutes three articulations with the axis: the medial atlantoaxial joint and the bilaterally expressed lateral atlantoaxial joints. These joints are important for head rotation. It must be mentioned that the atlas as well as the axis are special types of vertebrae, so-called rotational vertebrae. The atlas has no longer a vertebral body. This material fuses with the axis and comprises the characteristic feature of the axis, the dens axis. In addition, it must be mentioned that the tip of the dens axis contains the body of the proatlas. This proatlantic material appears in fetuses as ossiculum terminale (Bergmann) and is also present in young children.[65]

Essential Variations

In the craniocervical region a great number of different osseous variations may occur and these can be classified into the assimilation of the atlas and the manifestation of the occipital vertebra.[25] The manifestations of the occipital vertebra may lead to different entities of isolated ossicula, osseous bumps, or crests. The differential diagnosis of these elements is discussed intensively in literature.[25,65,66] Only some of these entities are important for endoscopic surgery. In particular, variations that make approaches to the brainstem difficult must be mentioned.

Assimilation of the Atlas

The assimilation of the atlas appears in less than 1% of individuals and is therefore a rare condition. It is important that not all cases with an osseous fixed atlas are real assimilations. According to Pfitzner[67] this term should only be used if the atlas loses its typical shape and identity and merges completely to the occipital bone, so that a new structure is formed. Cases where the atlas is only fused to the occiput, for example by a paracondyloid process, should be classified as occipitalization of the atlas. The assimilation of the atlas is a clinically relevant malformation, because vertebral vestibular crises originating from the assimilation are frequently observed as well as a progressive atlantoaxial subluxation, which develops in about 50% of cases.[68] Furthermore, a torticollis osseus can often be seen, due to the fixed malrotation of the assimilated atlas. In many cases the assimilation of the atlas is combined with other irregularities of the craniocervical junction; for example, a basilar impression, gaps of the dorsal arch, or a Klippel–Feil syndrome.

Processus Basilares

Basilar processes are small bony bumps located at the anterior margin of the foramen magnum. These excrescences may occur unilaterally or bilaterally, be firmly attached, or form accessory ossicles.[25,66,69] The basilar processes can be observed in with a frequency of about 4%. Etiologically the basilar processes derive from the hypochordal blastema of the proatlas. If exhaustive basilar processes fuse in the midline, this should not be confused with a third condyle. The osseous mass resulting from the fusion of basilar processes is usually perforated by an osseous canal, termed the canalis intrabasilaris Kollmanni. This canal does not exist in third condyles. The basilar processes do not seem to have any clinical significance beside differential diagnosis.

Condylus Tertius

The condylus tertius (third condyle) results if the hypochordal blastema of the proatlas persists in its medial part, whereas the lateral parts diminish. The typical third condyle is an osseous process positioned in the median sagittal plane at the anterior margin of the foramen magnum.[25,66,69] In some cases an articulation occurs with the tip of the dens axis or the anterior arch of the atlas.[70] The third condyle represents a clinically significant variation because it may cause serious disturbances of skull motility.[65] Rarely the third condyle can be misinterpreted as a nasopharyngeal tumor.[71]

Os Odontoideum and Ossiculum Terminale Bergmann Persistens

Both entities are variations of the dens axis. If the ossiculum terminale Bergmann is not fused with the dens axis, the ossiculum terminale Bergmann persistens occurs. This small droplike element can be positioned at the tip of the dens axis (orthotopic position) or at the anterior margin of the foramen magnum (dystopic position). These entities may form osseous bumps or even isolated accessory ossicles. For the difficult differential diagnosis of various entities, such as the orthotopic so-called os odontoideum, the dystopic os odontoideum, or the isolated third condyle, specialized literature must be consulted.[25,66,69]

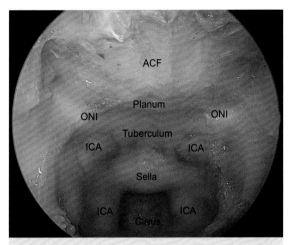

Fig. 2.21 Panoramic endoscopic view of the sphenoid sinus on a cadaveric specimen.
ACF, anterior cranial fossa; ICA, internal carotid artery; ONI, optic nerve impression.

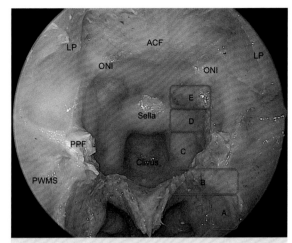

Fig. 2.22 Panoramic view of the sphenoid sinus on a cadaveric specimen with a didactic depiction of the endoscopic classification of the internal carotid artery territories in red (A, parapharyngeal; B, petrous; C, paraclival; D, parasellar; E, paraclinoid).
ACF, anterior cranial fossa; LP, lamina papyracea; ONI, optic nerve impression; PPF, pterygopalatine fossa; PWMS, posterior wall of the maxillary sinus.

2.2 Vessels and Nerves

Leo F. S. Ditzel Filho, Danielle de Lara, Daniel M. Prevedello, Domenico Solari, Bradley A. Otto, Amin B. Kassam, Ricardo L. Carrau

2.2.1 Introduction

Recent advances in skull base surgery, especially with the development of endoscopic techniques,[72] have led to an explosion of new approaches and management strategies.[72,73,74,75,76,77,78,79,80,81,82,83,84,85,86,87,88,89,90,91,92,93,94,95,96,97,98,99,100] Paramount for the modern skull base surgeon who wishes to offer his patients these novel treatment options is the proper understanding and knowledge of the ventral skull base anatomy from an endoscopic standpoint.[101] Within this new perspective on anatomy, special attention must be given to the vessels and nerves that traverse this intricate region (▶ Fig. 2.21).

Major vessels and their branches are accessed during endoscopic skull base surgery; complete awareness of their location and course is extremely important. Cranial nerve injury is another feared source of complications and morbidity in skull base surgery. In fact, the position of the cranial nerves in relation to the lesion at hand often dictates which approach is most appropriate.

In this section, we describe the surgical anatomy of the vessels and nerves that travel within the ventral skull base from an endoscopic point of view; surgical pitfalls and pearls related to these structures are also discussed.

2.2.2 Vessels

Internal Carotid Artery

The ICA is responsible for the major supply of blood to the brain. It arises from the common carotid artery, which bifurcates into internal and external carotid arteries, at the level of the third cervical vertebra. From its origin, the ICA runs superiorly to reach several areas of the brain and skull base.[102]

The ICA is classically divided in four segments, named according to the region or anatomic structure through which it is traversing: the cervical segment (C1), the petrous segment (C2), the cavernous segment (C3), and the supraclinoidal segment (C4). In terms of endoscopic skull base surgery, it is interesting and strategic to further divide the ICA into parapharyngeal, petrous, paraclival, parasellar, paraclinoid, and supraclinoidal segments (▶ Fig. 2.22). We believe that this second classification is more applicable to the endoscopic surgical strategy within the ventral skull base since it correlates with anatomical compartments that are amenable to endoscopic access; namely the parapharyngeal/infratemporal fossae, the petrous bone, the clivus, the cavernous sinus, sella turcica, and finally the suprasellar/supraclinoid areas.

The cervical segment begins at the common carotid artery bifurcation, where the ICA presents a structural enlargement, the carotid bulb. The artery runs cephalad inside the carotid sheath, medial to the internal jugular vein and anterior to the vagus nerve; it then enters the skull through the carotid canal in the petrous portion of the temporal bone, placed anterior to the jugular foramen.

The petrous segment of the ICA travels inside the petrous part of the temporal bone. This segment is divided into three portions: the ascending or vertical portion, the genu, and the horizontal portion. The petrous segment leaves the carotid canal on top of the foramen lacerum, medial to the trigeminal nerve and the petrolingual ligament. Its upward course is parallel to the clival recess; in fact the clival region itself is bound laterally by the two ascending ICAs. The paraclival ICA is considered to be inside the cavernous sinus. The paraclival ICA is what was originally called the posterior vertical component of the cavernous sinus ICA.

In the parasellar region of the cavernous sinus, the ICA constitutes its most medial wall. The ICA then continues up to the posterior clinoid process, returns forward to the anterior sphenoid bone and to the medial side of the anterior clinoid process, where the abducens nerve is located on its lateral side. The main branches of the intracavernous carotid are the lateral clival, the meningohypophyseal trunk, and the infralateral trunk, in ascending order. The ICA then contacts the optic strut as it curves posteriorly, forming the carotid siphon. At this level, a thickening of the periosteum projects around the ICA forming the proximal ring, which encases the segment of the ICA from the optic strut to the middle clinoid. From the distal aspect of the optic strut and under the anterior clinoid, a second complete ring, the distal ring, surrounds. The paraclinoid ICA is that segment located between the rings. At this level the McConnell capsular arteries originate. The paraclinoid ICA also gives rise to the superior hypophyseal artery that then travels from the carotid cave into the subarachnoid space to supply the pituitary stalk and gland as well as the cisternal segment of the optic nerves and chiasm.

The supraclinoid segment begins where the artery perforates the dura mater medial to the anterior clinoid process and below the optic nerve. This portion is divided in three segments based on the site of origin of the ophthalmic, posterior communicating, and anterior choroidal arteries. The ophthalmic artery arises at the beginning of the supraclinoid segment, usually at the superior surface of the ICA, at the medial side of the anterior clinoid process, and runs toward the optic canal, inferior and lateral to the optic nerve.

The posterior communicating artery is the second branch of the supraclinoid segment. It arises from the posteromedial surface of the ICA and runs medially above the sella turcica and the oculomotor nerve to join the posterior cerebral artery. Some perforating arteries arise from the posterior communicating artery, at its superior and lateral aspects, to penetrate the tuber cinereum, the floor of the third ventricle, the posterior perforated substance, and the optic tract. The major branch of the posterior communicating artery is the premamillary artery.

The anterior choroidal artery (usually more than one vessel) arises from the ICA lateral to the optic tract, and is directed posteromedial behind the ICA. It runs medially, passing below the medial side of the optic tract to reach the lateral edge of the cerebral peduncle and geniculate body. It turns laterally, through the crural cistern, to reach the uncus and the choroidal fissure and arrive at the choroidal plexus at the temporal horn. The ICA then divides into its two terminal branches: the anterior and middle cerebral arteries.

Hypophyseal Arteries

The superior hypophyseal arteries can arise from the ophthalmic segment of the supraclinoidal carotid artery; however, more often we see them originating inside the carotid cave proximal to the distal ring and then passing into the subarachnoid space medially to reach the suprasellar space. This group of small branches supplies mainly the pituitary stalk and anterior lobe of pituitary gland, but also the optic nerves, chiasm, and the floor of third ventricle (▶ Fig. 2.23). The arteries usually arise from the medial side of the ICA and travel medially to reach the pituitary stalk and chiasm. When approaching lesions of the sellar and suprasellar compartments, the surgeon must have full knowledge of this anatomy to prevent pituitary failure and visual loss of ischemic origin. In tuberculum sellae meningiomas these arteries tend to be pushed posteriorly since the tumor arises ventrally; conversely, in craniopharyngiomas, which originate from the pituitary stalk region, the arteries tend to be pushed anteriorly by the posteriorly located tumor and are encountered early in the procedure.

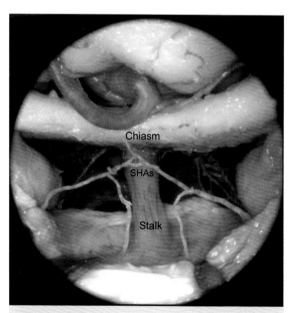

Fig. 2.23 Endoscopic view of the suprasellar region on a cadaveric specimen. Observe the relation of the superior hypophyseal arteries (SHAs) to the optic chiasm.

The inferior hypophyseal artery is a branch of the meningohypophyseal trunk of the parasellar segment of the ICA. It is directed medially to supply the posterior lobe of the pituitary gland and periosteum.

Vertebrobasilar System

The vertebrobasilar system is responsible for supplying blood to the posterior part of the circle of Willis. It is composed of the two vertebral arteries and the basilar artery (▶ Fig. 2.24).

The vertebral arteries arise from the subclavian arteries and enter the C6 transverse foramen to ascend through the foramina, in front of the cervical nerve roots, until they reach the laterally placed transverse foramen of C1. The arteries then run medially, penetrating the dura below the foramen magnum. They pass through the foramen in front of the dentate ligament and accessory nerve to reach the anterior portion of the medulla. On its pathway, the intradural portion of the vertebral arteries faces the occipital condyles, the hypoglossal rootlets and the jugular tubercles. Near the pontomedullary sulcus the vertebral arteries join to form the basilar artery. The main branches of the vertebral arteries are the anterior spinal arteries and the posteroinferior cerebellar artery (PICA).

The basilar artery arises from the junction of both vertebral arteries at the pontomedullary sulcus. It travels upward, in a shallow midline longitudinal groove (the basilar sulcus), at the anterior surface of the pons and behind the clivus. During its course at the prepontine cistern, the artery gives rise to the anteroinferior cerebellar arteries (AICAs). The AICAs pass around the pons, below or between the fascicles of the abducens nerve.

They form a ventral and a caudal loop. The ventral loop often enters the internal acoustic canal supplying the facial and vestibulocochlear nerves. They then reach the surface of the middle cerebral peduncle and supply the petrosal surface of the cerebellum at the cerebellopontine cistern.

The superior cerebellar artery (SCA) arises from the vertebral artery at the pontomesencephalic sulcus. The SCA passes through the crural and ambient cisterns, coursing below the trochlear nerve and above the trigeminal nerve. The artery then encircles the midbrain to supply the cerebral peduncles and the tentorial surface of the cerebellum.

The apex of the basilar artery is situated at the interpeduncular cistern, where it bifurcates to give rise to both of the posterior cerebral arteries (PCAs). The PCA runs around the midbrain, passes above the oculomotor and trochlear nerves, and supplies the occipital and the posteromedial temporal lobes. The PCA anastomoses with the posterior communicating artery in each side to complete the circle of Willis.

From an endoscopic endonasal perspective, the posterior circulation is accessed through the clivus. A partial clivectomy can be performed in three different levels: upper, middle and inferior, or a combination of the two for a total resection or panclivectomy. An upper clivectomy requires a pituitary transposition[103] or resection of the pituitary gland (in cases of panhypopituitarism). Once a dorsectomy (removal of the posterior clinoids) is performed and the dura is incised then the premesencephalic cistern is opened and the Liliequist membrane is visualized. The third cranial nerves are lateral to the Liliequist membrane located at the crural cistern running parallel to the posterior communicating arteries. The mammillary bodies can be seen posteriorly with the perforators. The SCA can be seen originating from the basilar artery below the level of the third cranial nerve. If the dural opening is extended inferiorly performing a middle clivectomy, then the pons can be seen with the basilar artery running in the prepontine cistern. Often the basilar artery is off center. Cranial nerves VI ascend from the pontomedullary sulcus above the vertebrobasilar junction laterally in the direction of the Dorello canals. An inferior clivectomy, below the level of cranial nerves VI, exposes the premedullary cistern all the way to the level of the foramen magnum. If a medial condylectomy is performed then cranial nerve XII can be seen entering the hypoglossal canal arising posterior to the vertebral artery. The ventral root of C1 can be visualized inferiorly traveling ventral to the vertebral artery.

Maxillary Artery

The so-called "internal" maxillary artery is the largest branch of the external carotid artery. Its mandibular segment, or proximal portion, runs forward and horizontal along the lower border of the lateral pterygoid muscle.

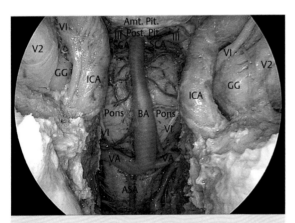

Fig. 2.24 Endoscopic view of a panclivectomy with exposure of the vertebrobasilar system. Observe the relation to the sella and to the carotid system.
ASA, anterior spinal artery; Ant. Pit., anterior pituitary; BA, basilar artery; GG, gasserian ganglion; ICA, internal carotid artery; III, third cranial nerve; Post. Pit., posterior pituitary; SCA, superior cerebellar artery; VA, vertebral artery; VI, abducens nerve; V2, maxillary nerve.

The second, or pterygoid portion, runs next to the ramus of the mandible and the surface of the lateral pterygoid muscle. It exits the infratemporal fossa through the pterygomaxillary fissure entering the pterygomaxillary fossa, which is located between the posterior maxillary wall and the pterygoid process. The third, or pterygopalatine portion, lies on the pterygopalatine fossa ventral to the nerve contents. Its terminal branches enter the posterosuperior part of the nasal cavity through the sphenopalatine foramen.

The maxillary artery and its branches supply the tympanic membrane, the mandibular muscles, oral and nasal cavity, and maxillary sinus.

The most important branch of the maxillary artery from an endoscopic endonasal skull base surgery perspective is the sphenopalatine artery, its terminal branch. It runs through the sphenopalatine foramen to reach the medial wall of nasal cavity and supply the posteroinferior part of the nasal septum.

Septal Arteries

The sphenopalatine artery gives rise to the posterior lateral nasal branches and to the posterior septal branches, which will anastomose with the ethmoidal, superior labial, and descending palatine arteries to assist supplying the frontal, maxillary, ethmoidal, and sphenoidal sinuses.

The posterior septal artery is of particular importance to endoscopic skull base surgery, since it gives rise to the nasoseptal artery that supplies the nasoseptal flap,[104] the primary reconstruction method utilized in the vast majority of cases.

Ethmoidal Arteries

The anterior and posterior ethmoidal arteries are branches of the ophthalmic artery. They rise under the superior oblique muscle and pass through the anterior and posterior ethmoidal canals, located at the frontoethmoidal suture, running to the cribriform plate (▶ Fig. 2.25).

The anterior ethmoidal artery runs near the anterior edge of the cribriform plate and supplies the mucosa of the anterior and middle ethmoidal sinuses and the dura covering the cribriform plate and the planum sphenoidale.

The posterior ethmoidal artery runs anterior to the orbital end of the optic canal. It supplies the mucosa of the posterior ethmoidal sinus and the dura of the planum sphenoidale.

These arteries are of strategic importance when dealing with tumors of the anterior cranial fossa, especially olfactory groove meningiomas.[99] They provide the major blood supply to these lesions; therefore, obliterating them in the early stages of the approach will deprive the tumor of blood and account for a safer resection. However, one must be careful while attempting to ligate these vessels; if not properly exposed they can retract into the

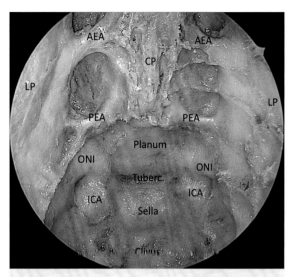

Fig. 2.25 Endoscopic view of the anterior cranial fossa on a cadaveric dissection.
AEA, anterior ethmoidal artery; CP, cribriform plate; ICA, internal carotid artery; LP, lamina papyracea; ONI, optic nerve impression; PEA, posterior ethmoidal artery; Tuberc., tuberculum.

lamina papyracea and cause a vision threatening retroocular hematoma.

Cavernous Sinus

The cavernous sinus is as dural envelope, located near the center of the skull base, which surrounds a venous space containing the cavernous segment of the ICA, cranial nerves, and venous confluences (▶ Fig. 2.26).[105]

The cavernous sinus is composed of anterior, posterior, and medial and lateral walls as well as a roof. From superior to inferior, the oculomotor, trochlear, and ophthalmic nerves course in the lateral wall of the sinus. The third and fourth nerves are close and run together at the sinus roof to reach the superior orbital fissure. The abducens nerve has the most medial site of entry among the nerves coursing inside the cavernous sinus and runs medial and parallel to the ophthalmic nerve (V_1) and lateral to the ICA (▶ Fig. 2.27).

The cavernous sinuses can be approached anteriorly and medially through ventral endoscopic routes[94]; this is especially relevant when dealing with pituitary adenomas. In these cases the tumor displaces the sinus laterally, along with its contents. Entry into the sinus usually does not generate any bleeding since the tumor blocks it. Once the tumor is resected and the sinus is unplugged, copious venous bleeding ensues, which can be controlled with powdered gelatin and thrombin or collagen powder. Continuous neurophysiological monitoring helps to avoid a cranial nerve or other neurologic injury. Adenomas that invade the cavernous sinuses are notoriously difficult to remove; however, the medial compartment of the

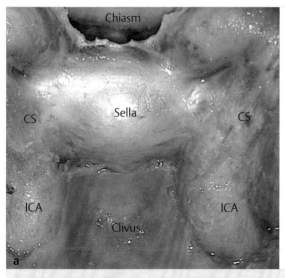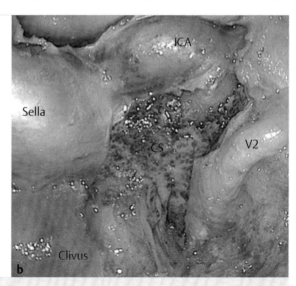

Fig. 2.26 a, b Anterior endoscopic view of the sellar/parasellar/cavernous sinus region on a cadaveric specimen dissection. (a) Anterior view of the left cavernous after bone removal, prior to dural opening. (b) Lateral view of the left cavernous sinus with a 30° endoscope after dural opening. Observe the rich venous confluence.
CS, cavernous sinus; ICA, internal carotid artery; V2, maxillary nerve.

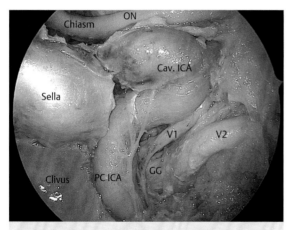

Fig. 2.27 Anterolateral view of the left cavernous sinus with a 30° rod-lens endoscope after removal of the venous confluences.
Cav. ICA, cavernous internal carotid artery; GG, gasserian ganglion; ON, optic nerve; PC ICA, paraclival internal carotid artery; VI, abducens nerve; V2, maxillary nerve.

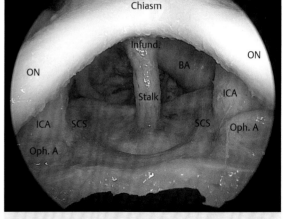

Fig. 2.28 Endoscopic view of the upper sellar region.
BA, basilar artery; ICA, internal carotid artery; Infund., infundibulum; ON, optic nerve; Oph. A, ophthalmic artery; SCS, superior circular sinus.

cavernous components can be safely cleaned through this approach.

The two cavernous sinuses communicate through the anterior, inferior, and posterior intercavernous sinuses and through the basilar sinus. The cavernous sinuses are also connected to the orbit, cerebral hemispheres, and posterior fossa through several venous channels.

Circular Sinus

The cavernous sinuses are connected across the midline by the intercavernous sinuses.[105] There is an anterior (to the pituitary gland) sinus and a posterior one (or superior and inferior). The anterior sinus is usually the largest and may cover the whole anterior wall of the sella. The structure formed by the connections of both the anterior and posterior intercavernous sinuses is named the circular sinus, a venous circle around the pituitary gland (▶ Fig. 2.28).

The anterior intercavernous sinus always ligated on endoscopic skull base surgery when approaching sellar lesions with suprasellar extension as craniopharyngiomas and when performing a pituitary transposition[103] to address lesions in the interpeduncular cistern. This step

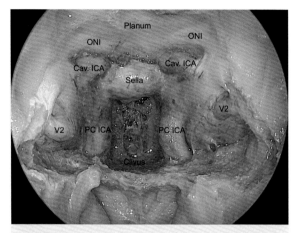

Fig. 2.29 Anterior endoscopic view of the clivus after partial bone removal and opening of the anterior dural leaflet. Observe the rich venous plexus (blue).
Cav. ICA, cavernous internal carotid artery; ONI, optic nerve impression; PC ICA, paraclival internal carotid artery; V2, maxillary nerve.

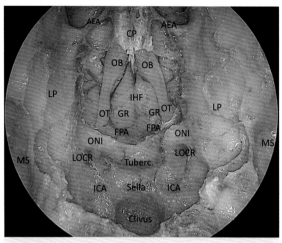

Fig. 2.30 Endoscopic view of the anterior cranial fossa on a cadaveric specimen after removal of the planum sphenoidale. AEA, anterior ethmoidal artery; CP, cribriform plate; FPA, frontopolar artery; GR, gyrus rectus; ICA, internal carotid artery; IHF, interhemispheric fissure; LOCR, lateral opticocarotid recess; LP, lamina papyracea; MS, maxillary sinus; OB, olfactory bulb; ONI, optic nerve impression; OT, olfactory tract; Tuberc., tuberculum.

can be safely performed, without major consequences to pituitary or cranial nerve function. On the other hand, lesions that originate exclusively from the suprasellar space, such as tuberculum sellae meningiomas, can be directly approached without the need to sellar opening or coagulation of the superior intercavernous sinus.

Basilar Plexus

The clival or basilar plexus is a large intercavernous venous connection located between the layers of dura posterior to the clivus (▶ Fig. 2.29). It extends across the back of the dorsum sellae and communicates with the inferior petrosal sinuses laterally, the cavernous sinuses superiorly, and the marginal sinus inferiorly. It creates a large venous confluence along the cavernous sinus posterior wall.

The abducens nerve often enters the posterior part of the cavernous sinus by running through the basilar plexus at the level of the confluence with the inferior petrosal sinus.

This anatomy is of particular interest to avoid abducens nerve injury when performing a clivectomy. Particularly when approaching clival chordomas,[106] attention is required because this specific tumor invades the space of the basilar plexus and surrounds cranial nerve VI in its interdural segment. Neurophysiological monitoring is very helpful for determining the nerve position.

Bleeding can be a major problem when approaching intradural lesions that have no skull base involvement. In cases where the clivectomy is performed in normal tissue

that is not compromised by tumor, the bleeding from the basilar plexus can be copious and life threatening. In this situation the use of bipolar forceps can be problematic as their use frequently results in greater damage of the superficial layer; thus, increasing the bleeding. Any type of coagulation attempt must have the goal of welding the two layers of dura, which can be achieved with modern bipolar devices with flat surface (Aquamantys; Medtronic Corporation, Jacksonville, Florida, United States); or filling the space between the layers with thrombotic substances such as gelfoam and thrombin pastes and/or collagen powder.

2.2.3 Nerves

Olfactory Nerve

The olfactory nerve (first cranial nerve) has its origin at the olfactory epithelium of the upper segment of the nasal cavity. Anterior to the sphenoethmoidal recess, numerous sensory nerve fibers arise and project through small foramina at the cribriform plate of the ethmoid bone to the olfactory bulb.

Placed over the cribriform plate at the olfactory groove, the olfactory bulb is the site of origin of the olfactory tract, which is intimately related to the inferior surface of the frontal lobes (▶ Fig. 2.30). The olfactory tracts lie at the olfactory sulci, which bound the rectus and orbital gyri, above the orbital plate of the frontal bones. At the posterior part of the orbital gyrus, the olfactory tract is enlarged and becomes the olfactory trigone.

The trigone base is placed in front of the anterior perforated substance while the tract bifurcates into lateral and medial olfactory stria. Through the olfactory stria, axons connect posteriorly to the limbic system, especially to the uncus and amygdala at the temporal lobe.

In endoscopic skull base surgery the olfactory nerves are typically addressed when dealing with anterior cranial fossa pathology. The most common scenarios are in olfactory groove meningiomas, esthesioneuroblastomas, and planum sphenoidale meningiomas. Esthesioneuroblastomas are malignant tumors that originate from the olfactory epithelium and consequently the resection of the olfactory nerve is mandatory. The dura is opened and the olfactory bulbs and tracts are dissected from the frontal lobes posteriorly. The olfactory tracts are then transected as posterior as possible above the planum sphenoidale to achieve oncological resection with tumor-free margins. In large olfactory groove meningiomas, olfaction preservation can become an issue; however, in cases of smaller tumors that affect predominantly one side of the anterior fossa, it is possible to perform the dural opening and resection solely on one side of the cribriform plate through a mononostril approach, thus preserving the patient's sense of smell. Planum sphenoidale meningiomas are more posterior and olfactory preservation is possible as long as the exposure and resection is limited to the roof of the sphenoid and the posterior ethmoidal arteries are kept as the limit of the planectomy anteriorly.

Optic Nerve

Responsible for transmitting visual information from the retina to the brain, the optic nerves are the second pair of cranial nerves. They are composed of retinal ganglion cell axons and leave the eye bulb and orbit through the optic canal at the sphenoid bone. At the optic canal, the optic nerve is enclosed in the optic sheath and passes just below the elevator and superior rectus muscles, through the medial part of the annular tendon. The ophthalmic artery enters the canal at the lateral side of the optic nerve and crosses above it medially.

When entering the cranial space, each optic nerve runs superior and medially toward the optic chiasm. The ICA passes below the optic nerve and crosses posterior and superior to reach the lateral surface of the chiasm (▶ Fig. 2.31). The optic chiasm is located just above and anterior to the pituitary gland and the anterior cerebral arteries course above it. Together with the anterior commissure and lamina terminalis, they compose the anterior wall of the third ventricle.

From the optic chiasm, fibers continue posteriorly and laterally in the optic tract, passing through the thalamus and the lateral geniculate body, turning into the optic radiation until they reach the visual cortex at the occipital lobe. The optic radiation is separated by the tapetum from the temporal horn of the lateral ventricle.

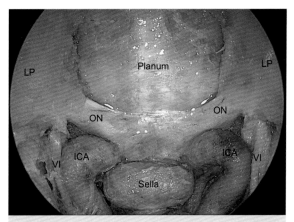

Fig. 2.31 Endoscopic view of the sellar region and the anterior cranial fossa after removal of the sellar anterior bone wall, tuberculum, planum, and partial opening of the optic canal. ICA, internal carotid artery; LP, lamina papyracea; ON, optic nerve; VI, abducens nerve.

The anatomy of the optic nerves is critical when dealing with several pathologies that are amenable to endoscopic endonasal management: pituitary adenomas with suprasellar extension, craniopharyngiomas and other sellar cystic lesions, and especially tuberculum sellae meningiomas. Meningiomas are tumors that often invade the optic canals; therefore, to improve visual outcomes, the periosteum must be opened posteriorly for proper tumor removal and appropriate optic nerve decompression.

Oculomotor Nerve

The oculomotor nerve is responsible for the vast majority of the eye's movements and for the innervation of the ciliary and pupillary sphincter muscles. It exits the midbrain at the oculomotor nucleus and the Edinger–Westphal nucleus.

The third pair of cranial nerves arises behind the mamillary bodies, below the posterior part of the floor of the third ventricle. It directs anteriorly at the interpeduncular fossa, passing over the superior cerebellar artery and under the posterior cerebral artery (▶ Fig. 2.32), crosses anteriorly and lateral to the posterior clinoid process, through the tentorial edge, where it is medial to the uncus and lateral to the posterior communicating artery. The nerve pierces the dura on the roof of the cavernous sinus at the oculomotor triangle to lie on the lateral wall of the cavernous sinus, above the other orbital nerves.

At the level of the posterior part of the superior orbital fissure, the oculomotor nerve splits in an upper and lower division and then enters the fissure through the oculomotor foramen in the annular tendon. The superior branch passes upward to innervate the superior rectus and elevator muscles, while the inferior branch innervates the medial and inferior rectus and inferior oblique muscles and gives rise to the motor root to the ciliary ganglion.

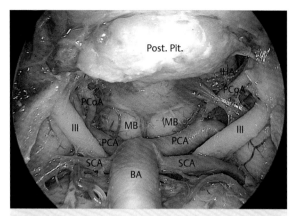

Fig. 2.32 Endoscopic view of the upper clival region after removal of the dorsum sellae in a cadaveric specimen with a 30° rod-lens endoscope pointed cephalad.
BA, basilar artery; IHA, inferior hypophyseal artery; III, third cranial nerve; MB, mammillary body; PCA, posterior cerebral artery; PCoA, posterior communicating artery; Post. Pit., posterior pituitary; SCA, superior cerebellar artery.

The third nerve can be jeopardized in lesions that affect the upper clivus/superior orbital fissure regions, especially chordomas. Continuous neurophysiological monitoring is crucial to prevent oculomotor injury while resecting these tumors endonasally. They are less susceptible to injury in endoscopic endonasal surgery to cavernous sinus lesions due to its lateral position.

Trochlear Nerve

The fourth cranial nerve is purely motor; it is also the thinnest cranial nerve. It arises from the dorsal aspect of the midbrain, below the inferior colliculi and runs laterally and anteriorly to enter the ambient cistern. The nerve runs through the subarachnoid space, passing between the superior cerebellar artery and the posterior cerebral artery and pierces the dura next to the free edge of the tentorium.

The trochlear nerve enters the cavernous sinus at its lateral wall and travels between the oculomotor and ophthalmic nerves toward the orbit (▶ Fig. 2.33), entering through the superior orbital fissure where it passes above and outside the annular tendon. The nerve runs medially above the levator oculi muscle to innervate the superior oblique muscle.

The trochlear nerve is rarely injured in endoscopic endonasal skull base surgery due to its intrinsic characteristics. It is extremely lateral in the crural cistern and can be only visualized through a transclival approach when an angled-lens rod-lens endoscope is used. Once in the cavernous sinus it is also very lateral and can be injured only when more radical resection of intracavernous sinus lesion is pursued. However, one must be care-

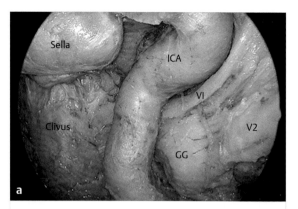

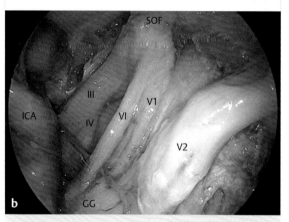

Fig. 2.33 a, b Cadaveric endoscopic dissection of the left cavernous sinus. **(a)** Anterior view. **(b)** Lateral displacement of the carotid artery to expose the cranial nerves.
GG, gasserian ganglion; ICA, internal carotid artery; III, third cranial nerve; IV, fourth cranial nerve; SOF, superior orbital fissure; V1, ophthalmic nerve; V2, maxillary nerve; VI, abducens nerve.

ful with supraorbital approaches due to the fact that the trochlear nerve assumes a very medial position in that region. Endoscopic endonasal removal of the medial superior roof of the orbit can result in cranial nerve IV palsy due to excessive periorbital retraction to reach lateral on the anterior skull base.

Trigeminal Nerve

The trigeminal nerve is mostly a sensory nerve, but also has motor functions. The large sensory root and the small motor root arise from the pons, near the superior limb of cerebellopontine fissure. The sensory roots join the trigeminal ganglion in a depression at the middle fossa floor, near the apex of the petrous part of the temporal bone, the Meckel cave.

At the cave, the trigeminal nerve trifurcates into three major branches (▶ Fig. 2.34), the ophthalmic, maxillary, and mandibular branches, distal to the trigeminal ganglion.

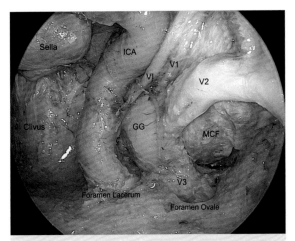

Fig. 2.34 Endoscopic cadaveric dissection of the left cavernous sinus/Meckel cave regions.
GG, gasserian ganglion; ICA, internal carotid artery; MCF, middle cranial fossa; V1, ophthalmic nerve; V2, maxillary nerve; V3, mandibular nerve; VI, abducens nerve.

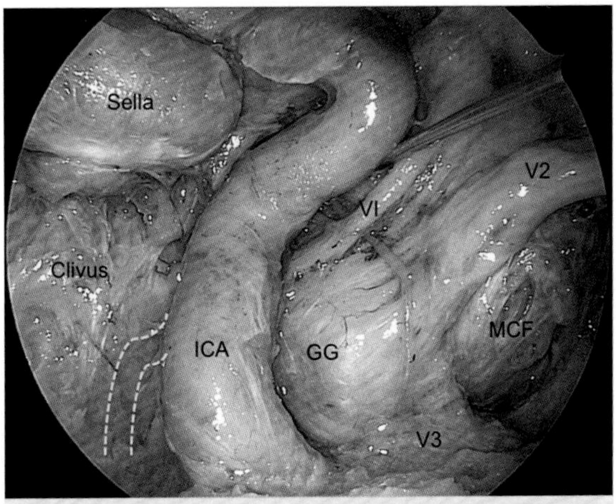

Fig. 2.35 Cadaveric specimen dissection depicting the left sixth cranial nerve trajectory from the posterior fossa to the cavernous sinus (dashed yellow lines).
GG, gasserian ganglion; ICA, internal carotid artery; MCF, middle cranial fossa; V2, maxillary nerve; V3, mandibular nerve; VI, abducens nerve.

The ophthalmic nerve supplies branches to portions of the eyes, the skin of eyelids, forehead, nose, and part of the nasal cavity. It leaves the Meckel cave and passes forward in the lateral wall of the cavernous sinus, with the oculomotor and trochlear nerves, to converge on the superior orbital fissure. The nerve splits just behind the annular tendon into lacrimal, frontal, and nasociliary nerves.

The maxillary nerve passes in the lower part of the cavernous sinus, gives rise to a meningeal branch, and exits the skull base through the foramen rotundum, in the greater wing of the sphenoid, to enter the pterygopalatine fossa. There, it gives communicating rami to the pterygopalatine ganglion and contributes the zygomatic, infraorbital, and palatine nerves to innervate the skin of the central part of the face, the nasal cavity, the sinuses, and the maxillary teeth.

The mandibular nerve is sensory and motor. It carries sensory information from the mandible, lower teeth and gums, external ear, tympanic membrane and chin, as well as from the meninges of the cranial convexity. The motor root supplies the pterygoids, temporalis, masseter, mylohyoid, anterior belly of digastric, tensor tympani, and tensor palatini muscles.

The mandibular nerve arises at the trigeminal ganglion and exits the middle cranial fossa through the foramen ovale. It enters the infratemporal fossa, located medial to the temporal fossa and below the greater sphenoid wing, and splits in four main branches: lingual, inferior alveolar, buccal, and auriculotemporal nerves.

The trigeminal nerve can be involved in several skull base pathologies, whether directly (trigeminal schwannomas) or indirectly (nasal malignancies with trigeminal branch infiltration). It is also an important landmark

(along with the ICA and cranial nerve VI) during endonasal approaches to the middle fossa through the quadrangular space.

Trigeminal schwannomas can be approached endonasally through the enlarged Meckel cave.[107] Sinonasal malignancies can often infiltrate the trigeminal branches and use the nerves as pathways to intracranial dissemination; in these cases the nerves must be dissected and sacrificed to ensure oncologic resection margins.

Abducens Nerve

The abducens nerve is a motor nerve. It arises from the pontomedullary junction, near the midline, and travels anteriorly through the pontine cistern. The nerve runs upwards and pierces the dura mater to then travel between the dura and the periosteum of the clivus (inside the basilar plexus as pointed earlier in this chapter) in a laterosuperior orientation that ends just lateral to the dorsum sellae. When passing at the ridge of the petrous temporal bone, it turns sharply and runs under the petrosphenoid ligament (Gruber ligament), forming the roof of the Dorello canal, to enter the cavernous sinus (▶ Fig. 2.35).

At the cavernous sinus, the abducens nerve passes below and lateral to the ICA and medial to the ophthalmic nerve. It enters the orbit through the lower part of the superior orbital fissure, passing below the ophthalmic nerve, to reach and innervate the lateral rectus muscle.

Cranial nerve VI is commonly injured in two different settings: tumors infiltrating the clivus, such as chordomas,[106] and tumors infiltrating the medial compartment of the cavernous sinus, such as pituitary adenomas. As with other cranial nerves, neurophysiological monitoring

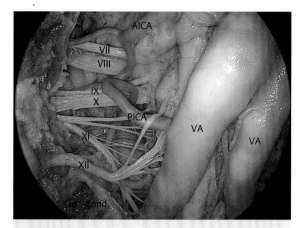

Fig. 2.36 Endoscopic "far-medial" approach to the lower clivus with partial right condylectomy on a cadaveric specimen, exposing the lower cranial nerves.
AICA, anterior inferior cerebellar artery; IX, glossopharyngeal nerve; Occ. Cond., occipital condyle; PICA, posterior inferior cerebellar artery; VA, vertebral artery; VII, facial nerve; VIII, vestibulocochlear nerve; X, vagus nerve; XI accessory nerve; XII, hypoglossal nerve.

is essential to prevent nerve damage; this is especially true in clival chordomas that infiltrate and distort the basilar plexus making it very difficult to visualize the nerve during surgery.

The VII and VIII Nerve Complex

The facial nerve, cranial nerve VII, is responsible for innervating the muscles of facial expression and for providing the special sensory information of the anterior two-thirds of the tongue and oral cavity. It arises from the cerebellopontine angle and runs through the posterior cranial fossa until it reaches the internal acoustic meatus.

The vestibulocochlear nerve is a sensory nerve responsible for balance and hearing. It arises at the end of the pontomedullary sulcus, lateral to the facial nerve, and crosses laterally to enter the internal acoustic meatus with the seventh nerve.

The VII and VIII nerve complex is seldom approached or visualized during endoscopic skull base surgery; cases such as large clival chordomas or meningiomas with lateral extension the resection may lead the surgeon away from the midline and the complex may come into sight (▶ Fig. 2.36).

Glossopharyngeal Nerve

The glossopharyngeal nerve has sensory and motor functions. It arises from the medulla, between the olive and the inferior cerebellar peduncle, rostral to the vagus nerve at the postolivary sulcus. The ninth nerve leaves the skull base through the jugular foramen (▶ Fig. 2.36) and passes through the intrajugular portion of the foramen on the medial side of the intrajugular process.

At the jugular foramen, the nerve passes on the medial side of jugular bulb. Then, it exits the foramen, turning forward along the lateral surface of ICA. The nerve gets enlarged at the site of its superior (jugular) and inferior (petrosal) ganglia.

The glossopharyngeal nerve descends deep to the styloid process in the neck to give sensory supply to the oropharynx, posterior part of the tongue, carotid sinus and carotid body, motor supply to the stylopharyngeus muscle, and send parasympathetic fibers to parotid gland.

Vagus Nerve

Cranial nerve X is composed of both motor and sensory roots and is also the longest. It leaves the medulla and the skull, passing through the neck, chest, and abdomen, contributing to laryngeal, pharyngeal, and autonomic visceral innervations.

Vagus nerve rootlets arise from the medulla at the postolivary sulcus and pierce the dura of the intrajugular process (▶ Fig. 2.36), at the vagus meatus, to reach the medial wall of internal jugular vein at the jugular foramen. The rootlets enter the jugular foramen just behind the glossopharyngeal nerve.

The vagus nerve has two sensory ganglia: one placed inside the foramen, the superior (or jugular) ganglion, and other placed below it, the inferior (or nodose) ganglion. At the superior ganglion the nerve communicates with the accessory nerve and also gives rise to the auricular branch. The inferior ganglion is located at the level of the atlanto-occipital joint. The vagus nerve descends in the carotid sheath to give rise to its branches to pharynx, larynx, heart, and abdominal viscera.

Accessory Nerve

The accessory nerve is composed of a spinal and a cranial root. The cranial component arises just caudal to the vagal fibers, at the postolivary sulcus, and runs toward the jugular foramen (▶ Fig. 2.36), entering the foramen through the vagal meatus, to join the vagus ganglia. It runs together with cranial nerve X and helps innervate, mainly, the superior laryngeal and pharyngeal branches of the vagus nerve.

The spinal accessory nerve emerges from the upper five segments of spinal cord, between the dorsal spinal nerve roots and dentate ligament. It ascends, entering the posterior cranial fossa through the foramen magnum and meets the accessory cranial fibers to emerge at the jugular foramen.

After exiting the skull base, the spinal accessory nerve runs backward in front of the internal jugular vein and turns down obliquely to reach and innervate the sterno-cleidomastoid and trapezius muscles.

Hypoglossal Nerve

The rootlets of the hypoglossal nerve emerge at the preolivary sulcus, between the olive and the pyramid. The nerve passes behind the vertebral artery to enter the hypoglossal canal (▶ Fig. 2.36), located below and medial to the jugular foramen, at the occipital bone.

The hypoglossal nerve exits the hypoglossal canal and travels behind the vagus nerve, running between the ICA and the internal jugular vein, in the carotid sheath. At the level of the atlas (C1), it turns forward, passing below the digastric muscle, and loops around the occipital artery to reach the submandibular region and the tongue.

Cranial nerve XII is essentially motor and innervates the intrinsic muscles of tongue. It also receives motor fibers from C1.

The anatomy of the hypoglossal nerve and the hypoglossal canal is especially useful while performing "far-medial" approaches to the lower clivus for tumors such as chordomas and meningiomas with significant lateral extension.

Vidian Nerve

The vidian nerve is formed by parasympathetic fibers of the greater superficial petrosal nerve from the middle cranial fossa as well as sympathetic fibers of the deep petrosal nerve.[108] It is usually accompanied by the vidian artery, a branch from the petrous ICA that anastomoses with branches from the internal maxillary artery within the vidian canal, though this specific vascular anatomy has been found to be variable.[108] A vidian vein is also usually present.

These neurovascular structures traverse the vidian canal, sometimes referred to as the pterygoid canal. It is formed at the junction between the body of the sphenoid bone and the pterygoid process.[109] It transports the vidian nerve from its formation at the carotid canal to the pterygopalatine fossa, where the nerve ends at the pterygopalatine ganglion.

Due to this posterior to the anterior trajectory and its intimate relation to the anterior genu of the petrous ICA, the vidian nerve and its canal have been identified as a safe and consistent landmark during endoscopic skull base approaches.[103,107,108] Knowledge of this anatomy is invaluable especially when dealing with large bone-deforming tumors, such as chordomas, which cause disruption of the normal anatomy and may significantly increase the risk of injury to the ICA. By drilling the vidian canal and following its path posteriorly, the surgeon will invariably reach the petrous ICA at its genu, before it becomes the paraclival carotid, thus enabling a safe approach to middle third of the clivus.

We believe that whenever possible the nerve must be preserved; this can be accomplished by transposing it superiorly after the opening of the canal.[110] Once it has been drilled and the nerve is fully freed, it may be mobilized according to the surgeon's needs during the remainder of the approach and the tumor resection. In some cases in which these measures are not feasible the nerve may be resected; in these instances patients may develop ipsilateral dry eye and diminished emotional tearing.

2.3 Endoscopic Glance at the Skull Base

Manfred Tschabitscher, Iacopo Dallan

2.3.1 Introduction

Describing the anatomy of the skull base and related structures is a complex and challenging task, particularly if the anatomy has to be depicted from an endonasal endoscopic surgical perspective. For this reason, we have decided to use the concept of "windows" as a teaching tool in this chapter. By opening one window it is possible to see what lies behind and this model can be reproduced endlessly during dissection. In this sense, the paranasal sinuses (especially the ethmoid and sphenoid sinuses) can be considered the endoscopic gateways to the ventral and lateral skull base. Obviously, knowledge of the surgical landmarks is mandatory to safely perform every approach to the skull base. Furthermore, it is paramount to have the best possible view of a dynamic working box when entering this area to deal with such surgery. It is the opinion of the authors that in every moment the surgeon should realize where he/she is going and have perfect knowledge of the boundaries of the box in which he/she is working. As the surgery proceeds, the box changes and the surgeon must consequently and dynamically get re-oriented with every change. Based on this instructional model, the first chambers to be described (and which the surgeon encounters) are the nasal fossae. They can be considered like a corridor, with different walls and, into which, many rooms open. The medial and lateral walls of each corridor are the nasal septum and the lateral nasal wall, respectively. Anatomically the medial wall is quite easy to understand, and, while it is important especially for reconstructive purposes, the anatomy of the lateral nasal wall is far more complex.

Endoscopically, the first structures encountered are the heads of the inferior and middle turbinates. The inferior turbinate is an independent bone attached to the medial maxillary wall, while the middle and superior turbinates (and sometimes the supreme one) belong to the ethmoidal complex. This anatomical structure is composed of bony cells that appear to grow with a superior-to-inferior direction like saddle bags.[111] These thin-walled chambers are situated in a space that is limited laterally by the lamina papyracea and medially by the sagittal portion of the middle and superior turbinates. The ethmoidal cells are divided into two groups by the ground lamella of the middle turbinate.

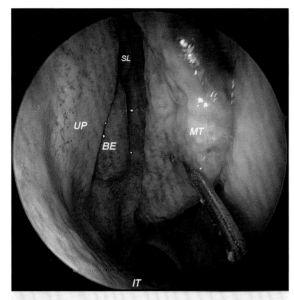

Fig. 2.37 Right nasal fossa, endoscopic view. The middle turbinate is medialized.
BE, bulla ethmoidalis; IT, inferior turbinate; MT, middle turbinate; SL, sinus lateralis; UP, uncinate process.

2.3.2 Anterior Ethmoid Cells

The anterior ethmoid cells open below the middle turbinate, into the middle meatus. Once the middle turbinate is removed, the middle meatus can be explored. The uncinate process, bulla ethmoidalis, and agger nasi are visible in front of the middle turbinate (▶ Fig. 2.37). Between the bulla ethmoidalis and the uncinate process, a boomerang-shaped cleft, namely the hiatus semilunaris, can be seen. The frontal recess forms the apex of this space.

The bulla ethmoidalis is the largest air cell in the anterior ethmoid sinuses; it is rarely nonpneumatized and in this case it is named torus ethmoidalis. The height of the bulla ethmoidalis is variable; if it does not reach the ethmoidal roof, a space varying in shape is present above the bulla: the supraretrobullar recess or sinus lateralis of Grünwald. If the bulla reaches the ethmoidal roof, it forms the posterior aspect of the frontal recess.

The uncinate process is a sagittal-oriented thin bony lamella, which usually runs parallel to the anterior surface of the bulla ethmoidalis. The anterior convex margin of the uncinate process bifurcates at the frontal maxillary process. The uncinate process can fuse with the agger nasi superiorly and with the ethmoidal process of the inferior turbinate.[112] Pneumatization of the agger nasi is quite variable but it is usually in close relationship with the lacrimal bone and consequently with the lacrimal sac.

2.3.3 Frontal Sinus

The paired frontal sinuses are roughly pyramidal in shape oriented with their bases placed inferiorly. An intersinus septum divides the two sinuses, rarely in a symmetric or equal fashion, and forms their medial wall. Their anterior walls correspond to the anterior frontal sinus table while the posterior walls have a vertical and a horizontal portion that are almost perpendicular to each other. This bone is approximately 1 mm thick. Their inferior wall (orbito-ethmoid-nasal) has an orbital section and a nasoethmoidal section, both lying in the horizontal plane but at different levels. The orbital portion is made up of a slim lamella of cortical bone, concave below and convex above, surmounting the orbit. The nasoethmoidal portion, named fovea ethmoidalis, is located at a lower level than the orbital section; it is made up of a quadrilateral lamella of sturdy, cortical bone. Its inferior plane is fused with the lateral portion of the cribriform plate, which in turn forms the insertion of the basal lamella of the middle turbinate. The medial aspect of the ethmoidal roof is formed by the lateral lamella of the cribriform plate, which is the site at greatest risk for iatrogenic cerebrospinal fluid leaks. The lateral lamella may show significant anatomic variations due to differences in size and orientation. It may also show anatomical asymmetries in its length and orientation on both sides. The highest point of the ethmoidal roof may surpass the cribriform plate by even 17 mm.[112,113]

Endoscopically, the frontal sinus opening is usually visualized at the most slanted site of the nasoethmoidal section. The opening, in the upper part of the frontal recess, is located at the junction of the frontal sinus and the ethmoid sinus. Its margins are made up of ethmoid components. With respect to the frontal opening, the frontal recess is a three-dimensional space located between independent bones that define its boundaries, form, and dimensions. The lateral lamella of the cribriform plate, which is fused with the sagittal portion of the basal lamella of the middle turbinate, composes the medial wall of the frontal recess. The lamina papyracea largely forms its lateral portion. The bulla ethmoidalis forms its posterior wall, but only if it reaches the ethmoidal roof. Most often, however, the bulla does not reach the ethmoidal roof and the frontal recess communicates posteriorly with the sinus lateralis. The agger nasi cells form the anterior wall.

2.3.4 Maxillary Sinus

This pyramidal-shaped sinus has its apex placed laterally and its base medially (corresponds to the lateral nasal wall). Its anterolateral wall corresponds to the face and the zygomatic process. Its posterior wall opens into the pterygopalatine and infratemporal fossa while the superior one represents the floor of the orbit. Its inferior wall of the maxillary sinus corresponds to the alveolar process. In an isolated maxillary bone, the medial wall of the maxillary sinus has a wide opening; in vivo, this opening is partially closed by the ethmoidal structures, palatine bone, and, to a lesser extent, by the lacrimal bone. The roof of the maxillary sinus transmits, within the infraorbital canal, the infraorbital bundle. Haller cells are a variation of ethmoid cells within the maxillary sinus, under the orbital floor. The natural ostium of the maxillary sinus usually opens into the caudal third of the ethmoidal infundibulum, inferolateral portion to the bulla ethmoidalis. The anterior and posterior fontanelle (anterior and posterior to the natural ostium, respectively) form the remaining part of the medial maxillary wall. Most frequently, the posterior fontanelle is dehiscent; thus, giving rise to an accessory ostium.

2.3.5 Posterior Ethmoid

The posterior ethmoidal complex is variable in shape, given the fact that the anterior and posterior walls can show different shapes and orientation. Functionally, the posterior ethmoidal cells drain above the middle turbinate, in the superior meatus. Its anterior wall is the ground lamella of the middle turbinate, while the sphenoid sinus borders it posteriorly. Paraseptally, the sphenoethmoidal recess represents the door leading to the natural ostium of the sphenoid. In about 10% of patients, there is an Onodi cell, which is a posterior ethmoidal cell that invades the sphenoid sinus laterally and/or superiorly. In some patients, the optic nerve and even the ICA can be in contact with the Onodi-Grünwald cell.[113] Laterally, the junction between the posterior ethmoid and the sphenoid sinus is at the level of the optic ring, the narrowest point of the optic canal.

2.3.6 Sphenoid Sinus

In a coronal plane, the sphenoid sinus is rectangular, usually larger laterolaterally than craniocaudally. Three types of sinuses can be distinguished based on their pneumatization: conchal, sellar, and presellar. In well-pneumatized sinuses, various landmarks can be recognized on the lateral wall of the sinus. Three prominences are visible in a superior-to-inferior direction including the canals of the optic nerve, ICA, and maxillary nerve (V_2). Between these prominences, it is possible to see some recesses and grooves (▶ Fig. 2.38). The lateral opticocarotid recess (lOCR) is a niche formed by the optic nerve superiorly and the ICA inferiorly, and it is viewed better if there is pneumatization of the optic strut. The medial opticocarotid recess (mOCR) represents the lateral aspect of the tuberculum sellae, which is the area of contact between the point of origin of the optic canal medially and the posterior margin of the parasellar carotid artery. In other

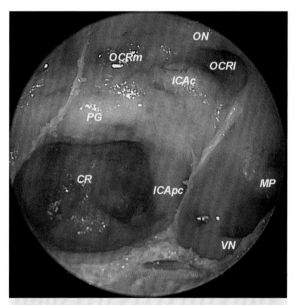

Fig. 2.38 Sphenoid sinus, endoscopic view. CR, clival recess; ICAc, cavernous portion of the internal carotid artery; ICApc, paraclival portion of the internal carotid artery; MP, maxillary prominence; OCRl, lateral opticocarotid recess; OCRm, medial opticocarotid recess; ON, optic nerve; PG, pituitary gland; VN, vidian nerve.

words, the tuberculum sellae connects with the mOCR on both sides.

The vidian nerve prominence is visible in the lateral portion of the inferior wall. On the posterior wall, the pituitary prominence lies above the clival recess, a wide groove that corresponds to the sphenoidal portion of the clivus. Furthermore, the space within the sphenoid bone is usually divided by one or several septa. On the anteroinferior wall of the sphenoid sinus lies the sphenoidal rostrum, which represents the inferior border of the sphenoidal floor. The pneumatisation of the sinus may occasionally extend anteriorly through the rostrum into the septum. As a rule, the more the rostral pneumatization is extended, the more lateral the natural ostium will be.

Superiorly, the planum sphenoidalis, the prechiasmatic sulcus, and the tuberculum sellae are visible from anterior to posterior. Sometimes the planum sphenoidalis has a lateral extension, the medial clinoid process. In about 10% of patients, it is possible to see the carotid-clinoid foramen (Henle foramen)[111] formed by the ossification of a bridge of dura mater between the anterior and medial clinoid process. The dorsum sellae and posterior clinoids border the sella turcica posteriorly and the cavernous sinuses comprise the lateral borders. The lamina papyracea forms the lateral border of the planum sphenoidalis. A downward sloping wall named the tuberculum sellae forms the anterior wall and the body of the sphenoid bone forms the floor.

2.3.7 Vascularization

Nasal vascularization is principally through the spheno-palatine artery and the ethmoidal arteries. Endoscopically, the anterior ethmoidal artery can be identified at the level of the first foveola, posterior to the opening of the frontal sinus, while the ethmoidal roof usually contains the posterior ethmoidal artery mail. The sphenopalatine artery runs between the orbital and the sphenoidal process of the palatine bone at the posterior edge of the maxillary sinus. Anterior to this foramen, the descending palatine artery runs through the palatine bone (posterior to the accompanying greater palatine nerve). The palato-vaginal artery is visible posteriorly, but only after the inferior displacement of the mucosa of the upper naso-pharyngeal wall. This vessel is one of the terminal branches of the maxillary artery.

2.3.8 Cribriform Plate Window

The anterior cranial fossa floor comes into view after complete removal of the ethmoidal complex and the nasal septum. The fovea ethmoidalis, lateral lamella of the cribriform plate, and the cribriform plate proper form the floor of the anterior cranial fossa. The relationship between the horizontally oriented cribriform plate and its lateral lamella is variable in shape, according to the different geometrical orientation and extension of the lateral lamella. The level of the cribriform plate is often lower than the rest of the anterior skull base. Even from a sagittal point of view, the anterior cranial base presents a concave shape with the deepest point usually localized in the middle. After removal of the septum and stripping of the mucosa over the nasal vault, it is possible to see the fila olfactoria, which are transmitted by the little openings in the cribriform plate (▶ Fig. 2.39).

The anterior and posterior ethmoidal neurovascular bundles exit the orbit and run medially toward the anterior cranial fossa transmitted by their corresponding foramina and canals, in close relationship with the floor of the anterior cranial fossa. These foramina are bordered by the frontal bone superiorly and the ethmoidal complex inferiorly. Usually, the anterior ethmoidal neurovascular bundles are easily identifiable posterior to the frontal sinus recess, at the level of the first foveola. In a well-pneumatized sinus, the bundle may run free within the ethmoidal complex and not within a canal in the skull base. Conversely the posterior ethmoidal artery runs almost constantly within the ethmoidal roof. It is common to see a middle ethmoidal neurovascular bundle as well. Commonly, the anterior ethmoidal neurovascular bundle can ramify at any point in the skull base.

By removing the bone of the median anterior cranial base, the crista galli becomes apparent. Laterally, a dural

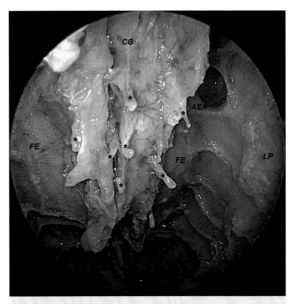

Fig. 2.39 Anterior cranial base, endoscopic view. AEA, anterior ethmoidal artery; CG, crista galli; FE, fovea ethmoidalis; LP, lamina papyracea. *Stars*, fila olfactoria.

plane is visible from orbit to orbit. The crista galli can extend to a variable depth into the cranial cavity, and is situated between the frontal bones. Usually it is a thick bony structure and is rarely pneumatized. To remove the crista galli, it is necessary to drill internally until it becomes eggshell thin; then, it can be removed easily. The falx cerebri can be seen in close proximity to the crista galli. This structure is a large fold of the dura in the sagittal plane, running in the midline between the cerebral hemispheres. As stated, it is attached anteriorly to the crista galli, mainly on its posterior border, and to the adjacent anterior skull base. At this level, the beginning of superior sagittal sinus is located just behind the frontal sinuses. When drilling the crista galli, venous bleeding can arise from the most inferior part of superior sagittal sinus or from the veins lying on the cribriform plate. From this point, the superior sagittal sinus runs superiorly in a shallow groove of the inner surface of the calvaria, with its lateral walls given by two laminae of the falx cerebri. In rare cases, it may communicate with the veins of the nasal cavity through the foramen cecum. At this level, it is sometimes possible to see the anterior falcine artery, a branch of the anterior ethmoidal artery.

By removing the falx cerebri and the dural plane, the basal surface of the frontal lobes and the inter-hemispheric fissure become evident. In the paramedian position, it is possible to locate the olfactory bulbs and, for posteriorly, the olfactory tract (▶ Fig. 2.40). The basal surface of the frontal lobes is divided by the olfactory sulcus into a medial compartment, the gyrus rectus, and a larger portion, the orbital gyri. Laterally, the orbital sulcus divides this latter portion into anterior, medial, lateral,

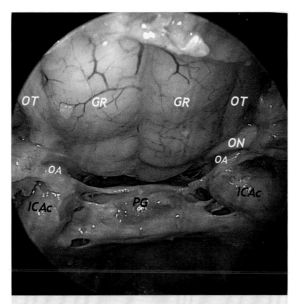

Fig. 2.40 Anterior cranial fossa, endoscopic view. The anterior cranial base and the dura mater have been removed.
GR, gyrus rectus; ICAc, cavernous portion of the internal carotid artery; OA, ophthalmic artery; ON, optic nerve; OT, olfactory tract; PG, pituitary gland.

and posterior groups. Endoscopically, this latter classification is of limited significance.

There is a rich vascularization coming from the anterior cerebral artery (ACA) in close relationship to the olfactory

bulb. This latter supplies the medial part of the orbital gyrus, the gyrus rectus, and the olfactory bulb and tract[114] on the basal surface. From an endoscopic point of view, only the orbitofrontal and frontopolar arteries are truly significant. These vessels usually arise from A2. The orbitofrontal artery is almost constantly present and arises usually from A2 (seldom arises from A1). From its point of origin, it passes downward and forward toward the floor of the anterior cranial fossa to reach the level of the planum sphenoidalis. The frontopolar artery arises usually from A2 and passes anteriorly along the medial surface of the hemisphere toward the frontal pole. Development of the venous network is far less constant. It is usually possible to recognize the frontopolar, anterior and posterior fronto-orbital veins, and the olfactory veins. All together, these veins drain the basal surface of the frontal lobe. The anterior fronto-orbital veins empty into the anterior part of the superior sagittal sinus; whereas, the posterior fronto-orbital veins empty into the veins below the anterior perforated substance that subsequently converge on the anterior end of the basal vein (▶ Fig. 2.41).[115]

2.3.9 Sphenoidal Window

A complete anterior sphenoidotomy exposes the gate to the middle and posterior cranial fossa. More specifically, the sellar, suprasellar, and cavernous regions, as well as the superior portion of the posterior cranial fossa, can be accessed through this window. Every landmark should be

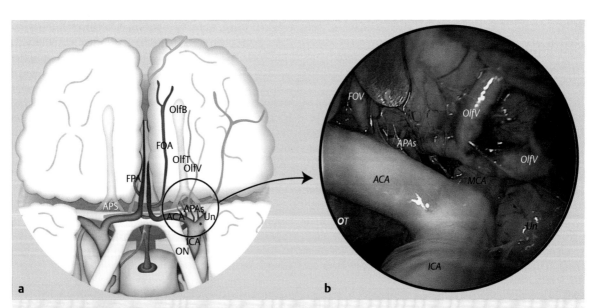

Fig. 2.41 a, b Three-dimensional reconstruction of the anterior cranial fossa and sellar region (a). Left anterior perforate substance, endoscopic view (b).
ACA, anterior cerebral artery; APAs, the anterior perforate substance arteries; APS, anterior perforate substance; FOA, fronto-orbital artery; FOV, fronto-orbital vein; FPA, frontopolar artery; ICA, internal carotid artery; MCA, middle cerebral artery; OlfB, olfactory bulb; OlfT, olfactory tract; OlfV, olfactory vein; OT, optic tract; Un, uncus. *Star*, middle cerebral artery.

recognized before proceeding. The sellar floor with the pituitary prominence is usually evident in the posterior part of the roof posterior to the planum sphenoidalis. The clival recess, a space bordered laterally by the paraclival ICA prominences and superiorly by the pituitary prominence, is below the sellar floor. As previously discussed, according to the degree of its pneumatization, various prominences and grooves can be easily identified on the lateral wall. From superior to inferior we find the prominences formed by the canals of the optic nerve, the ICA, and the maxillary nerve. After removal of the overlying bone, the periosteal and dural layers become evident. At this point, the close relationship between the optic pathways and the pituitary gland becomes clearer.

Sellar Compartment

Macroscopically, the pituitary gland is attached to the median eminence of the tuber cinereum of the hypothalamus through the infundibular stalk. The superior limit of the sellar compartment is provided by the diaphragma sellae (DS), which is the quadrilateral lamella with an opening through which the infundibular stalk passes. The borders of the DS are: anteriorly, the dural insertion on the tuberculum sellae; posteriorly, the dural insertion on the dorsum sellae; and laterally, the point where the medial wall of the cavernous sinus meets the superior wall. The lateral and superior portions of the pituitary gland are protected by the dura mater superiorly and the subdiaphragmatic cistern inferiorly while anteroinferiorly it is covered by bone. The capsule of the gland is in direct contact with the dural layers. Endoscopically, a superior and an inferior intercavernous sinus are easily identified. This complex vascular network lies within the dural layers (▶ Fig. 2.42). At the level of the inferior aspect of the pituitary gland, the inferior intercavernous sinus can be seen as well. Occasionally, these sinuses can be united, completely covering the anterior surface of the gland.

Small arteriolar branches can be found on the dural surface. Removal of the dural layer exposes the pituitary gland. A very close relationship between the cavernous portion of the ICA and the pituitary gland is present, but it is quite variable even in the absence of pathology. Below the body of the pituitary gland, it is possible to see the terminal ramification of the inferior hypophyseal artery bilaterally. By superiorly transposing the body of the pituitary gland, the dorsum sellae and the posterior clinoids are visible with the diaphragma sellae connecting the posterior gland to the dorsum sellae.

Supraretrosellar Compartment

Macroscopically, the suprasellar region can be compared with an equilateral pyramid,[116] with the sellar diaphragm as base. The anterior side contains the lamina terminalis, the optic chiasm, the paired optic nerves, and the anterior

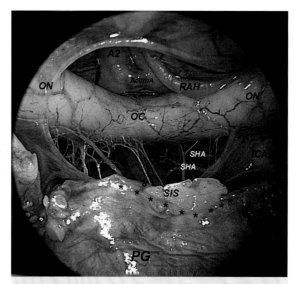

Fig. 2.42 Suprasellar region, endoscopic view.
A2, anterior cerebral artery (second segment); AcomA, anterior communicating artery; ICAi, intracranial portion of the internal carotid artery; OC, optic chiasm; ON, optic nerve; PG, pituitary gland; RAH, recurrent artery of Heubner; SHA, superior hypophyseal artery; SIS, superior intracavernous sinus. *Black circle*, inner layer of the dura mater; *stars*, outer layer of the dura mater.

communicating artery complex. Laterally, we find the optic tract, the ICA, the posterior communicating artery, the anterior choroidal artery, and the third cranial nerve. The posterior side contains the interpeduncular fossa, the basilar tip with P1 segments and superior cerebellar arteries, and the exit of the third cranial nerves. The infundibulum and the pituitary stalk mark the apex of the pyramid.[116] Endoscopically, the optic chiasm is clearly evident above and in front of the pituitary gland. The pituitary stalk can also be seen passing posterior to the optic chiasm. A rich arterial network coming from the internal carotid arteries is present all around the pituitary stalk. This network is provided by the superior hypophyseal arteries, which usually arise from the supraclinoid portion of the ICA. Rarely, these vessels can arise from the cavernous portion of the ICA. Sometimes it is possible to see a "crown" of arteries around the superior aspect of the pituitary stalk, from which coaxial vessels run downward to reach the body of the anterior lobe of the pituitary gland (▶ Fig. 2.43). On the inferomedial surface of the optic nerves, it is possible to see the ophthalmic artery, normally arising as the first branch of the supraclinoid ICA, and entering the optic canal a short distance from its origin. The ophthalmic artery, the optic nerve, and the olfactory tract are in close relationship.

Superolateral to the optic chiasm, the supraclinoid segment of the ICA can be seen running upward on the lateral side of the optic tract, where it then divides into the ACA and the middle cerebral artery (MCA) just below

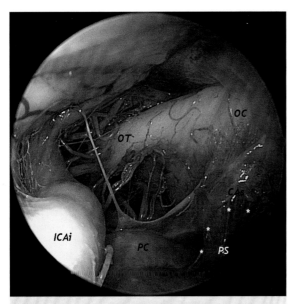

Fig. 2.43 Right suprasellar region, endoscopic view. CAs, circuminfundibular arteries; ICAi, intracranial portion of the internal carotid artery; OC, optic chiasm; OT, optic tract; PC, posterior clinoid; PS, pituitary stalk. *Stars*, coaxial branches.

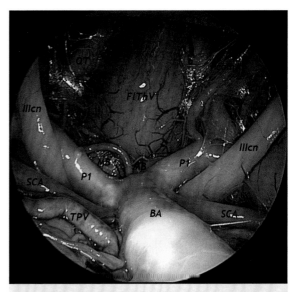

Fig. 2.44 Basilar tip region, endoscopic view from below. AchA, anterior choroidal artery; BA, basilar artery; FlThV, floor of the third ventricle; IIIcn, oculomotor nerve; MB, mammillary body; OT, optic tract; P1, posterior cerebral artery (first segment); PcomA, posterior communicating artery; SCA, superior cerebellar artery; TPV, transverse pontine vein.

the anterior perforate substance. There is a large arterial complex at this level, where the branches are known, overall, as anterior perforating arteries. By definition, this is a group of arteries that enter the anterior perforated substance; they originate from the ICA, the ACA, the MCA, and the anterior choroidal artery. The veins from the frontal lobes (such as the olfactory veins and the orbital veins) converge at this area (▸ Fig. 2.41).

One can see the anterior communicating artery complex with the first segments of ACA (A1 and A2) as well as the lamina terminalis in the midline, above the chiasm (▸ Fig. 2.42). Slightly more anterior lies the posterior portion of the olfactory tracts, as well as the gyri recti. The olfactory vein is usually identifiable close to the olfactory tract, while the anterior cerebral vein, which has been joined by the paraterminal veins coming from the interhemispheric fissure, is generally visible over the chiasm. At this level, the anterior communicating vein can be seen as well. By passing infrachiasmatically or by transposing the pituitary gland, the basilar apex network with its close relationship with the oculomotor nerves is evident. These nerves pass inferior and slightly lateral to the posterior communicating artery (PcomA) in cases of normal configuration, while in cases of fetal configuration the nerve runs beneath or medial to PcomA. The oculomotor nerves arise in the interpeduncular cistern, on the medial side of the cerebral peduncle and run anterolaterally to reach the roof of the cavernous sinus. The Liliequist membrane, an arachnoidal structure, is attached superiorly to the oculomotor nerves and anteriorly to the dorsum sellae. Anteriorly, the oculomotor nerves pierce the roof

of the cavernous sinus. As stated before, in the anterior incisural space below the floor of the third ventricle, the posterior part of the circle of Willis is exposed (▸ Fig. 2.44). At the level the interpeduncular cistern, below the mammillary bodies, the peduncular veins are visible. More superiorly and laterally, it is possible to see the basal vein running on the lateral surface of the mesencephalon in the ambient cistern.

Ventricular Compartment

The lamina terminalis is easily recognized passing above the optic chiasm. This is a thin layer of gray matter and pia mater that fills the space between the anterior commissure and the optic chiasm. After opening the lamina terminalis, the front door to the third ventricle is opened and, by means of a 30° lens endoscope, a panoramic view of the third ventricle is gained. The mammillary bodies are visible in the anterior part of the floor of the third ventricle, as well as the infundibular recess. Above them, the massa intermedia, a bridging structure between thalami, is usually visible. Proceeding distally, the posterior commissure and the beginning of the aqueduct below are visible. The suprapineal recess, the habenular commissure, the pineal recess, and body complete the posterior wall of the third ventricle. Above this portion, the thalamic prominences are visible with the choroid plexus above them. The foramina of Monro are visible when turning the lens upward. By doing so, the central portion of the lateral ventricle can be explored.

Cavernous Compartment

The cavernous sinus with its neurovascular contents lies on the lateral surface of the pituitary gland. Its dural walls surround a venous-filled space, through which a segment of the ICA, the abducens nerve, and the sympathetic plexus run. The sinus extends from the superior orbital fissure anteriorly to the area lateral to the dorsum sellae posteriorly.[117] The lateral and medial walls join anteriorly along the superior orbital fissure and inferiorly along the upper border of the maxillary nerve.

The cavernous ICA can be divided into a parasellar and a paraclival segment; more correctly named the intracavernous trigeminal portion (because it is in close relationship to V_2). The first segment forms the shape of a "C" with medial concavity. Below V_2, the ICA presents another short segment, which is paraclival but extracavernous. This supralacerum portion is delimited superiorly by V_2 and inferiorly by the petrolingual ligament (▶ Fig. 2.45). Endoscopically, the most identifiable nervous structure visible within the cavernous sinus is the abducens nerve, with its typical inferior-to-superior and medial-to-lateral course.

A rich neural network can be seen between the sympathetic fibers of the ICA and the abducens nerve. The nerve passes lateral to the ICA and enters the cavernous sinus below the superior petrosphenoidal ligament. Within the cavernous sinus, it runs almost parallel to the ophthalmic nerve (V_1). The artery of the inferior cavernous sinus, also known as the inferolateral trunk, is slightly more distal to the meningohypophyseal trunk (MHT) and nearly always passes above the abducens nerve, ending more or less in the area of the Meckel cave. Lateral to the abducens nerve plane (sixth cranial nerve), the oculomotor nerve (third cranial nerve), the trochlear nerve (fourth cranial nerve), V_1 and inferiorly V_2 can be seen. Typically, the trochlear nerve is accompanied by its homonymous artery, which is similar in size to the nerve. Endoscopically, different fibrous-dural septations can be observed within the cavernous sinus, thus apparently creating a common space with different venous lacunae, in which the terminal branches of the inferolateral trunk run with variable shapes. While the inferolateral trunk is easy to see, the McConnell capsular artery, when present, is somewhat difficult to identify. On the roof of the cavernous sinus, the close relationship with the optic nerve is very evident.

The ophthalmic artery usually arises at the supraclinoid portion of the ICA above the dural roof of the cavernous sinus, but in less than 10% of patients it can originate from the cavernous portion. The dural sheath of the optic nerve is closely related to the cavernous sinus dura. The meningohypophyseal trunk is usually visible at the posterior vertical segment of the ICA and usually arises at the medial aspect of this. Other branches of the MHT are the dorsal meningeal artery, for the dura of the posterior cranial fossa, and the Bernasconi-Cassinari artery, for the tentorium.

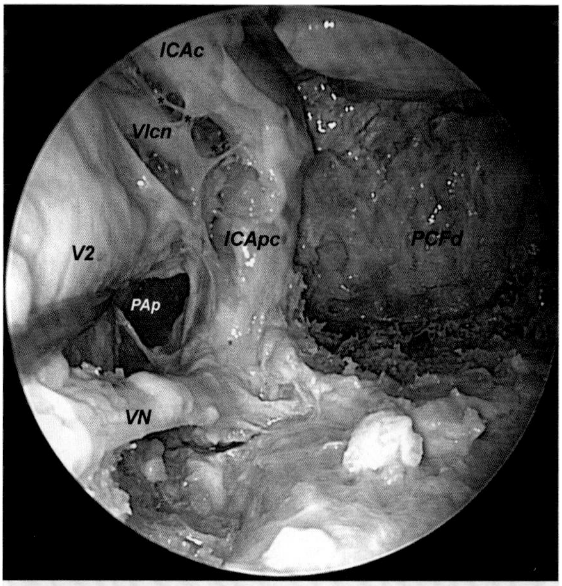

Clival Compartment

Below the body of the pituitary gland lies the pituitary fossa; once it is removed, the dura of the posterior cranial fossa becomes evident. The terminal ramification of the dorsal meningeal artery can usually be appreciated in the superior portion. Once the first dural layer is removed, the basilar plexus is evident. This represents the most constant venous connection between the cavernous sinuses.

The posterior cranial fossa is exposed upon opening the dural window (see clival window).

Clival and Craniocervical Windows

This gateway leads to the posterior cranial fossa and the upper spine. Depending upon the degree of pneumatization of the sphenoid sinus, the sphenoidal floor will endoscopically divide the sphenoidal portion of the clivus from the nasopharyngeal portion, in variable proportions. In some cases, the pneumatization is so extensive that it reaches the basilar part of the occipital bone. The bony segments of these windows are the sphenoidal body and the basilar part of the occipital bone. In the superior portion of the window, the paraclival segment of the ICA and the vidian nerves represent the lateral limit of the corridor.

Fig. 2.45 Right Meckel cave region, endoscopic view. ICAc, cavernous portion of the internal carotid artery; ICApc, paraclival portion of the internal carotid artery; PAp, petrous apex; PCFd, posterior cranial fossa dura; V2, maxillary nerve; VIcn, abducens nerve; VN, vidian nerve. *Stars*, anastomosis between sympathetic fibers and abducens nerve.

By removing the vomer and the sphenoidal floor, the sphenoidal and rhinopharyngeal portions of the clivus are united and a mucosal layer covers the deeper structures. In a superior and deeper plane, the pharyngobasilar membrane is attached to the basisphenoid, covering the upper clivus, and represents the upper limit of the superior constrictor muscle. Below the level of the carotid artery (lacerum foramen), the dissection can be extended laterally as far as the parapharyngeal portion of the ICA.[118] It must be stressed that the position of this portion of the ICA is extremely variable and that sometimes it can be on the posterior wall of the nasopharynx.[77]

The clival bone appears when the pharyngobasilar membrane and the longus capitis, one of the prevertebral muscles, are removed. The longus capitis usually originates at the level of the midclivus. Once the clival bone has been removed, the basilar plexus (the most extensive series of intracavernous connections) is visible. The inferior petrosal sinuses join this plexus laterally. In the lateral aspects of this region, the abducens nerve passes at a variable level through the basilar plexus in its own canal,[113] and then enters the posterior wall of the cavernous sinus. This nerve passes through the basilar plexus near the paraclival portion of the ICA. Close to the abducens nerve, the inferior hypophyseal artery (usually a branch of the MHT) is visible. Other arteries include the dorsal meningeal artery and the Bernasconi-Cassinari artery. Moreover, the dorsal meningeal artery can be very close to the abducens nerve at the dura of the posterior cranial fossa. The inferior portion of the clivus, which belongs to the occipital bone, represents the anterior margin of the foramen magnum.

As previously stated, the longus capitis muscles are attached at various levels in the median inferior clivus, while at C1 level we find the longus colli muscles. These muscles are covered by nasopharyngeal mucosa. In the upper part, the pharyngobasilar membrane represents the first layer under the mucosa, while below we find the superior portion of the superior constrictor muscle. More caudally, the external cover of the superior constrictor muscle is the buccopharyngeal fascia. Once the muscular plane (given principally by the longus colli and longus capitis) is removed, the anterior longitudinal ligament, and below it the atlanto-occipital membrane, become apparent. By removing these two connective layers, the inferior two-thirds of the clivus, C1 and C2, are exposed. To view the dens (part of the second cervical vertebra, C2), the anterior arch of the first cervical vertebra (C1) must be removed. Complete removal of the anterior arch of C1 allows viewing the occipital condyles at the lateral borders of the foramen magnum.

The dens is attached to the inferior border of the occipital bone by means of tenacious ligaments, the apical and the alar ligaments. To free the dens, all these ligaments and the transverse ligament must be removed. In this manner, a wide corridor to the anterior portion of the foramen magnum is created.

After opening the dura mater, all the neurovascular structures become visible. In the inferior portion, the vertebral arteries can be seen at their exit from the vertebral canal. The posterior inferior cerebellar artery and the anterior spinal artery are also visible. There is a close relationship between the lower cranial nerves and PICA at this level. The hypoglossal nerve can be identified above the first tract of the intradural vertebral artery; usually, this nerve arises (in the preolivary sulcus) as a series of rootlets that converge on the dural orifices of the hypoglossal canal where a significant venous network lies (▶ Fig. 2.46).

In the superior portion, the basilar tip region in front of the midbrain is visible behind the pituitary gland. The posterior cerebral artery arises directly from the basilar artery as terminal branches, usually with a perpendicular orientation. The first segment of the posterior cerebral artery is termed P1 before joining the PcomA; thereafter, it is known as P2. Below the posterior cerebral arteries, the superior cerebellar arteries originate from the lateral aspect of the basilar artery: usually just one vessel from each side. More than one superior cerebellar artery from one side is rarely seen. Normally, the superior cerebellar artery crosses below the oculomotor nerve and runs posteriorly below the trochlear nerve and above the trigeminal nerve. Occasionally, the lateral loop reaches the entry zone of root of the trigeminal nerve. The arterial network from the posterior cerebral artery is usually well visible in front of the cerebral peduncles. It is possible to see the thalamic perforating arteries that arise from P1 and enter the brain by passing through the posterior perforated substance and the medial part of the cerebral peduncles in the area behind the mammillary bodies. Endoscopically, they are indistinguishable from the premamillary arteries, which are branches from the posterior communicating artery entering the same area. With respect to the thalamic perforating arteries, the thalamogeniculate arteries arise directly from the P2 beneath the lateral thalamus and penetrate part of the roof of the ambient cistern. At this level, it is usually possible to see the peduncle vein running posteriorly around the cerebral peduncle, above the PCA and below the thalamus (▶ Fig. 2.46).

The pontotrigeminal vein arises on the superior and cerebellar peduncles and passes rostrally to the trigeminal nerve. The anterior, medial, and lateral pontomesencephalic veins can also be seen at this level. Transverse pontine veins are a group of veins that transverse the pons at various levels. They run laterally above or below the trigeminal nerve to drain into the superior petrosal vein, the pontotrigeminal vein, or the vein of the cerebellopontine fissure. At the mesencephalic level, the lateral anterior pontomesencephalic vein may anastomose with

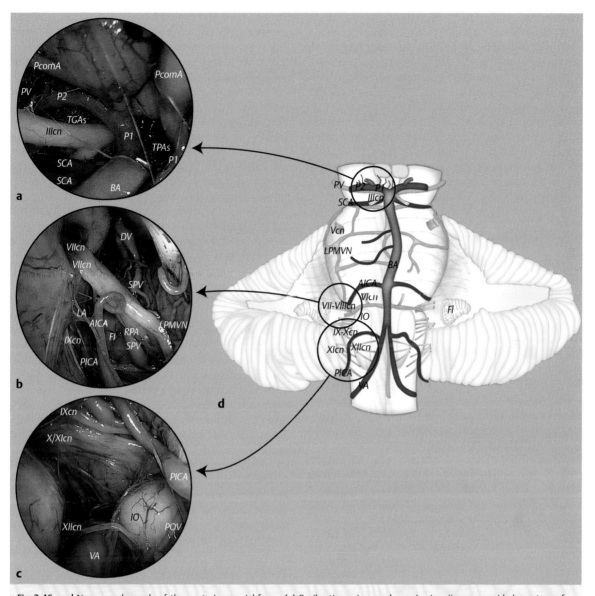

Fig. 2.46 a–d Nerves and vessels of the posterior cranial fossa. **(a)** Basilar tip region, endoscopic view (image provided courtesy of Professor P. Castelnuovo). **(b)** Right cerebellopontine angle, endoscopic view from anterior. **(c)** Right laterobulbar region, endoscopic intracranial view. **(d)** Three-dimensional reconstruction of the posterior cranial fossa.
AICA, anteroinferior cerebellar artery; BA, basilar artery; DV, Dandy's vein; Fl, flocculus; IIIcn (CS), intracavernous portion of the oculomotor nerve; IIIcn, oculomotor nerve; IO, inferior olive; IXcn, glossopharyngeal nerve; IX–X, glossopharyngeal and vagus nerves; LA, labyrinthic artery; LPMVN, lateropontomesencephalic vein network; P1, posterior cerebral artery (first segment); P2, posterior cerebral artery (second segment); PcomA, posterior communicating artery; PICA, posteroinferior cerebellar artery; POV, preolivary vein; PV, peduncular vein; RPA, recurrent perforating artery; SCA, superior cerebellar artery; SPV, superior petrosal vein; TGAs, thalamogeniculate arteries; TPAs, thalamoperforating arteries; VA, vertebral artery; Vcn, trigeminal nerve; VIcn, abducens nerve; VII–VIIIcn, facial nerve and vestibuloacoustic nerve; VIIcn, facial nerve; VIIIcn, vestibuloacoustic nerve; X/XIcn, vagus and accessory nerves; XIcn, accessory nerve; XIIcn, hypoglossal nerve.

the basal and peduncular vein and the vein of the pontomesencephalic sulcus. Caudally, at pons level, it joins the transverse pontine vein (usually in the midpons) and the pontomedullary sulcus vein in close proximity to the abducens nerve. A close relationship between AICAs and veins is present.

More laterally, in the cerebellopontine angle it is possible to see a complex neurovascular network, given principally by the superior petrous veins (SPVs), the AICA and its branches, and cranial nerves V to VIII. The SPVs are divided into medial, intermediate, and lateral groups depending on whether they enter the middle, intermediate, or lateral third of the superior petrosal sinus, respectively.[119] The SPV is formed approximately at trigeminal nerve level by the transverse pontine vein, the pontotrigeminal veins, the cerebellopontine fissure veins, and the vein of the middle cerebellar peduncle. A close view of the area around the internal acoustic meatus, by means of a 45° lens, allows clear identification of the labyrinthine artery that nearly always arises from the AICA. In two-thirds of patients, there are two or three branches.[120] Recurrent perforating arteries, arising from the AICA, run along the facial and vestibulocochlear nerves to reach the brainstem, surrounding the entry zones of these nerves (▶ Fig. 2.46).

2.3.10 Orbital Window

A standard sphenoethmoidectomy completely exposes the lamina papyracea. In this way it is possible to see relevant anatomical elements: the anterior and posterior ethmoidal foramina, which transmit the anterior and posterior ethmoidal neurovascular bundles, and, on the orbital floor, the infraorbital bundle. The lamina papyracea forms the medial wall of the orbit. By removing this thin bony layer, the periorbita is exposed. Removal of the periorbita allows identification of the extraconal medial orbital fat.

Once this fat is removed, the medial muscular wall becomes visible. This wall is mainly composed of the medial rectus muscle and, to a lesser extent, the inferior rectus muscle inferiorly and the superior oblique muscle superiorly. The anterior and posterior ethmoidal neurovascular bundles passing between the medial rectus muscle and the superior oblique muscle are evident. A variable amount of intraconal fat between the muscles is visible also. To view the intraconal structures, the medial rectus muscle must be displaced. The intraconal portion of the orbital fat fills the space. By gentle dissection, the fat is removed and the anatomical elements become evident step after step.

Within the fat, it is usually possible to see a branch of the ophthalmic artery for the inferior rectus muscle with its superior-to-inferior direction. The venous network presents a less constant distribution and for this reason an accurate description of the venous network is of limited significance. Only the medial collateral vein seems to be quite constant in its presentation.[121]

In the upper part of the intraconal space, the nasociliary nerve, a branch of the ophthalmic nerve (V_1), is visible. This nerve enters the intraconal orbital cavity lateral to the optic nerve, passes above it, and runs obliquely beneath the superior rectus muscle and superior oblique muscle to reach the superomedial orbital quadrant. While crossing the optic nerve, it gives rise to the long ciliary nerves, small branches that contain sympathetic fibers to the dilator pupillae muscle. The long ciliary nerves, given their size, should be sought with care in endoscopic dissection. The anterior and posterior ethmoidal nerves emerge from the nasociliary nerve and can be easily detected. The nasociliary nerve becomes the infratrochlear nerve distally to the origin of the anterior ethmoidal nerve. Furthermore, the first part of this nerve can be visible transnasally (▶ Fig. 2.47).

The ophthalmic artery is very close to the nasociliary nerve and enters the optic canal in its inferolateral portion, and passes over the optic nerve to reach the medial wall of the orbit running beneath the inferior border of the superior oblique muscle (▶ Fig. 2.48). Endoscopically, the relationship between the ophthalmic artery and nasociliary nerve is quite constant. The artery gives rise to the anterior and posterior ethmoidal arteries, and these vessels are easily identifiable even intra-orbitally. Other branches of the ophthalmic artery, and the supraorbital and supratrochlear arteries, are not usually visible transnasally.

Near the ophthalmic artery and the nasociliary nerve it is usually possible to identify the superior ophthalmic vein. This vessel is one of the most constant in the intra-orbital venous network and is probably the main venous trunk of the orbit. Compared with the superior ophthalmic vein, the inferior ophthalmic vein is less constant and not always identifiable. When present as a single trunk, it usually communicates through the inferior orbital fissure with the pterygoid venous plexus. A venous trunk usually links superior ophthalmic vein and inferior ophthalmic vein. The superior ophthalmic vein is located typically below the belly of the superior rectus muscle. In this sense, this muscle represents the roof of the intraconal space. However, the levator palpebrae superioris muscle is bove the superior rectus muscle. The superior division of the oculomotor nerve lies under the superior rectus muscle; however, it has no significant or constant relationship with the muscle. However it does send a branch to the muscle itself along its course.

Going below the medial rectus muscle, the intraorbital portion of the optic nerve becomes evident after removing the fat completely. The optic nerve runs with its characteristic course in an anterolateral to posteromedial direction toward the orbital apex and the optic chiasm, dividing the intraconal orbit in four quadrants. At its more distal end, it is covered by the ciliary arteries, branches of the ophthalmic artery, for the vascular supply of the eyeball. These vessels are usually well identifiable in endoscopic dissection.[122] The long ciliary nerves lie in close proximity to the ciliary arteries. These structures can be seen upon delicate dissection (▶ Fig. 2.47).

2.3.11 Maxillary Window to the Infratemporal Fossa and the Upper Parapharyngeal Space

The posterior maxillary wall represents the front door to the infratemporal fossa. Once removed, the thin periosteum becomes apparent and, below it, a complex vascular

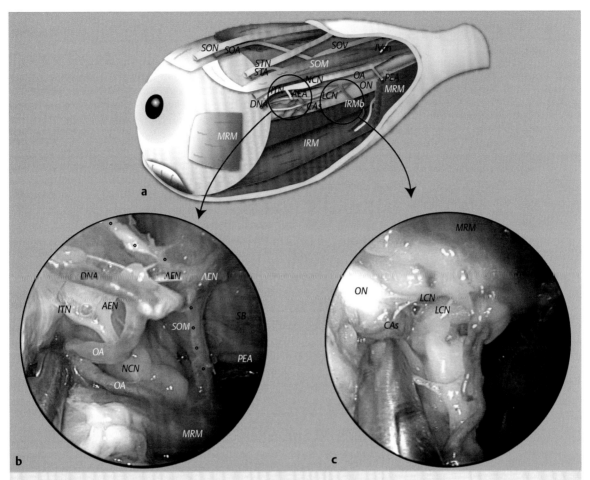

Fig. 2.47 a–c Contents of the orbita. **(a)** Reconstruction of the medial aspect of the orbit. **(b)** Right orbit, endoscopic view of the upper part of the anterior medial intraconal space. **(c)** Right orbit, endoscopic view of the medial intraconal space.
AEA, anterior ethmoidal artery; CAs, ciliary arteries; DNA, dorsal nasal artery; IRM, inferior rectus muscle; IRMb, branch for the inferior rectus muscle; ITN, infratrochlear nerve; IVcn, trochlear nerve; LCN, long ciliary nerve; MRM, medial rectus muscle; NCN, nasociliary nerve; OA, ophthalmic artery; ON, optic nerve; PEA, posterior ethmoidal artery; SB, skull base; SOA, supraorbital artery; SOM, superior oblique muscle; SON, supraorbital nerve; SOV, superior ophthalmic vein; STA, supratrochlear artery; STN, supratrochlear nerve. *Black circles,* periorbit.

network given by the terminal branches of the maxillary artery is evident. This arterial network is fully exposed after the removal of the periosteum. Endoscopically, it is usually possible to recognize the inferior alveolar, the sphenopalatine, the descending palatine, the palatovaginal, and the infraorbital arteries. Of these, the palatovaginal artery can be better viewed in the roof of the nasopharynx once the mucosa has been dissected away from the basisphenoid. Below the vascular plane, it is possible to identify the lateral pterygoid muscle (LPM) horizontally oriented and, caudal to it, the medial pterygoid muscle (MPM) with a slight superior-to-inferior direction. The inferior alveolar nerve and the lingual nerve are visible on the lateral surface of the MPM (▶ Fig. 2.49). A corridor between the LPM, MPM, and temporalis muscle can be identified, leading to the mandibular condyle.

Pterygopalatine Corridor

The first structure is represented by the palatine bone, which in turn represents the posterior margin of the middle antrostomy. The descending palatine artery and the infraorbital bundles can be identified within the palatine bone and in the roof of the maxillary sinus, respectively. The sphenopalatine arteries and nerves pass through the sphenopalatine foramen, formed by the orbital and sphenoidal process of the palatine bone and closed superiorly by the sphenoidal bone.

The pterygoid bone complex lies posterior to the palatine bone. The medial pterygoid plate represents the lateral wall of the choana. By drilling in a lateral direction where the pterygoid plate joins the basisphenoid, the vidian canal can be identified.[123,124]

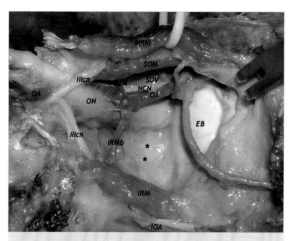

Fig. 2.48 Left orbit, macroscopic vision of the medial intraconal space.
EB, eyeball; IIIcn, oculomotor nerve; IOA, infraorbital artery; IRM, inferior rectus muscle; IRMb, branch for the inferior rectus muscle; MRM, medial rectus muscle; NCN, nasociliary nerve; OA, ophthalmic artery; ON, optic nerve; PEA, posterior ethmoidal artery; SOM, superior oblique muscle; SOV, superior ophthalmic vein. *Stars,* long ciliary nerves.

This nerve is a landmark to the ICA, at the level of the supralacerum portion (first genu) (▶ Fig. 2.45). Slightly laterally, the upper part of the pterypalatine fossa is addressed by tracing the infraorbital nerve posteriorly. Among the fat it is possible to see the maxillary nerve and, slightly behind, the foramen rotundum. A complex network of vessels and nerves lies within the pterypalatine fossa. The pterygopalatine ganglion is usually well identifiable, as well as the communicating nerves between V_2 and the pterygopalatine ganglion. The pterygopalatine ganglion receives the vidian nerve. The zygomatic nerve usually exits the pterygopalatine fossa to enter the infratemporal fossa. The greater and lesser palatine nerves and descending palatine artery descend into the pterygopalatine fossa and pass through their homonymous canals to reach the oral cavity. The artery for the foramen rotundum, coming from the maxillary artery, usually follows the maxillary nerve to the cavernous sinus, anastomosing with the terminal branches of the posterolateral trunk coming from the cavernous portion of the ICA. With the vidian nerve and the V_2 under vision, the bone of the great sphenoidal wing is drilled out; therefore, opening the door to the gasserian ganglion and cavernous sinus.[107]

Medial Corridor

Behind the lateral pterygoid muscle, in the medial aspect of the infratemporal fossa, it is possible to see the tensor and the levator veli palatini muscles. The tensor muscle is closely related to the lateral surface of the superior constrictor muscle while the levator runs medially to the superior constrictor muscle and reaches the nasopharyngeal surface of the soft palate. Together, these muscles create a plane that drives directly to the parapharyngeal portion of the ICA. The ascending pharyngeal artery lies slightly anterior to the ICA. The internal jugular vein, covered laterally by the styloid process, lies closely related to the ICA. At this level, the styloid muscles can be seen running inferiorly. The venous network within the infratemporal fossa is extremely variable in shape and forms the so-called pterygoid plexus. By deepening the medial dissection, passing between the parapharyngeal portion of the ICA and the prevertebral muscle, the hypoglossal nerve and (sometimes) the superior sympathetic ganglion can be seen on the lateral surface of the upper vertebrae. By moving upwards, the hypoglossal canal at the basiocciput can be seen as well.

Lateral Corridor

Slightly lateral to the tensor veli palatini muscle, the mandibular nerve (V_3) emerges from the skull base and passes through the foramen ovale (▶ Fig. 2.49). This nerve divides after a short course into anterior and posterior trunks. The posterior trunk divides further into three branches (auriculotemporal, inferior alveolar, and lingual nerves) while the anterior one usually generates two or three branches for the temporal muscle (buccal and masseteric nerves plus the nerve for the lateral pterygoid muscle). Very close to the skull base, the mandibular nerve gives rise to three to four branches to supply the middle cranial fossa dura, medial pterygoid muscle, tensor tympani muscle, and tensor veli palatini muscle. These nerves are difficult to detect because they are within a venous plexus around V_3. While running laterally, the auriculotemporal nerve encounters and envelops the middle meningeal artery, dividing temporarily into two branches. This vessel, a branch of the maxillary artery, runs vertically to enter the skull through the foramen spinosum, slightly posterior and lateral to the foramen ovale. The deep temporal arteries (anterior and posterior), the buccal artery and other minor vessels that feed the surrounding soft tissues are not easy to recognize in the infratemporal fossa. In fact, their position is quite variable within the infratemporal fossa; therefore, their identification requires a careful dissection.

In the upper aspect of the infratemporal fossa, close to the skull base, the mandibular nerve lies on the lateral surface of the Eustachian tube, which descends from the middle ear inferiorly, anteriorly, and medially to open into the lateral wall of the nasopharynx. The intimate relationship between the ICA, the Eustachian tube, and V_3 must be strongly underlined. The Eustachian tube is of paramount importance for detecting the superior portion of the parapharyngeal ICA and consequently the jugular foramen area. It is like an arrow pointing to the parapharyngeal ICA that enters the carotid foramen.[125] Unfortunately, the position of the parapharyngeal portion

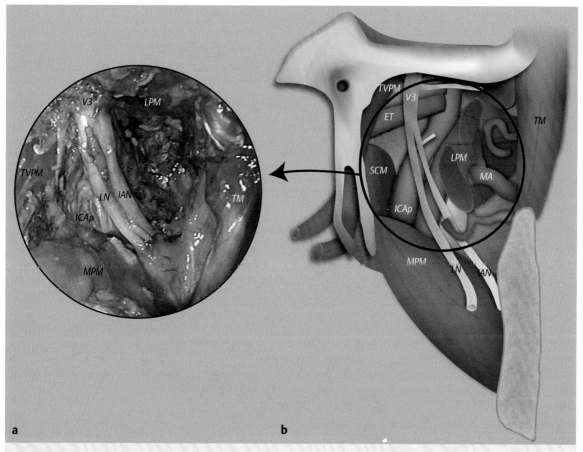

Fig. 2.49 a, b Left infratemporal fossa. **(a)** Endoscopic view. **(b)** Three-dimensional reconstruction.
ET, Eustachian tube; IAN, inferior alveolar nerve; ICAp, parapharyngeal portion of the internal carotid artery; LN, lingual nerve; LPM, lateral pterygoid muscle; MA, maxillary artery; MPM, medial pterygoid muscle; SCM, superior constrictor muscle; TM, temporalis muscle; TVPM, tensor veli palatini muscle; V3, mandibular nerve.

of the ICA is unpredictable below this foramen and no definitive anatomical landmark can be given. What is certainly true is that this segment presents a close relationship with the wall of the pharynx, more commonly the lateral one but rarely the posterior one. Furthermore, the presence of arterial looping or kinking makes any attempt to describe this position rather limited in value.

Acknowledgments

Special thanks to Elena Bacci for her expertise and patience in producing the three-dimensional reconstructions, and to Shona Dryburgh for her assistance in revising the manuscript.

References

[1] Schmidt HM. Mass and level differences of the media structures of the anterior cranial fossa of the people [in German]. Gegenbaurs morph Jahrb Leipzig 1974; 120: 538–559

[2] Kaplan HA, Browder A, Browder J. Nasal venous drainage and the foramen caecum. Laryngoscope 1989; 83: 327–329

[3] Sieglbauer F. Textbook of Normal Human Anatomy [in German]. Berlin, Vienna: Urban & Schwarzenberg; 1943

[4] Dressler L. About the hyperostosis of the frontal bone [in German]. Beitr path Anat 1927;78: 332–363

[5] Prescher A, Schick B. The evolutionarily explainable defects of the skull base [in German]. In: Mühling J, Schweigert HG, eds. Zehnte Jahrestagung der Deutschen Gesellschaft für Schädelbasischirurgie. Niebüll, Verlag videel OHG 2003: 15–20

[6] Brors D. Bone and dura structures of the sella region: an anatomical and radiological study of microsurgical view [in German]. Inaug.-Diss. Aachen; 1998

[7] Prescher A, Brors D, Adam G. Contribution to the knowledge of the posterior clinoid processes [in German]. In: Lanksch WR, Lehmann L, eds. Die hintere Schädelgrube und der kraniozervikale Übergang. Reinbek: Einhorn-Presse Verlag; 1998:162–168

[8] Gruber W. Contributions to the anatomy of the sphenoid and temporal bone [in German]. Imperatorskaja Akademija Nauk (St. Petersburg) 1859; 1: 3–14

[9] Destrieux C, Velut S, Kakou MK, Lefrancq T, Arbeille B, Santini JJ. A new concept in Dorello's canal microanatomy: the petroclival venous confluence. J Neurosurg 1997; 87: 67–72

[10] Prescher A, Brors D, Schick B. Topographic anatomy of the petrous apex and the Dorello channel [in German]. In: Bootz F, Strauss G, eds.

Die Chirurgie der lateralen Schädelbasis. Berlin: Springer 2002: 31–35

[11] von Spee F. Graf. Skeleton teaching, II: head [in German]. In: von Bardeleben K, ed. Handbuch der Anatomie des Menschen. Jena: Gustav Fischer; 1896: 1–280

[12] Lang J. Head, Part B: brain and skull eyes [in German]. Berlin Heidelberg New York: Springer; 1979

[13] Tisch-Rottensteiner K. Openings and varieties of the middle cranial fossa [in German]. Med. Diss. Würzburg; 1975

[14] Faure A, Masse H, Gayet-Delacroix M et al. What is the arcuate eminence? Surg Radiol Anat 2003; 25: 99–104

[15] Goerke M. The otitic diseases of the meninges [in German]. In: Denker A, Kahler O, eds. Handbuch der Hals-Nasen-Ohrenheilkunde, Bd 8 Teil 3. Berlin: Springer; Munich: Bergmann; 1927:1–54

[16] Gruber W. Contributions to the development of the cranial reason, I [in German]. Memoires de L'Academie Imperiale des Sciences de St. Petersbourg. 1869; 1–34

[17] Rutz KP. Shape, dimensions and curves of the skull channels: carotid canal, condylar canal, mastoid foramen, "Emissarium occipital" and the shape and size of the sphenoid lingula [in German]. Med. Diss. Würzburg; 1975

[18] Platzer W. [Anatomy of taenia interclinoidea and its relation to the internal carotid artery] Fortschr Geb Rontgenstr Nuklearmed 1957; 87: 613–616

[19] Platzer W. The variability of the internal carotid artery in the cavernous sinus in relation to the variability of the skull base [in German]. Gegenbaurs Morpholisches Jahrbuch 1957; 98: 227–243

[20] Hauser G, De Stefano GF. Epigenetic variants of the human skull. Stuttgart: Schweizerbart; 1989

[21] Sternberg M. A not previously described channel in sphenoid human [in German]. Anat Anz 1888; 3: 784–785

[22] Schick B, Brors D, Prescher A. Sternberg's canal—cause of congenital sphenoidal meningocele. Eur Arch Otorhinolaryngol 2000; 257: 430–432

[23] Virchow R. Studies on the development of the skull in the ground healthy and morbid condition and the influence thereof on the skull shape, facial features and brain construction [in German]. Berlin: Reimer; 1857

[24] Ingelmark BE. About the craniovertebral border region in humans [in German]. Acta Anat Suppl (Basel) 1947; 6: 461

[25] Prescher A. The craniocervical junction in man, the osseous variations, their significance and differential diagnosis. Ann Anat 1997; 179: 1–19

[26] Prescher A, Brors D. The various shapes of the paries jugularis and the frequency of additional ducts in the fossa jugularis as further factors influencing the spread of pathological processes. Eur Arch Otorhinolaryngol 1995; 252: 26–29

[27] Oehmke HJ. The importance of the canal basilar artery and its representation in the radiograph [in German]. Gegenbaurs Morphol Jahrb 1963; 104: 459–475

[28] Le Double AF. Focuses on changes in the skull bones of man [in French]. Paris: Vigot Freres; 1903

[29] Klaus E. The basilar impression [in German]. Leipzig: S Hirzel; 1969

[30] Graf von Keyserlingk D, Prescher A. Basilar impression [in German]. Eur Arch Otorhinolaryngol Suppl 1993; 1: 365–372

[31] Wullstein HL, Wullstein SR. Injuries of the rhino and otobasis from the aspect of the pneumatic system in the skull [in German]. Chirurg 1970; 41: 490–494

[32] Lang J. Clinical Anatomy of the Nose, Nasal Cavity and Sinuses [in German]. Stuttgart, New York: Thieme; 1988a

[33] Lang J. Posterior ethmoid cells and their relation to the optic canal [in German]. HNO 1988b; 36: 49–53

[34] Stammberger H, Hosemann W, Draf W. Anatomic terminology and nomenclature for paranasal sinus surgery [in German]. Laryngorhinootologie 1997; 76: 435–449

[35] Grünwald L. Descriptive and topographic anatomy of the nose and sinuses [in German]. In: Denker A, Kahler O, eds. Handbuch der Hals-Nasen-Ohrenheilkunde Vol1,1. Berlin: Springer; 1925:1–95

[36] Blumenbach JF. Decas collectionis suae craniorum diversarium gentium illustrata. Göttingen: Dieterich; 1790

[37] Krmpotic-Nemanic J, Draf W, Helms J. Surgical Anatomy of the Head and Neck Region [in German]. Berlin, Heidelberg, New York, Tokyo: Springer; 1895

[38] Kaufmann E. About a typical form of mucosal tumor (lateral mucosal swelling) on the outer wall of the nose [in German]. Monatsschr Ohrenheilk 1890; 24: 13–19

[39] Zuckerkandl E. Normal and Pathological Anatomy of the Nasal Cavity and its Pneumatic Attachments [in German]. Vienna: Braumüller; 1893

[40] van Alyea OE. Ethmoid labyrinth; anatomical study, with consideration of the clinical significance of its structural characteristics. Arch Otolaryngol 1939; 29: 881–902

[41] Lang J, Schlehahn F. Ethmoid foramina and ethmoid canals [in German]. Verh Anat Ges 1978; 72: 433–435

[42] Minnigerode B. On the anatomy and clinical significance of the canalis ethmoidalis [in German]. Z Laryngol Rhinol Otol 1966; 45: 554–559

[43] Keros P. [On the practical value of differences in the level of the lamina cribrosa of the ethmoid] Z Laryngol Rhinol Otol 1962; 41: 809–813

[44] Boege K. On the anatomy of the frontal sinus: frontal sinuses [in German]. Diss. Königsberg; 1902

[45] Gerber PH. The Complications of Sinusitis [in German]. Berlin: Karger; 1909

[46] Boenninghaus G. The operation on the sinuses of the nose [in German]. In: Katz L, Preysing H, Blumenfeld F, eds. Handbuch der speziellen Chirurgie des Ohres und der oberen Luftwege. Vol 3, 1 edn. Würzburg: Kabitzsch; 1913: 69–250

[47] Tonndorf W. On the anatomy of the cribriform plate and the olfactory Crista [in German]. Beitr Anat Physiol Ohr Nase 1926; 23: 654–667

[48] Killian G. On the anatomy of the nose of human embryos [in German]. Arch Otorhinolaryngol 1895; 3: 17–47

[49] Vogt K, Schrade F. Anatomical variations of frontal sinus duct system. results of radioresistometric examinations (author's transl) [in German]. Laryngol Rhinol Otol (Stuttg) 1979; 58: 783–794

[50] Highmore N. Corporis Humani disquisitio anatomica. Broun; 1651

[51] Lang W. Traumatic enophthalmos with retention of perfect acuity of vision. Transact Ophthalmol. Soc. 1889; 9: 41–43

[52] Schicketanz HW, Schicketanz W. Indirect and direct tooth damage following surgery of the maxillary sinus [in German]. HNO 1961; 9: 169–175

[53] Underwood AS. An inquiry into the anatomy and pathology of the maxillary sinus. J Anat Physiol 1910; 44: 354–369

[54] Hardy J. Surgery of the pituitary gland, using the trans-sphenoidal approach. Comparative study of 2 technical methods [in French]. Union Med Can 1967; 96: 702–712

[55] Draf W. Surgical treatment of the inflammatory diseases of the paranasal sinuses. Indication, surgical technique, risks, mismanagement and complications, revision surgery [in German]. Arch Otorhinolaryngol 1982; 235: 133–305

[56] Prescher A, Brors D. A rare variety of the course of the internal carotid artery and rarefying hyperostosis of the cranial vault. Surg Radiol Anat 1994; 16: 93–96

[57] Lang J, Sakals E. Spheno-ethmoidal recessus, the nasal aperture of the nasolacrimal duct and the hiatus semilunaris [in German]. Anat Anz 1982; 152: 393–412

[58] Forschner L. About the risk of bleeding during operations on the sphenoidal [in German]. Arch Ohren Nasen Kehlkopfheilkd 1950; 158: 271–275

[59] Wareing MJ, Padgham ND. Osteologic classification of the sphenopalatine foramen. Laryngoscope 1998; 108: 125–127

[60] Jacobsson M, Davidsson A, Hugosson S, Tjellström A, Svendsen P. Aberrant intratympanic internal carotid artery: a potentially hazardous anomaly. J Laryngol Otol 1989; 103: 1202–1205

[61] Lewin L. The presence of persistence of the stapedial artery in humans and the comparative anatomy and phylogenetic significance of this phenomenon [in German]. Arch Ohrenheilk. 1906; 70: 28–44

[62] Lo WWM, Solti-Bohman LG, McElveen JT, Jr. Aberrant carotid artery: radiologic diagnosis with emphasis on high-resolution computed tomography. Radiographics 1985; 5: 985–993

[63] Bauer U. Anatomical variants of the sigmoid sinus, the fomane jugular vein and the jugalaris [in German]. Z Anat Entwicklungsgesch 1971; 135: 35–42

[64] Lang J, Weigel M. Nerve-vessel relations in the region of the jugular foramen. Anat Clin 1983; 5: 41–56

[65] von Torklus D, Gehle W. The Upper Cervical Spine [in German]. Stuttgart: Thieme; 1975

[66] Prescher A. The differential diagnosis of isolated ossicles in the region of the dens axis. Gegenbaurs Morphol Jahrb 1990; 136: 139–154

[67] Pfitzner W. Contributions to the knowledge of the human skeleton extremities, VIII: the morphological elements of the human hand bones [in German]. Morph Anthrop 1900; 2: 77–157

[68] Brocher JEW, Willert HG. The occipito-cervical region [in German]. Thieme: Stuttgart; 1980

[69] Prescher A, Brors D, Adam G. Anatomic and radiologic appearance of several variants of the craniocervical junction. Skull Base Surg 1996; 6: 83–94

[70] von Lüdinghausen M, Palm M, Prescher A et al. Accessory joints between basiocciput and atlas/axis in the median plane. Clin Anat 2005; 18: 558–571

[71] Will CH. Condylus tertius, mistaken for a naso-pharyngeal tumor [in German]. Rofo 1980; 133: 557–558

[72] Kassam A, Snyderman C, Carrau R. An evolving paradigm to the ventral skull base. Skull Base 2004: 14

[73] Kassam A, Snyderman CH, Mintz A, Gardner P, Carrau RL. Expanded endonasal approach: the rostrocaudal axis. Part II. Posterior clinoids to the foramen magnum. Neurosurg Focus 2005; 19: E4

[74] Kassam A, Snyderman CH, Mintz A, Gardner P, Carrau RL. Expanded endonasal approach: the rostrocaudal axis. Part I. Crista galli to the sella turcica. Neurosurg Focus 2005; 19: E3

[75] Kassam A, Thomas AJ, Snyderman C et al. Fully endoscopic expanded endonasal approach treating skull base lesions in pediatric patients. J Neurosurg 2007; 106 Suppl: 75–86

[76] Kassam AB, Engh JA, Mintz AH, Prevedello DM. Completely endoscopic resection of intraparenchymal brain tumors. J Neurosurg 2009; 110: 116–123

[77] Kassam AB, Gardner P, Snyderman C, Mintz A, Carrau R. Expanded endonasal approach: fully endoscopic, completely transnasal approach to the middle third of the clivus, petrous bone, middle cranial fossa, and infratemporal fossa. Neurosurg Focus 2005; 19: E6

[78] Kassam AB, Gardner PA, Snyderman CH, Carrau RL, Mintz AH, Prevedello DM. Expanded endonasal approach, a fully endoscopic transnasal approach for the resection of midline suprasellar craniopharyngiomas: a new classification based on the infundibulum. J Neurosurg 2008; 108: 715–728

[79] Cappabianca P, Alfieri A, Colao A et al. Endoscopic endonasal transsphenoidal surgery in recurrent and residual pituitary adenomas: technical note. Minim Invasive Neurosurg 2000; 43: 38–43

[80] Prevedello DM, Kassam AB, Snyderman C et al. Endoscopic cranial base surgery: ready for prime time? Clin Neurosurg 2007; 54: 48–57

[81] Prevedello DM, Thomas A, Gardner P, Snyderman CH, Carrau RL, Kassam AB. Endoscopic endonasal resection of a synchronous pituitary adenoma and a tuberculum sellae meningioma: technical case report. Neurosurgery 2007; 60 Suppl 2: E401, discussion E401

[82] Cappabianca P, Buonamassa S, Cavallo LM, Mariniello G, de Divitiis O. Neuroendoscopy: present and future applications. Clin Neurosurg 2004; 51: 186–190

[83] Cappabianca P, Cavallo LM, Colao A et al. Endoscopic endonasal transsphenoidal approach: outcome analysis of 100 consecutive procedures. Minim Invasive Neurosurg 2002; 45: 193–200

[84] Cappabianca P, Decq P, Schroeder HW. Future of endoscopy in neurosurgery. Surg Neurol 2007; 67: 496–498

[85] Carrau RL, Jho HD, Ko Y. Transnasal-transsphenoidal endoscopic surgery of the pituitary gland. Laryngoscope 1996; 106: 914–918

[86] Carrau RL, Snyderman CH, Kassam AB, Jungreis CA. Endoscopic and endoscopic-assisted surgery for juvenile angiofibroma. Laryngoscope 2001; 111: 483–487

[87] Castelnuovo PG, Delù G, Sberze F et al. Esthesioneuroblastoma: endonasal endoscopic treatment. Skull Base 2006; 16: 25–30

[88] Cavallo LM, Cappabianca P, Galzio R, Iaconetta G, de Divitiis E, Tschabitscher M. Endoscopic transnasal approach to the cavernous sinus versus transcranial route: anatomic study. Neurosurgery 2005; 56 Suppl: 379–389; discussion 379–389

[89] Cavallo LM, de Divitiis O, Aydin S et al. Extended endoscopic endonasal transsphenoidal approach to the suprasellar area: anatomic considerations - part 1. Neurosurgery 2007; 61: 24–34

[90] Cavallo LM, Messina A, Cappabianca P et al. Endoscopic endonasal surgery of the midline skull base: anatomical study and clinical considerations. Neurosurg Focus 2005; 19: E2

[91] Cavallo LM, Messina A, Gardner P et al. Extended endoscopic endonasal approach to the pterygopalatine fossa: anatomical study and clinical considerations. Neurosurg Focus 2005; 19: E5

[92] Cavallo LM, Prevedello DM, Solari D et al. Extended endoscopic endonasal transsphenoidal approach for residual or recurrent craniopharyngiomas. J Neurosurg 2009; 111: 578–589

[93] Doglietto F, Prevedello DM, Jane JA, Jr, Han J, Laws ER, Jr. Brief history of endoscopic transsphenoidal surgery—from Philipp Bozzini to the First World Congress of Endoscopic Skull Base Surgery. Neurosurg Focus 2005; 19: E3

[94] Frank G, Pasquini E. Endoscopic endonasal approaches to the cavernous sinus: surgical approaches. Neurosurgery 2002; 50: 675

[95] Frank G, Pasquini E, Doglietto F et al. The endoscopic extended transsphenoidal approach for craniopharyngiomas. Neurosurgery 2006; 59 Suppl 1: 75–83; discussion 75–83

[96] Frank G, Pasquini E, Mazzatenta D. Extended transsphenoidal approach. J Neurosurg 2001; 95: 917–918

[97] Gardner PA, Kassam AB, Rothfus WE, Snyderman CH, Carrau RL. Preoperative and intraoperative imaging for endoscopic endonasal approaches to the skull base. Otolaryngol Clin North Am 2008; 41: 215–230, vii.

[98] Gardner PA, Kassam AB, Snyderman CH et al. Outcomes following endoscopic, expanded endonasal resection of suprasellar craniopharyngiomas: a case series. J Neurosurg 2008; 109: 6–16

[99] Gardner PA, Kassam AB, Thomas A et al. Endoscopic endonasal resection of anterior cranial base meningiomas. Neurosurgery 2008; 63: 36–52, discussion 52–54

[100] Gardner PA, Prevedello DM, Kassam AB, Snyderman CH, Carrau RL, Mintz AH. The evolution of the endonasal approach for craniopharyngiomas. J Neurosurg 2008; 108: 1043–1047

[101] Snyderman C, Kassam A, Carrau R, Mintz A, Gardner P, Prevedello DM. Acquisition of surgical skills for endonasal skull base surgery: a training program. Laryngoscope 2007; 117: 699–705

[102] Rhoton AL, Jr. The supratentorial arteries. Neurosurgery 2002; 51 Suppl: S53–S120

[103] Kassam AB, Prevedello DM, Thomas A et al. Endoscopic endonasal pituitary transposition for a transdorsum sellae approach to the interpeduncular cistern. Neurosurgery 2008; 62 Suppl 1: 57–72, discussion 72–74

[104] Hadad G, Bassagasteguy L, Carrau RL et al. A novel reconstructive technique after endoscopic expanded endonasal approaches: vascular pedicle nasoseptal flap. Laryngoscope 2006; 116: 1882–1886

[105] Rhoton AL, Jr. The cavernous sinus, the cavernous venous plexus, and the carotid collar. Neurosurgery 2002; 51 Suppl: S375–S410

[106] Stippler M, Gardner PA, Snyderman CH, Carrau RL, Prevedello DM, Kassam AB. Endoscopic endonasal approach for clival chordomas. Neurosurgery 2009; 64: 268–277, discussion 277–278

[107] Kassam AB, Prevedello DM, Carrau RL et al. The front door to Meckel's cave: an anteromedial corridor via expanded endoscopic endonasal approach—technical considerations and clinical series. Neurosurgery 2009; 64 Suppl: ons71–ons82, discussion ons82–ons83

[108] Kassam AB, Vescan AD, Carrau RL et al. Expanded endonasal approach: vidian canal as a landmark to the petrous internal carotid artery. J Neurosurg 2008; 108: 177–183

[109] Osawa S, Rhoton AL, Jr, Seker A, Shimizu S, Fujii K, Kassam AB. Microsurgical and endoscopic anatomy of the vidian canal. Neurosurgery 2009; 64 Suppl 2: 385–411, discussion 411–412

[110] Prevedello DM, Pinheiro-Neto CD, Fernandez-Miranda JC et al. Vidian nerve transposition for endoscopic endonasal middle fossa approaches. Neurosurgery 2010; 67 Suppl Operative: 478–484

[111] Tschabitscher M, Galzio RJ. Endoscopic anatomy along the transnasal approach to the pituitary gland and the surrounding structures. In: De Devitiis E, Cappabianca P, eds. Endoscopic Endonasal Transsphenoidal Surgery. Vienna, New York: Springer-Verlag; 2003:21–39

[112] Castelnuovo P. Endoscopic Cadaveric Dissection of the Nose and Paranasal Sinuses. Tuttlingen, Germany: Endo-Press; 2002

[113] Lang J. Clinical Anatomy of the Nose, Nasal cavity and Paranasal Sinuses. New York, NY: Thieme; 1989

[114] Rhoton AL Jr. The supratentorial arteries. In: Rhoton AL Jr, ed. Cranial Anatomy and Surgical Approaches. USA: Lippincott Williams & Wilkins; 2003:81–148

[115] Rhoton AL Jr. The cerebral veins. In: Rhoton AL Jr, ed. Cranial Anatomy and Surgical Approaches. USA: Lippincott Williams & Wilkins; 2003: 187–232

[116] Perneczky A, Tschabitscher M, Resch KDM. Endoscopic Anatomy for Neurosurgery. Stuttgart, New York: Thieme; 1993

[117] Yasuda A, Campero A, Martins C, Rhoton AL, Jr, de Oliveira E, Ribas GC. Microsurgical anatomy and approaches to the cavernous sinus. Neurosurgery 2005; 56 suppl 1: S4–S27

[118] Cavallo LM, Messina A, Cappabianca P et al. Endoscopic endonasal surgery of the midline skull base: anatomical study and clinical considerations. Neurosurg Focus 2005; 19: E2

[119] Rhoton AL Jr. The posterior fossa veins. In: Rhoton AL Jr, ed. Cranial Anatomy and Surgical Approaches. USA: Lippincott Williams & Wilkins; 2003:501–24

[120] Rhoton AL Jr. The cerebellar arteries. In: Rhoton AL Jr, ed. Cranial Anatomy and Surgical Approaches. USA: Lippincott Williams & Wilkins; 2003:461–500

[121] Gürkanlar D, Gönül E. Medial microsurgical approach to the orbit: an anatomic study. Minim Invasive Neurosurg 2006; 49: 104–109

[122] Rhoton AL Jr. The orbit. In: Rhoton AL Jr, ed. Cranial Anatomy and Surgical Approaches. USA: Lippincott Williams & Wilkins; 2003:331–62

[123] Cavallo LM, Messina A, Gardner P et al. Extended endoscopic endonasal approach to the pterygopalatine fossa: anatomical study and clinical considerations. Neurosurg Focus 2005; 19: E5

[124] Vescan AD, Snyderman CH, Carrau RL et al. Vidian canal: analysis and relationship to the internal carotid artery. Laryngoscope 2007; 117: 1338–1342

[125] Dallan I, Bignami M, Battaglia P, Castelnuovo P, Tschabitscher M. Fully endoscopic transnasal approach to the jugular foramen: anatomic study and clinical considerations. Neurosurgery 2010; 67 Suppl Operative: ons1–ons7, discussion ons7–ons8

Chapter 3

Etiology, Biology, and Pathology of Skull Base Tumors

3 Etiology, Biology, and Pathology of Skull Base Tumors

Gerhard Franz Walter

3.1 Introduction

In this chapter, the properties of tumors of the skull base which can or possibly could be treated by endonasal endoscopic surgery are dealt with from a neuropathological point of view. The aim is to provide a quick orientation for endoscopic surgeons interested in macroscopic and microscopic pathomorphology, rather than to replace the comprehensive information to be found in the World Health Organization (WHO) classification handbooks.

The relevant international reference for the classification of tumors is the series of classification books edited by the WHO. For skull base tumors, three of the books are of special interest: WHO Classification of Tumours of the Central Nervous System,[1] WHO Classification of Head and Neck Tumours,[2] and WHO Classification of Tumours of Soft Tissue and Bone.[3] The description of tumor entities used in this chapter follow the WHO handbooks to a great extent.

For practical reasons, I have chosen to divide the chapter on skull base tumors into four subchapters with regard to histogenetic principles, four subchapters with regard to anatomic regions, and a short subchapter dedicated to metastatic tumors:

- Meningeal tumors
- Tumors of the peripheral, autonomous, and central nervous systems
- Tumors of the hematopoietic system
- Germ cell tumors and dysontogenetic tumorlike cysts
- Tumors of the sellar region
- Tumors of the nasal cavity and paranasal sinuses
- Tumors of the osseous skull base
- Tumors of orbit and eye
- Metastatic tumors

Each subchapter begins with a table on classification (typing) and dignity from benign to malignant (grading) followed by a more detailed description of the presented tumor entities including brief information on age and sex distribution, and on incidence. The main intention is to provide a wide scale of pathomorphological images enabling clinicians to better interpret the value and the limitations of histopathological findings.

3.2 Definitions

3.2.1 Etiology

The etiology of any incipient tumor is based on either one or a cascade of several mutations within a cell of origin; thus, the tumor begins with a single mutated cell losing its growth control. In short, mutations of growth regulating and enhancing oncogenes and/or growth inhibiting suppressor genes as well as mutations of repair genes may lead to less controlled or uncontrolled tumor growth and progression.

3.2.2 Classification

Typing

The naming of tumors is based on their cell or tissue of origin regarding ontogenetic derivations. In few cases, historic names are still in habitual use.

Grading

The biological potential and behavior including clinical prognosis is different for tumors of the central nervous system and tumors of other locations. For tumors of the central nervous system, a scale with increasing malignancy from benign grade I tumors to malignant grade IV tumors is used. Criteria comprise, for example, cellular atypia, mitotic activity, microvascular proliferation, and necrosis. For tumors outside the central nervous system, several grading systems based on various histological parameters have been published and proved to correlate with prognosis. Parameters comprise differentiation of tissue, mitotic activity, necrosis, and also several decisive pathohistological patterns for the tumor entity in question. For instance, the two most widely used systems for tumors of soft tissue and bone are the NCI system (National Cancer Institute, United States) and the FNCLCC system (Fédération Nationale des Centres de Lutte Contre le Cancer, France). For these entities, I have chosen a simplified grading overview indicating only benign, intermediate and malignant behavior.

Staging

Determination of the spreading of tumors throughout the body incorporates histological grade as well as tumor size and depth, regional lymph node involvement, and distant metastasis. The relevant classification source for staging of tumors outside the central nervous system is the TNM (tumor size, node involvement, and metastatic status) Classification of Malignant Tumours[4] edited by the Union for International Cancer Control (UICC). Since primary tumors of the central nervous systems regularly do not involve lymph nodes or give rise to distant metastasis, these tumors are not incorporated in the TNM system.

3.2.3 Prognosis

The survival time and rate are based on empirical and statistical data for any specific tumor entity. However, for the individual patient there is a mere estimate. Prognostic data, as provided by tumor grading, also present information pertaining the natural history of disease, and, therefore, the probability of disease relapse and durability of remission. Molecular properties of a tumor such as specific mutations may improve the possibility for a meaningful prognosis. For instance, the allelic loss of chromosomal arms 1p and 9q is associated with a markedly improved clinical course in patients with histologically confirmed anaplastic oligodendroglioma,[5] a finding that has been corroborated in a large number of scientific articles.

3.2.4 Prediction

The probability of response to a specific therapeutic agent or modality is based on molecular testing by means of predictive markers. Molecular properties of a tumor or molecular differences within a single tumor entity are identified as being decisive for a desirable response to a specific therapy. For example, the primary mechanism of action of temozolomide (Temodal, MSD Merck Sharp & Dohme, Haar, Bavaria, Germany) is the addition of methyl groups to the O_6 position of guanine to produce lethal methylguanine adducts. The DNA repair enzyme O_6-methylguanine-DNA methyl transferase (MGMT) reverses this process by repairing methylguanine adducts. A multinational collaborative trial reported that *MGMT* gene silencing enhanced benefits in glioblastoma patients treated concurrently with radiotherapy and temozolomide.[6] Conversely, patients with tumors not methylated at the MGMT promoter did not benefit from this therapy compared with radiotherapy alone. The MGMT promoter methylation status (▶ Fig. 3.1) can be evaluated via methylation-specific polymerase chain reaction (PCR) with primers specific to either the methylated or the unmethylated sequences in routine laboratory testing, and can be used on DNA from formalin-fixed paraffin-embedded (FFPE) tumor tissue. For another example, deletions of chromosomal arms 1p and 19q are not only associated with a markedly improved clinical course in cases of anaplastic oligodendroglioma, but combined 1p19q loss as well as loss of 1p are also associated with enhanced chemosensitivity to the procarbazine–lomustine–vincristine (PVC) chemotherapy regimen. By means of fluorescence in situ hybridization (FISH, ▶ Fig. 3.2) the 1p19q status of a tumor can easily be assessed. Fluorescent probes are hybridized directly to FFPE tissue sections, permitting direct microscopic evaluation of chromosomal copy number in tumor cells.

For optimal postoperative treatment by an oncologist, every protocol of a histopathological examination has to document the complete actual typing, grading, and

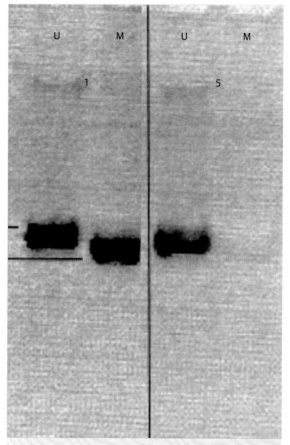

Fig. 3.1 Comparison of two cases of glioblastoma for MGMT methylation status: case 1, methylated (a band for the unmethylated sequence is also present because of nontumorous cells within the tumor such as blood vessels); case 5, unmethylated. The band of the PCR product of the unmethylated sequence is 122 bp long (upper line), that of the methylated sequence is 129 bp (lower line). Polyacrylamide gel electrophoresis of a methylation-specific PCR.

staging of the tumor, including the results for predictive markers where appropriate.

Frozen section diagnosis in intraoperative consultation can provide a fast diagnosis. In the majority of cases, within approximately 20 minutes after the surgical biopsy, reliable and accurate information on the principle typing (for instance glioma versus lymphoma versus metastasis), the most probable grading (benign versus malignant), and the completeness of the resection of tumor tissue (still within the tumor tissue versus tumor-free surrounding tissue) should be possible. However, it has to be kept in mind that under certain circumstances the histological quality of frozen tissue may be inferior to the quality of paraffin-embedded tissue. Furthermore, the staining techniques for intraoperative consultation usually are restricted to hematoxylin and eosin (H&E) staining. Therefore, correction of the diagnostic information given by frozen sections may be necessary after

Fig. 3.2 Oligodendroglioma cells showing loss of chromosome 1p as illustrated by the single red dot (1p probe) in comparison to two green signals (1q probe) per cell. Dual-color 1p FISH.

Table 3.1 Classification and grading of meningeal tumors

Type		WHO grade
Meningioma		
	Meningothelial	I
	Fibrous (fibroblastic)	I
	Transitional (mixed)	I
	Psammomatous	I
	Angiomatous	I
	Microcystic	I
	Secretory	I
	Lymphoplasmacyte-rich	I
	Metaplastic	I
	Chordoid	II
	Clear cell	II
	Atypical	II
	Papillary	III
	Rhabdoid	III
	Anaplastic (malignant)	III
Hemangiopericytoma		II
	Anaplastic	III
Hemangioblastoma		I
Leptomeningeal melanocytic lesions		
	Diffuse melanocytosis	Intermediate
	Melanomatosis	Malignant
	Melanocytoma	Benign/intermediate
	Malignant melanoma	Malignant

definitive and detailed histological examination with a broad spectrum of methods available.

3.3 Meningeal Tumors

Classification and grading of meningeal tumors are shown in ▶ Table 3.1.

3.3.1 Meningiomas

Meningiomas represent about 25% of all primary intracranial tumors. All ages, with a peak incidence in the fifth to seventh decades, are affected. Benign meningiomas are found predominantly in females, whereas no sexual prevalence can be found in malignant variants. There is a correlation between pregnancy and rapid tumor growth. About 90% of meningiomas have progesterone receptors, 40% have estrogen receptors, and 40% have androgen receptors. Meningiomas may be induced by radiation therapy with an average time interval of about 20 to 35 years, the latter depending from the radiation dose.

At the skull base, the olfactory grooves, the parasellar area and tuberculum sellae, and the sphenoidal ridges are involved, and rarely the meningeal sleeve of the optic nerve. Extensions of intraventricular meningiomas to the skull base are possible. Grossly, meningiomas grow in a nodular spherical or dumbbell-shaped growth type or in an "en plaque" growth type expanding in a diffuse carpetlike fashion. Meningiomas en plaque tend to permeate adjacent bony structures causing hyperostosis (▶ Fig. 3.3).

Histology

Meningiomas (▶ Fig. 3.4) derive on one hand from neuroectodermal cells of the arachnothelial layer, the arachnoidal cap cells, on the other hand from mesenchymal cells of subarachnoidal blood vessels, and from fibroblasts of the subarachnoidal connective tissue. The composition of these histological elements is responsible for the principal different subtypes of meningiomas. However, the histological patterns of the different subentities of meningioma are manifold, and even a mixture of patterns is frequent.

WHO Grade I

- Meningothelial meningiomas form epithelioid syncytial cell clusters with oval pale nuclei that contain little chromatin and pseudoinclusions. Few whorls or psammoma bodies may be encountered (▶ Fig. 3.5).
- Fibrous meningiomas are arranged in intersecting fascicles and are composed of spindled fibroblasts producing collagenous fibers between elongated strands of meningothelial tissue (▶ Fig. 3.6).

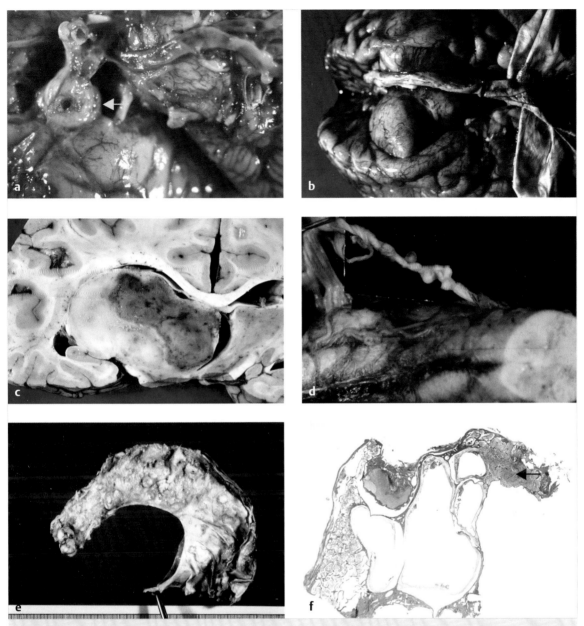

Fig. 3.3 a–f Meningiomas. **(a)** Nodular meningioma surrounding the internal carotid artery (*arrow*). **(b)** Large bilateral meningioma of the falx compressing the surrounding brain tissue. **(c)** Anaplastic intraventricular meningioma with extended necrosis. **(d)** Micromeningiomas along the pars spinalis of the glossopharyngeal nerve. **(e)** En plaque meningiomatosis of the falx. **(f)** Skull base with clivus, sella turcica, pituitary gland, and ethmoidal sinus. Note the meningioma en plaque in the olfactory region (*arrow*) (Elastica van Gieson).

- Transitional meningiomas show a pronounced tendency to form whorls as predominant histological feature (▶ Fig. 3.7).
- Psammomatous meningiomas are sparsely cellular and contain abundant calcified round psammoma bodies (▶ Fig. 3.8).
- Angiomatous meningiomas exhibit a vascular component of large and small blood vessels that exceeds 50% of the tumor volume (▶ Fig. 3.9).

- Microcystic meningiomas grossly appears soft with a glistening cut surface ("humid meningioma") and forms microcysts containing pale-eosinophilic mucinous fluid (▶ Fig. 3.10).
- Secretory meningiomas usually resemble meningothelial meningioma, which contains small round periodic acid–Schiff (PAS)-positive hyaline inclusions, the pseudopsammoma bodies (▶ Fig. 3.11).

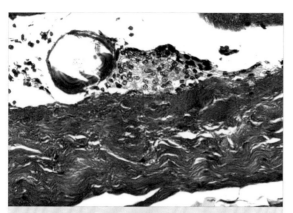

Fig. 3.4 Dura (blue) with incipient meningioma and round psammoma body (Masson trichrome).

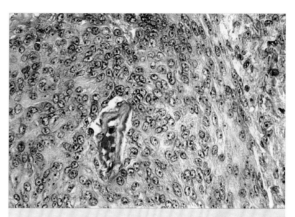

Fig. 3.5 Meningothelial meningioma with syncytially arranged tumor cells and typical pale nuclei containing only few chromatin (Goldner trichrome).

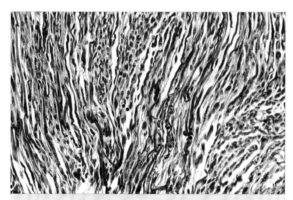

Fig. 3.6 Fibrous meningioma characterized by proliferation of collagenous fibers (blue) in between the meningothelial tumor cells (violet) (Masson trichrome).

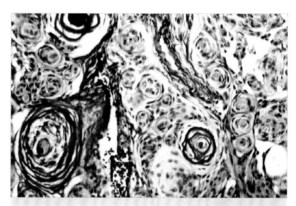

Fig. 3.7 Transitional meningioma with abundant meningothelial and fibrous whorl formation (Masson trichrome).

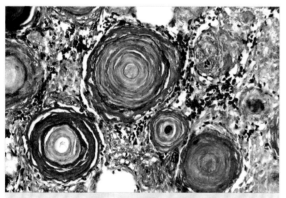

Fig. 3.8 Psammomatous meningioma with abundant calcified psammoma bodies (Masson trichrome).

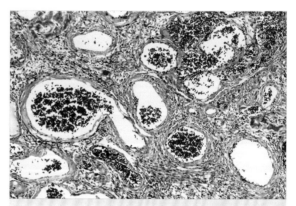

Fig. 3.9 Angiomatous meningioma with abundant blood vessels within the tumor (Masson trichrome).

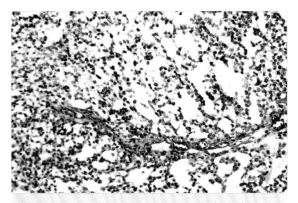

Fig. 3.10 Microcystic meningioma (Masson trichrome).

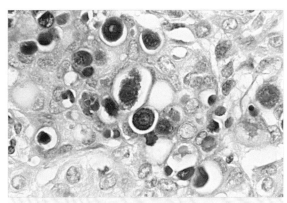

Fig. 3.11 Secretory meningioma with pseudopsammoma bodies rich in glycogen (PAS).

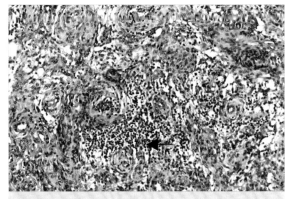

Fig. 3.12 Lymphoplasmacyte-rich meningioma (H&E). Note the lymphocytic infiltration (*arrow*).

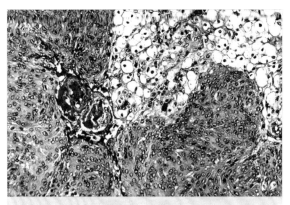

Fig. 3.13 Metaplastic meningioma with xanthomatous differentiation characterized by foci of foamy xanthoma cells (Masson trichrome)

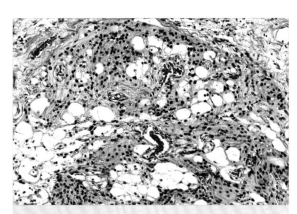

Fig. 3.14 Metaplastic meningiomas with lipoblastic differentiation with scattered lipocytes (Masson trichrome).

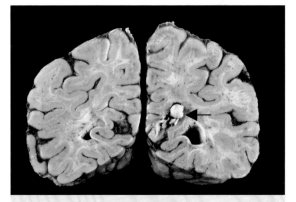

Fig. 3.15 Metaplastic meningioma with osteoblastic differentiation characterized by bone formation in form of a "brain stone" (*arrow*).

- Lymphoplasmacyte-rich meningiomas show dense lymphocytic infiltrates intermingled with meningothelial nests (▶ Fig. 3.12).
- Metaplastic meningiomas show focal xanthomatous (▶ Fig. 3.13), lipomatous (▶ Fig. 3.14), osseous (▶ Fig. 3.15), or cartilaginous areas (▶ Fig. 3.16), singly or in combination.

All subentities of tumors described above are benign.

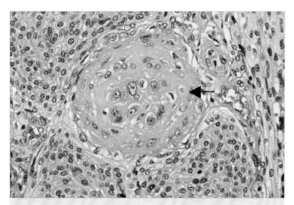

Fig. 3.16 Metaplastic meningioma with chondroblastic differentiation characterized by foci of cartilage (*arrow*) (H&E).

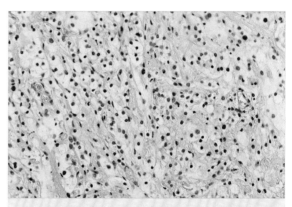

Fig. 3.17 Clear cell meningioma with glycogen-rich cytoplasm; the glycogen is washed out (H&E).

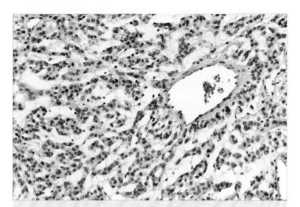

Fig. 3.18 Chordoid meningioma with strands of tumor cells in a mucous-rich matrix (H&E).

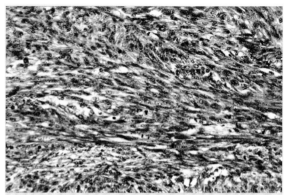

Fig. 3.19 Atypical meningioma with increased mitotic rate (Masson trichrome).

WHO Grade II

- Clear cell meningiomas show polygonal uniform glycogen-rich cells that, in conventional histology, appear "clear" when the glycogen is washed out (▶ Fig. 3.17).
- Chordoid meningiomas resemble the histological features of chordoma and are composed of eosinophilic, epithelioid, and vacuolated cells forming trabeculae. In some cases, chordoid meningioma is associated with Castleman disease, a benign local or generalized angiofollicular hyperplasia of lymph nodes[7] (▶ Fig. 3.18).
- Atypical meningiomas combine increased mitotic activity of 4 or more mitoses per 10 high-power fields with increased cellularity and other signs of histological pleomorphism (▶ Fig. 3.19).

Chordoid, clear cell, and atypical meningiomas are classified as WHO grade II because of a much higher rate of recurrence than WHO grade I meningiomas.

WHO Grade III

- Papillary meningioma is characterized by a predominant perivascular pseudopapillary pattern. The young patients, including children, suffer from local invasion in the brain, recurrences, and even metastases mostly to the lung (▶ Fig. 3.20).
- Rhabdoid meningioma (rare) contains either patches or sheets of plump rhabdoid cells with eosinophilic cytoplasm and large eccentric nuclei.
- Anaplastic (malignant) meningioma exhibits malignant histological features and a markedly elevated mitotic activity of 20 or more mitoses per 10 high-power fields. Local invasion in the brain is a common feature (▶ Fig. 3.21). Note that invasion of the dura and adjacent bone is not to be seen as sign of malignancy.

3.3.2 Hemangiopericytoma

- Meningeal hemangiopericytoma is a not uncommon mesenchymal tumor mainly occurring in younger

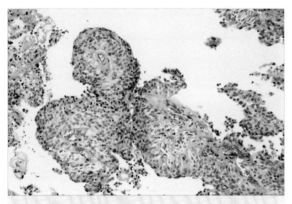

Fig. 3.20 Papillary meningioma with focal necrosis (H&E).

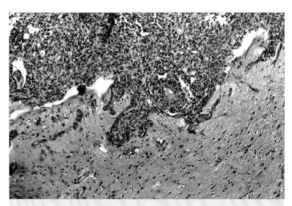

Fig. 3.21 Anaplastic (malignant) meningioma invading the adjacent brain tissue (H&E).

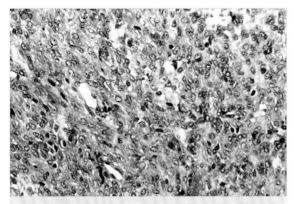

Fig. 3.22 Hemangiopericytoma characterized by high cellularity and jumbled arrangement of spindle cells (Masson trichrome).

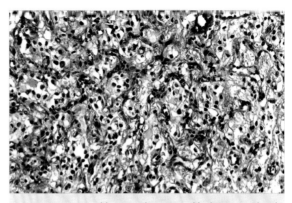

Fig. 3.23 Hemangioblastoma characterized by large vacuolated stromal cells and capillaries (Masson trichrome).

adults and slightly more often in men than in women. It is almost always attached to the dura, and is therefore somewhat similar on imaging to meningiomas. Histologically, the hemangiopericytoma is composed of tightly packed tumor cells with a rich network of reticulin fibers and with numerous slitlike vascular channels and branching staghorn-type vessels (▶ Fig. 3.22).

- Anaplastic hemangiopericytoma has a high tendency to recur and to late metastasis to bone and lung. Histologically, it shows nuclear atypia, increased mitotic activity, necroses and hemorrhage.

3.3.3 Hemangioblastoma

Hemangioblastoma (synonyms capillary hemangioblastoma, Lindau tumor) is a benign, relatively rare, highly vascular, and often cystic tumor of angiomesenchymal origin.[8] In its sporadic form, it is observed in adults with an approximately equal male:female ratio.

In association with von Hippel-Lindau syndrome (VHL), it occurs in significantly younger patients. VHL is an autosomal dominant disorder caused by germline mutations of the *VHL* gene on chromosome 3p. Different mutations of the *VHL* gene are correlated with different phenotypes. In VHL next to hemangioblastomas of the central nervous system and the retina, extraneural manifestations such as clear cell renal carcinoma, pheochromocytoma and paragangliomas, epididymal cystadenoma, neuroendocrine tumors and microcystic adenomas of the pancreas, and endolymphatic sac tumors can be observed.

In the posterior fossa, the cerebellar hemispheres, the vermis, and the fourth ventricle, most often in the area postrema, are affected. Unusually it may occur in the suprasellar region. The tumor is sharply demarcated from the adjacent brain tissue. Histologically, hemangioblastoma is characterized by two components, namely large, vacuolated, foamy stromal cells containing lipid droplets, and a rich network of thin-walled small vessels (▶ Fig. 3.23).

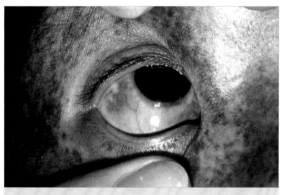

Fig. 3.24 Nevus of Ota with extensive melanotic pigmentation of the skin and the sclera.

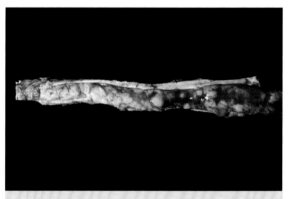

Fig. 3.25 Malignant melanomatosis surrounding the spinal cord spreading from the skull base along the CSF pathways.

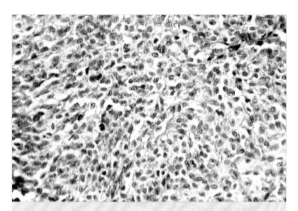

Fig. 3.26 Malignant melanoma characterized by brown-pigmented tumor cells (H&E).

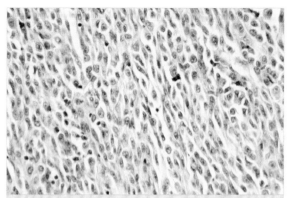

Fig. 3.27 Amelanotic malignant melanoma without melanotic pigmentation (H&E).

3.3.4 Leptomeningeal Melanocytic Lesions

Primary melanocytic lesions of the meninges are rare. They arise from melanocytes found in the pia mater. Diffuse and circumscribed, benign and malignant, and melanotic and amelanotic variants occur. It is important to distinguish melanocytic lesions from histogenetically different tumor entities undergoing melanization such as schwannoma, medulloblastoma, or paraganglioma:[9]

- The diffuse melanocytosis (melanosis) involves the leptomeninges including those of the skull base by a proliferation of leptomeningeal melanocytes within the Virchow-Robin spaces but without gross tumor formation and without invasion of the brain. It may be associated with the congenital nevus of Ota[10] (▶ Fig. 3.24).

The malignant change to melanomatosis (▶ Fig. 3.25) is characterized by invasion into the adjacent brain parenchyma.
- The melanocytoma is a solitary circumscribed tumor deriving from leptomeningeal melanocytes. It does not invade surrounding structures.
- The primary leptomeningeal malignant melanoma has to be distinguished from metastatic malignant melanoma. It is a highly aggressive tumor and may metastasize along the cerebrospinal fluid pathways and to remote organs (▶ Fig. 3.26 and ▶ Fig. 3.27).

Histologically, leptomeningeal melanocytic lesions are composed of spindle cells or epithelioid cells similar to melanocytic tumors arising in other sites.

Table 3.2 Classification and grading of tumors of the peripheral, autonomous, and central nervous systems

Tumor type	WHO grade
Peripheral nerve sheath tumors	
• Schwannoma	I
• Plexiform schwannoma	
• Melanotic schwannoma	Potentially malignant
• MPNST	II, III, or IV
• Epithelioid MPNST	
• MPNST with mesenchymal differentiation	
• Glandular MPNST	
Jugulotympanic paraganglioma (chemodectoma)	I
• Glomus jugulare tumor	
• Glomus tympanicum tumor	
Pilocytic astrocytoma	I
Pilomyxoid astrocytoma	II
Ependymoma	II or III

MPSNT, malignant peripheral nerve sheath tumor.

3.4 Tumors of the Peripheral, Autonomous, and Central Nervous Systems

Classification and grading of peripheral, autonomous, and central nervous system tumors are shown in (▶ Table 3.2).

3.4.1 Schwannomas

Schwannomas derive from Schwann cells that form the myelin sheath in peripheral nerves. With the exception of the olfactory and optic nerves being entirely invested by central myelin formed by oligodendrocytes, the peripheral portion of the other cranial nerves is invested by peripheral myelin formed by Schwann cells (▶ Fig. 3.28). Schwannomas account for approximately 7% of all primary intracranial tumors. All ages, with a peak incidence in the fourth to sixth decades, are affected. The tumor occurs more often in women, the female:male ratio is 2:1.

About 90% of intracranial schwannomas are vestibular schwannomas (synonyms acoustic neuroma, acoustic neurinoma). Vestibular schwannomas arise from the vestibular branch of the eighth cranial nerve. The tumor growth regularly commences in the internal auditory canal followed by an expansion into the cerebellopontine angle (▶ Fig. 3.29). Bilateral vestibular schwannomas are pathognomonic for neurofibromatosis 2 (NF2) (▶ Fig. 3.30).

Schwannomas of the trigeminal nerve arising from the trigeminal root, the gasserian ganglion, and the three major trigeminal roots are rare, all other locations are extremely rare.

Grossly, schwannomas are usually encapsulated, globoid lesions with a soft texture. Histologically, schwannomas often show a biphasic pattern of elongated cells in interlacing fascicles (Antoni A areas, ▶ Fig. 3.31) and of clear areas of fatty degeneration (Antoni B areas) (▶ Fig. 3.32).

The variant of cellular schwannoma with a high cellularity remains benign (▶ Fig. 3.33). The plexiform and melanotic variants are not typical for skull base schwannomas.

3.4.2 Malignant Peripheral Nerve Sheath Tumors

Malignant peripheral nerve sheath tumors (MPNSTs) of the vestibular nerve are rare.[11,12] They are characterized by a fascicular pattern similar to cellular schwannoma and numerous mitoses (▶ Fig. 3.34). Extremely rare variants with a potentially malignant course comprise, on the one hand, the malignant triton tumor with rhabdomyoblastic cells[13,14] reminiscent of the triton tumor observed in neurofibromatosis 1, and the melanotic schwannoma[15] on the other hand. However, there is a debate as to whether melanocytic tumors of the cerebellopontine angle mimicking vestibular schwannomas might be actually malignant melanomas.[16]

Immunohistochemically, melanotic schwannomas are reactive for Schwann cell markers (such as S-100 protein) as well as melanoma markers (such as HMB-45 or Melan A). About 50% of the psammomatous variant of melanotic schwannoma is associated with the Carney complex, an autosomal dominant disorder characterized by lentiginous facial pigmentation, cardiac myxoma, and endocrine overactivity. Melanotic nonpsammomatous trigeminal schwannoma, as the first manifestation of Carney complex, has been reported postulating that the absence of psammoma bodies or cranial localization does not exclude this diagnosis.[17]

3.4.3 Jugulotympanic Paraganglioma

Paragangliomas (synonym chemodectoma) are benign neuroendocrine tumors producing catecholamine. They derive from autonomous nervous cell complexes. Intracranial paragangliomas are rare. They show a female predilection and a peak in the fifth and sixth decades of life. At the skull base, they may be situated either in relation to the jugular bulb (glomus jugulare tumor) or under the mucosa of the middle ear (glomus tympanicum tumor).

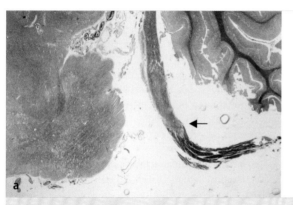
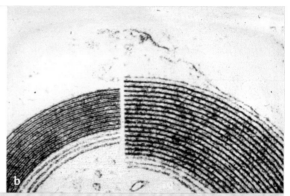

Fig. 3.28 a, b Myelin sheaths. **(a)** Cerebellopontine angle with transition (*arrow*) between the central portion of the acoustic nerve with myelin sheaths formed by oligodendroglial cells (turquoise) and the peripheral portion with myelin sheaths formed by Schwann cells (dark violet) (Luxol fast blue–PAS). **(b)** Ultrastructural difference between peripheral myelin with a major dense line and a smaller intermediate line (left) and central myelin only with a major dense line (right). Transmission electron micrograph.

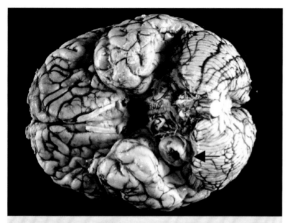

Fig. 3.29 Vestibular schwannoma in the cerebellopontine angle (*arrow*).

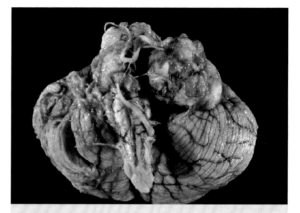

Fig. 3.30 Bilateral vestibular schwannoma in neurofibromatosis 2 after surgical removal of the smaller one in the right cerebellopontine angle. The remaining larger vestibular schwannoma leads to compression of the pons and the cerebellum.

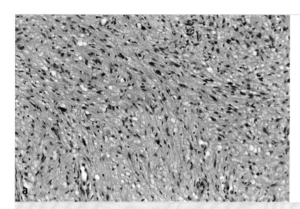
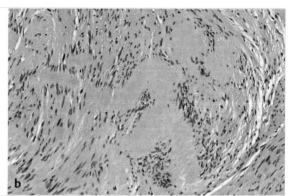

Fig. 3.31 a, b Antoni A areas of schwannomas. **(a)** Loose fascicular pattern of elongated tumor cells with spindle-shaped nuclei (Antoni A) (H&E). **(b)** Typical palisading of tumor cell nuclei (H&E).

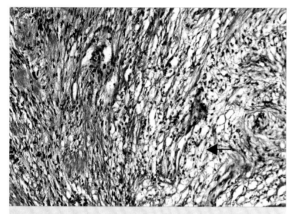

Fig. 3.32 Vestibular schwannoma with dense Antoni A areas and clear Antoni B areas with fatty degeneration (*arrow*).

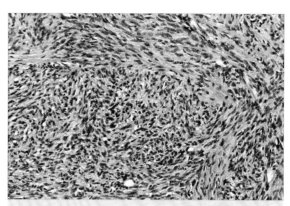

Fig. 3.33 Dense fascicular pattern of cellular schwannoma (H&E).

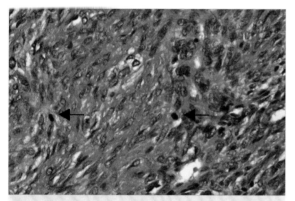

Fig. 3.34 Malignant peripheral nerve sheath tumor characterized by fascicular pattern, polymorphous tumor cells, and mitotic figures (*arrows*) (H&E).

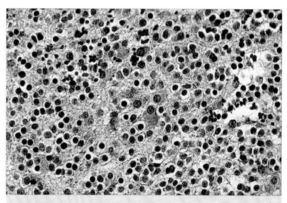

Fig. 3.35 Jugulotympanic paraganglioma with "Zellballen" arrangement of chief cells (Masson trichrome).

Histologically, paragangliomas are composed of well-defined groups of cells forming clusters or "Zellballen." Epithelioid monomorphic chief cells, which express synaptophysin and chromogranin immunohistochemically, are supported by sustentacular cells (▶ Fig. 3.35).

3.4.4 Pilocytic Astrocytoma

The pilocytic astrocytoma derives from glial cells of phylogenetical old brain structures. It occurs in children and young adults. There is no sex predilection. Preferred sites include the optic nerve and the chiasmatic and hypothalamic region, as well as the brain stem and cerebellum. Histologically, bipolar "hairlike" cells with Rosenthal fibers are typical (▶ Fig. 3.36).

3.4.5 Pilomyxoid Astrocytoma

The pilomyxoid astrocytoma is closely related to pilocytic astrocytoma. It occurs typically in the first year of life. There is no sex predilection. The chiasmatic and hypothalamic region is the most common location (▶ Fig. 3.37).

Histologically, the tumor is characterized by bipolar tumor cells that show an angiocentric arrangement in a myxoid matrix (▶ Fig. 3.38).

3.4.6 Ependymoma

Ependymomas derive from ependymal cells. At the skull base, infratentorial ependymomas of the fourth ventricle (▶ Fig. 3.39) occur in children, with a mean age of 6.4 years.

Histologically, the well-demarcated tumor shows cells arranged radially around blood vessels with perivascular anuclear zones (pseudorosettes), and ependymal rosettes (▶ Fig. 3.40). Variants such as the papillary ependymoma, the clear cell ependymoma, and the tanycytic ependymoma occur; the latter variant is most common in the spinal cord. The semimalignant anaplastic ependymoma is relatively frequent in children, particularly in the posterior fossa location.

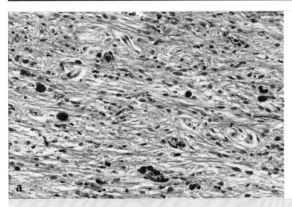 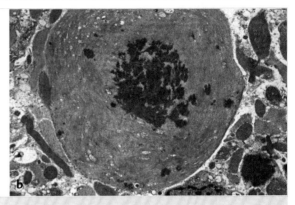

Fig. 3.36 a, b Pilocytic astrocytoma. (a) Bipolar hairlike piloid cells showing numerous Rosenthal fibers (red) (Masson trichrome). (b) Large centrally degenerated Rosenthal fiber (transmission electron micrograph).

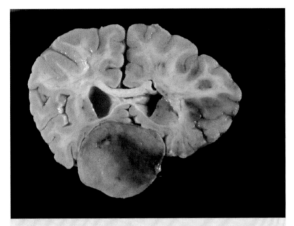

Fig. 3.37 Pilomyxoid astrocytoma of the optic nerve with prominent myxoid matrix.

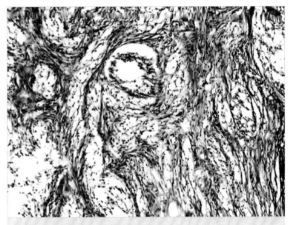

Fig. 3.38 Pilomyxoid astrocytoma with tumor cells in a myxoid matrix (Masson trichrome).

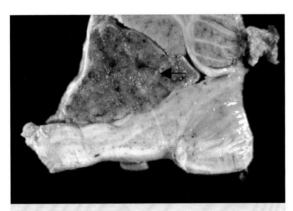

Fig. 3.39 Ependymoma of the fourth ventricle (arrow).

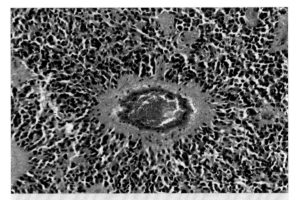

Fig. 3.40 Ependymoma with typical perivascular pseudorosette (H&E).

3.5 Tumors of the Hematopoietic System

Classification and grading of tumors of the hematopoietic system are shown in ▶ Table 3.3.

3.5.1 Primary Central Nervous System Lymphomas

Malignant lymphomas arising primarily in the central nervous system and also affecting the skull base region must be differentiated from secondary involvement in systemic lymphomas as well as in meningeosis lymphomatosa. They affect all ages with a peak incidence in immunocompetent patients during the sixth and seventh decades of life. The male:female ratio is 3:2. In cases of immunodeficiency, young patients may be involved.

Histologically, as in other anatomic locations, malignant lymphomas are classified according to the WHO classification, respecting the Revised European-American Lymphoma (REAL) classification.[18] More than 90% of primary lymphomas of the central nervous system are diffuse large B-cell lymphomas (▶ Fig. 3.41).

Table 3.3 Classification and grading of tumors of the hematopoietic system

Tumor type	WHO grade
Primary central nervous system lymphomas	Malignant
Langerhans cell histiocytosis	
• Unifocal	Benign
• Multifocal	Intermediate to malignant
Non-Langerhans cell histiocytosis	Benign to malignant

3.5.2 Langerhans Cell Histiocytosis

Langerhans cell histiocytosis (LCH) was previously referred to as histiocytosis X embracing eosinophilic granuloma and Hand–Schüller–Christian disease.

LCH typically occurs in children under 15 years of age. There is no sex predilection. The most common form is a solitary monostotic osteolytic lesion of the skull in the form of an eosinophilic granuloma. Multifocal, thus polyostotic, manifestations have a poor outcome with a mortality rate up to 20%. The cerebral LCH with principal involvement of the hypothalamus and posterior pituitary has been referred to as Hand–Schüller–Christian disease.

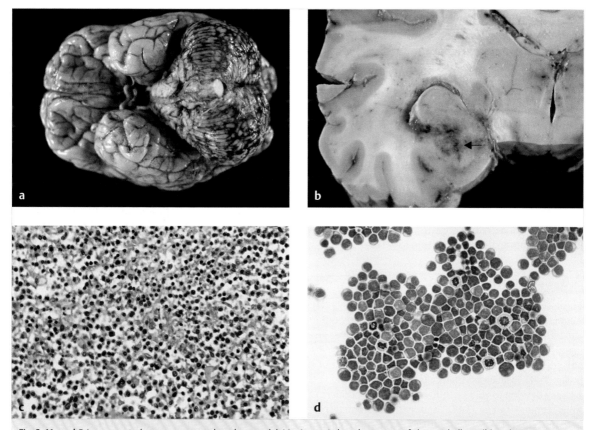

Fig. 3.41 a–d Primary central nervous system lymphomas. **(a)** Meningeosis lymphomatosa of the cerebellum. **(b)** Malignant non-Hodgkin lymphoma in the hippocampal region (*arrow*). **(c)** Diffuse B-cell non-Hodgkin lymphoma composed of primarily transformed lymphocytes (H&E). **(d)** CSF fluid cytology of a malignant non-Hodgkin lymphoma of diffuse large B-cell type (May–Grünwald–Giemsa).

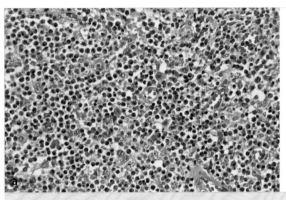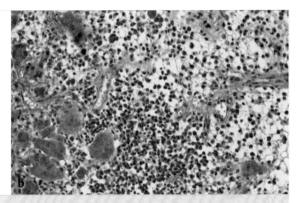

Fig. 3.42 a, b Langerhans cell histiocytosis. (a) LCH (eosinophilic granuloma) composed of primarily eosiniphilic cells (H&E). (b) LCH composed of plasma cells, lymphocytic, eosinophilic and Langerhans histiocytic cells, and multinucleated Touton giant cells (H&E).

Histologically, tumor cell infiltrates are composed of Langerhans cells, macrophages, lymphocytes, and plasma cells, typically often with a variable fraction of eosinophils and Touton giant cells (▶ Fig. 3.42).

3.5.3 Non-Langerhans Cell Histiocytosis

Non-LCH in adults includes Rosai-Dorfman disease with dural-based solitary or multiple masses and Erdheim-Chester disease with involvement of cerebellum, cerebellopontine angle, choroid plexus, pituitary, meninges, and orbit. In young children, intracranial juvenile xanthogranuloma may occur in the brain or the meninges.

Histologically, emperipolesis is typical; that is, well preserved lymphocytes and plasma cells taken in the cytoplasm of macrophages.

3.6 Germ Cell Tumors and Dysontogenetic Tumorlike Cysts

Classification and grading of germ cell tumors and dysontogenetic tumorlike cysts are shown in ▶ Table 3.4.

3.6.1 Germ Cell Tumors

Germ cell tumors are highly malignant dysontogenetic tumors that derive from undifferentiated or poorly differentiated germ cells. Primordial germ cells themselves give rise to germinoma (▶ Fig. 3.43). Cells with early embryonic differentiation give rise to embryonal carcinoma (▶ Fig. 3.44). Extraembryonal cells deriving from the yolk sac may develop to yolk sac tumor (synonym endodermal sinus tumor) (▶ Fig. 3.45), and extraembryonal cells deriving from the placenta may develop to choriocarcinoma (▶ Fig. 3.46). Mixed tumors occur. Germ cell tumors may be encountered along the midline of the brain, the pineal region, and also extend to the skull base.

3.6.2 Teratoma and Tumorlike Dysontogenetic Cysts

Tumorlike dysontogenetic cysts such as epidermoid and dermoid ontogenetically may be seen as incomplete teratomas that are not differentiated into all three germ layers.

- The *epidermoid* derives from differentiated cells of the ectodermal germ layer forming cysts with squamous epithelial-lined wall.
- The *dermoid* derives from differentiated cells of the ectodermal germ layer forming cysts with squamous epithelial-lined wall and derivatives from skin appendices such as hair follicles and hairs, and sebaceous glands (▶ Fig. 3.47).
- *Teratomas* derive from all three germ layers and comprise a varying tissue mixture of all kinds of immature and mature tissue. Although the vast majority of these tumors are benign, teratomas with malignant transformation of one of the tissue components, for example, teratocarcinoma, can occur (▶ Fig. 3.48).

Table 3.4 Classification and grading of germ cell tumors and dysontogenetic tumorlike cysts

Tumor type	WHO grade
Germ cell tumors	
Germinoma	Malignant
Embryonal carcinoma	Malignant
Yolk sac tumor	Malignant
Choriocarcinoma	Malignant
Teratoma	
Mature teratoma	Benign
Immature teratoma	Intermediate
Teratoma with malignant transformation	Malignant
Tumorlike dysontogenetic cysts	
Epidermoid cyst	
Dermoid cyst	

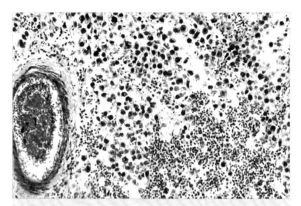

Fig. 3.43 Germinoma with biphasic appearance of large tumor cells and small lymphocytes due to a typical inflammatory reaction (H&E).

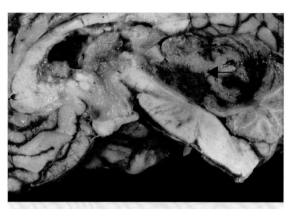

Fig. 3.44 Embryonal carcinoma of the pineal region (*arrow*).

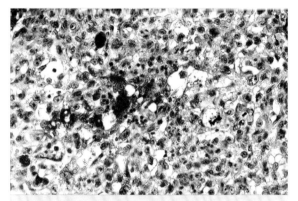

Fig. 3.45 Yolk sac tumor with α-fetoprotein (AFP)-positive tumor cells (red) (APAAP technique, alkaline phosphatase–antialkaline phosphatase).

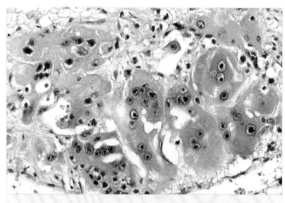

Fig. 3.46 Choriocarcinoma with placenta-derived syncytiotrophoblastic giant cells (H&E).

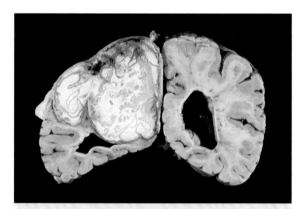

Fig. 3.47 Large dermoid cyst filled with fatty cell debris and hairs.

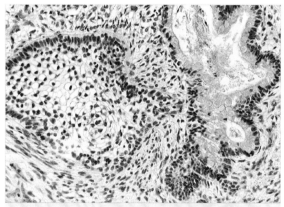

Fig. 3.48 Mature teratoma with a mixture of unevenly distributed different mature tissue components (H&E).

Table 3.5 Classification and grading of tumors of the sellar region

Tumor type	WHO grade
Pituitary adenoma	Benign
Pituitary carcinoma	Malignant
Spindle cell oncocytoma of the adenohypophysis	I
Pituicytoma	I
Granular cell tumor of the neurohypophysis	I

Craniopharyngioma
  Adamantinomatous craniopharyngioma
  Papillary craniopharyngioma
	I

3.7 Tumors of the Sellar Region

Classification and grading of tumors of the sellar region are shown in (▶ Table 3.5).

3.7.1 Pituitary Adenoma

Pituitary adenomas derive from adenohypophysial cells (▶ Fig. 3.49) and represent up to 25% of all intracranial tumors. Their prevalence increases with advancing age. Whereas microadenomas are still growing within the intrasellar adenohypophysis, macroadenomas show an often impressive suprasellar extension (▶ Fig. 3.50). These lesions may compress or infiltrate neighboring structures. Hormone excess syndromes can occur.

Histologically, the traditional classification of chromophobic (▶ Fig. 3.51), acidophilic, and basophilic adenomas has been abandoned in favor of an immunohistochemical classification based on hormone content. There are hormonally functioning adenomas (▶ Fig. 3.52) and nonfunctioning adenomas, with the latter accounting for approximately one-third of all pituitary adenomas. For the morphological determination of hormone excretion, transmission electron microscopy is useful in clinically symptomatic patients. After enhanced extrusion of hormone granules, sparsely granulated adenomas are observed in electron microscopy, whereas no hormone positivity can be seen in immunohistochemical examination of these patients.

3.7.2 Pituitary Carcinoma

Pituitary carcinomas are rare and characterized by marked polymorphism and mitoses. Distant metastases may occur but they are extremely rare.

3.7.3 Spindle Cell Oncocytoma of the Adenohypophysis

The spindle cell oncocytoma of the adenohypophysis is a rare benign tumor. There is no sex predilection. The tumor has no endocrine activity. Macroscopically, the tumor is indistinguishable from pituitary adenomas. Histologically, the tumor is composed of interlacing fascicles of cells with eosinophilic oncocytic cytoplasm.

3.7.4 Pituicytoma

The pituicytoma is a benign and extremely rare tumor that originates in the neurohypophysis or infundibulum. It occurs in adults of the fifth to seventh decades with a male:female ratio of 1.6:1. Histologically, the tumor consists of elongated spindle cells.

3.7.5 Granular Cell Tumor of the Neurohypophysis

The granular cell tumor is a benign and rare tumor that arises from the neurohypophysis or infundibulum. It is observed in adults, with a female predominance of 2:1. The usually circumscribed tumor occurs in a sellar and suprasellar localization. Histologically, the tumor cells are characterized by an abundant granular eosinophilic cytoplasm.

3.7.6 Craniopharyngioma

Craniopharyngiomas derive from remnants of the Rathke pouch epithelium and the craniopharyngeal duct. They occur in adults above 40 years of age and, in cases of the adamantinomatous variant, also in children. Craniopharyngiomas have a suprasellar localization with a minor intrasellar component (▶ Fig. 3.53).
- Adamantinomatous craniopharyngioma is characterized by strands and lobules of squamous epithelium bordered by tumor cell palisades and nodules of "wet keratin" (▶ Fig. 3.54).
- Papillary craniopharyngioma is characterized by papillae of squamous epithelium (▶ Fig. 3.55).

3.8 Tumors of the Nasal Cavity and Paranasal Sinuses

Classification and grading of tumors of the tumors of the nasal cavity and paranasal sinuses are shown in (▶ Table 3.6).

3.8.1 Schneiderian Papilloma

Schneiderian papillomas derive from ciliated respiratory mucosa lining the nasal cavity and paranasal sinuses. They occur typically in adults with a clear predilection for males, with the exception of oncocytic papilloma being equally distributed between the sexes.

Inverted papilloma shows an endophytic invagination of hyperplastic ribbons of basement-membrane enclosed

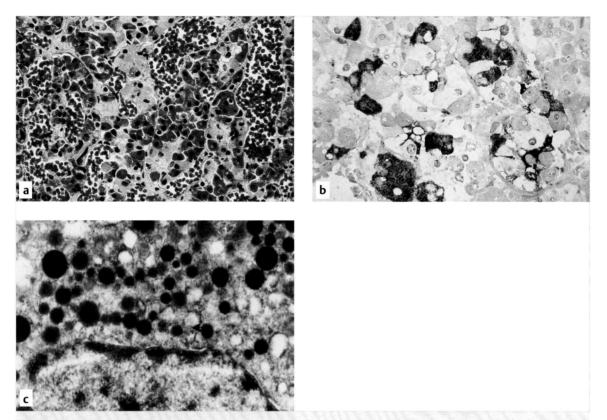

Fig. 3.49 a–c Cells of the pituitary gland. (a) Nontumorous pituitary gland with a mixture of chromophobic, eosinophilic, and few basophilic cells (Masson trichrome). (b) Nontumorous pituitary gland with large growth hormone (GH)-secreting cells (brown) and folliculostellate cells (black) (immunohistochemical double staining GH-DAB, S-100 protein PAP technique). (c) Densely granulated growth-hormone-secreting cell. Note the electron-dense round hormone granules next to the nucleus (*arrowhead*) (transmission electron micrograph).

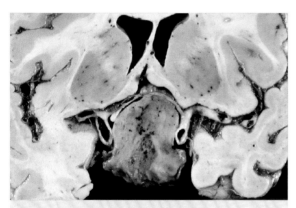

Fig. 3.50 Pituitary macroadenoma with infrasellar and suprasellar growth.

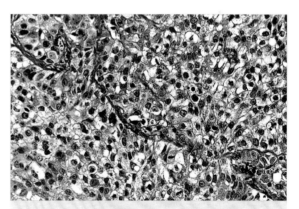

Fig. 3.51 Chromophobic adenoma (Masson trichrome).

epithelium into the underlying stroma (▶ Fig. 3.56). Characteristically they arise from the lateral nasal wall in the middle turbinate or ethmoid recesses, and often extend into the sinuses. About 10% are complicated by carcinomas.[19]

Oncocytic papilloma is composed of both endophytic and exophytic growth of multiple layers of columnar cells with oncocytic features characterized by swollen, finely granular cytoplasm (▶ Fig. 3.57). Malignant change is seen in more than 10% of cases.[20]

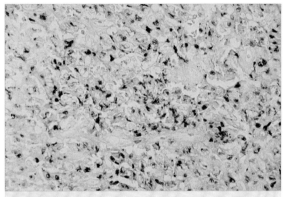

Fig. 3.52 Prolactin (PRL)-secreting cells in a prolactinoma (PRL-DAB immunohistochemistry).

Table 3.6 Classification and grading of tumors of the nasal cavity and paranasal sinuses

Tumor type	WHO grade
Schneiderian papilloma	
• Inverted papilloma	Benign; malignant change possible
• Oncocytic papilloma	Benign; malignant change possible
• Exophytic papilloma	Benign; malignant change exceptional
Sinonasal squamous cell carcinoma	Malignant
Nasopharyngeal angiofibroma	Benign
Nasal glioma	Benign
Esthesioneuroblastoma (olfactory neuroblastoma)	Malignant

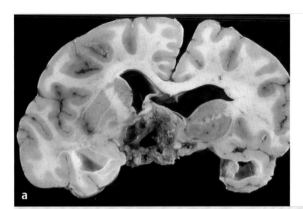
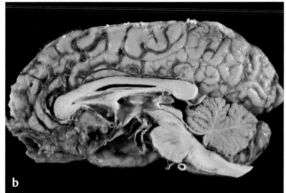

Fig. 3.53 a, b Craniopharyngioma (a) Poorly demarcated cystic craniopharyngioma invading the third ventricle and the basal ganglia. (b) Brownish resorption-wall of brain tissue a long time after surgical resection of a craniopharyngioma.

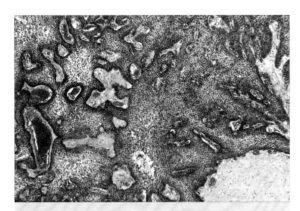

Fig. 3.54 Adamantinous craniopharyngioma with squamous epithelium bordered by cell palisades (H&E).

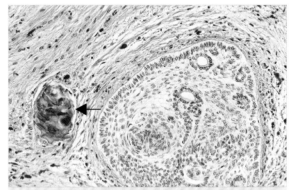

Fig. 3.55 Nodule of "wet keratin" (*arrow*) representing remnants of pale nuclei embedded within a keratinous mass next to squamous epithelium bordered by cell palisades (Masson trichrome).

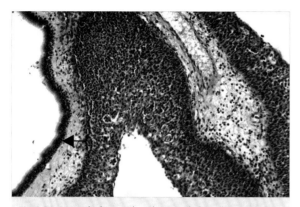

Fig. 3.56 Beneath the regular ciliary epithelium (*arrow*) an epithelial island of inverted Schneiderian papilloma enclosed by fibrous stroma (H&E).

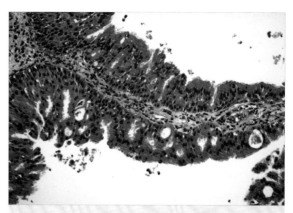

Fig. 3.57 Exophytic growth of stratified multilayered columnar epithelium in oncocytic Schneiderian papilloma characteristically containing numerous small cysts filled with mucin (H&E).

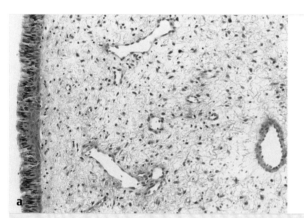

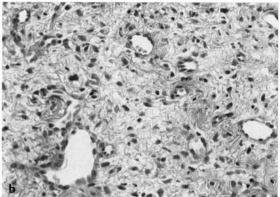

Fig. 3.58 Nasopharyngeal angiofibroma. (a) Nasopharyngeal angiofibroma under an intact respiratory epithelium (Masson trichrome). (b) Nasopharyngeal angiofibroma with thin-walled vessels surrounded by loose fibrous connective tissue (Masson trichrome).

Exophytic papilloma is characterized by exophytic papillary growth of multiple layers of epithelial cells. Malignant change is exceptional.

3.8.2 Sinonasal Squamous Cell Carcinoma

Sinonasal squamous cell carcinoma originates from the mucosal epithelium of the nasal cavity or paranasal sinuses. It occurs most frequently in the maxillary sinus and the nasal cavity, and more rarely in the ethmoid, sphenoid, and frontal sinuses. Risk factors include exposure to nickel, chlorophenols, and textile dust, smoking, and a history of sinonasal Schneiderian papilloma. The tumor can invade adjacent sites.

Histologically, the nonkeratinizing type is characterized by a plexiform or ribbonlike growth pattern. The keratinizing type is identical to squamous cell carcinoma of other sites.

3.8.3 Nasopharyngeal Angiofibroma (Juvenile Nasopharyngeal Angiofibroma)

Nasopharyngeal angiofibroma is a benign highly vascularized mesenchymal tumor in juvenile males. A testosterone-dependent puberty-induced polypoid tumor growth in the posterolateral nasal wall or the nasopharynx is observed.

Histologically, thin-walled, slitlike vessels are surrounded by relatively dense fibrous stroma (▶ Fig. 3.58). Long-standing lesions show increased keloidlike fibrosis. Local aggressive growth with recurrences can occur.

3.8.4 Nasal Glioma

Nasal glioma is not a tumor in the strict sense but a congenital malformation. It consists of a mass of heterotopic neuroglial tissue usually measuring up to 3 cm and

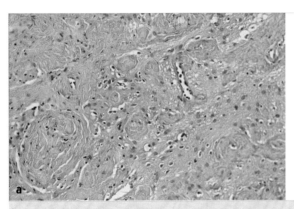
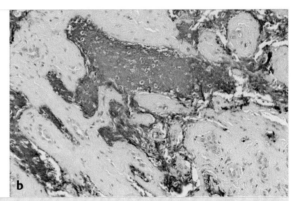

Fig. 3.59 a, b Nasal glioma. (a) Nasal glioma with glial islands in turquoise fibrous matrix. Masson trichrome. (b) Nasal glioma with positivity for glial fibrillary acidic protein (GFAP) within the glial islands. GFAP.

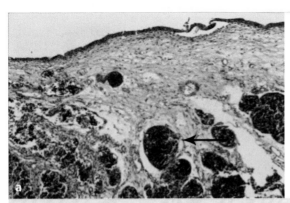
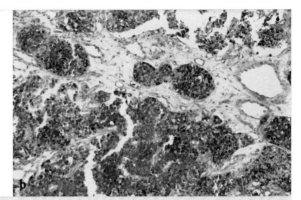

Fig. 3.60 a, b Esthesioneuroblastoma. (a) Esthesioneuroblastoma with tumor lobules separated by a vascular stroma under the olfactory epithelium (arrow) (H&E). (b) Esthesioneuroblastoma with a strong immunohistochemical expression of synaptophysin within the tumor lobules (Synaptophysin).

presenting within the nasal cavity or near the bridge of the nose. There may be communication between the intranasal and extranasal components through a defect in the nasal bone. It is present at birth and in most patients diagnosed by the age of 2 years. There is no sex predilection.

Histologically, the nasal glioma is composed of islands of glial tissue surrounded by bands of vascularized connective tissue (▶ Fig. 3.59). Being a malformative lesion there is no local aggressive behavior or malignant potential.

3.8.5 Esthesioneuroblastoma (Olfactory Neuroblastoma)

The esthesioneuroblastoma is a rare neuroectodermal tumor originating from the olfactory membrane of the sinonasal tract. The common site is in the upper nasal cavity in the region of the cribriform plate. Ectopic tumors in the lower nasal cavity or within the paranasal sinuses are possible. A bimodal age distribution with peaks in the second and sixth decades of life can be noted. There is no sex predilection.

Histologically, the tumor consists of circumscribed submucosal lobules separated by vascularized fibrous stroma (▶ Fig. 3.60). The tumor cells exhibit characteristics of neuroblastic cells. A grading system with four grades has been proposed.[21]

3.9 Tumors of the Osseous Skull Base

Classification and grading of tumors of the osseous skull base are shown in (▶ Table 3.7).

3.9.1 Plasma Cell Myeloma

Plasma cell myeloma (synonyms: multiple myeloma, Kahler disease, plasmacytoma) is a malignant immunosecretory tumor that derives from a single clone of immunoglobulin secreting end-stage B cells. Bence Jones protein

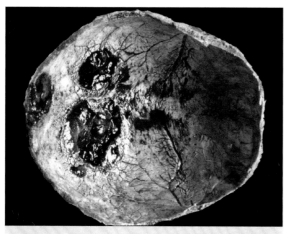

Fig. 3.61 Osteolytic lesions of plasma cell myeloma of the skull.

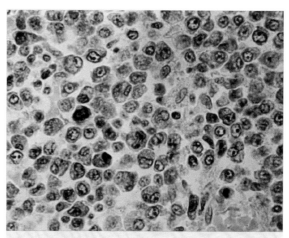

Fig. 3.62 Plasma cell myeloma with transformed immature plasma cells (May–Grünwald–Giemsa).

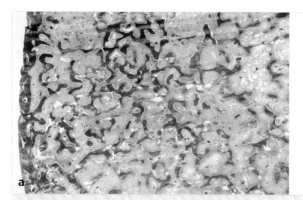

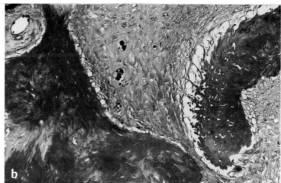

Fig. 3.63 a, b Fibrous dysplasia. (a) C-shaped bony spicules and hypocellular fibrous stroma (Masson trichrome). (b) Osseous component (red) with woven (not lamellar) bone (Masson trichrome).

is found in the urine in 75% of patients. The multifocal bone-marrow-based tumor shows skeletal destruction with osteolytic lesions including the skull location (▶ Fig. 3.61). Localized solitary plasmacytoma of the skull may occur.

Histologically, aggregates of immature plasma cells are characteristic (▶ Fig. 3.62).

Table 3.7 Classification and grading of tumors of the osseous skull base

Tumor type	WHO grade
Plasma cell myeloma	Malignant
Fibrous dysplasia	Benign
Ossifying fibromyxoid tumor	Potentially malignant
Osteoblastoma	Benign
Osteosarcoma	Malignant
Chondroblastoma	Benign
Chondrosarcoma	Malignant
Chordoma	Malignant

3.9.2 Fibrous Dysplasia

Fibrous dysplasia is a benign medullary fibro-osseous lesion and may be monostotic (MFD) involving one bone, or polyostotic (PFD) involving several bones. MFD and PFD are mainly diagnosed in children and young adults. There is no general sex predilection in MFD; however, with regard to the skull base manifestation there is a predilection for males. In contrast the female:male ratio is 3:1 for PFD.

The tympanic, mastoid, squamous, or petrous temporal bones may be involved. Unusual sites include the internal auditory canal, the lateral semicircular canal, and the ossicles. PFD may manifest in infants in the setting of McCune-Albright syndrome caused by mutations in the GNAS1 gene and associated with café-au-lait spots and hyperfunctioning endocrinopathies. Malignant transformation occurs, but rarely.

The bone shows local grayish and firm expansions where the marrow is replaced by an intramedullary proliferation of trabecular woven bone admixed with fibrous tissue (▶ Fig. 3.63). The lesion arises abruptly from a bland spindle cell stroma.

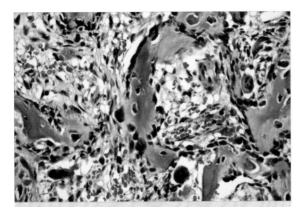

Fig. 3.64 Osteoblastoma with irregular islands of osteoid, osteoblasts, and osteoclastlike multinucleated giant cells (H&E).

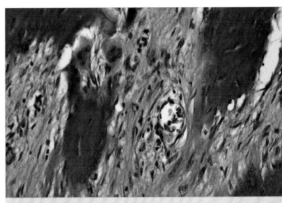

Fig. 3.65 Osteosarcoma with fusiform spindle cells around an osseous matrix (dark red) (H&E).

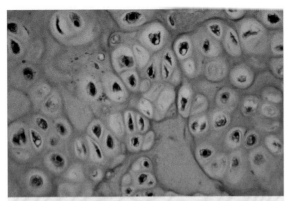

Fig. 3.66 Chondroblastoma with well-defined cytoplasmic borders (H&E).

3.9.3 Ossifying Fibromyxoid Tumor

Ossifying fibromyxoid tumor is a rare tumor and even rarer in the skull base region. Recurrences are common. Cords of ovoid tumor cells are embedded in a fibromyxoid matrix, often surrounded by a shell of lamellar bone. A nonossifying variant in the nasopharyngeal region has been reported.[22]

3.9.4 Osteoblastoma

Osteoblastoma is a rare benign bone forming tumor. Sites of involvement include the spine, particularly the posterior elements, and the jaw (cementoblastoma).

Histologically, it has identical features to osteoid osteoma producing woven bone spicules that are lined by a single layer of osteoblasts (▶ Fig. 3.64). Diffusely scattered osteoclast-type multinucleated giant cells are often present.

3.9.5 Osteosarcoma

A skull location of osteosarcoma is very rare, but involvement of skull tends to increase with age. There is a male predominance. In older patients, a predisposing condition such as Paget disease of the bone or postradiation sarcoma should be considered.

Histologically, the typical tumor is composed of fusiform spindle cells around an osseous matrix (▶ Fig. 3.65). Subtypes include osteoblastic, chondroblastic, and fibroblastic osteosarcoma.

3.9.6 Chondroblastoma

Chondroblastoma is a rare benign bone tumor that occurs in adults in the fifth decade of life. There is a male predominance. At the skull base, the temporal bone is most frequently affected. Grossly, a whitish tumor is seen.

Histologically, sheets of chondroblasts with well-defined cytoplasmic borders are characteristic (▶ Fig. 3.66).

3.9.7 Chondrosarcoma

Chondrosarcoma is a malignant tumor that is extremely rare in craniofacial bones. It occurs in adults in the fifth to seventh decades of life. Grossly, chondrosarcomas have a translucent white color.

Histologically, the cartilaginous tumor cells with ill-defined borders permeate between pre-existing bony trabeculae (▶ Fig. 3.67).

3.9.8 Chordoma

Chordoma is a malignant bone tumor that recapitulates notochord. It occurs in adults with a male predominance. At the skull base, chordomas are typically located in the clivus (▶ Fig. 3.68). A small proportion may involve the nasopharynx and/or paranasal sinuses. They extend into the surrounding structures and may often form large tumor masses. Metastases may occur.

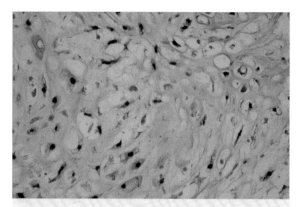

Fig. 3.67 Chondrosarcoma G2 with ill-defined cytoplasmic borders (H&E).

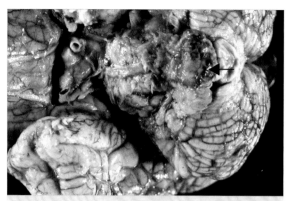

Fig. 3.68 Expansively growing chordoma of the skull base arising from the clivus (*arrow*).

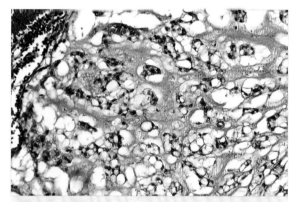

Fig. 3.69 Chordoma cords of physaliphorous tumor cells in a myxoid matrix (Masson trichrome).

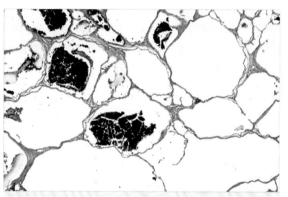

Fig. 3.70 Cavernoma of the orbit with small and large thin-walled cavernous vessels (Masson trichrome).

Histologically, chordomas are lobulated tumors with tumor cells arranged in cords within a myxoid stroma (▶ Fig. 3.69).

3.10 Tumors of Orbit and Eye

Classification and grading of tumors of the orbit and eye are shown in (▶ Table 3.8).

3.10.1 Tumors of the Orbit

Vascular Tumors

The most frequent tumors of the orbit (~10–15%) are of vascular origin and benign:
- Capillary hemangioma (juvenile hemangioendothelioma) can be observed in 1 to 2% of the newborn. It is mainly localized in the upper nasal part of the orbit. Spontaneous regression is observed in about two-thirds of the cases.
- Cavernomas (cavernous hemangiomas) occur in the second to fourth decades of life and are mainly localized behind the eye bulb (▶ Fig. 3.70).

Pilocytic Astrocytoma

Pilocytic astrocytoma (optic glioma) of the intraorbital optic nerve occurs in the first two decades of life and is frequently combined with a generalized neurofibromatosis type 1 (NF1, von Recklinghausen disease).

Meningioma

The primary meningioma of the orbit derives from the meningeal sheath of the optic nerve and can be seen mainly in middle-aged women and in children, again frequently combined with NF1. An extension of an olfactory meningioma into the orbit is possible.

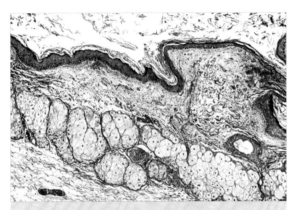

Fig. 3.71 Dermoid cyst of the orbit with keratinizing epithelium and subepithelial sebaceous glands surrounded by a fibrous matrix (Masson trichrome).

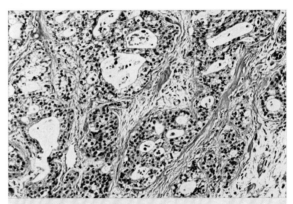

Fig. 3.72 Adenoid cystic carcinoma of the lacrimal gland with microcystic spaces (H&E).

Table 3.8 Classification and grading of tumors of orbit and eye

Tumor type	WHO grade
Orbit	
Capillary hemangioma (juvenile hemangioendothelioma)	Benign
Cavernoma (cavernous hemangioma)	Benign
Pilocytic astrocytoma (optic glioma)	I
Meningioma	I–III
Dermoid cyst	Benign
Adenoid cystic carcinoma of the lacrimal gland	Malignant
Lymphoma	Malignant
Embryonal sarcoma	Malignant
Rhabdomyosarcoma	Malignant
Chondrosarcoma	Malignant
Osteosarcoma	Malignant
Eye	
Retinoblastoma	Malignant
Melanoma	Malignant

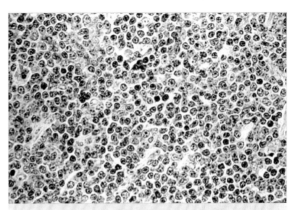

Fig. 3.73 Small lymphocytic lymphoma (SLL) of the orbital ocular adnexae (Giemsa).

Dermoid Cyst

The dermoid cyst predominates among teratoid tumors of the orbit. Histologically, it is identical to intracerebral dysontogenetic dermoid (▶ Fig. 3.71).

Adenoid Cystic Carcinoma

Adenoid cystic carcinoma of the lacrimal gland is the most frequent malignant primary orbital tumor in adults. There is no sex predilection.

Histologically, it resembles the adenoid cystic carcinoma of the salivary glands, characterized by a cribriform pattern of epithelial cells with microcystic spaces filled with mucoid material (▶ Fig. 3.72).

Lymphomas

The orbital ocular adnexae may occasionally be involved as an extranodal site of malignant lymphomas, which behave as in other anatomic locations (▶ Fig. 3.73). The lymphomatous infiltration must be differentiated from the pseudolymphoma which appears as an inflammatory pseudotumor. An inflammatory pseudotumor can also occur in Graves disease, being responsible for exophthalmus in Basedow trias.

Sarcomas

Sarcomas of the orbit are rare. However, the embryonal sarcoma is the most frequent malignant primary orbital tumor in childhood. Further, the orbit is one of the sites of predilection for mesenchymal chondrosarcoma. In some cases of survivors of retinoblastoma who have received radiation to the orbit, a neoplastic sequel in the form of osteosarcoma is observed.

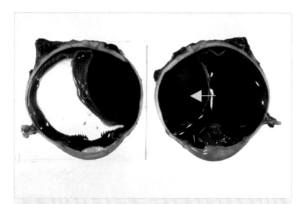

Fig. 3.74 "Black" malignant melanoma (*arrow*) of the pigmented choroid layer of the retina.

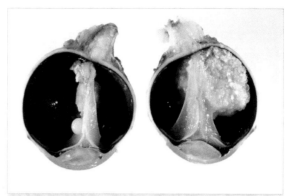

Fig. 3.75 "White" endophytic growth pattern of retinoblastoma.

Metastatic Tumors

About 5 to 10% of orbital tumors are metastatic. In children, in the first 3 years of life, neuroblastoma is the most frequent metastatic tumor.

3.10.2 Tumors of the Eye

For skull base surgeons, primary tumors of the eye bulb warrant special interest when the tumor transcends the sclera and infiltrates the neighboring orbital tissue.

Malignant Melanoma of the Uvea

Malignant melanoma of the uvea is the most frequent malignant primary tumor of the eye bulb (1 tumor per 100,000 population per year). It arises mainly in the retinal/choroid pigmented epithelium, but can also arise in the pigmented epithelium of the iris or ciliary body. It occurs in the sixth to seventh decades; melanomas of the iris are also seen in younger patients. The typical growth pattern is nodular ablating and pushing the retina into

the vitreous humor. Invasion into the orbit is possible. Pigmented and amelanotic forms occur (▶ Fig. 3.74).

Retinoblastoma

Retinoblastoma derives from retinal nerve cells and is the most frequent malignant primary tumor of the eye bulb in childhood (1 tumor per 1 million per year). Typically it is diagnosed between the first and second years of life. Familial cases tend to affect both eyes.

The tumor shows either an exophytic growth diffusely infiltrating the retina and the subretinal space or an endophytic growth toward the vitreous humor (▶ Fig. 3.75). In premature neonates, exophytic retinoblastoma should be differentiated from retrolental fibroplasia (retinopathia praematurorum) caused by oxygen deficit (▶ Fig. 3.76).

3.10.3 Metastatic Tumors

Of course all kinds of metastatic tumors spreading from carcinomas, sarcomas, melanomas, or lymphomas can be encountered in all parts of the central nervous system as

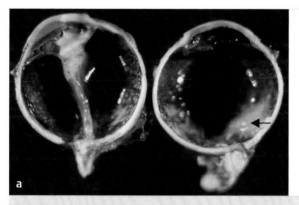
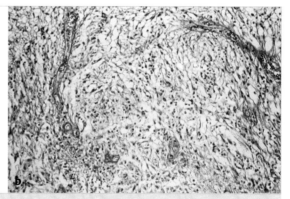

Fig. 3.76 a, b Retrolental fibroplasia. **(a)** Retrolental fibroplasia with "exophytic" retinal fibrosis (*arrow*). **(b)** Nontumorous retrolental fibroplasia (Masson trichrome).

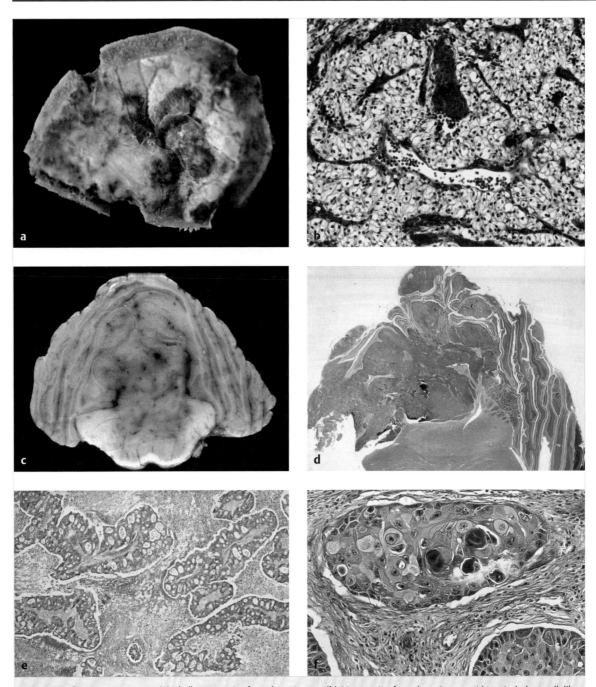

Fig. 3.77 a–f Metastatic tumors. **(a)** Skull metastasis of renal carcinoma. **(b)** Metastasis of renal carcinoma with typical plant-cell–like appearance of tumor cells (Masson trichrome). **(c)** Cerebellum with metastasis of rhabdomyosarcoma. **(d)** Cerebellum with metastasis of rhabdomyosarcoma (H&E). **(e)** Metastasis of a colorectal adenocarcinoma (Masson trichrome). **(f)** Metastasis of a squamous cell carcinoma of the lung with keratinizing nodules (red) (Masson trichrome).

well as in the meninges and the osseous skull base. Mainly circumscribed solid metastases with more or less distinct borders toward the surrounding tissue occur, but diffusely growing tumors may be observed also. Histologically, the metastases may often but not always exhibit a striking resemblance to the primary tumor, thus allowing a specific typing (► Fig. 3.77).

Metastatic tumor cells may also diffusely spread in the arachnoid forming meningeosis carcinomatosa, sarcomatosa, or lymphomatosa(► Fig. 3.41a). A meningeal

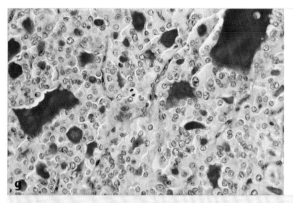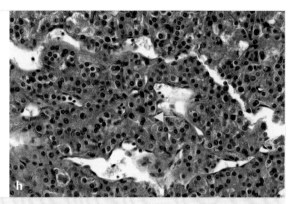

Fig. 3.77 (*Continued*) **g-h** Metastatic tumors. **(g)** Metastasis of a thyroid carcinoma with colloid-secretion (PAS). **(h)** Metastasis of a hepatocellular carcinoma with discrete greenish gall secretion (*arrow*) (H&E).

metastatic spread of malignant melanoma is possible, but the differential diagnosis of a diffuse benign meningeal melanocytosis or a malignant meningeal melanomatosis has to be kept in mind. Rarely, a carcinosis of the dura can be observed.

References

[1] Louis DN, Ohgaki H, Wiestler OD, Cavenee WK, eds. World Health Organization Classification of Tumours of the Central Nervous System. Lyon: IARC Press, 2007

[2] Barnes L, Eveson JW, Reichart P, Sidransky D, eds. World Health Organization Classification of Tumours. Pathology and Genetics of Head and Neck Tumours. Lyon: IARC Press, 2005

[3] Fletcher DM, Unni KK, Meterns F, eds. World Health Organization Classification of Tumours. Pathology and Genetics of Tumours of Soft Tissue and Bone. Lyon: IARC Press, 2002

[4] Sobin LH, Gospodarowicz MK, Wittekind C. TNM Classification of Malignant Tumours. 7th ed. New York: John Wiley & Sons, 2009

[5] Cairncross JG, Ueki K, Zlatescu MC et al. Specific genetic predictors of chemotherapeutic response and survival in patients with anaplastic oligodendrogliomas. J Natl Cancer Inst 1998; 90: 1473–1479

[6] Hegi ME, Diserens AC, Gorlia T et al. MGMT gene silencing and benefit from temozolomide in glioblastoma. N Engl J Med 2005; 352: 997–1003

[7] Kepes JJ, Chen WY, Connors MH, Vogel FS. "Chordoid" meningeal tumors in young individuals with peritumoral lymphoplasmacellular infiltrates causing systemic manifestations of the Castleman syndrome. A report of seven cases. Cancer 1988; 62: 391–406

[8] Stein AA, Schilp AO, Whitfield RD. The histogenesis of hemangioblastoma of the brain. A review of twenty-one cases. J Neurosurg 1960; 17: 751–761

[9] Brat DJ, Giannini C, Scheithauer BW, Burger PC. Primary melanocytic neoplasms of the central nervous systems. Am J Surg Pathol 1999; 23: 745–754

[10] Balmaceda CM, Fetell MR, O'Brien JL, Housepian EH. Nevus of Ota and leptomeningeal melanocytic lesions. Neurology 1993; 43: 381–386

[11] Kudo M, Matsumoto M, Terao H. Malignant nerve sheath tumor of acoustic nerve. Arch Pathol Lab Med 1983; 107: 293–297

[12] Mrak RE, Flanigan S, Collins CL. Malignant acoustic schwannoma. Arch Pathol Lab Med 1994; 118: 557–561

[13] Best PV. Malignant triton tumour in the cerebellopontine angle. Report of a case. Acta Neuropathol 1987; 74: 92–96

[14] Han DH, Kim DG, Chi JG, Park SH, Jung HW, Kim YG. Malignant triton tumor of the acoustic nerve. Case report. J Neurosurg 1992; 76: 874–877

[15] Miller RT, Sarikaya H, Sos A. Melanotic schwannoma of the acoustic nerve. Arch Pathol Lab Med 1986; 110: 153–154

[16] Piedra MP, Scheithauer BW, Driscoll CL, Link MJ. Primary melanocytic tumor of the cerebellopontine angle mimicking a vestibular schwannoma: case report. Neurosurgery 2006; 59: E206; discussion E206

[17] Carrasco CA, Rojas-Salazar D, Chiorino R, Venega JC, Wohllk N. Melanotic nonpsammomatous trigeminal schwannoma as the first manifestation of Carney complex: case report. Neurosurgery 2006; 59: E1334–E1335; discussion E1335

[18] Jaffe ES, Harris NL, Stein H, Vardiman JW. World Health Organization Classification of Tumours. Pathology and Genetics of Tumours of Haematopoietic and Lymphoid Tissues. Lyon: IARC Press, 2001

[19] Barnes L. Schneiderian papillomas and nonsalivary glandular neoplasms of the head and neck. Mod Pathol 2002; 15: 279–297

[20] Maitra A, Baskin LB, Lee EL. Malignancies arising in oncocytic schneiderian papillomas: a report of 2 cases and review of the literature. Arch Pathol Lab Med 2001; 125: 1365–1367

[21] Hyams VJ, Batsakis JG, Michaels L, eds. Tumors of the upper respiratory tract and ear. 2nd series. Washington: Armed Forces Institute of Pathology, 1988

[22] Thompson J, Castillo M, Reddick RL, Smith JK, Shockley W. Nasopharyngeal nonossifying variant of ossifying fibromyxoid tumor: CT and MR findings. AJNR Am J Neuroradiol 1995; 16: 1132–1134

Chapter 4

Imaging Assessment and Endovascular Treatment

4

4 Imaging Assessment and Endovascular Treatment

4.1 Advanced Diagnostic Imaging of Skull Base Tumors

Bernhard Schuknecht, Erich Hofmann

4.1.1 Introduction

Imaging studies are of paramount importance in the diagnostic work-up of skull base tumors. Imaging is performed to obtain information regarding the origin and extent of a lesion and its relationship toward anatomic structures relevant for treatment. Assessment of the individual anatomy is essential prior to surgical treatment.[1]

Imaging does not replace definitive histological, pathological, or microbiological analyses. In a small subset of lesions, however, imaging may provide a tissue-specific appearance; therefore, provide a diagnosis without the need for sampling of the lesion. Limitations of imaging, however, include the recognition of tumor infiltration beyond macroscopic visibility following perineural, fascial, or dural planes, and recognition of micrometastases.

Imaging delineates the location and extension of a lesion, and helps to identify bone involvement, which are invaluable factors to stratify patients for a treatment option and to support the surgical resection. In a considerable number of lesions, high-resolution imaging aids to establish a diagnosis or support the pathologist to substantially narrow the differential diagnosis.

Computed tomography (CT) and magnetic resonance (MR) are the principal imaging techniques when assessing tumors related to the skull base. Positron emission tomography (PET)/CT has gained importance for the staging of neoplasms, distinguishing a recurrence from postoperative changes, and in a small subset of patients detecting the location of a concealed primary malignancy.

CT and MR are occasionally supplemented by digital subtraction angiography (DSA). However, DSA is rarely required for diagnostic purposes. In patients with tumors that display a high degree of vascularization and that have been shown to affect the internal carotid artery by CT or MR, DSA provides a the means to complete a preoperative embolization or to assess the collateral circulation.

Conventional X-rays have been entirely replaced by CT at the skull base. Radiograms (plain films) such as the Water's view offer limited sensitivity for the detection of disease in the maxillary (67.7%), frontal (1.9–54%), and ethmoid sinuses (0–58.9%).[2] These numbers justify abstention from any kind of conventional X-rays in favor of cross-sectional CT or MR assessment.

4.1.2 Goals of Imaging

Goals of imaging include the identification or verification of the presence of a lesion and to distinguish a tumor from other processes such as inflammation or malformation. Imaging findings should provide supportive criteria that enable the categorization of a lesion as a malformation, an infectious or inflammatory process, or a neoplasm (soft tissue or bone tumor, or a potential metastasis). Imaging studies need to be focused on the anatomic region of interest and tailored to specific questions raised before treatment, or after therapy on follow-up examinations.[1,3]

Imaging studies need to scrutinize a lesion with respect to its origin, relationship with relevant anatomic structures, and the presence of infiltration of the osseous skull base, dura, or periorbita.[4] Anatomical relationships with the internal carotid artery and the cavernous sinus are of particular importance. The examination should distinguish the tumor margins from surrounding fluid and mucosal swelling. In conclusion, imaging should be highly accurate establishing the preoperative extent of a lesion and the scope of the required surgery.[5]

In benign lesions, such as inverted papilloma and meningioma, adherence of the tumor to the periosteum or dura and subtle hyperostosis may indicate the actual tumor origin. Recognition and delineation of these structures by imaging, followed by surgical removal, may prevent recurrence.[6] Imaging should also address the degree of vascularization of a lesion. Advanced techniques such as time-resolved MR angiography provide this information noninvasively.

In malignancy, any perineural disease extension needs to be ascertained.[7] Adequate staging requires an accurate identification of the local extent of disease, regional lymph node involvement, and systemic metastases prior to treatment.[8]

Examinations after treatment aim to recognize any early or late complications, assess the presence of residual tumor, and differentiate recurrent tumor from scar or reconstructive soft-tissue flaps. Close collaboration among the neuroradiologist, the otolaryngologist–head and neck surgeon, the radio-oncologist, and the pathologist is mandatory to best accomplish the above-mentioned goals. CT and MR morphologic imaging may be supplemented by advanced imaging techniques. These should be employed using radiation sparing, cost-effective, and tailored techniques, and provide supportive information for the diagnosis and/or treatment. Examples are three-dimensional (3D) CT in the case of craniofacial lesions or CT angiography to delineate the intracranial and cervical vasculature. MR angiography allows a noninvasive assessment demonstrating blood flow within major extracranial and intracranial vessels. Time-resolved MR angiography provides images of the arterial, capillary, and venous phases; thus, allowing the assessment of vascularization with a high temporal resolution (0.7 seconds).

MR diffusion-weighted imaging (DWI), spectroscopy, and perfusion studies provide further information regarding the tissue characteristics of a lesion. Morphologic imaging should be performed in a way that permits data integration into an image-guidance system, to be used for intraoperative navigation or as a planning tool for radiotherapy.[9]

CT and MR imaging (MRI) provide different information. CT excels at evaluating osseous anatomy and cortical bone changes, while MR better depicts soft tissue, including differentiation of tissue composition (i.e., fluid), perineural spread, and bone marrow alteration. Important considerations to order CT or MR include the primary focus of interest on either bone or soft-tissue information. In fact, taking advantage of the complimentary role of CT and MR, both modalities are frequently ordered. Obtaining both CT and MR does not only serve diagnostic purposes but is also increasingly used in a therapeutic regimen. CT–MR image fusion yields composite images that combine features of each component imaging modality.[10]

The information provided by CT and MRI and by particular advanced imaging techniques in different tumors is detailed in the following sections.

4.1.3 Inverted Papilloma

Based on CT and MRI findings, inverted papilloma may be subdivided into tumors that arise within the nasal cavity and those that originate from the maxillary or ethmoid sinus with or without nasal extension.[11] The majority of inverted papilloma confined to the nasal cavity in a series of 55 tumors was centered within the middle meatus and tended to obstruct the osteomeatal complex.[12] Tumors originated less frequently within the maxillary sinus (25.0%), anterior ethmoid (21.1%), sphenoid sinus (6.6%), frontal sinus (6.6%), septum (2.6%), and posterior ethmoid (2.6%). The skull base was affected in 7%.[13]

Unilateral tumor involving the lateral nasal wall, the maxillary or ethmoid sinus with a lobulated surface is typical of inverted papilloma on CT. CT and MR may allow staging of inverted papillomas based on location and extension within the nasal cavity (T1), the superomedial maxillary or ethmoid sinus ± nasal cavity extension (T2), and the remainder of the maxillary sinus, or sphenoid, or frontal sinus ± ethmoid or nasal cavity extension (T3). T4 tumors extend outside the confines of the nose and/or paranasal sinuses.[14]

A "columnar"[15] or "convoluted cerebriform pattern"[16,17] is a valuable imaging feature on MR (▶ Fig. 4.1a). T2-weighted (T2W) images depict alternating hypointense (dark) and hyperintense (bright) striations throughout the tumor. Pathologic–radiologic correlation showed that metaplastic squamous epithelium, loosely fibrous stroma, and intervening gaps between tissue folds create this appearance on MR.[16] A "convoluted cerebriform pattern" provided a sensitivity of 100% in 30 patients with inverted papilloma; however, 17 of 128 malignant sinonasal tumors (13.3%) also harbored this feature, accounting for a specificity of 87%. The positive predictive value, negative predictive value, and accuracy of this sign were 64, 100, and 89%, respectively. A convoluted cerebriform pattern was diffusely present in 26/30 (86.7%) of inverted papillomas, while a focal "convoluted pattern" presentation prevailed in 65% in sinonasal malignancy.

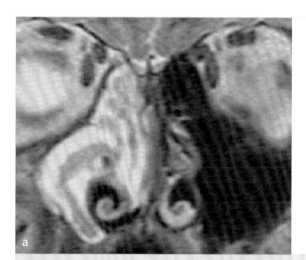
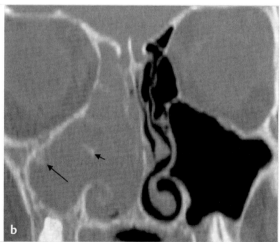

Fig. 4.1 a, b Inverted papilloma of the maxillary sinus. **(a)** Extension into the nasal cavity and anterior ethmoid with typical "convoluted cerebriform pattern" on the T2W coronal MR image. **(b)** High-resolution bone window algorithm CT reveals a focal hyperostosis at the roof of the maxillary sinus indicating the site of tumor origin (*long arrow*). Remaining bone (*short arrow*) of the medial wall, and not calcification, is visible below the enlarged maxillary sinus ostium.

In 29 cases of inverted papilloma, bone involvement was visible on CT as thinning (93%) or as a bowing (79%).[13] Similarly, MR demonstrated bone remodeling in 19 of 23 tumors (82.6%). Bone alterations did not correlate with the size of the inverted papilloma.[15] Focal and intermediate size erosions, were found in MR in 17.4% of patients. Conversely, extensive erosion was present in 92.3% of sinonasal malignancies.

Bone resorption at the cribriform plate, fovea ethmoidalis, and the sphenoid sinus walls commonly simulates aggressive bone destruction rather than bone remodeling. This is a site finding, which may be found in conjunction with inverted papilloma, polyposis, and in a mucocele; thus, it is not a sign of malignancy.[18]

Focal hyperostosis on CT adjacent to the inverted papilloma (▶ Fig. 4.1b) shows a high correlation with the point of origin of sinonasal inverted papilloma[12] and supports the need for subperiosteal removal and bone drilling.[6] CT determination of focal hyperostosis corresponded to the actual tumor origin in 89.1% of 55 cases.[12] On MR, this sign of attachment is commonly not visible (▶ Fig. 4.1a). Focal hyperostosis corresponded to the site of attachment in every instance of inverting papilloma arising in the maxillary, frontal, posterior ethmoid, and sphenoid sinuses. Two patterns of focal hyperostosis were observed: a plaquelike manifestation that involved the lateral wall of the nasal cavity, and a cone-shaped bone thickening (▶ Fig. 4.1b) that was seen only in the walls of the paranasal sinuses or at the bony septum.

Entrapped bone related to the inferior and middle turbinates was more common (34.8%) than true calcifications (▶ Fig. 4.1b). Calcifications were noted in 5 of 29 primary tumors (17%) and in 11% of recurrent tumors. Remarkably, two out of five cases with calcifications were associated with malignancy. Rarely, inverted papillomas may consist of a bony mass surrounded by polypoid soft tissue.[19]

> **Note**
>
> Typical imaging signs that suggest an inverted papilloma include a columnar or convoluted cerebriform pattern on T2 W MRI, and bone erosion, as well as focal hyperostosis at the site of origin on CT.

Inverted papillomas have an association with malignancy and an ability to destroy bone. Focal loss of the "convoluted cerebriform pattern" or columnar pattern may point to malignant transformation: this was the case in four of eight patients reported by Jeon et al.[17] Bone erosion was found on CT in 12 of 29 inverted papillomas (41%), but malignant transformation was found in only four.[13] More reliable signs indicating malignancy are aggressive bone destruction and extrasinonasal tumor extension.

Inverted papillomas have a tendency to recur following excision, despite their benign nature. Recurrence presents as a new growing mass that is localized at least partly within the same region as the primary tumor. Compared with the location of the primary lesion, recurrent tumors more frequently affect the frontal sinuses (61%) and the orbit (43%).[13] Imaging patterns of recurrent inverted papilloma are identical to those of the initial tumors regarding a lobulated surface pattern and internal structure.

In a systematic review of 10 studies focusing on radiologic assessment of inverted nasal papilloma, Karkos et al concluded that preoperative evaluation of inverted papillomas involves the use of both CT and MRI.[20]

CT is the imaging modality of choice to identify focal hyperostosis as the site of origin of inverted papilloma, delineation of the individual anatomy, and identification of bone destruction as a sign of potential malignancy. MR overcomes the limited ability of CT to distinguish tumor from inflammation; therefore, MR allows better delineation of tumor extension. This is particularly important in areas such as the supraorbital recess of the frontal sinus or the lateral recess of the maxillary sinus, which present limited endoscopic access and where mucosal inflammation may further obscure the tumor. MR is more sensitive to detect recurrent tumor.

4.1.4 Osteoma

Osteomas are benign lesions composed of mature bone. On CT, osteomas are frequently encountered incidentally as densely ossified smoothly marginated, well-defined tumors associated with the ethmoid or frontal sinuses. The frontal sinus is most commonly affected (57%).[21] CT precisely localized the osteoma in relation to the frontonasal duct in 37% of patients, followed by locations above and lateral to the ostium of the frontal sinus in 21%. The maxillary sinus was affected in approximately 20% and the sphenoid sinus was rarely involved.

Frontoethmoid osteomas frequently have a size of only a few millimeters. Larger osteomas may cause obstruction of sinus drainage when the ostium is affected or when a major part of the frontal sinus lumen is filled by the tumor.

> **Note**
>
> High-resolution CT with bone algorithm images represents the "gold standard" for radiologic assessment of paranasal sinus osteomas.

CT demonstrates their anatomic location and extension, and the attachment of the tumor pedicle.[22] CT facilitates surgical planning and in anatomically difficult locations may be used for intraoperative image guidance to support endoscopic surgery or other forms of minimally invasive surgery. Furthermore CT best distinguishes the typical appearance of an osteoma from other fibro-osseous tumors such as ossifying fibroma and fibrous dysplasia, and malignant tumors such as chondrosarcomas and osteosarcomas.

MR is advocated in addition to CT when complications such as a mucocele,[23] cerebral abscess,[24,25] tension pneumocephalus,[26,27,28] and cranial nerve or orbital apex compromise[29] are present. CT is best suited to plan the ideal site for a sinusotomy or ethmoidectomy and to assess drainage patency.[22] Osteotomies of fronto-orbital or nasal bone flaps and outer table grafts are best visualized with CT.[30] Postoperative control to assess the site of removal, particularly any remaining bone shell, is based on CT. MR is preferred over CT for follow-up imaging after removal of an intracranial complication such as a mucocele or subepidural abscess or in case of any suspected cerebral intracranial complication.

4.1.5 Fibrous Dysplasia

Fibrous dysplasia affects the skull and facial skeleton in 25% of patients in the monostotic form and in 40 to 60% of cases who harbor the polyostotic variant.[31]

High-resolution bone window algorithm CT images show an expansile lesion with replacement of cancellous bone by poorly organized fibro-osseous tissue. Fibrous dysplasia may display a typical CT appearance known as "ground glass appearance" (▶ Fig. 4.2a). However, an homogeneous sclerotic hazy texture is present on CT in only 25% of lesions, a mixed density pattern prevails in 50%, and a lucent "pseudo"-cystic appearance is seen in 25% of tumors.

> **Note**
>
> CT for fibrous dysplasia typically shows thinning and displacement of cortical bone caused by expansion of the medullary bone space with an abrupt transition to the adjacent normal bone.

Fibrous dysplasia predominantly affects the external bone contour; thus, the bone surface directed toward the intracranial space is less affected. Three-dimensional CT may be beneficial to depict the extent of craniofacial and

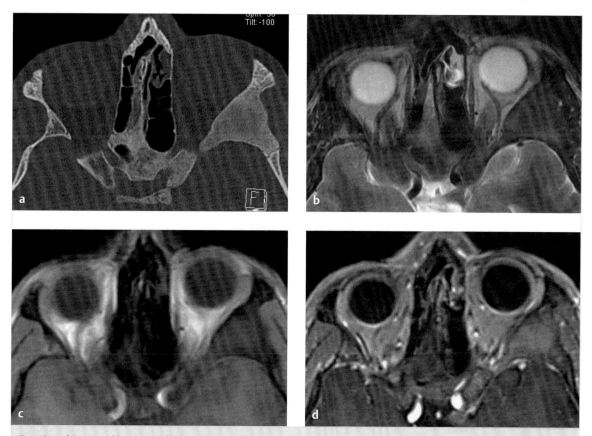

Fig. 4.2 a–d 24-year-old man with fibrous dysplasia of the greater and lesser wing of the sphenoid bone. (a) The CT displays bone expansion with typical "ground glass appearance," thinning of cortical bone, reduction of orbital volume, and slight narrowing of left optic canal. T2 W (b), T1 W noncontrasted (c), and T1 W gadolinium-enhanced fat suppressed images (d) depict left exophthalmos and homogeneous low signal of the fibro-osseous tissue with mild contrast enhancement and signal increase indicating low activity fibrous dysplasia.

orbital distortion. CT displays multiple bone involvement (on average 3.2) by extension of the lesion over adjacent sutures. Only 30% of patients show disease limited to a single bone.[32] In a series of 21 patients diagnosed by CT and MR,[33] the ethmoid bone was most commonly affected (71%), followed by the sphenoid (43%), frontal (33%), maxilla (29%), temporal (24%), parietal (14%), and occipital (5%) bones.

Clinical relevance of fibrous dysplasia lies on the narrowing of neural foramina, fissures and canals (e.g., optic nerve), and cosmetic deformities. Additional factors are a reduction of orbital (▶ Fig. 4.2) and intracranial volume and the possibility albeit low potential (0.5%) for sarcomatous transformation.

MRI is most useful in assessing the impact of the fibro-osseous lesion on adjacent cranial nerves, vessels, orbital contents, and brain parenchyma.[34] On MR, fibrous dysplasia has a low T2 and T1 signal intensity (▶ Fig. 4.2b, c). A correlation of MR and histopathologic findings in five patients showed "inactive" fibrous dysplasia to harbor a low signal on T2W and T1-weighted (T1W) images and slight or missing enhancement on T1W images (▶ Fig. 4.2d). "Active" lesions contain high signal areas on T2W images, spontaneous high signal regions on unenhanced T1W images and enhance strongly after contrast administration.[31] Pathologic examination in another study performed in 13 patients[35] revealed less cellularity, fewer bone trabeculae and collagen fibers, and a variable degree of cystic changes and hemorrhage in areas of T2 signal increase.

Cysts and hemorrhage may point to a potential common pathogenesis of the occasional association of fibrous dysplasia and an aneurysmal bone cyst.[34] The hypothesis for this association relies on initiation of intraosseous hypervascularity by fibrous dysplasia as the primary bone lesion leading to reactive aneurysmal bone cyst formation with characteristic intralesional hemorrhagic cysts.[36] A combination of CT and MR is best suited to detect and localize this association as a sinonasal manifestation of fibrous dysplasia as well.[36]

4.1.6 Ossifying Fibroma

Ossifying fibroma is a rare, benign fibro-osseous lesion of the craniofacial skeleton. Ossifying fibromas of the sinonasal tract present on CT as expansile, multiloculated lesions delineated by a thick bony wall. Occasionally an eggshell-thin rim of bone may be present. The psammomatoid type is more common in the sinonasal tract, while the trabecular variant predominantly affects the mandible and maxilla.

The internal structure consists of an area of low density that may contain septations[37] or striations of calcification. A low attenuation center may show increased density following intravenous contrast administration.[37] CT defines the location which most commonly affects the ethmoid

and sphenoid sinus and the relationship with the orbital walls and skull base.[37]

> **Note**
>
> Ossifying fibromas of the sinonasal tract present on CT as expansile, multiloculated lesions delineated by a thick bony wall.

On MR, fibro-osseous lesions show a low-to-intermediate signal intensity on T1W images and variable signal intensity on T2W sequences.[37,38] The bony margins and central calcification are typically hypointense relative to gray matter on T2W sequences. Nonossified regions, cystic areas, or the rare occurrence of an associated mucocele display increased T2 signal intensity on MR.[39] Fluid levels on T2W images are an exceptional finding in sinonasal ossifying fibromas.[40] Following intravenous administration of contrast agent, the thick outer layer of the lesion and internal septations enhance intensely.[37]

MR best delineates involvement of the dura, periorbita, optic, and other cranial nerves by fibro-osseous lesions. However, it is the CT appearance of a thick outer rim and hypoattenuated, septated or calcified center that provides some specificity to the imaging findings.[37]

4.1.7 Schwannomas

Schwannomas of the sinonasal tract are rare tumors that, as in other areas of the body, arise from Schwann cells of the nerve sheath. An estimated 4% of head and neck schwannomas affect the nasal cavity and paranasal sinuses. The ethmoid, maxillary sinuses, nasal fossa, and sphenoid sinus are involved in decreasing order of frequency.[41] CT findings consist of an expansile lesion causing pressure, erosion, and bone remodeling, which may be attributed to one of the divisions of the trigeminal nerve (▶ Fig. 4.3a). A soft-tissue algorithm CT depicts mild and patchy contrast enhancement with areas of little enhancement indicating cystic components (▶ Fig. 4.3b).

Nasal cavity schwannomas may arise along autonomic nerves along the septum and lateral wall and evoke pressure erosion of the adjacent walls and of the cribriform plate.[42] Reports are conflicting on whether schwannomas located within the olfactory rim or groove may originate from olfactory nerve components.[43,44] Occasionally, erosion and destruction of ethmoid cells and dehiscence of the cribriform plate on CT may simulate an aggressive lesion probably attributable to the fact that sinonasal schwannomas—in contrast to other locations—are not encapsulated.[45] The MR appearance of sinonasal schwannomas resembles schwannomas in other locations. Schwannomas are oval or rounded, well-defined, and tend to remodel adjacent bone (▶ Fig. 4.3a, b). Their signal intensity is hypointense on T1W and heterogeneous

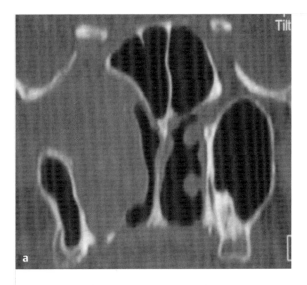
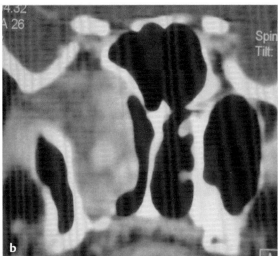
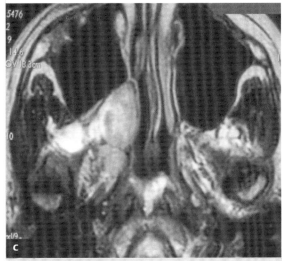

Fig. 4.3 a–c Sinonasal schwannoma along the course of the greater palatine nerve protruding into the posterior nasal cavity. (a) CT depicts bone remodeling of the pterygopalatine fossa and enlargement of the sphenopalatine foramen. (b) Patchy enhancement is visible on soft-tissue CT. (c) Axial MR T2 W image shows a multilobulated tumor with cystic and solid components without any vessels as features to distinguish it from an angiofibroma.

to hyperintense on T2 W images (▶ Fig. 4.3c), with prominent enhancement after gadolinium administration. Heterogeneous contrast uptake and signal on T2 W images of schwannomas is usually associated with cystic changes.

> **Note**
>
> MR signal intensity is not specific for schwannomas and may be duplicated by pleomorphic adenomas, low-grade adenoid cystic carcinomas, or esthesioneuroblastomas.

Schwannomas along the septum may appear as solid mass lesions[42] or as partly cystic, pedunculated tumors.[46]

In a review of the literature, 10 cases[46] were evenly distributed along the anterior and posterior septum.

MRI defines the outlines and internal structure of the tumors better than CT. MR is helpful in differentiating tumor from retained secretions.[45] In two patients with intracranial growth, reported in a series of five patients, orbital extension and preservation of the dura were well delineated. Malignant schwannomas may occur as sporadic lesions but are more commonly associated with neurofibromatosis type 1. Patients with neurofibromatosis type 1 present benign and malignant peripheral nerve sheath tumors but usually do not provide specific imaging features. One must suspect malignant transformation or a neoplasm different from a neurogenic tumor when the lesion attains a very large size, is ill-defined, or depicts infiltration of the brain parenchyma.[47,48]

4.1.8 Angiofibroma

Angiofibroma is a benign lesion composed of angiomatous tissue within a fibrous stroma, lacking a capsule, and displaying locally invasion. Imaging depicts angiofibromas as tumors centered at the sphenopalatine foramen[49] (► Fig. 4.4a) with a variable though predictive pattern of extension into the nasopharynx, the posterior nasal cavity, pterygopalatine, and infratemporal fossae.[50] In addition, they may involve the orbit and intracranial space.

Imaging is invaluable to raise the suspicion of an angiofibroma, or diagnose the lesion, depict its location, and specify extracranial and potential intracranial extension.

CT depicts remodeling and erosion of cortical bone (► Fig. 4.4a) with progressive bone destruction in advanced tumors. Bone erosion and destruction is centered initially along the pterygopalatine fossa. Secondary extension commonly affects the sphenoid sinus (60%), the posterior maxillary (43%), and the ethmoid sinuses (35%). Skull base involvement has been previously estimated to occur in 5 to 20% of tumors; however, recent data suggest that it may be considerably more common (74%).[51]

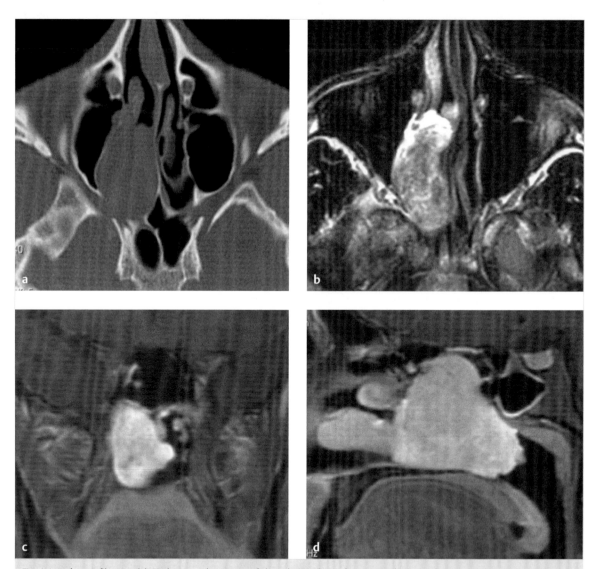

Fig. 4.4 a–d Angiofibroma. (a) CT depicts enlargement of the sphenopalatine foramen and pressure erosion of the osseous contour of the posterior nasal cavity. (b) Axial MR T2 W image indicates dilated vessels shown as punctuate spots ("flow voids") at the lateral tumor margin. (c) Slight erosion is visible at the base of the right pterygoid process on T1 W contrast-enhanced coronal image. (d) T1 W contrast-enhanced sagittal image shows extension toward the skull base within the posterior nasal cavity.

Based on CT, the first staging system was introduced in 1981.[52] The classification reflected the number of anatomic sites occupied by the lesion rather than the actual tumor size. Since then, several modifications have emerged.[53,54,55,56,57] In a recently revised staging system, the route of skull base extension and the vascularization pattern provided the best predictors of residual tumor and recurrence.[51]

In case of skull base infiltration, CT depicts extension along the vidian canal and the foramen rotundum into the base of the pterygoid plates, major wing, and body of sphenoid bone. High-resolution CT is advocated to identify the presence of infiltration of the basisphenoid, which is a predictor of recurrence in 93% of tumors.[58]

A contrasted CT shows dense homogeneous vascularization of the tumor. Marked contrast uptake is a distinguishing feature that differentiates it from other lesions such as antrochoanal polyp, meningoencephalocele, inflammatory polyp, or neoplasm.

On MR, angiofibromas display intermediate-to-high T2 signal and typically harbor punctuate to serpentine signal loss called "flow voids" as a sign of intratumoral vessels (▶ Fig. 4.4b). A homogeneous signal increase occurs following intravenous contrast administration (▶ Fig. 4.4c, d). Contrast-enhanced MR is particularly sensitive to recognize cancellous bone and intracranial infiltration. A prerequisite is a fat-suppressed contrasted technique and comparison with nonenhanced T1 W images centered on the anterior and central skull base. T2 W MR is superior to CT to distinguish tumor tissue from retention secondary to obstructed sinuses. MRI characteristics virtually differentiate any differential diagnosis.

MR angiography displays increased vascularity in the arterial phase when applied as a time-resolved technique. Enlarged maxillary and external carotid artery branches are present on contrasted MR angiography. Markedly improved MRA time resolution has contributed to replace digital subtraction angiography as a diagnostic technique and to consign interventional angiography to being a route for preoperative embolization.

> **Note**
>
> CT depicts bone erosion and destruction that is initially centered around the pterygopalatine fossa. High-resolution CT is advocated to identify infiltration of the basisphenoid, which is a predictor of recurrence. MR delineates extracranial and skull base extension and is complementary to CT. MR angiography displays increased vascularity in the arterial phase. DSA is used only for preoperative embolization.

Advances in imaging have led to improved surgical planning of angiofibromas. MR delineation of extracranial and skull base extension is supplementary to CT, which provides bony landmarks. In addition it may serve for image fusion and intraoperative image guidance. Follow-up imaging after tumor resection, or after adjuvant radiotherapy due to incomplete surgical excision, relies on MR.[59] An initial baseline examination is recommended 3 months after surgery when healing of postoperative changes has taken place. After this time, residual tumor components will become visible. However, areas of contrast enhancement that do not correspond to tumor may persist for up to 6 to 12 months. Possible explanations for subsequently disappearing "lesions" include residual hemorrhage, reaction along tissue flaps used for reconstruction, or prolonged reparative tissue reaction.

Follow-up examinations in higher staged angiofibromas require imaging to be focused on areas known for site-specific higher rates of occurrence. These comprise the basisphenoid, the cavernous sinus, and the infratemporal fossa.

4.1.9 Pituitary Adenoma

Imaging assessment of the sella relies on MR to attribute the origin of a lesion to the pituitary gland as in pituitary adenomas, to a derivative of the craniopharyngeal duct such as Rathke cyst or craniopharyngioma, or to the sphenoid sinus mucosa and bone. Pituitary microadenomas are usually well recognized due to optimal tumor and pituitary gland discrimination by high-resolution MR focused on the sella. Microadenomas, however, may display a signal that is identical to normal pituitary tissue in 20 to 30% of cases.

> **Note**
>
> Dynamic contrasted sequences are particularly useful to recognize microadenomas based on a slower rate of contrast uptake, a lower peak enhancement, and contrast retained within the microadenoma on late contrast-enhanced images.

Pituitary macroadenomas exceed 10 mm in size and commonly demonstrate sella enlargement, lateral extension into the cavernous sinus, or superior enlargement with elevation of the optic chiasm. Inferior infiltration of the basisphenoid occurs in 19% of tumors[60] and may mimic an invasive neoplasm on imaging (▶ Fig. 4.5).

T2 W images depict the relationship of the macroadenoma to the pituitary gland and dura, and the degree of skull base, cavernous sinus, and petrous apex invasion (▶ Fig. 4.5a). Images in the sagittal plane show the extent of clival infiltration and potential submucosal extension into the sphenoid sinus (▶ Fig. 4.5b). T2 W images best distinguish tumor tissue from retained fluid. Typical imaging findings in invasive adenomas consist of multilobulated upper margin, small intratumoral cysts (▶ Fig. 4.5a), or hemorrhage (10%).[61] T1 W contrast-enhanced images, preferentially with fat suppression technique, are additional

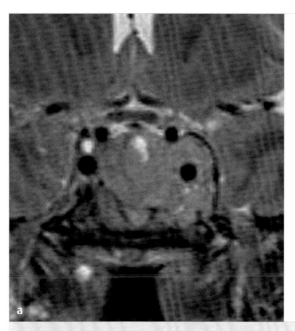 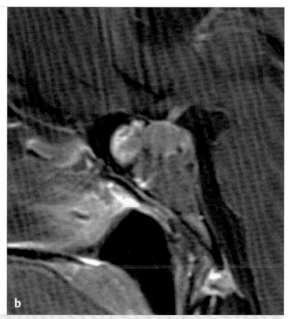

Fig. 4.5 a, b Nonfunctioning macroadenoma with invasion of the left cavernous sinus, sphenoid sinus and clivus shown on coronal T2 W (a) and sagittal contrast-enhanced T1 W (b) MR images. The origin from the left lateral and inferior pituitary gland leads to infiltration of the sphenoid body and well-discernable elevation of the gland on the sagittal image. Notice marked mucosal enhancement covering an anterior part of the tumor that protrudes into the sphenoid sinus.

images required to detect intraosseous or cavernous sinus involvement. In conjunction with T2 W sequences, contrasted T1 W sequences better differentiate intraclival macroadenomas from chordoma, chondrosarcoma, plasmacytoma, metastasis, or sphenoid sinus tumors, and inflammatory pseudotumor of the skull base.

Macroadenomas are fibrous in 12% of cases.[62] Their resultant hard consistency may represent a challenge to endoscopic tumor resectability. In an MRI–pathological correlation in 22 patients harboring a macroadenoma, hard tumor consistency correlated with increased collagen content, elevated apparent diffusion coefficient (ADC) values, and T2 W signal intensity.[63] Therefore, a combination of morphologic T2 W images with diffusion imaging may provide an estimate of the macroadenoma consistency in a noninvasive fashion. Additional preoperative information may be gained from quantitative proton spectroscopy. A study on 16 macroadenomas showed a strong positive linear correlation between concentrations of a choline metabolite on spectroscopy and the MIB-1 proliferative cell index.[64]

CT complements MR, as it depicts bony landmarks, bone remodeling, and sphenoid erosion. Depending on the size and direction of tumor extension, CT delineates the macroadenoma encroaching upon the sphenoid sinus roof, posterior ethmoid, the petrous carotid canal, and apex. For adequate surgical exposure of the sella floor, CT provides the basis for a checklist of normal anatomy: the degree of sphenoid sinus pneumatization (e.g., presellar type), septal insertion on the posterior wall and/or insertion on the carotid prominence and optic nerve canal, and medial extension of the cavernous sinus. Intraoperative neuronavigation may confirm alterations of individual anatomy. Intraoperative imaging reliably assesses the extent of resection. Intraoperative MR or CT may reveal suspicious or definite tumor remnants; thus leading to an extended resection to increase the percentage of tumor removal.

> **Note**
>
> For pituitary adenomas, CT may complement the MR, depicting bony landmarks, bone remodeling, and sphenoid sinus anatomy.

Postoperative follow-up MR assesses the degree of removal and depicts any residual tissue within the cavernous sinus or suprasellar cistern. The first examination is not scheduled before 3 months, unless a complication like a cerebrospinal fluid (CSF) fistula requires urgent imaging. Follow-up after additional radiotherapy also relies on MR as the preferred imaging modality to depict regression of tumor tissue.

4.1.10 Craniopharyngioma

Craniopharyngiomas present as expansile, commonly infrachiasmatic tumors with a tendency to expand into

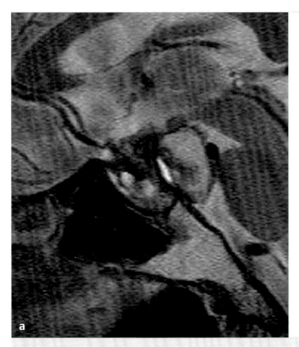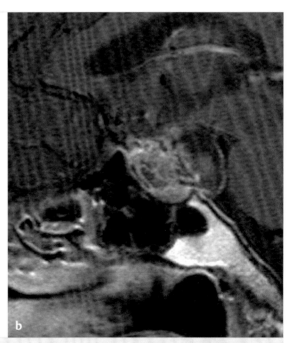

Fig. 4.6 a, b Papillary infrachiasmatic craniopharyngioma with a solid partially calcified component and a retrosellar cystic part in a 26-year-old male. The T2 W sagittal (**a**) and T1 W contrast enhanced (**b**) MR images show dark and heterogeneous enhancement, partially calcified solid tumor in close contact to the chiasm that displays contrast uptake (**b**) indicating—surgically confirmed— adhesions. The cystic part causes displacement of the basilar artery.

the suprasellar cistern. Characteristic CT findings corresponding to the adamantinous histologic type comprise a partially calcified and partially cystic lobulated, predominantly suprasellar lesion in a child or adolescent. The papillary or squamous type commonly affects adults and displays a round, mainly solid appearance, and rarely harbors calcified components.[65] Since calcification and cyst formation are characteristic findings, CT may be more specific than MR in the diagnosis of craniopharyngiomas.[66]

MR distinguishes the adamantinous variant by the presence of T1 hyperintense large cysts, which are likely to contain cholesterol, blood degradation products, or proteinaceous fluid.[65] Conversely, cysts in papillary or squamous craniopharyngiomas are smaller and, commonly, hyperintense (bright) on T2 images only (▶ Fig. 4.6**a**). Contrast enhancement produces strong signal increase within the cyst wall and is typically heterogeneous in the solid areas of the tumor (▶ Fig. 4.6**b**). Notably, most intraventricular craniopharyngiomas harbor a significant solid component.[67] Vessel encasement may be shown noninvasively by MR angiography and is more frequent in the adamantinous type.

MR precisely depicts the intrasellar and suprasellar portions of the craniopharyngioma.[68] Suprasellar extension predominates; however, craniopharyngiomas occa-

sionally display marked extension into the posterior (12%), anterior, or middle cranial fossa. Signal increase of the optic chiasm and tract and adjacent brain parenchyma on T2 W, Flair, and T1 W contrast-enhanced images may represent edema or gliosis related to compression or tumor adhesion (▶ Fig. 4.6**a**, **b**). Despite high-resolution MR techniques, the degree of tumor adhesion to the chiasm cannot be anticipated accurately.

MR helps to elucidate the possible surgical routes of access, according to location and extent. Several classification systems have been proposed based on the relationship of the tumor with the diaphragma sella, the pituitary stalk, the chiasm, and the third ventricle. These structures must be identified relative to the tumor location, growth, and extension. Some authors have suggested that a transcranial approach is more suitable for craniopharyngiomas with suprasellar extension.[69] Conversely, craniopharyngiomas with limited preinfundibular and infrachasmatic extension seem more suited to an endoscopic-assisted approach. Craniopharyngiomas may rarely present as entirely extradural, infrasellar skull base lesions. Less than 12 cases have been reported with this presentation.[70] Contrary to intracranial craniopharyngiomas, an origin within, or extension into, the sphenoid sinus is not reliably identified by MR. In addition, benign conditions such as inflammatory sinus disease may mask tumors in this location.[71]

MR is superior to CT delineating the various components of intra- and suprasellar craniopharyngiomas; however, CT is often required to differentiate calcification and cystic lobulation, to assess the degree of skull base involvement, and to depict paranasal sinus anatomy.

Postoperative follow-up examinations to assess the degree of tumor removal and the location of any residual tumor are based on MR. In a retrospective analysis of postoperative findings in 10 patients, residual tumor was found at the third ventricle, the chiasm and pituitary stalk in decreasing frequency.[72] However, 6 of 10 patients showed progressive reduction in residual contrast enhancement on follow-up examinations, which according to the authors may indicate an initial overestimation of the residual tumor.

4.1.11 Meningioma

Meningiomas may secondarily extend into the nasal cavity from an intracranial lesion or (rarely) occur primarily at an extracranial site within the nasal cavity, paranasal sinuses, or nasopharynx.[73] Imaging delineates meningiomas of the anterior skull base as dural-based tumors, which may originate at a median location within the olfactory groove, the planum sphenoidale, or tuberculum sellae. Each of these locations corresponds to 5% of intra-cranial meningiomas. Medial sphenoid ridge meningiomas arise from the anterior clinoid process and the lesser wing of the sphenoid, and constitute 15 to 20% of intra-cranial meningiomas (▶ Fig. 4.7).

CT depicts meningiomas as extracerebral, well-defined, isodense to hyperdense homogeneous tumors that display marked and commonly homogeneous contrast uptake. Intratumoral calcifications may be present and may indicate the psammomatous histologic subtype. Their dural attachment is characterized by marked hyperostosis and bone sclerosis or by a localized elevation of the planum sphenoidale with "hyperpneumatization" of the sphenoid sinus.[74] These findings are also found on high-resolution MR images (▶ Fig. 4.7). Histologically, the hyperostosis associated with meningiomas corresponds to tumor invasion of the bone at the cranial base.[75]

In 15% of the meningiomas arising from the anterior cranial fossa one may find extracranial extension into the ethmoid sinuses or olfactory rim. High-resolution bone window images, reconstructed in three planes, are required to recognize concomitant ethmoid, sphenoid, or frontal sinus involvement.

CT data fused with MR 3D volume sequences for neuronavigation lends substantial intraoperative support to endoscopic endonasal surgery for skull base meningiomas.

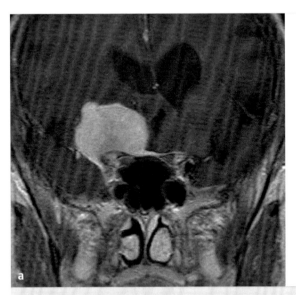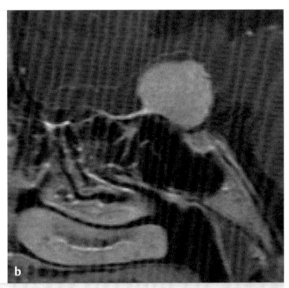

Fig. 4.7 a, b Meningioma of the anterior clinoid process with a "dural tail sign" extending along the planum sphenoidale shown on the coronal T1 W (**a**) and sagittal T1 W gadolinium-enhanced (**b**) MR images. There is focal hyperostosis of the superior surface of the anterior clinoid process and planum sphenoidale and slight contrast enhancement along the optic nerve (**a**). Note marked elevation of the brain parenchyma indicated by the course of the fronto-orbital artery (**b**) and precise anatomic delineation of the sphenoethmoid recess.

On MR, the dural attachment is depicted on postcontrast images with a linear extension as a "dural tail" adjacent to the area of hyperostosis (▶ Fig. 4.7**a**, **b**). Extracranial, orbital, and dural extensions are best demonstrated in T1 W gadolinium-enhanced fat-suppressed images and coronal thin T2 W 3D Space images.

Tuberculum sellae meningiomas are distinguished from pituitary adenomas by their bright homogeneous contrast enhancement, a suprasellar rather than a sellar epicenter, and a tapered extension into the anterior dural base.[76] Imaging delineation of the optic nerve and chiasm is crucial as visual decline and/or field defects are the most common manifestations (▶ Fig. 4.7**a**); thus, a surgical decompression will target these structures.[77] In large meningiomas a 3D contrast-enhanced MR angiography and 3D T1 W volume sequence (MPRAGE) may delineate displacement of the internal carotid artery and/or infiltration of the sphenoparietal and cavernous sinus.

Several histologic subtypes of meningiomas may display different signal intensity on T2 W MR sequences relative to cerebral gray matter depending on cellularity and collagen content. A correct histological subtype categorization was achieved in 80% of tumors and allowed stratification into fibroblastic or transitional meningioma, resulting in a hypointense appearance; and as meningotheliomatous or angioblastic subtypes, owing to hyperintense signal characteristics.[78]

Atypical or malignant meningiomas may exhibit irregular margins and heterogeneous appearance, brain parenchyma invasion with marked edema, and adjacent bone destruction. These neuroimaging features are more common than in typical meningiomas; although they are not unique or reliable. In a comparison of diffusion-weighted imaging and ADC values between 25 atypical/ malignant and 23 benign meningiomas, the mean ADC values of atypical/ malignant meningiomas were significantly lower.[79] Irrespective of the histological type, extensive resection of suspicious bone and dura, as indicated by CT and MRI, is a preventive measure and a crucial step in radical removal of these tumors.[80]

> **Note**
>
> CT depicts meningiomas as extracerebral, well-defined, isodense to hyperdense homogeneous tumors with homogeneous contrast uptake and, possibly, intratumoral calcifications. Dural attachment is characterized by marked hyperostosis and bone sclerosis. On MR, the dural attachment is depicted on postcontrast images as a "dural tail" adjacent to the area of hyperostosis. Extracranial, orbital, and dural extensions are best demonstrated in T1 W gadolinium-enhanced fat-suppressed images and coronal thin T2 W 3D Space images.

Postoperative occurrence of a CSF leak seems more common following the surgical resection of anterior skull base meningiomas. CT and MR examination may be necessary to delineate the osseous anatomy and identify the site of the leak. Heavily T2 W MR sequences may obviate the need for intrathecal contrast. The status and position of a previous nasoseptal flap or alternative method for reconstruction of the optic chiasm, pituitary gland, and the presence of herniated brain should be ascertained prior to surgical exploration.

The cranial base and nasal cavity are sites for potential recurrence of olfactory groove and tuberculum sellae meningiomas. Recurrence is commonly the result of an incomplete resection of hyperostotic bone or regrowth at the edge of a previous surgical field. Long-term surveillance using MR is necessary, following surgery or radiotherapy, to assess stability, regression, or regrowth (especially in partially resected lesions)

4.1.12 Esthesioneuroblastoma

Esthesioneuroblastomas are linked with the basal progenitor cells of the olfactory epithelium and therefore occur along the distribution of olfactory epithelium with a variable location, size, and imaging appearance. CT and MR provide evidence of an esthesioneuroblastoma when a unilateral pedunculated lesion is present within the superior nasal cavity or olfactory rim. Large esthesioneuroblastomas (▶ Fig. 4.8) may adopt a dumbbell shape centered at the cribriform plate, commonly cross midline, and they may show considerable intracranial extension.

CT, MRI, and PET/CT scanning play complementary roles in the detection and staging of esthesioneuroblastomas. CT findings consist of a soft-tissue tumor within the olfactory rim, at the cribriform plate or within the anterior cranial fossa. One percent of tumors may primarily involve the sphenoid sinus.[81] Osseous changes typically associated with esthesioneuroblastomas consist of expansion and bowing of bone, and focal osteolysis.[82] Bone destruction affects the cribriform and the perpendicular plate of the ethmoid bone by the midline (▶ Fig. 4.8**b**); and, with increasing tumor size, it eventually affects the lateral wall of the nasal cavity, the paranasal sinuses, and orbit.[83,84] On CT, esthesioneuroblastomas may exceptionally present with exuberant bony hyperostosis[85] or mimic fibrous dysplasia at the site of bone invasion.[86]

Intratumoral calcification is common in larger esthesioneuroblastomas (▶ Fig. 4.9**b**) and needs to be distinguished from remnants of bone erosion. Calcification may be diffusely distributed or affect the central tumor portion and is considered a relatively specific diagnostic feature.[83]

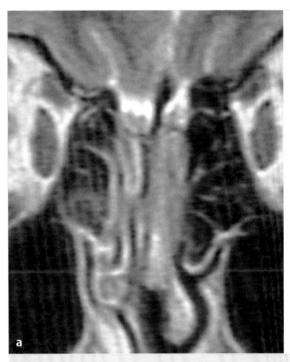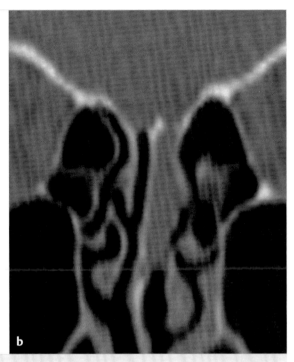

Fig. 4.8 a, b Small esthesioneuroblastoma. **(a)** Tumor within left olfactory rim in continuity with the olfactory bulb with linear vertical oriented (dark) blood vessel on T2 W image. **(b)** Coronal CT depicts mild expansion of the left olfactory cleft and erosion of the cribriform plate.

Note

Esthesioneuroblastomas show marked homogeneous contrast uptake unless areas of necrosis or calcification are present. The pattern of contrast enhancement does not differ from squamous cell carcinoma, sinonasal undifferentiated carcinoma, melanoma, or metastatic disease involving the same location.

MRI is helpful in defining tumor margins and possible intracranial extension (▶ Fig. 4.8a). MR demonstrated infiltration of the ethmoid cells in all of 15 patients.[87] MR signal characteristics and pattern of contrast enhancement are nonspecific. Esthesioneuroblastomas exhibit mild-to-marked contrast enhancement. A virtually pathognomonic sign is the presence of multiple cysts at the tumor–brain interface in the intracranial portion (▶ Fig. 4.9a).[88] On T2 W images, the presence of serpentine vertically oriented flow voids is a characteristic finding, which reflects the hypervascular nature of esthesioneuroblastomas.[89] Intratumoral hemorrhage may occur and was found by MR in 2 out of 11 tumors.[90]

Intracranial extension has been categorized based on MR as cranionasal and cranio-orbital-nasal, and extracranial extension as naso-orbital.[90] The extracranial portion typically shows a combined expansile and destructive growth pattern.

MR is important for tumor staging, as it delineates the extent of involvement of the intracranial space, the sinuses, and orbit to better advantage than does CT. MR aids in differentiating tumor from concurrent obstructive sinus infection. Initial staging requires CT as well to assess the degree of bone involvement, to depict the individual anatomy, and to obtain a dataset for potential intraoperative navigation.[1]

Based on imaging, esthesioneuroblastomas are precisely staged by the Kadish classification or alternative classifications such as the modified TNM (tumor size, node involvement, and metastasis status) staging introduced by Dulgerov and Calcaterra. The principal purpose is better prognostic differentiation to derive at therapeutic recommendations. Imaging findings such as infiltration of the dura, periorbita, brain parenchyma, and orbit determine the degree of resectability and represent relevant predictors of recurrence.

As esthesioneuroblastomas can metastasize via lymphatic and hematogenous routes, imaging should cover the neck to assess the presence of cervical lymph node metastases. This will be present in 5 to 20% of patients. Furthermore 10 to 30% of patients will develop distant metastases. Staging is increasingly performed by PET/CT that may reveal otherwise occult lymph node and systemic metastasis.[91]

Routine surveillance with regular follow-up imaging is recommended for several years. CT and MRI appearance

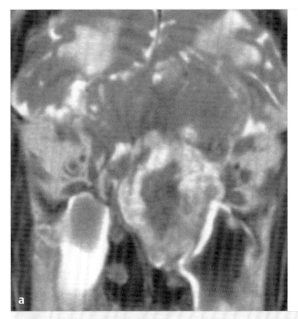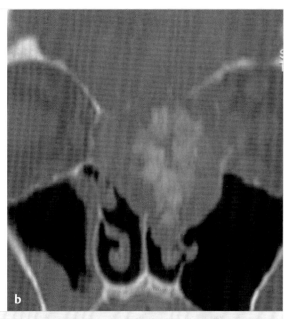

Fig. 4.9 a, b Large esthesioneuroblastoma extending into the anterior cranial fossa causing brain edema as shown. (a) Coronal T2 W image. Few marginal bright cysts delineate the superior contour of the tumor from the adjacent brain parenchyma. (b) Coronal CT depicts destruction of the anterior skull base and of the left lamina papyracea by a tumor that harbors marked calcification within the nasal portion.

of recurrent esthesioneuroblastoma does not differ from tumors imaged at initial presentation.[92] Recurrence commonly presents as tumor nodules at resection margins, but may rarely involve diffuse subdural spread.[93]

> **Note**
>
> As esthesioneuroblastomas can metastasize via lymphatic and hematogenous routes, imaging should evaluate the neck better. Alternatively a PET/CT should be performed preoperatively.

Follow-up imaging also needs to include the cervical nodes. Attention has been drawn to lymph node metastasis in uncommon locations such as retropharyngeal nodes. In a retrospective analysis of 17 patients, retropharyngeal lymph node metastasis was present but overlooked at initial presentation in one patient and on follow-up occurred in an additional three patients.[94]

4.1.13 Chordoma

Imaging depicts chordomas as destructive median or paramedian skull base lesions that arise from remnants of the primitive notochord. Radiologic evaluation of chordoma infiltration of the skull base and assessment of the tumor relationships with the brainstem, sella, chiasm, cavernous sinuses, and internal carotid arteries require

both CT and MRI.[95] Depending on the location relative to the spheno-occipital synchondrosis, chordomas are classified as centroclival, superoclival and inferoclival, and paraclival tumors.

> **Note**
>
> CT and MRI are essential to ascertain the presence and location of clival chordomas.

Characteristic CT findings consist of a commonly median or paramedian located, circumscribed, expansile soft-tissue mass, associated with lytic bone destruction. Sclerosis at the margin of bone infiltration is missing.[96] Soft-tissue components include cystic nonenhancing areas and other moderate-to-marked contrast enhancing parts of the tumor. Nonenhancing tumor corresponds to myxoid and gelatinous material. Intratumoral hyperdense foci are invariably present on CT, and represent fragments of destroyed bone and, to a lesser degree, calcified tumor matrix.[95,97] High-resolution CT with bone window algorithm, (reconstructed in sagittal, coronal, and axial planes) provides exquisite anatomic detail regarding the center of the tumor with respect to the spheno-occipital and petro-occipital synchondroses in median and paramedian chordomas, respectively. CT better delineates the involvement of the osseous confines of the sella, sphenoid sinus, internal carotid canals, jugular foramina, and petrous apices.[95]

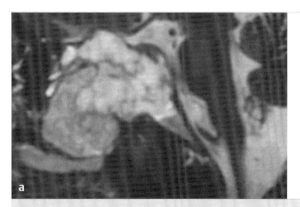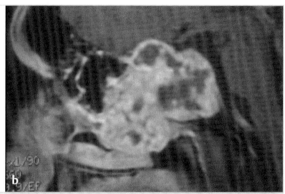

Fig. 4.10 a, b Chordoma arising superior to the spheno-occipital synchrondrosis, so-called "superoclival chordoma" with extension into the planum sphenoidale, and into the sphenoid and posterior ethmoid sinus and nasal cavity. The multilobulated cystic appearance with bright signal on the sagittal T2 W image (**a**) and partial "honeycomb" pattern of contrast enhancement on T1 W gadolinium-enhanced images (**b**) are typical features, though indistinguishable from a chondrosarcoma.

CT may aid in distinguishing classic chordomas from chondrosarcomas and the chondroid variant of chordomas. Matrix calcification may be more prominent in chondrosarcomas, which may also exhibit a variable stippled and amorphous appearance.[96,98]

> ### Note
>
> MR is superior to CT in defining the location and extent of the tumor relative to the brainstem, pituitary gland, optic chiasm, the cavernous sinuses, and nasopharynx, and delineation of displacement, and/or infiltration of the dura and prevertebral fascia.

T2 W images show a multiseptate, hyperintense lesion, which is sharply marginated and commonly displays a pseudoencapsulated appearance with a low-intensity rim. High signal is caused by watery gelatinous tumor matrix. Intratumoral T2 hypointense (dark) areas correspond to calcification, highly proteinaceous material, and rarely hemorrhage (▶ Fig. 4.10a). Low-to-intermediate tumor signal on T1 W images is easily recognized within the high signal intensity fat of the clivus on noncontrast sequences. Therefore, fat suppression is preferred to assess intraosseous, prevertebral, or orbital soft-tissue invasion. Following contrast material injection, chordomas exhibit moderate-to-marked signal increase.[99] A honeycomblike pattern of signal increase (▶ Fig. 4.10b) within a part or the entire tumor is a typical finding.[89] Contrast enhancement is occasionally minor or absent when large amounts of mucinous material, necrosis, or intratumoral hemorrhage prevail.[95]

The signal intensity of the chondroid variant of chordomas is reported to be lower on T2 W images due the predominant cartilaginous matrix, which causes T1 and T2 shortening.[100] Chondroid chordomas resemble chondrosarcomas in signal intensity. Chondroid chordomas and chondrosarcomas are more commonly found in a paramedian location along the petro-occipital synchrondrosis.[95] When present on CT or MR, linear, arclike, or globular calcifications in chondrosarcomas are a distinguishing feature lacking in intracranial chordomas.[97] However, in a comparison between 16 chordomas and 9 chondrosarcomas, Oot et al found no differentiating features on MRI.[99]

Rarely chordomas may display an entirely intradural location. The prepontine cistern is most frequently involved followed by the cerebellopontine angle and suprasellar cistern.[101]

Preoperative assessment of chordomas requires noninvasive angiography, as displacement and encasement of major vessels is common, occurring in up to 79% of chordomas with intracranial extension.[102] MR angiography shows displacement and encasement of the basilar and/or carotid arteries; therefore, it obviates the need for cerebral angiography for diagnostic purposes.

A combination of CT and MRI is best for posttreatment follow-up. An initial baseline examination may provide only an estimate of the degree of tumor removal and the location of any residual intraosseous or soft-tissue component. However, as postoperative changes within the commonly extensive areas of resection resolve, follow-up examinations will allow more precise determination of remaining tumor. Detailed knowledge on the kind of surgical approach—open microscopic, endoscope assisted, or fully endoscopic endonasal—and of the surgical report avoids mistaking postoperative changes at the site of resection and at the closure site. Follow-up imaging should conform to the techniques used for the preoperative imaging. Ideally high-resolution imaging with thin slices (0.4 to 0.9 mm) by 3D T2 W and T1 Gd enhanced sequences is performed to lend support to any potential additional treatment planning such as stereotactic radiotherapy, or intensity-modulated or proton beam radiotherapy.

Follow-up imaging has to take into consideration that tumor recurrence or dissemination may affect unusual sites. Therefore a high degree of clinical and imaging "suspicion" are required in order not to miss the rare incidence of intradural seeding[103] or lymph node metastasis derived from skull base chordomas.[95]

4.1.14 Sinonasal Malignant Tumors

Imaging of sinonasal malignancy is challenging due to the common advanced stages, and the proximity of the neoplasms toward the skull base, cranial nerves, and neural foramina. There is frequently a marked overlap of the imaging findings of different tumors on CT and MR, and this precludes a specific histological diagnosis.[7] Therefore, the contribution of the radiologist is to attribute a lesion to the category of a probable malignant tumor, to describe its location and extent, and to recognize involvement of anatomic structures that determine the treatment plan, the surgical approach, and/or the prognosis.

Imaging initially relies on CT to assess the extent of osseous destruction on bone algorithm images and to map the patient's individual anatomy. CT is more sensitive and accurate in delineating erosion of thin cortical bone like the cribriform plate, the ethmoid sinuses, and the lamina papyracea. A contrasted CT with soft-tissue window evaluates tumor spread beyond the paranasal sinuses and nasal cavity. MR is superior to CT to distinguish tumor from retained secretions and to show direct extension into soft tissue and cancellous bone, and infiltration of the dura and vessel walls.[4,104] The signal on T2W images is lower in malignancy than in benign lesions. A total of 69.1% of malignancies presented with a signal isointense to brain compared with 28.5% of benign tumors.[105] The distinction between sinonasal tumors and inflammatory tissues is best accomplished with T2W sequences. Ninety-five percent of sinonasal tumors have an intermediate T2 signal, while only 5% have bright T2 signal.[106] On gadolinium-enhanced MR images, tumors usually enhance less than mucosa and mostly show a solid enhancement pattern.[107]

> **Note**
>
> CT and MRI are mandatory to substantiate the suspicion of a malignancy. CT bone algorithm images show the extent of osseous destruction. MR is superior to CT to distinguish tumor from retained secretions and to delineate direct extension into soft tissue and infiltration of the dura and vessel walls.

4.1.15 Squamous Cell Carcinoma

CT findings suggestive of squamous cell carcinoma include a tumor origin within a paranasal sinus (70%),

most commonly in the maxillary sinus or the nasal cavity (30%). Origin in the ethmoid (10%), or frontal or sphenoid sinuses (2%) is rare.[104] Aggressive destruction or absence of adjacent bone is a conspicuous finding, which is present in 80% of patients (▶ Fig. 4.11a–c).[107] This finding may be subtler when the tumor is located within the ethmoid or frontosphenoid sinuses. On CT, contrast enhancement is more difficult to distinguish from adjacent inflammation than by MR.

Squamous cell carcinomas (SCCs) of the maxillary sinus tend to attain a large size before diagnosis; thus, patients may additionally harbor metastatic lymph nodes at presentation.[108] Therefore, CT imaging must assess the cervical lymph nodes as well (at least in T3 and T4 tumors).

> **Note**
>
> Since SCCs of the paranasal sinuses may show metastatic spread (most frequently lymph node infiltration) preoperative staging must include imaging of the neck and chest.

MR supplements CT when the tumor has reached the skull base, the periorbita, or dura, and when retroantral fat and the pterygopalatine fossa are infiltrated. Due to high cellularity and a prominent nuclear-to-cytoplasmic ratio, neoplasms exhibit low signal on T2W images (▶ Fig. 4.11a). T2W MR images aid to differentiate tumor from obstructed sinus secretions, which commonly show a high signal.

Direct extension to the dura, periorbita, and pterygopalatine fossa is better displayed by MR.[104] Contrast enhancement is mild to moderate, diffusely homogeneous and does not include areas of necrosis. When the tumor abuts the skull base, linear enhancement of the dura does not necessarily imply infiltration. Eisen et al reported a specificity of 100% and greater sensitivity when there is adjacent pial enhancement (50%), thickness of dural enhancement greater than 5 mm, (75%) and the presence of focal dural nodules (88%) (▶ Fig. 4.11b).

To recognize the extent of soft-tissue invasion, bone marrow infiltration, and perineural spread, one must compare precontrast and fat-suppressed contrasted sequences (▶ Fig. 4.11b).[4] Reliable identification of subtle tumor extension requires a focused high-resolution study.[109]

4.1.16 Adenocarcinomas

Adenocarcinomas may present on CT as well as poorly defined soft-tissue density masses associated with bone remodeling and destruction. A greater number of adenocarcinomas (63%) occupy the upper part of the nasal cavity and the ethmoid cells.[106] Among neoplasms of the ethmoid, adenocarcinoma is the most frequent histology

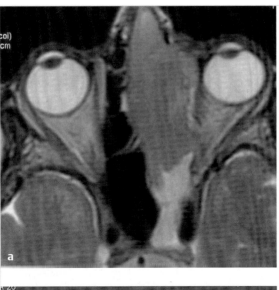
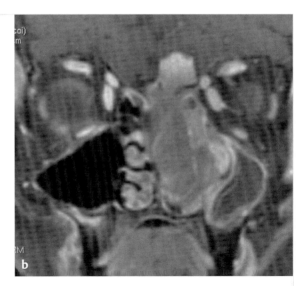
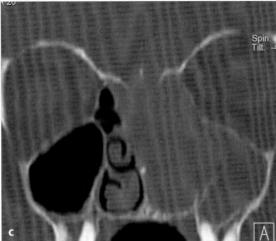

Fig. 4.11 a–c Squamous cell carcinoma of the left nasal cavity with low signal on the axial T2 W MR image indicating a highly cellular tumor. Infiltration is visible causing obstruction of left sphenoid sinus (**a**). The tumor abuts the lamina papyracea and invades the anterior cranial fossa by a nodular component shown on the coronal T1 W contrast-enhanced image performed with fat suppression (**b**). There is only mild contrast enhancement except for the intradural tumor portion and the remainder of the middle turbinate. Note tumor extension along the dura above the orbital roof on the left (**b**) and osteolysis of the septum, cribriform plate, and inferior turbinate shown by high-resolution CT (**c**). A false "benign pattern" is bowing of the lateral wall of the nasal cavity with retained secretions in the left maxillary sinus.

(49.7%) followed by SCC (10.4%) and adenoid cystic carcinoma (7.6%).[110] Low-grade adenocarcinomas have a propensity to arise from the septum (▶ Fig. 4.12), while high-grade adenocarcinomas tend to present with a wide range of sinus involvement.[111]

MR is the most sensitive imaging modality to determine their primary location and to distinguish an exophytic growth pattern (▶ Fig. 4.12a, b) from a solid, infiltrative growth associated with areas of necrosis. MR may show the lesion extending extracranially from the ethmoid sinuses into the olfactory rim (▶ Fig. 4.12a, b) or intracranially into the frontal lobes, where it may occasionally cause bifrontal hemorrhages.[112]

CT may show continuous tumor extension from a nasoethmoidal, or rarely a frontal or sphenoid sinus, origin with bowing or focal destruction of the septum (▶ Fig. 4.12c), cribriform plate, adjacent sinuses, and orbital walls. Inferring the degree of differentiation based on bone window CT is usually not possible unless marked osteolysis of the skull base is present.

In a retrospective review of MR findings[105] 87.5% of adenocarcinomas displayed a signal on T1 W sequences that was hypointense relative to brain; this was significantly higher than SCCs (21.4%). According to the histologic type and degree of differentiation of the nonintestinal adenocarcinomas, the T2 signal was isointense and

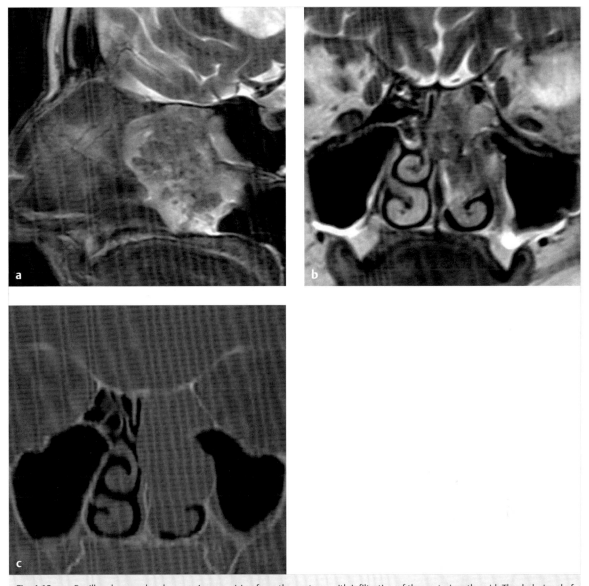

Fig. 4.12 a–c Papillary low-grade adenocarcinoma arising from the septum, with infiltration of the posterior ethmoid. The dark signal of the papillary structure of the tumor is well visualized on T2 W sagittal (**a**) and coronal (**b**) sequences that depict extension toward the cribriform plate and ethmoid roof. Mucosal swelling is shown along the inferior border (**a**) and fluid retention within left posterior ethmoid (**b**). Focal erosion of the septum is indicated on the coronal T2 W image and confirmed by CT, which depicts otherwise intact osseous structures (**c**). Note the visibility of normal septal vessels (**a**) on high-resolution 3 Tesla MR.

more heterogeneous in the majority of tumors (55%); followed in frequency by a hyperintense (33%) or hypointense (11%) appearance.[105] However, distinction between different histologic types is not reliably feasible by MRI. Rather than signal characteristics, the location within the ethmoid and upper nasal cavity, with infiltration of the anterior skull base, should raise the suspicion of an adenocarcinoma.

> **Note**
>
> Among neoplasms of the paranasal sinuses, adenocarcinoma is the most frequent histology followed by SCC. Distinction between different histologic types is not feasible by imaging alone.

4.1.17 Adenoid Cystic Carcinoma

Adenoid cystic carcinomas may present on CT as a soft-tissue lesion that commonly arises from the hard palate, the nasal cavity, or the maxillary sinus. Origin in the ethmoid, frontal, and sphenoid sinuses, or nasopharynx is less common.[113,114] A frequent feature in adenoid cystic carcinomas is a propensity for perineural extension even with early stage tumors. Perineural extension is also associated with squamous cell and basal cell carcinoma, lymphoma, and melanoma; however, CT findings of perineural extension in conjunction with a small strongly enhancing tumor should raise suspicion for an adenoid cystic carcinoma. CT with bone window algorithm shows enlargement and erosion of nerve canals and foramina, obliteration of fat planes along cranial nerves, and soft-tissue expansion of the cavernous sinus and Meckel cave.[115]

MR is the imaging modality of choice to depict the primary location and the pathways of spread of adenoid cystic carcinoma.[116] MR findings, however, are not specific in differentiating adenoid cystic carcinoma from other neoplasms. A T2 hypointense appearance has been reported in one-third of adenoid cystic carcinomas. However, the majority of adenoid cystic carcinomas have been found to present with a T2 hyperintense appearance.[105] Low T2 signal correlated with highly cellular tumors (solid subtype), which carry a poorer prognosis, while high T2 signal tumors corresponded to less cellular subtype of adenoid cystic carcinoma (cribriform or tubular subtype) associated with a better prognosis.[117]

Contrary to the indirect signs of perineural spread shown by CT, MR enables direct recognition of tumor extension along cranial nerves, dura, and fascia planes. Typical findings consist of nerve enlargement and contrast enhancement, perineural fat and bone marrow infiltration, and invasion of dura, cavernous sinus, and gasserian ganglion.[115,118] MR is also more sensitive to recognize denervation of the muscles of mastication as an indicator of mandibular nerve infiltration.[116] By delineation of the macroscopic borders of the tumor extension, MR may alter the treatment regimen and provide an indication for additional radiotherapy.

Note

Adenoid cystic carcinomas arise most commonly from the hard palate, the nasal cavity, or the maxillary sinus. Perineural spread leads to nerve enlargement and contrast enhancement, perineural fat and bone marrow infiltration, and invasion of dura, cavernous sinus, and gasserian ganglion, all of which are better delineated by MRI.

Follow-up MR examinations are required at close intervals in patients with adenoid cystic carcinoma as they have a significant risk of local recurrence.[114] In advanced stage disease or after treatment of tumor recurrences, imaging needs to assess the cervical lymph nodes and lungs to recognize potential lymph node infiltration and distant metastases.

4.1.18 Sinonasal Undifferentiated Carcinoma

Sinonasal undifferentiated carcinomas are uncommon, highly aggressive neoplasms arising within the ethmoid sinuses and superior nasal cavity. On imaging, sinonasal undifferentiated carcinomas are difficult to distinguish from other poorly differentiated sinonasal carcinomas and nonepithelial neoplasms. CT findings in 11 patients comprised a large tumor size exceeding 4 cm in eight patients. High aggressiveness was apparent by the bone destruction and invasion of the paranasal sinuses in 10 patients and by extension into the anterior cranial fossa and orbit in seven and four patients, respectively.[119] Contrast enhancement on soft-tissue CT was variable.

MR images of sinonasal undifferentiated carcinoma show an isointense to hyperintense appearance on T2 W images and heterogeneous contrast enhancement. Examination of 20 patients revealed that 50% presented with dural invasion, 30% had invasion of the cavernous sinus, and the orbit was involved in another 30%.[120] Coronal T1 W contrast-enhanced MR images reveal frequent invasion into the orbits and adjacent sinuses.[121] The commonly advanced local disease in these patients requires both CT and MRI.[122] In addition, MRI of the neck is recommended due to the propensity for nodal metastasis at presentation.[122]

Other poorly differentiated carcinomas of the sinonasal cavity include SCCs, sinonasal neuroendocrine carcinomas, and rhabdomyosarcomas. Imaging cannot differentiate between these highly aggressive neoplasms.[118]

Follow-up imaging after aggressive multimodality treatment of sinonasal undifferentiated carcinomas relies on MR to exclude surgical complications and to monitor treatment response.[122] Close imaging surveillance is particularly relevant because patients are prone to locoregional recurrence or may develop distant metastasis[123] including the rare occurrence of intradural drop metastasis.[124]

4.1.19 Neuroendocrine Carcinoma

Neuroendocrine carcinoma encompasses a spectrum of neoplasms that are classified into three subtypes:
- Typical carcinoid tumor (well-differentiated neuroendocrine carcinoma).
- Atypical carcinoid tumor (moderately differentiated neuroendocrine carcinoma).
- Small cell carcinoma (poorly differentiated neuroendocrine carcinoma).[107]

In a 20-year review encompassing 72 patients, a common location was shared by sinonasal neuroendocrine carcinomas, sinonasal undifferentiated carcinomas, small cell carcinomas, and esthesioneuroblastomas.[125]

Sinonasal endocrine carcinoma is an uncommon neoplasm with imaging manifestations that consisted of extensive nasal cavity and paranasal sinus involvement in 10 patients and extension beyond the nasal cavity with concomitant orbital and intracranial infiltration in another 11 patients.[126]

CT and MR depict an expansile lesion with erosion of the nasal septum and adjacent skull base[107] and common involvement of the sphenoid sinus.[127] Kanamalla et al reported three patients with sinonasal neuroendocrine carcinoma.[128] Imaging findings in two patients showed a mass that involved the sphenoid sinus in one patient and maxillary sinus in the other. Bone erosion and expansion were common features in both cases on CT. Minimal heterogeneous contrast enhancement was shown in the only tumor examined by MR. The third patient presented with a metastasis within the superficial lobe of the parotid gland.

Neuroendocrine carcinomas appear to have no distinctive CT or MRI findings[126,128]; however, a median tumor with involvement of the sphenoethmoid area causing expansion and destruction of the skull base could indicate the rare basaloid type of squamous cell carcinoma or a histology different from SCC.

> **Note**
>
> There are no specific imaging criteria for sinonasal neuroendocrine carcinomas. These malignancies are prone to metastatic spread and have high rates of locoregional failure and distant metastases. Preoperative staging must include CT imaging of the neck and the chest or PET/CT.

Patients with sinonasal neuroendocrine carcinoma and undifferentiated carcinoma have high rates of locoregional failure and distant metastases despite aggressive surgery and despite the frequent use of chemoradiation therapy.[125] MR surveillance needs to cover the skull base and neck and should also include the brain, as neuroendocrine carcinomas develop intracranial metastases even as an isolated distal site.[125] PET/CT is gaining increasing importance as an initial tool for staging and follow-up surveillance.

4.1.20 Sinonasal Malignant Melanoma

Sinonasal malignant melanoma on CT presents as a lobulated or polypoid lesion with a predilection for the lower nasal cavity (▶ Fig. 4.13). The lateral nasal wall, septum, middle and inferior turbinates, and vestibule are the primary sites of origin in decreasing frequency.[7] Melanomas located within the paranasal sinuses affect the maxillary sinus more commonly than the ethmoid and frontal sinuses. Primary melanoma of the sphenoid sinus is extremely rare and only few cases have been reported.[129]

Precise attribution of the lesions to a specific anatomic location within the nasal cavity and paranasal sinuses contributes to stratify surgical approaches and to derive prognostic factors. Melanomas derived from the septum and nasal cavity appear to have a better prognosis. Conversely, maxillary and ethmoid sinus locations were found to be adverse factors for disease-free survival.[130]

Diffuse tumor enhancement is shown on contrast-enhanced soft-tissue algorithm CT images. Unless endoscopy raises the suspicion of a melanoma or bone window high-resolution CT images depict bone remodeling or erosion, the imaging appearance is nonspecific and may resemble a polyp or mucosal swelling or other neoplasms. CT is important for delineation of involvement of the skull base, the orbit, or the walls of the nasal cavity and paranasal sinuses. Furthermore, knowledge of the integrity of the nasal vault and hard palate and of the individual anatomy is of paramount importance prior to endoscopic tumor removal.

> **Note**
>
> Malignant melanoma is nonspecific and may resemble a polyp or mucosal swelling or other neoplasms; thus, endoscopy is more specific. It has a predilection for the lower nasal cavity.

On MR, malignant melanomas of the nasal cavity and paranasal sinuses may show a characteristic signal, which is mainly attributable to the degree and distribution of melanin pigmentation and partly attributable to hemorrhage.[131] Melanotic melanomas may present with hyperintense (bright) signal on noncontrast T1W images due to paramagnetic effects exerted by melanin and/or hemorrhage (▶ Fig. 4.13a). Amelanotic melanomas present in 30 to 40% of tumors and have intermediate signal intensity.

According to their CT appearance, melanomas seem more commonly expansile than infiltrating.[131] However, the outlines of tumor invasion need to be scrutinized (▶ Fig. 4.13b) to provide an estimate of tumor extension into the floor of the nasal cavity, cartilage and into the skull base and orbit. MR is particularly supportive in amelanotic melanomas, where resection margins are more difficult to be determined endoscopically than in melanotic tumors.

T2 signal is heterogeneous with a tendency of melanotic melanomas to show a low signal (▶ Fig. 4.13c) and of amelanotic tumors to have high-signal intensity.[132] Additional features are lines of low signal on T2W images or enhancing linear structures (▶ Fig. 4.13c) that

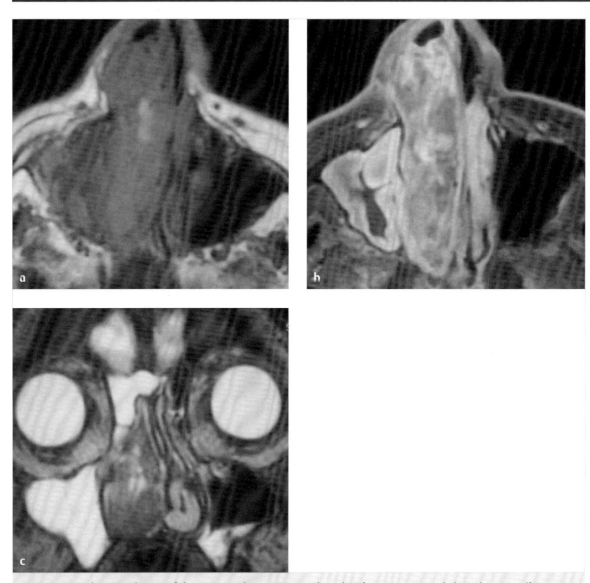

Fig. 4.13 a–c Melanotic melanoma of the septum with extension into the right inferior meatus, vestibule, and anterior olfactory rim. **(a)** An area of intratumoral hemorrhage is shown with high signal on the axial T1 W image. **(b)** There is focal lack of contrast enhancement in this location of the tumor that shows moderate contrast uptake. Bright enhancing mucosal rim delineates the margins of the tumor except for areas of mucosal infiltration at the anterior septum and lateral wall of vestibule. **(c)** Differentiation of the expansile rather than infiltrative tumor from retained secretions is best appreciated on the T2 W image.

histopathologically correlate with intratumoral vessels or fibrous septa.[131]

After contrast administration, sinonasal melanomas exhibit a moderate-to-marked increase in signal intensity (▶ Fig. 4.13b). Their imaging appearance is nonspecific for amelanotic tumors and may resemble SCC, adenocarcinoma, and sinonasal undifferentiated carcinoma. Melanotic melanomas may harbor a more specific MRI appearance; however, other lesions that may present hemorrhage need to be excluded including hemangioma, juvenile angiofibroma, and hemorrhagic metastasis.

Note

Sinonasal malignant melanomas are highly aggressive and have dismal prognosis with short survival rates. A significant difference from their cutaneous counterpart is their primary tendency to hematogenous spread. Therefore, preoperative staging must comprise PET/CT. MR is preferable for follow-up surveillance and to assess local tumor control. Imaging of lymph nodes and the search for distant metastases is also required and best achieved by PET/CT.

4.1.21 Lymphoma

Sinonasal lymphoma commonly presents on CT as soft-tissue lesions with increased density on noncontrast studies. The nasal cavity is the predominant location in T-cell and natural killer cell/T-cell lymphoma. These tumors were previously known as midline (lethal) granuloma or angiocentric lymphoma, and may present within the nasal cavity as bulky tumors or as soft-tissue lesions without apparent mass effect.[133] In contrast to T-cell lymphomas, sinus involvement without nasal disease is common in B-cell lymphoma.[134]

> **Note**
>
> The nasal cavity is the predominant location in T-cell and natural killer cell/T-cell lymphoma, whereas B-cell lymphoma show sinus involvement without nasal disease.

CT is useful for staging of lymphomas and assessing bone involvement. These tumors remodel rather than erode the adjoining bone unless infiltration affects the adjacent sinuses, more commonly the medial wall of the maxillary sinus and ethmoid cells.[135] Within the nasal cavity, bone erosion first affects the nasal septum, a finding that is typical but not specific for non-Hodgkin T-cell lymphomas.[133] However, based on an analysis of seven patients the same authors deny the presence of any distinguishing imaging features between non-Hodgkin T-cell lymphoma and Wegener granulomatosis. Skull base destruction on CT with concomitant brain involvement was noted in 7 out of 24 patients (29.2%) with extranodal non-Hodgkin lymphoma of the sinonasal tract.[136] Nonseptal bone erosion affects the sinus walls and hard palate and is commonly associated with T-cell lymphomas.[133]

B-cell lymphomas are more likely to affect the paranasal sinuses, invade the orbit (▶ Fig. 4.14), and skull base. With 2.2% of all patients with sinonasal tract tumors, the sphenoid sinus is a rare primary location. Non-Hodgkin B-cell lymphomas were the second most common tumors within the sphenoid sinus in a review of 23 neoplasms, superseded only by combined adenocarcinomas and SCCs in 26%. Following in frequency were adenoid cystic carcinomas (17.5%), sarcomas and sinonasal undifferentiated carcinomas in 8.8% each, and endocrine carcinomas, melanoma, plasmocytoma, and malignant hemangiopericytoma with 4.4% each.[137]

MRI is performed to assess the soft-tissue extension of lymphomas especially orbital, infratemporal, and intracranial involvement.[135,138] Lymphomas appear low in signal intensity on T1 W images and isointense to hyperintense on T2 W images (▶ Fig. 4.14 **a,b**). Lymphomas of the nasal cavity commonly present as soft-tissue lesions centered on the septum and turbinates with variable paranasal sinus extension. In nine patients reported by Ooi et al,[139] the tumor was confined to the nasal cavity in two, showed extension into the paranasal sinuses in an additional four patients, and infratemporal infiltration in one case. Superior nasal cavity location led to involvement of the ethmoid, orbit, and maxillary sinuses in another two cases.

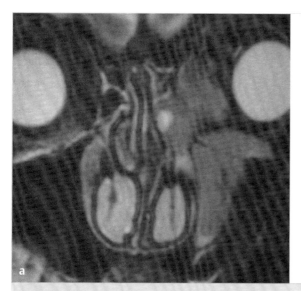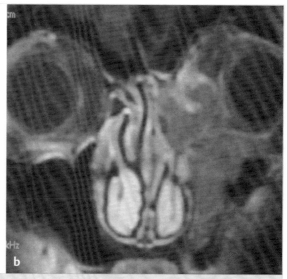

Fig. 4.14 a, b Sinonasal B-cell lymphoma with maxillary sinus and anterior ethmoid location, middle meatus, and orbital invasion. **(a)** The lymphoma is shown as a moderately bright tumor on T2 W fat-suppressed image. It is well delineated and distinguished from bright signal of mucosa and retained fluid. **(b)** The tumor displays enhancement on the surface on T1 W contrast-enhanced fat-suppressed image. Fat suppression technique is performed in both T2 W and T1 W sequences to distinguish the orbital tumor component and surface enhancement from the otherwise bright—now suppressed—orbital fat signal.

Lymphomas arising from the maxillary sinus appear as solid mass lesions.[140] However, a minority may display mucosal thickening only, which requires MRI to be distinguished from inflammatory tissue.[140]

MR aids in distinguishing tumor from adjacent mucosa, fluid retention (▶ Fig. 4.14 **a**), and granulation tissue.[141] Enhancement following intravenous contrast administration is usually much lower than in carcinomas and shows a tendency to predominantly demarcate the surface mucosa from the underlying submucosal tumor location (▶ Fig. 4.14 **b**). PET/CT has emerged as an important imaging modality for initial staging, follow-up investigations under therapy, and in the course of follow-up surveillance.[142]

> **Note**
>
> Lymphomas appear on CT as soft-tissue lesions with increased density on noncontrasted studies. MR shows a low in signal intensity on T1 W images and isointense to hyperintense on T2 W images. PET/CT is the preferred imaging modality for initial staging as well as in follow-up surveillance.

4.1.22 Metastases

Imaging is required to depict the location, extension, and potential multiplicity of metastases that may affect the skull base. Skull base metastasis is usually a late event in the course of a malignancy; however, it may be the first sign of cancer in up to 29% of patients.[143]

> **Note**
>
> Skull base metastases display a predilection for the clivus, major and lesser wing of the sphenoid, and the vicinity of the jugular foramen.

Because of hematogenous spread, skull base metastases are primarily centered within cancellous bone. Skull base metastases display a predilection for the clivus (▶ Fig. 4.15), major and lesser wing of the sphenoid, and the vicinity of the jugular foramen.[144] Due to higher sensitivity to depict bone marrow changes, MR is superior to CT in detecting cancellous bone infiltration (▶ Fig. 4.15a).

Metastases affecting the sinonasal tract are uncommon and imply a primary tumor location within the kidney, lung, or gastrointestinal tract. CT best delineates the osseous destruction caused by metastases in this location.[145]

CT better distinguishes cortical bone erosion and cancellous bone infiltration caused by metastases (▶ Fig. 4.15**b**) from expansion and replacement due to bone abnormalities such as fibrous dysplasia, or tumors such as osteochondroma.[144] Furthermore CT is more accurate than MR in differentiating metastasis from Paget disease or an intraosseous meningioma.[133]

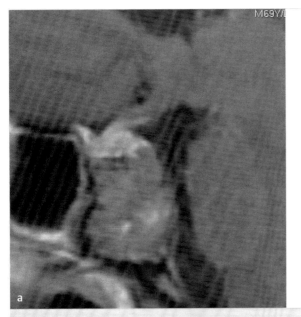 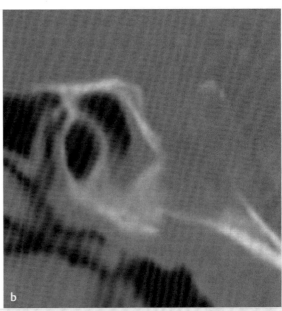

Fig. 4.15 a, b Metastasis from carcinoma of the breast within the clivus in a 44-year-old patient with double vision due to VI nerve palsy. **(a)** Infiltration of cancellous bone of the clivus is depicted by a metastasis that shows diminished contrast uptake on the sagittal T1 W contrast-enhanced fat-suppressed image. **(b)** Elevation of the pituitary gland is found due to infiltration of the sella floor shown on the sagittal CT image. Note destruction of posterior cortical bone at the dural border and preservation of the anterior and inferior cortical bone toward the sphenoid sinus and roof of the epipharynx.

Based on the density shown on CT, metastases appear as osteolytic, osteoblastic, or mixed density lesions. CT identification of an osteoblastic type of metastases may allow narrowing of the potential primary site of malignancy.

MR is more precise to define the extent of tumor invasion into the bone marrow (▶ Fig. 4.15a) and is more sensitive to delineate infiltration of adjacent dura, cranial nerves, and vessels.[7] MR supplements CT in distinguishing a metastasis from a plasmacytoma,[31] amyloid deposition,[146] and inflammatory myofibroblastic "pseudo" tumor[147] by a typical, although not specific, signal decrease on T2 W images. MR also distinguishes metastasis from direct extension by neoplasms that infiltrate the skull base such as nasopharyngeal carcinoma, SCC, sinonasal undifferentiated carcinoma, adenocarcinoma, neuroendocrine carcinoma, esthesioneuroblastoma, or melanoma.

Tumor location is a significant factor for the particular yield provided by CT and MR in recognizing infiltration of bone and bone marrow in the skull base.[148] Contrary to the anterior skull base, MR surpasses CT in the clivus and vicinity of the jugular foramen due to increased marrow content of the adjacent sphenoid and occipital bone.[4]

Comparing precontrast T1 W MR images and T1 fat-suppressed sequences, following intravenous administration of contrast material, best shows the extent of bone marrow invasion. Some metastases have slight contrast uptake (▶ Fig. 4.15a); therefore, comparing precontrast images and gadolinium-enhanced fat-suppressed sequences is essential.

Obstruction of adjacent paranasal sinuses, infiltration of the brain, and optic nerve compression are best depicted on T2 W images. Hypervascular metastases originating from the kidney, thyroid, or malignant melanoma may mimic hypervascular tumors such as hemangiopericytoma, paraganglioma, and angiofibroma. Time-resolved MR angiography with a high temporal resolution (currently feasible 0.7 seconds) is a noninvasive means to define the degree of vascularity and provide an indication for preoperative embolization.

4.2 Endovascular Interventional Procedures of Skull Base Pathologies

Ralf Siekmann, Erich Hofmann

4.2.1 Introduction

This section deals with techniques, treatment strategies, and indications for vascular interventional neuroradiology in the face and neck region. It especially addresses skull base surgeons and other surgeons who may not be familiar with the methods and applications of endovascular interventions. Endovascular therapies cannot be neatly divided into neurointerventions of the brain, spine, and skull base, or other procedures of the head and neck region, either anatomically or based on vascular territories; the scope of the chapter is to cover those procedures that are of clinical and practical interest to physicians who perform extradural skull base surgery and otolaryngology–head and neck surgery.

Basic principles of angiographic and interventional techniques and strategies are described in this section; however, readers who want to explore the subject more deeply or are interested in specific areas should consult standard works in this field.[149,150,151,152] This section does not tackle percutaneous biopsies for histologic differentiation of indeterminate masses, or percutaneous therapeutic procedures to decompress or obliterate cystic lesions. This section focuses on diseases that are treatable via endovascular approaches, (transarterial or, less commonly, transvenous embolization) using catheter-based techniques. Exceptions are those lesions that can be embolized by direct puncture, such as paragangliomas or capillary venous hemangiomas. Thus, the contents of this chapter are limited based on clinical criteria and technical aspects.

The great majority of vascular procedures pertaining to otolaryngology–head and neck surgery are interventional procedures in the territory of the external carotid artery (ECA). At the turn of the century, Dawbarn performed the first embolization in this vascular territory, using hot liquid wax to embolize malignant tumors of the neck and face. However, the experimental and clinical work regarding the vascular anatomy and physiology of the ECA by Djindjian and his students laid the groundwork for a comprehensive system. Using vascular diagnoses and pathology, it provided the basis for a rational therapeutic approach to vascular lesions in the head and neck. In the 1970s, this school established the basic principles of interventional techniques in this vascular territory that remain valid.[153] Development of improved catheters, embolization materials, and techniques in the 1980s and 1990s represent another milestone for interventional neuroradiology. This development continues today, making it reasonable to expect future improvements and expansions of endovascular field in the skull base region. Striking new developments in interventional and embolization materials (e.g., new fluid embolic materials, stents, flow diverters) and DSA technology (biplanar angiography units, 3D rotational angiography), along with advances in our understanding of the physiology and pathophysiology of vascular diseases, have led to rapid worldwide expansion of neurointerventional techniques. As a result, endovascular treatment strategies have become an integral part of the overall treatment plan for vascular pathologies in skull base surgery and an essential tool in many routine clinical situations.

4.2.2 Basic Principles of Embolization and Techniques

Most endovascular procedures start with the puncture and catheterization of the common femoral artery, which has significant advantages compared with other approaches. First and foremost, it gives access to all relevant vascular territories in the head and neck region. It also provides the examiner and other personnel with a high degree of radiation safety. One disadvantage is the need for long catheters, which may be difficult to control in those elderly and atherosclerotic patients with extreme vessel elongation. In these patients or when the access route is obstructed or extremely narrowed (usually in the pelvic arteries and occasionally at the lumbar aortic level), the common carotid artery or other cervical vessel can be punctured directly or catheterized via a transbrachial approach. Since the external carotid artery is prone to vasospasms, direct puncture of that vessel is an acceptable option only when other approaches cannot be used. On the other hand, direct puncture of the external carotid artery is an important last resort when no other access is possible due, for example, to previous surgical ligation or radiotherapy exposure. A large number of catheters with a special curve at their distal end (e.g., vertebral, sidewinder, multipurpose catheters) are available and specially designed for catheterizing the cervical supra-aortic vessels.

Every intervention should be preceded by a comprehensive angiographic work-up of all head and neck vessels. For some elective interventions, diagnostic angiography and the intervention can be done at separate times. This staged approach is easier for patients to tolerate and gives the examiner time to discuss with other clinicians; thus, resulting in better planning of the interventional strategy. Currently, a high-quality, biplanar DSA-capable angiography unit has become a basic necessity for embolizations in the skull base, as well as the face and neck regions. It allows the visualization of vessels in all planes and significantly reduces radiation exposure, contrast volumes, and examination time, which will increase the efficacy and safety of the intervention procedure.

High-quality, low-osmolar nonionic contrast medium is particularly recommended for the facial region to minimize the pain caused by the contrast material. Vascular interventions in the head and neck region can generally be performed under local anesthesia. Neuroleptanalgesia or general anesthesia may be indicated in patients who are anxious, uncooperative (e.g., severe trauma, children, confused patients) or where a longer procedure time is expected. Ordinary sedative procedures are often insufficient to achieve this goal. General endotracheal anesthesia increases the safety of the examination by allowing rapid catheterization of the vessels.

Another important aspect of external carotid artery angiography should be considered. Because of its nerve supply, this vessel, unlike the internal carotid artery, often undergoes a severe vasospasm in response to mechanical irritants, chemical agents, and pain-induced host reactions. Vasospasms may have several adverse effects:

1. They may prevent an adequate angiographic study and may block access to the desired catheter position for the embolization.
2. The angiographic series may distort the vascular and hemodynamic situation and, for example, may fail to show potentially dangerous anastomoses between the external carotid artery/ophthalmic artery and other arteries supplying the brain.
3. Every vasospasm increases the risk of embolization, including the danger of embolic agent refluxing into potentially "dangerous anastomoses" or directly into arteries that supply the eye or brain.
4. They may decrease the effectiveness of the procedure due to reduced flow in feeding arteries.

Besides the rapid and precise catheterization of vessels, the best way to prevent vasospasm is by administering general anesthesia, which will produce a deeper analgesic and vasoplegic effect than neuroleptanalgesia. However, the inability to assess neurologic status in the unconscious patient is a disadvantage. If vasospasm still occurs, the intra-arterial injection of lidocaine or nitrate solution can reduce the duration and severity of luminal narrowing. Lidocaine can also be used along with contrast medium for functional, preinterventional testing of the brain and cervical nerves. When the test result is interpreted, however, it should be noted that the hemodynamic situation may change in response to embolization and that nerve deficits are detectable for only a short time after the lidocaine injection.

Another important danger is the risk of thromboembolic complications. This risk correlates directly with the duration of catheterization for diagnosis and therapy, patient age, and the extent of atherosclerotic vascular changes. Intravenous heparinization is recommended for the prevention of thromboembolism. Regimens stated in the literature range from 10 to 40 IU/kg/hour with or without a single bolus injection. It is desirable to increase the partial thromboplastin time (PTT) to at least double the normal value. Instruments that can monitor PTT or activated clotting time (ACT) in relative units based on multiple readings in the angiography room are available commercially. Many vascular laboratories use coagulation test kits to determine the effect not only of heparin but also of aspirin and clopidogrel. Their value and necessity are controversial, however, and we cannot yet make a definitive evaluation or general recommendation. The following simple method has proven valuable for routine use: check the coagulation factors prior to the angiography and intervention. Inject a single bolus of 3,000 to 5,000 IU heparin before the procedure. Add the same amount for every 500 mL of electrolyte solution used to flush the catheter and sheath system. If there is a danger of hemorrhage, the heparin dosage should be reduced or eliminated depending on the estimated risk. Unlike aspirin and clopidogrel, the effects of heparin can be reversed by the intravenous administration of protamine sulfate.

Blood pressure and electrocardiogram (ECG) should be monitored throughout the intervention. A decrease in blood pressure may reduce flow through the catheter and increase the risk of reflux during embolization. The contrast agent itself can be a cause for hypotension; thus, it is recommended that the intervention should be performed at a slightly hypertensive blood pressure level.

As mentioned above, a large number of specially shaped catheters are available for catheterization. Selective, usually bilateral diagnostic angiography of all supra-aortic vessels is performed, depending on the specific vascular pathology. This will give the examiner a rapid and comprehensive overview of the vascular anatomy, hemodynamics, and pathology in the entire head and neck region. The presence of stenoses, occlusions, collateral pathways, and anatomic vascular variants is important and their assessment constitutes essential information prior to any intervention. Diagnostic catheter sizes of 4 or 5 Fr should be used. Larger catheters and wires of various size and flexibility may be used as needed in patients with extensive vascular elongation. Prior to interventions in the external carotid artery system, the internal carotid artery territory should also be imaged due to the close anatomical and functional relationships between the two vascular systems. They communicate chiefly through branches of the OphA and numerous vessels arising directly from the carotid siphon of the internal carotid artery. For the same reason, the vertebral artery and its anastomoses via cervical muscle branches with the occipital artery and ascending pharyngeal artery should be selectively catheterized and imaged in patients with lesions near the skull base in the posterior upper neck. The subclavian artery, thyrocervical trunk, and ascending cervical artery should also be selectively catheterized and imaged in patients with more deeply situated neck lesions.

The intervention itself is performed with a large-bore guide catheter. A 5 or 6 Fr catheter size is usually adequate in the external carotid artery system. The guide catheter allows for continuous and better vascular imaging during the intervention, while the indwelling microcatheter controls the embolization. It is introduced with a microwire using a coaxial technique. "Road mapping" before catheterization greatly facilitates the navigation of the vessels. The risk of external carotid vasospasm can be reduced by placing the guide catheter in the common carotid artery and catheterizing the external carotid artery and its branches with the microcatheter system. Modern guide catheters with a soft tip allow for a safer and less traumatic technique, even in the external carotid artery. The angiographic survey view of the external carotid artery is an essential part of the angiographic

protocol. Except for the auricular region, the external carotid artery territory is not a terminal vascular bed. It is more like a network of anatomical and functional vascular units that intercommunicate via numerous vertical, horizontal, and transverse anastomoses and regulate cervicofacial vascularity by maintaining a hemodynamic balance. The internal carotid artery, vertebral artery, and subclavian artery are integrated into this system through numerous side branches.

One of the greatest dangers and risks of interventional procedures in the skull base, and face and neck regions is the unwanted embolization of embolic material into vessels supplying the brain. This may occur through existing vascular connections, through anastomoses that open during the embolization, or through undesired reflux. Any acute occlusion of a vessel by the embolic material, for example, will produce a hemodynamic change that may cause pre-existing vascular connections (i.e., present but functionally inactive anastomoses) to open. This is one reason why surgical vascular ligations, including individual branches of the external carotid artery, sometimes are not as successful as expected and may fail to arrest bleeding or prevent recurrent bleeding despite ligation of the main trunk. On the other hand, one advantage of this special feature of external carotid artery angioarchitecture and hemodynamics is that embolization generally does not cause necrosis of the skin or mucosa. This complication most often results from the use of liquid embolic material (e.g., 96% ethanol), microspheres, very small polyvinyl alcohol particles (smaller than 50 µm in high dilution), or in patients with severe preexisting skin or mucosal damage such as in Rendu–Osler–Weber syndrome.

4.2.3 Embolization Materials

Since the beginning of interventional endovascular therapy in the skull base and head and neck region, many different embolic materials have been tested and used for vascular occlusion. A large percentage of these materials are purely of historical interest today. Unfortunately an embolic material that fulfills every requirement does not yet exist. The number of agents in current clinical use has dwindled to manageable proportions. This chapter deals with the most important materials used for embolizations in the face and neck region.

All embolic materials can be classified by their physical characteristics as solid (embolic particles, balloons, coils) or liquid, and by their biological characteristics as absorbable or nonabsorbable. Another important aspect is the biological tolerance of embolic materials. Sometimes other devices can be additionally and technically helpful; these include detachable or nondetachable balloons, electrolytically detachable platinum coils, various number of stents and flow diverters, which are also occasionally used for embolizations in the face and neck region, but they are not as important in that region as they are in the treatment of intracranial cerebral aneurysms, and arteriovenous and intracranial or extracranial stenoses.

Balloons can temporarily occlude the vessel to prevent the spread of embolic material and undesired reflux. Detachable coils as used for intracranial aneurysm therapy are a technically simpler option to produce a controlled, circumscribed vascular occlusion or decrease in flow at the desired site. Another way to accomplish this goal in smaller vessels is by the use of gelatin sponges (e.g., Gelfoam; Pfizer Inc., New York, United States). This is rarely necessary, however, when microcatheters are used and small vessels are selectively catheterized using the correct technique. Electrolytically detachable microcoils are a technically simpler option that can produce a controlled, circumscribed vascular occlusion at the desired site. Nondetachable microcoils (Berenstein liquid coils, Topaz coils) can be used proximally (proximal protection) to reduce blood flow in a vessel that has been embolized distally with a particulate agent. Larger pieces of gelatin sponges may also be used for this purpose. The most important embolic materials are listed and reviewed below.

Polyvinyl Alcohol

Polyvinyl alcohol (PVA) belongs to the category of non-absorbable, water-insoluble particulate embolic agents. PVA is produced by reacting vinyl alcohols with a formaldehyde catalyst. Available particle sizes currently range from less than 50 µm up to 1,000 µm. PVA particles are suspended in contrast medium because they are not radio-opaque by themselves. During the embolization, it is important to keep the particles as homogeneously suspended as possible and not to dilute them too much to reduce the aggregation tendency of the PVA and to prevent catheter occlusion by the embolic material, especially when larger particles and smaller-gauge catheters are used. This has prompted some authors to recommend the use of microspheres. These agents are deformable, do not clump, and have a well-defined penetration depth. They have very little aggregation tendency, so there is no risk of catheter clogging. One disadvantage is their higher cost as compared with PVA particles. The risk of microcatheter occlusion is significantly reduced when PVA particles are injected in accordance with user guidelines (homogeneity, dilution of the PVA suspension).

Although PVA particles are not absorbable, the vascular occlusion caused by these agents is not permanent. Histologic studies have shown that in addition to mechanical obstruction of the vessel lumen (primary occlusive mechanism), the particles induce local platelet aggregation. This thrombus may partially or completely dissolve and lead to stable recanalization of the vessel lumen by re-endothelialization, as in spontaneous thrombosis of the arterial or venous limb. The efficacy and duration of the

vascular occlusion depends mainly on the secondary occlusion mechanism of platelet aggregation. Particle size, dilution, vessel size, and collateralization are the critical factors that determine the relationship between the primary and secondary occlusion mechanisms, thus making it controllable to some degree. The indications for using PVA particles in the skull base, and face and neck regions are derived from their properties. Indications include preoperative or palliative embolization of vascularized tumor, hemorrhage, and aneurysm occlusion in the territory of the external carotid artery. Provided that there are no larger arteriovenous shunts in vascularized tumors, PVA is very efficacious.

A major advantage of PVA particles is that they rarely cause necrosis of the skin or mucosa.[154] The particle size is determined by the integrity of the arterial–capillary barrier.[155] If the barrier is compromised due to an arteriovenous fistula or arteriovenous malformation larger particles or other embolic materials should be used to produce effective occlusion. Generally speaking, however, PVA particles are not the material of choice for the embolization of arteriovenous fistulas or malformations. The selection of particle size and its dilution should be varied during the course of the procedure. Initially, small particles can be used at high dilution to obtain deeper tissue penetration. This allows the embolic material to reach the precapillary level and produce distal vascular occlusion. This is followed by the use of larger and/or less diluted particles to occlude larger, more proximal vessels. Proximal protection of the embolization using microcoils is recommended in larger branches of the external carotid artery after the embolization has been completed, especially in preoperative interventions.

In summary, PVA particles are widely used because they are easy to control and are available commercially at relatively low cost. They produce effective, long-lasting vascular occlusion without cytotoxic effects.

Microspheres

Trisacryl gelatin microspheres (Embosphere; BioSphere Medical, Rockland, Massachusetts, United States) provide an alternative to PVA particles.[156,157] Unlike PVA, the microspheres have a smooth, uniform surface. They cannot aggregate in microcatheters or in the bloodstream, and this has two important advantages:
1. No danger of catheter clogging.
2. Level of vascular occlusion can be reliably predicted in advance.

It is still uncertain whether these theoretical advantages have significant practical value in the control of bleeding, for example. Otherwise it has been shown that less blood loss occurs after the preoperative embolization of meningiomas with microspheres in comparison with PVA particles.[158] Microspheres are available in sizes from 40 to 1,200 µm.

Microcoils

Coils used in interventional neuroradiology can be classified into two groups. The first group consists of coils used in the treatment of predominantly intracranial true ("berry") aneurysms. Since their introduction by Guglielmi in 1990 (Guglielmi detachable coils), they have undergone rapid technical advances and have revolutionized the treatment of these aneurysms. They are less important for endovascular procedures in the skull base and face and neck regions due to the different pathologies found in these vascular territories as well as economic factors. For these reasons they will not be discussed further in this section.

The second group consists of microcoils and platinum coils of various diameters, lengths, and configurations that can be placed with a microcatheter but do not have a special detachment system. They are released into the vessel lumen using a pushwire or simple saline (pressure) injection. The coils are manually introduced at the proximal end of the microcatheter through the catheter hub. Thrombogenicity can be increased by using microcoils coated with Dacron fibers (fibered coils).[159] These coils have two main indications in the skull base and face and neck regions: following the successful distal occlusion of a vascular territory using particulate embolic material, the proximal vascular segment is occluded with microcoils, which support the distal particle embolization by decreasing perfusion (principle of proximal protection). A second important indication is the occlusion of a vessel distal to the microcatheter tip that should not be embolized ("protective occlusion") before the particles are introduced. This principle has been in practice for some time and was formerly accomplished with small gelatin sponge pieces or other materials. Despite having no detachment system, microcoils can usually be placed with precision, especially when a pushwire is used; thus, their use in the external carotid artery territory is considered safe and effective.

Gelatin Sponges

Gelatin sponge (e.g., Gelfoam) is one of the oldest embolic materials and is still commonly used in neuroradiologic endovascular therapy.[160,161] Belonging to the class of absorbable particulate embolic agents, the gelatin sponge can be cut to size just before use or injected in powder form (100 and 1,000 µm). Even the smallest particles will not enter the venous side of the circulation as long as the arteriocapillary boundary is intact and there are no arteriovenous shunts.

Because gelatin sponge is not radiopaque, a contrast medium is added so that the embolization can be fluoroscopically controlled. Just as with PVA particles, the occlusion mechanism is based on a primary mechanical obstruction of the vessel lumen followed by platelet aggregation. Gelatin sponge is characterized biologically by a high degree of tissue tolerance. A mild foreign-body reaction is very rarely observed, while moderate inflammatory changes in the vessel wall and surrounding tissue are somewhat more common. Because it is absorbable, gelatin sponge produces a temporary vascular occlusion. The recanalization rate depends on particle and vessel size and collateralization. Recanalization times range from 2 to 30 days. The arterial pressure in the embolized vessel significantly influences the recanalization rate. Therefore, whenever possible, distal embolization with gelatin sponge should be augmented by a proximal occlusion using larger microcoils or other materials. Gelatin sponge can also be used in cases that require temporary vascular occlusion. For example, if the catheter cannot be placed far enough distally for PVA embolization, or if it is necessary to prevent undesired reflux into a proximal vessel, that vessel can be occluded with a larger piece of gelatin sponge. If gelatin sponge is used preoperatively, the surgery should be performed within 2 to 3 days. Gelfoam is best suited for preoperative tumor embolization. Despite the particle size and temporary occlusion, gelatin sponge can induce perivascular tumor necrosis. Gelfoam is not suitable as a standalone measure for embolizing tumors due to the temporary nature of the occlusion.

Cyanoacrylates

Cyanoacrylates are a group of liquid, fast-curing tissue adhesives that are known for their surgical applications. The most commonly used cyanoacrylates are the two stereoisomers n-butyl-2-cyanoacrylate and isobutyl-2-cyanoacrylate, better known under the trade names Histoacryl and Bucrylate. Intravascular curing of the agent takes place as the monomers react chemically to form the polymer through a condensation process catalyzed by anions. Cyanoacrylates are not radiopaque in themselves. If they are not diluted with lipiodol, tantalum powder should be added for visualization. The curing time may be influenced by the addition of lipiodol and the proportion of Histoacryl to lipiodol. The more lipiodol is added, the more slowly the agent cures.[162]

Because saline solution, blood, or contrast medium can trigger the condensation reaction, the application catheter should be filled with an anionic binding agent (usually 10% glucose) prior to embolization. Cyanoacrylates have proven to be most effective in the treatment of arteriovenous malformations and arteriovenous fistulas.[163] Generally these agents are not used for the palliative or preoperative embolization of tumors. Cyanoacrylates have significantly higher tissue toxicity than PVA particles and gelatin sponge. They have also been shown to provoke a vascular and perivascular inflammatory response and foreign body reaction with associated granuloma formation. The neoplastic potential of the above cyanoacrylates is still unknown, but to date there is no definite proof of malignant tumor induction by either of the two agents.

Onyx

Onyx (Covidien, Mansfield, Massachusetts, United States) is a liquid embolic agent consisting of an ethylene vinyl alcohol copolymer (EVOH) dissolved in a dimethyl sulfoxide (DMSO) solution. It is mixed with large amounts of tantalum powder (~35%) so that it can be visualized. Onyx is available in concentrations of 18, 24, and 30 (corresponding to 6–8% EVOH). High-density Onyx HD-500 (20% EVOH) is used exclusively for the treatment of large intracranial aneurysms and will not be considered here. Onyx can be applied only through catheters specifically approved for that purpose and pretreated with DMSO. A major advantage of Onyx over cyanoacrylates is that it is nonadhesive, making it possible to use larger amounts of the embolic agent. The reflux of Onyx causes a "plug" to form on and around the microcatheter tip, at which point the embolic agent can be injected distally along the resulting pressure gradient.

Onyx is used mainly in the treatment of arteriovenous malformations. Other applications include the endovascular therapy of tumors and dural fistulas and the direct injection of the agent into paragangliomas. Its slow application rate (0.1–0.3 mL/min) makes it easy to control. Even when Onyx is used in vascular lesions with an arteriovenous shunt, any material that enters the venous circulation is less likely to cause venous occlusion than cyanoacrylates since the embolic material tends to spread along the vein wall.

Summarizing my own experience and the literature, Onyx can be recommended as a safe and clinically efficacious embolic agent in the endovascular management of vascular lesions in the head and neck region.[164]

4.2.4 Test Occlusion of Vessels—Applications, Principles, and Indications

The test occlusion of a vessel, meaning the temporary occlusion of a vessel lumen and its more distal branches, can be performed on numerous vessels in the skull base and neck regions. Test occlusions are most commonly performed on the internal carotid artery. Because the basic principles of test occlusion apply regardless of the vascular territory involved, the basic principles and techniques that apply to all test occlusions will be reviewed using the internal carotid artery as an example.

Acute ligation of the internal carotid artery leads to neurologic deficits in 20% of patients and historical data indicate rates as high as 50%.[165] The rationale for a temporary test occlusion is to determine whether a proposed occlusion of the internal carotid artery will cause neurologic deficits. Test occlusion is generally performed with a silicone balloon owing to its relatively gentle radial pressure, which will reduce or eliminate any unwanted angioplastic effect. The occlusion should last no longer than

30 minutes and should be discontinued at once by deflating the balloon if any neurologic deficits appear. The test is of high accuracy in predicting postocclusion deficits and is interpreted on the basis of clinical and angiographic criteria. According to the literature, the percentages of true-positive or true-negative results have not improved significantly despite numerous additional studies (such as EEG, HMPAO SPECT, xenon-133 CT, transcranial Doppler ultrasound, O15-H$_2$O PET, intravascular pressure measurement, MRI, and CT perfusion imaging).[166,167,168,169] Also, the additional studies often yield contradictory results during or after the test occlusion. There are various reasons for this, which are discussed at length in the literature. It is important to inform patients and surgical colleagues that there is always a marginal uncertainty to predict whether a patient will tolerate or not a definitive vascular occlusion.

Test occlusion is performed in the conscious, nonsedated patient, as a high degree of patient cooperation is required (▶ Fig. 4.16). A bilateral approach through the inguinal arteries is necessary. Generally it is sufficient to place a 4 or 5 Fr catheter one side and a 6 Fr catheter in the other side. The larger catheter is used to introduce a guide catheter and to inflatable balloon catheter into the common carotid or internal carotid artery. The diagnostic catheter is used for angiographic monitoring during the trial occlusion. If a guide catheter is used, it is positioned in the common carotid artery, external carotid artery, or internal carotid artery and a 3 or 8 mm balloon is introduced up to the occlusion level. The balloon should be of the proper size and material and should have good compliance, meaning that the pressure on the plunger during injection of the contrast medium and saline mixture should convert directly to balloon inflation, ideally in a 1:1 ratio. The 3 to 4 mm balloon is a good choice when the internal carotid artery will be temporarily occluded distal to the vascular pathology. An anesthesiologist should be present during the test to monitor the patient and to induce controlled hypotension during the last 10 minutes of the 30-minute test occlusion period. The blood pressure should be lowered to approximately two-thirds of the initial systolic value; that is, by approximately 25%. The method evaluated by the Buffalo group simulates a stressful situation by inducing blood pressure variations like those occurring in everyday situations.[170] Nitroprusside is administered to titrate the desired fall in blood pressure. Other groups of authors have published significantly better test occlusion outcomes with detectability rates for neurologic deficits of up to 20% during controlled hypotension, with only a 5% rate of false-negative results. Other groups rate the predictive value of controlled hypotension less highly.

As an additional note, the authors have found that the intravenous injection of 1,000 mg acetazolamide and HMPAO (hexamethyl propylene amine oxine) before or during the test occlusion provides valuable additional

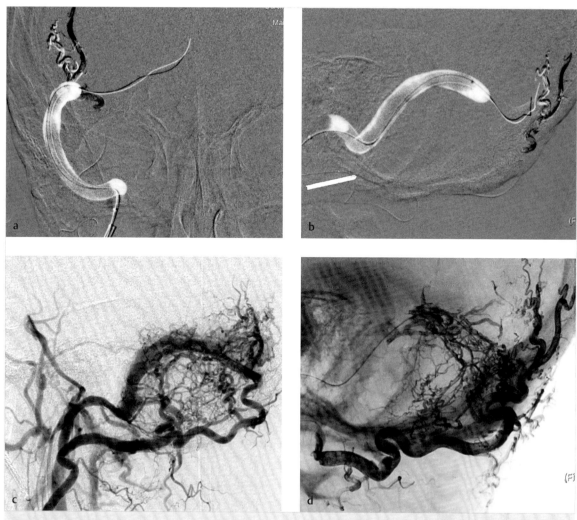

Fig. 4.16 a–d Temporary occlusion of the sigmoidal sinus with a transvenously placed balloon catheter. The principle of venous test occlusion is technically the same as temporary occlusion of this or another segment of the sinuses for transarterial embolization of a dural arteriovenous fistula for delivery a higher volume of embolic material and achieving better angiographic and clinical results. Placement of the balloon in the anteroposterior and lateral view after venous approach and placement of the guiding catheter in the internal jugular vein at the level of the skull base (**a, b**). Preinterventional angiogram of the dural arteriovenous fistula (**c**) and the cast (**d**) after arterial embolization with Onyx of different weights.

information for predicting outcomes in our patients. The test occlusion is followed by a 99mTc-HMPAO SPECT examination, which clearly demonstrates the cerebral reserve capacity as well as side-to-side differences in blood flow during the occlusion.[169]

The patient should undergo a neurologic examination before the test occlusion, and the same neurologist should examine the patient during and after the occlusion. Neurologic tests are repeated several times during the occlusion and should at least cover motor and sensory function, speech and speech recognition. Both clinical and angiographic criteria should be used in interpreting the results. Vascular occlusion by the balloon is followed by the angiographic documentation and assessment of collateral flow through the ipsilateral external carotid artery and contralateral internal carotid artery. Flow from the vertebrobasilar system via the posterior communicating artery may also be assessed. When contrast medium is injected into the contralateral internal carotid artery, a delay of the capillary venous phase greater than 1 to 2 seconds in the ipsilateral cerebral vessels predicts that the patient will not be able to tolerate the vascular occlusion.

After the test occlusion is completed, the balloon is deflated and postocclusion angiograms are obtained. These images should demonstrate the extracranial and intracranial vessels to exclude any vessel wall dissections and local vascular dilatations (angioplastic effect). There should be no evidence of thromboembolic complications in the intracranial vessels. The examination is performed with full heparinization and monitoring of ACT values. The complication rate is very low with an appropriate preparation and a cooperative patient. Complication rates in the literature are about 7%, with a range from 1 to 13%, and correlate with publication dates (general experience and improved methodology, advances in catheter and balloon technology) and with the number of additional methods used to interpret the test. Adequate anticoagulation is obvious. The predictive value of temporary vascular occlusion is high when compared with the rate of neurologic deficits that are expected to occur spontaneously without testing.[171]

Tests can also be performed on the venous side of the vascular system in the same way as on the arterial side. One method is to temporarily occlude the transverse and sigmoid sinuses and evaluate collateral flow through a second arterial approach. Surgical indications would include tumors that have invaded these venous structures and should be removed to accomplish a radical resection. Temporary testing may also be necessary during the intervention in cases where the endovascular occlusion of the transverse or sigmoid sinus, for example, is proposed for the treatment of a dural arteriovenous fistula and it is uncertain whether the patient can tolerate the procedure. Clinical testing is not possible in these cases due to the delayed manifestation of symptoms. The test is interpreted by carefully analyzing the angiographic series obtained during the venous occlusion.[172,173]

In summary, a test occlusion should be performed before any planned ligation of large extracranial and intracranial vessels. The result provides a basis for obtaining adequate informed consent prior to surgery. Test occlusion should be performed even in cases where the mere possibility of vascular ligation is being considered during preoperative planning. The result of the test occlusion is an important aid in planning the operation, evaluating alternative modalities of therapy, and for medicolegal reasons. Therefore all surgeons should be cognizant of advantages of an occlusion test and consider its indications during their preoperative planning.

4.2.5 Applications of Endovascular Therapy

Bleeding in the Head and Neck Region

Bleeding in the head and neck region is one of the main indications for endovascular therapy in otorhinolaryngology.[174] Bleeding can be classified etiologically as primary (epistaxis) or secondary. The secondary group includes all bleedings that results from a known underlying disease. This category includes vascular injuries, benign and malignant tumors, postoperative or postirradiation bleeding, Rendu–Osler–Weber syndrome, the full spectrum of vascular malformations and tumors, diseases of the hematopoietic system, and inflammatory changes with vascular erosion.

Besides this initial differentiation between primary and secondary cause of bleeding, which relies on a detailed patient history and modern imaging, the treatment strategy also depends on the urgency of treatment (that is, whether the intervention must be done as an emergency procedure or can be performed electively).

Idiopathic Epistaxis

Epistaxis is classified as idiopathic if it has no demonstrable cause other than general risk factors such as hypertension and generalized atherosclerosis. Approximately 60% of the population experiences this event at least once during their lifetime. Most cases involve a single innocuous bleed that does not require medical treatment. Most of these mild nosebleeds result from the vulnerability of the Kiesselbach plexus in the anterior part of the nasal septum and usually follow a trivial injury. However, about 2 to 6% of nosebleeds are significant events that require medical attention.[175] The majority of these cases can be controlled by simple physical measures and occasionally require anterior or posterior intranasal packing. Unlike simple nosebleeds, these complicated bleeds originate mainly from the posterior portion of the nose.[176] If the foregoing measures are not sufficient to produce hemostasis, the condition is classified as intractable epistaxis.[177] In some cases this may become a life-threatening event. Several options are available to the surgeon in this situation:

1. Posterior nasal packing may be repeated, usually using the Bellocq method, and may be combined if necessary with superficial electrocautery of the nasal mucosa. Packing works by exerting pressure on the nasal mucosa to stop the bleeding without causing necrosis of the mucosa. The incidence of necrosis correlates with the intensity and duration of the pressure, which is why the packing should remain in place no more than a few days. Superficial electrocautery should not be too extensive for the same reason.
2. If the bleeding originates from the upper nose; thus, arising from the anterior or posterior ethmoidal branches of the ophthalmic artery, the source of the bleeding can be obliterated by surgical exposure and electrocautery of the bleeding vessels.
3. With bleeding from the posterior part of the nasal septum, the surgical option of last resort is vascular ligation.

Endovascular hemostatic therapy provides an alternative to surgical treatment and is an option in patients with recurrent bleeding (▶ Fig. 4.17). Selective visualization of the internal carotid artery is recommended initially to detect or exclude bleeding from the anterior or posterior ethmoidal artery. The external carotid is defined next. Although the internal maxillary artery is the principal source of intractable posterior epistaxis, the territories of the facial artery (lateral nasal artery, ascending palatine

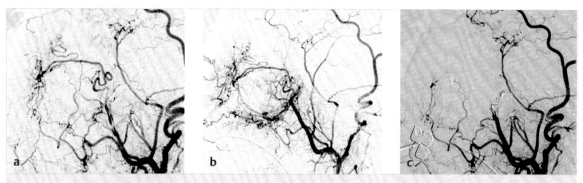

Fig. 4.17 a–c Idiopathic intractable epistaxis. A 55-year-old man with severe epistaxis and several treatments prior to the embolization (repeated anterior and posterior nasal packing, cauterizations). The angiogram of the external carotid artery demonstrates no visible extravasation of contrast agent in the early (**a**) and late (**b**) arterial phase. There are some irregularities and zones of high vascularity in the distal territory of the infraorbital artery, sphenopalatine arteries and the descending palatine artery, probably due to the packing and the prior treatment. Despite this "normal" angiogram the patient suffered from severe life-threatening epistaxis, which stopped immediately after embolization with PVA particles from small size (50–150 μm) in high dilution to medium size (150–300 μm) in lower dilution after PVA administration. The interventional procedure was finished with a proximal occlusion of the distal internal maxillary artery with placement of microcoils (**c**).

artery) and superficial temporal artery (transverse facial artery) should also be defined angiographically as potential bleeding sites. Some authors always include selective bilateral vascular imaging in their angiographic protocol.[178] However, it is reasonable to deviate from this protocol if clinical findings definitely localize the bleeding to a particular side.

Angiograms rarely provide direct evidence of bleeding by showing contrast extravasation. Increased vascular density on angiograms results mainly from the compression effect of intranasal packing on the mucosa. However, there are frequent indirect signs of a bleeding vessel such as caliber variations in the distal branches of the internal maxillary artery, collateralization, looping, or an increased vascular blush. The most common angiographic finding associated with intractable bleeding is a more or less normal angiogram.

Following coaxial insertion of the microcatheter system (larger-gauge systems are recommended when PVA particles will be used), embolization should be performed from a distal position. Swift placement of the coaxial system is important in emergency situations and is technically straightforward in most cases. Combined microcatheter–microwire systems have proven useful in these situations. If the bleeding originates from the internal maxillary artery, as is generally the case, the catheter tip should always be placed distal to the origin of the middle meningeal artery, or preferably in the pterygopalatine fossa proximal to the division of that vessel into the descending palatine artery, infraorbital artery, and sphenopalatine artery. A more distal placement by selective catheterization of the sphenopalatine artery, for example, is often not possible and is not advisable due to collateralization and carries a significant risk of vasospasm. The distal vascular territories can still be embolized from a

catheter placed in the pterygopalatine fossa. This is the major difference from clipping that vessel at the same location.

Small PVA particles in the 50 to 150 μm range make a suitable embolic agent and should be used in a highly diluted form. The particles can be suspended in a mixture of saline and contrast medium. As the embolization proceeds, the dilution should be decreased and larger particles (150–300 μm) should be used. In special cases when treating patients with Rendu–Osler–Weber syndrome a higher particle size and lower dilutions are recommended. Small gelatin sponge particles or gelatin sponge powder can be used as an alternative to PVA particles, although they provide only temporary vascular occlusion. Ultimately, gelatin sponge particles offer no real advantage over PVA. Angiographic series should be obtained during the procedure to document the progress of the embolization at intervals of 10 to 20 minutes. The intervals should shorten toward the end of the embolization, when there is greater likelihood that reflux will occur from the distal embolization and that preexisting collaterals to the intracranial vessels will be opened.

When the embolization is complete, angiography should demonstrate a patent internal maxillary artery past the origin of the middle meningeal artery. Finally a new survey angiogram of the external carotid artery should be obtained. If it shows no signs of early collateralization, the intervention is completed and the Bellocq packing may be removed in the angiography suite or not later than the following day. The success rate of this procedure is high and approaches 100% for intractable epistaxis and the complication rate is low. Unlike surgical ligation, the embolization may be repeated if bleeding should recur. For this reason, microcoils should not be placed proximally (e.g., in the internal maxillary artery) as they might be for a preoperative tumor embolization, to maintain access for recatheterization in the event that bleeding recurs.

The complications of this treatment are identical to those of cerebral angiography, which is why the procedure should be used cautiously in patients with severe atherosclerotic changes. Midfacial pain occurs as a side effect in about 25% of cases but is usually controllable with standard analgesic therapy. Necrosis of the skin or the mucosa is extremely rare even after bilateral embolization and the use of PVA particles in the 50 to 150 μm size range. Of course, embolization should not be too extensive in bilateral cases.

In summary, embolization therapy is a reasonable alternative to vessel ligation in the treatment of idiopathic intractable epistaxis. It provides distal occlusion at the precapillary level when embolized from the internal maxillary artery in the pterygopalatine fossa.[179,180,181] An additional advantage compared with surgery is that the treatment can be repeated if bleeding recurs.

Traumatic Bleeding

Posttraumatic bleeding in the face and neck region can generally be controlled by manual compression. Hemostasis is further supported by the soft-tissue swelling that often occurs in severely injured patients. If the patient continues to bleed despite all efforts, the bleeding vessel must be ligated as quickly as possible. Concomitant extensive swelling, especially in the midfacial region, can occasionally make it difficult or impossible to locate the vessel requiring ligation or determine the exact location of the bleeding site.

In this situation, angiography is helpful for locating the source of the bleeding and occlusion of the vessels by embolization in the same sitting. The angiographic findings will dictate the best embolization strategy, although individual cases may be influenced by various other factors such as the condition of the patient, pending operations that are more urgent, associated injuries, and the extent of blood loss. Larger particles in the 150 to 500 μm range are generally used in these emergency situations, and particles as large as 500 μm are sometimes used in hemodynamically unstable patients, as it is common to find large vascular cutoffs and time is a limiting factor when blood loss is severe. If neck injuries are present, both subclavian arteries and the vertebral arteries should always be imaged. If the vertebral artery or internal carotid artery is ruptured, the vessel should be occluded with a detachable balloon or coils. Before this is done, angiography should confirm that the contralateral arteries could deliver adequate collateral flow.

Because neither angiography nor clinical findings during test occlusion of the vertebral artery (unlike test occlusion of the internal carotid artery) can reliably predict the hemodynamic and functional impact of vertebral artery occlusion, the decision whether to perform this measure should be made in consultation with clinical colleagues based on the vital threat to the patient. In elective occlusion tests, it is helpful to add electrophysiologic monitoring, which would be too time consuming in emergency situations.

Another important point in the endovascular therapy of traumatic facial lesions relates to the treatment of posttraumatic aneurysms. Generally an interval of 10 days to 3 weeks passes from the trauma to the detection of the aneurysm. Because these lesions are generally pseudoaneurysms, which differ from true aneurysms by the absence of a vessel wall and a broad area of contact with the parent vessel, endovascular occlusion of the aneurysm and parent vessel is recommended.[182] The occlusion can be induced by PVA particles, as in idiopathic epistaxis, but the selection of particle size should be based on the size of the aneurysm and parent vessel. Generally there is no need to use small particles. Gelfoam particles are another option, although there is an increased risk of recurrence due to the temporary nature of the occlusion. Mechanical coils or detachable balloons are not advantageous even for occluding large aneurysms because, while the parent vessels remains intact, these devices are less reliable for obliterating the aneurysm and carry a risk of rebleeding due to recanalization.

Rendu–Osler–Weber Disease

Rendu–Osler–Weber disease, known also as hereditary hemorrhagic telangiectasia (HHT), is inherited as an autosomal dominant trait. A dysplastic disease of the vessel wall, it predominantly involves vessels and may therefore be manifested in all organs. HHT is compatible with life in heterozygous individuals only. The diagnosis is based on the triad of telangiectasia, recurrent bleeding, and a positive family history. Involvement of the facial skin and mucosae is very common. Multiorgan involvement can lead to a diversity of possible clinical manifestations. The facial skin and mucosae are among the sites of predilection. Almost all patients have recurrent episodes of mild to severe epistaxis, and there is a high incidence of fatal hemorrhage (4–27%) due to frequent and severe bleeding.[183]

Intranasal packing for hemostasis can be used only to a limited degree and at low pressure to avoid mucosal necrosis. Nd-YAG laser therapy reportedly has a positive influence on the course of HHT. In severe cases the anterior nasal mucosa can be replaced with a skin graft and this will affect the frequency and severity of the bleeds. Epistaxis is often accompanied by oral bleeding, but this condition rarely requires treatment and is even more rarely an indication for interventional therapy.

Embolization therapy can contribute to hemostasis in acute bleeds and will probably reduce the recurrence rate of epistaxis.[184] Interventional therapy is basically the same as the regimen described in the section on epistaxis, but a few special features should be noted. HHT patients with epistaxis have chronically deficient blood flow to the nasal mucosae and often have pre-existing areas of necrosis. For this reason, the use of standard amounts of small PVA particles may cause additional necrosis of the embolized mucosal areas and could actually promote the disease. Thus it is best to use embolization measures that are more limited in both the number and intensity of treatments. The use of medium- to large-sized particles at a lower dilution and smaller quantity produce the desired effects on hemostasis and recurrence rate while maintaining acceptable blood flow to the nasal mucosa. Gelatin sponge or other embolic materials are also suitable. Unfortunately, the overall progression of the disease is not influenced by embolization or any of the other therapies.

Embolization of Tumors

Tumor embolization has two principal goals. First, it may be part of the overall treatment strategy and can be used preoperatively to improve tumor clearance or even reduce a tumor to operable size. To achieve this goal, embolization must induce necrosis of the tumor bed and devascularization through the selection of a suitable embolic material and sufficiently selective catheterization of the tumor vessels. Generally this requires a comprehensive, preinterventional angiographic work-up and a careful analysis of the tumor angioarchitecture. Details on the treatment of paragangliomas and juvenile nasopharyngeal fibromas are presented below to illustrate tumor embolization in the face and neck region. Similar techniques are used on other hypervascular tumors of the face and neck, especially capillary hemangiomas, which are not described in this chapter.

The second fundamentally different goal of tumor embolization is the palliative treatment of tumors, most notably malignancies. In the face and neck region, this large group consists primarily of SCCs. With SCCs as with other tumors, embolization can induce necrosis and devascularization of the nonnecrotic portions of the tumor, although often this is not the primary goal. Since the treatment of most malignancies involves a combination of surgery and chemoradiation, embolization therapy is withheld at most centers to maximize response to radiotherapy, which correlates positively with the oxygen saturation of the tissue.

In most cases, then, interventional treatments for squamous cancers are limited to purely palliative hemostasis for tumor hemorrhage or isolated treatments for tumor reduction or pain relief when other forms of treatment are no longer appropriate. It should be noted, however, that tumor embolization provides very little pain relief. Percutaneous and peritumoral infiltration therapy with concentrated alcohol or other agents is preferred for this indication. This is rarely practiced today, however, owing to advances in pain management.

To illustrate these principles, the two sections below deal with two types of tumors suitable for embolization as a preoperative or standalone interventional therapy at many interventional centers.

Paragangliomas

Paragangliomas (formerly called chemodectomas when located at the carotid bifurcation) are benign tumors that contain cells derived from the neural crest and consequently are of neuroectodermal origin. Sometimes they are referred incorrectly as glomus tumors. They are known as paragangliomas because they arise from parasympathetic paraganglia. In addition to the common benign form, however, there are also malignant forms which invade surrounding tissues and metastasize.

Paragangliomas have four sites of predilection in the head and neck region. They are designated by their location as carotid paragangliomas (carotid body tumors, chemodectomas, ▶ Fig. 4.18), vagal paragangliomas (glomus vagale tumors), tympanic paragangliomas (glomus tympanicum tumors, ▶ Fig. 4.19), and jugular paragangliomas (glomus jugulare tumors, ▶ Fig. 4.20).[185] The tumors often grow slowly over a period of years, and initial complaints appear only after the tumor has reached considerable size. As with juvenile angiofibromas, preoperative embolization can allow for a safer and more radical surgical removal. This particularly applies to large, multicompartmental tumors. If the clinical symptoms are mild and the tumor is monocompartmental and shows very little progression over time, embolization alone may relieve the patient's complaints for years. As an isolated palliative measure, embolization is also recommended in patients for whom surgery would pose a high functional risk or who would be classified as high-risk patients due to age and comorbidity. Because these tumors are often multifocal and bilateral, their angiographic evaluation should include selective bilateral views of the vertebral artery, internal carotid artery, and external carotid artery, along with selective views covering at least the internal maxillary artery, occipital artery, ascending pharyngeal artery, and posterior auricular artery. Paragangliomas in this region are often supplied by branches of the external carotid artery and show a typical focal blush of rapid onset, which persists for some time and may be drained by various venous pathways. Arteriovenous shunts may appear along with the actual tumor vessels and are important in determining the embolization strategy and providing the surgeon with important preinterventional and preoperative information.

Encasement or infiltration of the internal carotid artery is often present, especially with large paragangliomas. Test occlusion of the internal carotid artery is recommended in these cases as described above. If the patient cannot

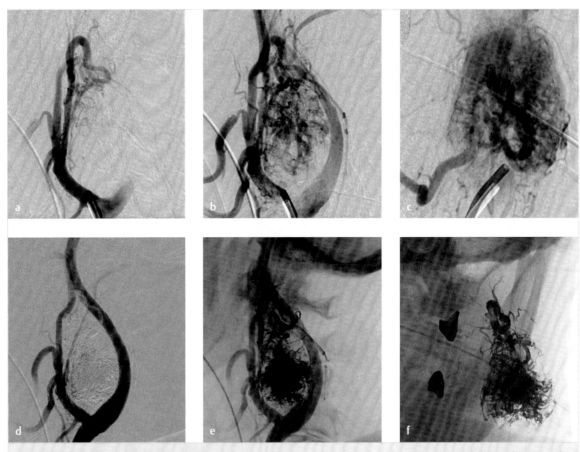

Fig. 4.18 a–f Carotid paraganglioma treated preoperatively with a direct approach. A 66-year-old woman with a typical angiographic appearance of a carotid paraganglioma. Note the very early and intensive inhomogeneous tumor blush (**a, b** lateral view), which stays long after the venous phase of the angiogram (**c**, anteroposterior view). The widening of the carotid bifurcation is typical for these tumors. After direct puncture of the tumor and delivery of Onyx 18, 21, and 34, there is no contrast agent visible in the tumor bed in the angiogram after the procedure (**d**). The unsubtracted digital angiogram (**e**) in the lateral view and the cast of the embolic material alone is demonstrated in anteroposterior view (**f**). Two days after the intervention the tumor was removed without any blood loss for the patient.

tolerate the test occlusion, the interventional and surgical strategy should be modified accordingly. If radical surgery is necessary, a high-flow bypass and the possibility of pre-operative stent insertion should be discussed before the procedure. The stent would be implanted into the internal carotid artery through the tumor-encased segment, and the surgeon could then remove the tumor as far as the stent, increasing the degree of tumor clearance.[186] One dis-advantage of this method is the waiting period between stent implantation and surgery. The surgeon must wait at least 6 to 8 weeks for endothelialization to occur as a neo-intima forms on the inner surface of the stent. A 3-month course of combined aspirin and clopidogrel therapy is also necessary to minimize the risk of stent thrombosis and thromboembolic complications both before and after stent implantation.

The embolization strategy is guided by the overall treatment plan and whether the intervention is pre-

operative or palliative. The goal in both cases is to occlude as many tumor compartments as possible by selective catheterization of their feeders and embolization of the tumor bed. Particle sizes from 100 and 300 μm are best for embolization. Since the goal of the embolization is to devascularize the tumor parenchyma rather than obliter-ate the tumor vessels, particle injection should be per-formed according to the principles described in the section on particulate agents. One principle is to start with the smallest particles at high dilution, then reduce the dilution, and finally increase the particle size. Some authors see major advantages in using microspheres, which are used with the same technique and in the same sizes. Following adequate distal embolization of the tumor parenchyma with particles, the procedure con-cludes with a proximal feeder occlusion using microcoils, for example. Another option is direct puncture of the tumor followed by injection of liquid polymers

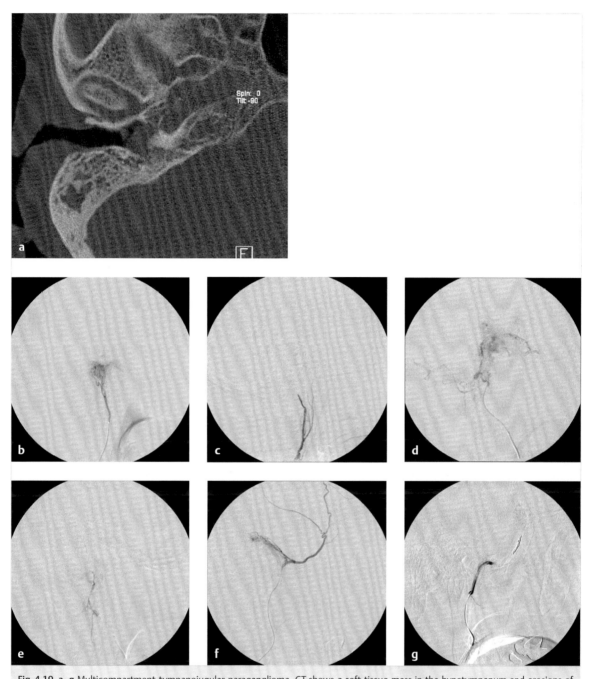

Fig. 4.19 a–g Multicompartment tympanojugular paraganglioma. CT shows a soft-tissue mass in the hypotympanum and erosions of the jugular bulb (**a**). A staged embolization through feeders supplied by the ascending pharyngeal artery (**b**), posterior auricular artery (PAA) (**c**), and middle meningeal arteries (**d**) was performed after selective catheterization of the feeders with a microcatheter using microspheres of 100 to 300 μm as embolic material. The postinterventional angiograms demonstrate a complete devascularization (**e–g**) of the tumor.

(cyanoacrylates)[187] or ethylene vinyl alcohol copolymers (Onyx) under fluoroscopic control.[188,189,190] At present we cannot offer a definitive recommendation on which strategy is best, and the decision will depend mainly on the experience and background of the interventionalist.

In summary, preoperative angiographic work-up is essential for paragangliomas. While not always necessary for making a diagnosis, angiography is of major importance in determining the interventional and surgical strategy. Test occlusion should always be considered in

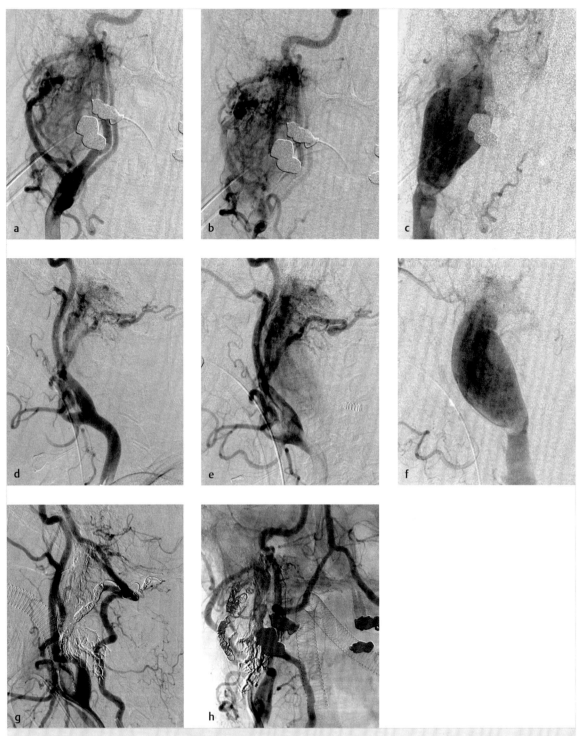

Fig. 4.20 a–h Jugular paraganglioma treated preoperatively with a transarterial approach. A 69-year-oldwoman with a giant jugular paraganglioma suffered only from swelling and a mild tinnitus. The angiogram in lateral (**a–c**) and anterior–posterior (**d–f**) view in different phases from early to late shows the intensive hypervascularized tumor. There was also supply from muscle branches of the vertebral artery (not shown). After transarterial embolization with Onyx and n-butyl-2-cyanoacrylate only a small amount a tumor vascularization at the dorsal upper part of the tumor is still visible. Demonstrated in a subtracted (**g**) and unsubtracted (**h**) lateral view after injection of contrast in the common carotid artery and vertebral artery simultaneously at the end of the procedure.

patients with large tumors and vascular encasement. The goals of endovascular therapy as well as the extent of tumor clearance should be defined between the neuroradiologist and operative surgeon according to the treatment goal and the extent of disease. The target site for devascularization is the tumor bed and not the vessels feeding the paraganglioma.

Juvenile Nasopharyngeal Angiofibromas

Juvenile nasopharyngeal angiofibroma (JNA) is a benign, locally destructive tumor that originates in the posterolateral roof of the nasopharynx. It predominantly affects young males. JNA is the most common benign tumor in adolescents. Because of its slow growth, the tumor may be asymptomatic for a long time and then present clinically with signs of nasal obstruction and epistaxis. Tumors at an advanced stage may cause unilateral or bilateral maxillary sinusitis, nasal discharge, swelling of deep and superficial facial structures, cranial nerve palsies, and exophthalmos. Intracranial extension, especially into the cavernous sinus, may incite symptoms of cavernous sinus syndrome with cranial nerve deficits, CSF rhinorrhea, altered mental status, and signs of increased intracranial pressure. Pathways of tumor spread into preexisting spaces and cavities and the locally destructive growth explain the clinical symptoms. Initially the tumor expands anteriorly into the nasal cavity and posteriorly into the nasopharynx. As this occurs, adjacent bony structures may be displaced (deviated nasal septum, anterior bulge in the posterior antral wall), or they may be partially or completely destroyed. These changes are a result of local pressure effects rather than bone invasion by the tumor. If it continues to grow unchecked, the tumor will expand into the pterygopalatine and infratemporal fossae and invade the orbit from below through the inferior orbital fissure. Intracranial extension occurs as the JNA grows through the nasal roof into the anterior cranial fossa, through the middle fossa via the foramen lacerum lateral to the cavernous sinus, or through the sella between the pituitary gland and internal carotid artery medial to the cavernous sinus.

JNA is hypervascular, which explains its intense enhancement on CT and MRI as well as the strong tumor blush that appears on angiograms in the early capillary phase and persists into the capillary and venous phases. The vascularity also explains the often severe hemorrhages that occur as the disease progresses. Since the tumor does not respect the facial midline or cranial cavity, preoperative and interventional angiographic studies should include selective views of the external carotid artery and internal carotid artery as well as superselective views of at least the internal maxillary artery, facial artery, and ascending pharyngeal artery on both sides. Because the tumor is hypervascular, preoperative embolization is always desired and should be an established part of tumor therapy. Embolization will reduce intraoperative blood loss, shorten the duration of surgery, and increase the degree of tumor clearance, resulting in a lower risk of recurrence. JNA has a recurrence rate of about 17%, which rises to 50% if intracranial extension has already occurred.

Tumor embolization with small or medium-sized PVA particles has proven effective. Changing from small to larger particles is recommended, depending on the timing of the proposed surgery, and is also recommended during the course of the embolization. Saline dilution of the particles is also changed from a high to lower dilution. Thus the embolization strategy is the same as that described for paragangliomas. Again, it may be prudent to occlude the proximal tumor feeders or internal maxillary artery prior to the operation. Multiple sessions are often required, and surgery should be scheduled from the next up to 5 days after the last embolization.

The embolization of large masses should start with branches of the external maxillary artery, generally the internal maxillary artery and ascending pharyngeal artery. If direct branches from the carotid siphon contribute to tumor vascularity, usually these vessels are small and cannot be directly catheterized. In these situations where the tumor is fed by branches of the internal carotid artery, it may be appropriate to consider direct particulate embolization from the internal carotid artery with temporary distal balloon protection, test occlusion of the internal carotid artery, and possible definitive occlusion of the internal carotid artery, depending on the clinical symptoms and tumor size and the desired degree of tumor clearance. Definitive occlusion of the internal carotid artery with embolization after prior test occlusion under neurologic control, once widely recommended, is practiced today only if surgical ligation of the vessel is planned. From an interventional standpoint, temporary supraophthalmic occlusion of the internal carotid artery is adequate to embolize the small vessels from the carotid siphon that supply the tumor. Major difficulties arise when the tumor is supplied by the ethmoidal branches of the ophthalmic artery. This situation justifies a wait-and-see approach to determine whether embolization of the internal maxillary artery will reduce or even eliminate ethmoidal tumor feeders detectable by angiography. If this is not the case, direct embolization via the ophthalmic artery is appropriate only if orbital tumor invasion has already caused a complete or near-complete loss of vision before the intervention. Otherwise electrocautery of the ethmoidal vessels can be performed immediately before the operation. In all cases the overall treatment strategy should be determined in closely with the surgeon.[191]

Vascular Malformations

Treatment of vascular malformations in the face and neck is an important part of endovascular interventional therapy and often is an important prelude to subsequent surgical resection. It can critically reduce lesion volume prior to surgical treatment. Even when used alone, it can often eliminate vascular pathology or is able to reach a cosmetically and medically acceptable result in inoperable or hard-to-reach facial regions and malformations. The angiographic work-up aids greatly in the classification of vascular malformations, although there is still no generally accepted classification scheme. This explains why so many classification systems are in current use. For clarity, we will classify vascular malformations based on angiographic criteria owing to their practical relevance. The following criteria are important in terms of treatment strategy, and the following questions should be answered by angiographic imaging (and MRI and CT if necessary) prior to every intervention and/or operation:

1. Is the lesion a vascular tumor, an arteriovenous fistula, or arteriovenous malformation?
2. Does the vascular pathology contain any arteriovenous shunts, and if yes, is the flow gradient across the shunt a low-, medium-, or high-flow connection?
3. How does the vascular pathology appear in the arterial, capillary, and venous phases (e.g., for distinguishing between an arterial and capillary–venous hemangioma)?
4. Does angiography show connections between the tumor vessels and intracranial vessels ("dangerous anastomoses")?
5. Do the arterial feeders have a significant impact on normal brain and facial circulation?
6. How is the collateral supply to the affected region?
7. What is the presumptive risk of intraoperative bleeding?
8. Is the preoperative or preinterventional test occlusion of one or more vessels necessary for making treatment decisions?

Answers to these questions, inferred from angiographic data, provide a rationale for the basic planning the interventional and/or operative strategy.

Arteriovenous Malformations

Arteriovenous malformations are abnormal communications between arterial and venous vessels that bypass the normal capillary bed. The arteriovenous malformations include a nidus of variable size and shape. Intracranial arteriovenous malformations most commonly arise from nonfunctional dysplastic tissue and thus do not pose a problem for endovascular interventional therapy or surgical measures. Along with the arteriovenous fistulas, they are the true vascular malformations. They should be described as malformations, not as angiomas, since they are not tumors in the true sense. Like tumors, they have a tendency to growth on the base of proliferative activity. This activity is based on hemodynamic factors, caused mainly by flow, and angiogenetic impact. For this reason the term "angioma" should be applied exclusively to true vascular tumors such as hemangiomas. There is no basic

hemodynamic difference between arteriovenous fistulas and arteriovenous malformations. However, arteriovenous malformations have a nidus that is not present in arteriovenous fistulas.

Arteries are usually dilated and open directly into a normal or pathologic vein. It is fairly common to find mixed patterns of vascular pathology in which arteriovenous malformations contain fistulous compartments. Both types of lesion require comprehensive angiographic study, since they may be supplied by multiple arterial feeders located far from the actual nidus or the point of the fistula, where it connects directly to the vein(s). Also, the presence of multiple arteriovenous malformations is not uncommon. Following the angiographic study, the treatment strategy should be discussed with the surgeon. The following questions should be addressed:

1. Is surgical treatment possible, and what is the presumed risk of intraoperative bleeding?
2. Which compartments would be most difficult for the surgeon in terms of location and anticipated blood loss?
3. How many preoperative endovascular sessions will be needed, and what would be the interval from the treatments to operation?
4. Is there a need for a preinterventional and/or preoperative test occlusion?
5. Is radiotherapy an option?
6. If surgery is not possible, is it reasonable to proceed with endovascular therapy alone? What is the goal—flow reduction or complete obliteration of the malformation?

Published data vary on the last point regarding the goals and benefits of endovascular therapy alone for arteriovenous malformations. Some authors maintain that a simple flow reduction and obliteration of certain compartments are helpful in reducing the bleeding risk, while others dispute this effect and even claim that the risk of bleeding is increased. On the whole, it is unlikely that partial occlusion will be of much benefit for arteriovenous malformations, although it may help to relieve the symptoms of some arteriovenous fistulas (e.g., it may improve tinnitus caused by a dural arteriovenous fistula). A detailed discussion of these interesting questions would exceed the scope of this survey article.

Many different embolic materials may be used in the setting of combination therapy (embolization and surgery). Onyx and cyanoacrylates have proven effective and are particularly recommended if monotherapy is the goal of the interventional procedure. The catheterization of arterial feeders is usually successful, at least to the intranidal level, using flow-directed microcatheters. Arteriovenous fistulas in the arteriovenous malformation and flow-related intracranial and extracranial aneurysms require a different strategy and treatment than arteriovenous malformations without these characteristics. Detachable and nondetachable microcoils, PVA particles, and other embolic agents can also be used, especially in the treatment of arteriovenous fistulas. Despite all the classification systems, this disease requires an individualized treatment concept based on the individual angioarchitecture, hemodynamics, and localization of the vascular pathology. The concept should be decided on an interdisciplinary basis before every treatment and should include the option of radiotherapy.

Arteriovenous malformations of the face and neck region, unlike intracranial arteriovenous malformations, are classified into three stages: quiescent, expansile (i.e., growing), and locally destructive. Two-thirds of malformations are located in the midfacial region and are particularly common in the cheek, ear, nose, and forehead. The cosmetic aspect of arteriovenous malformations in the face and neck region is a special issue that must be considered along with the danger of skin necrosis and the possibility of plastic surgery, and these considerations will influence the selection of embolic materials. For example, Onyx is as effective for facial arteriovenous malformations as it is intracranially, but with malformations that have extensive subcutaneous involvement, the shine-through effect of the black tantalum is cosmetically objectionable and would contraindicate its use in these patients.[192] While one or two sessions are usually adequate for the preoperative endovascular therapy of intracranial arteriovenous malformations, the size of facial and neck lesions will often require multiple sessions to achieve a cosmetically acceptable result or prepare for surgery.

Most malformations in the head and neck region are not associated with an arteriovenous shunt and are described as low-flow venous or capillary–venous malformations. They are usually treated with sclerosing agents administered by direct injection. A catheter-based angiographic study is usually not required and in most cases is done only to exclude arterial feeders. Patients present for medical treatment due to functional complains, recurrent bleeds, and especially for cosmetic reasons because arteriovenous malformations or hemangiomas in the craniofacial region are often disfiguring.

Because transarterial endovascular treatment is not possible, direct puncture of the venous malformation is an option in patients who have been selected for endovascular treatment. Numerous embolic agents with a sclerosing action are cited in the literature including ethanol, sodium tetradecyl sulfate, and many others. Regardless of which embolic agent is used, the section below lists a few basic treatment principles that should be followed. They are valid for all embolic agents that are injected directly into a compartment for devascularization.

After sterile draping of the site, a needle is introduced directly into the vascular lesion, followed by contrast injection and angiographic imaging. The angioarchitecture and hemodynamic profile are documented. Bolus injection is done to confirm or exclude significant centripetal venous drainage into the right atrium. If this drainage is present,

the embolic agent should be injected only after the drainage has been stopped. This is often accomplished in the face and neck region by manual compression of the draining vessels, dependent positioning of the upper body, or a Valsalva maneuver during the therapy to raise the intrathoracic pressure.

Repeated sessions are often necessary and require a cooperative patient, especially in cases where surgical removal is impossible or unacceptable for cosmetic reasons. Pain often occurs after embolization but responds well to simple analgesics. Postinterventional swelling is problematic, especially with large vascular lesions that are close to the upper airways. This may require patient monitoring in an intermediate care unit after the procedure or in an intensive care unit after general endotracheal anesthesia. Peri-interventional corticosteroid therapy is recommended in these cases, but its benefits are controversial.

A cosmetically favorable result or volume reduction is often achieved even with very extensive hemangiomas. Sometimes surgical resection actually becomes possible after endovascular therapy. With incurable hemangiomas, appropriate counseling and education about the importance of repeated sessions can be of tremendous benefit for patients and family members.

Dural arteriovenous fistulas and carotid-cavernous fistulas are the most common types of arteriovenous fistula. They are classified according to hemodynamic criteria and can be treated by transarterial and transvenous endovascular therapy (▶ Fig. 4.21). Carotid-cavernous fistulas are classified as direct or indirect. Indirect carotid-cavernous fistulas can also be treated with particles and microcoils, while direct carotid-cavernous fistulas often require the use of detachable balloons, transvenous treatment with detachable coils, as well as frequent occlusion of the internal carotid artery, which would require preinterventional test occlusion of that vessel.[193]

To summarize, vascular lesions are differentiated into vascular tumors and malformations. Their classification and treatment is complex and should be determined on an interdisciplinary basis. Regardless of the individual treatment concept, treatment should always be preceded by a comprehensive angiographic study.

Aneurysms

Aneurysms of the face and neck region are rarely congenital, unlike intracranial aneurysms, and are far less common than "berry aneurysms" in the circle of Willis. Rare entities, most of which have already been described, are traumatic aneurysms of the common carotid artery, internal carotid artery (extradural segment), and external carotid artery and their branches, especially after severe midfacial trauma, pseudoaneurysms after surgery (e.g., tonsillectomy) and/or irradiation. Other even rarer etiologies include flow-related aneurysms associated with

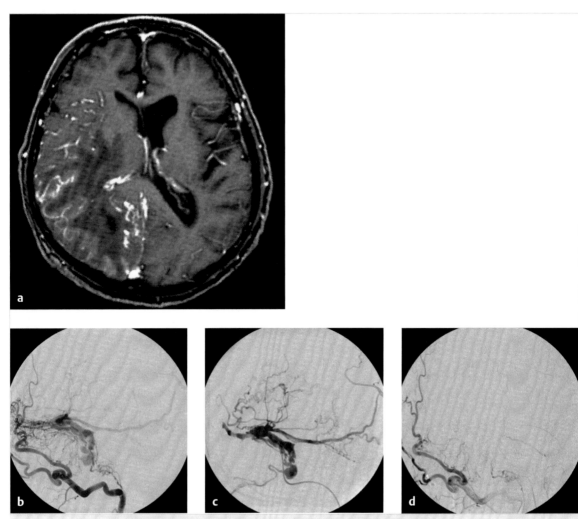

Fig. 4.21 a–d Type IV dural arteriovenous fistula (Classification of Cognard) leading to venous congestion. **(a)** T1 W MRI following contrast medium application depicts dilated draining pial veins and an interstitial brain edema. **(b)** Selective injection into the occipital artery shows a myriad of feeders converging into an isolated segment of the transverse sinus. Note the exclusively leptomeningeal drainage into veins of the temporal lobe. **(c)** A guiding catheter can be placed in the patent segment using a transvenous access. **(d)** Complete devascularization was achieved with packing of the segment with detachable platinum coils.

arteriovenous fistulas and malformations, mycotic aneurysms, and aneurysms in patients with angiodysplasia.

A characteristic feature of traumatic and postoperative pseudoaneurysms is that they may become symptomatic due to bleeding between 10 and 14 days after the trauma or the surgical procedure. Shorter intervals have not yet been reported. The aneurysms usually present clinically with epistaxis and postoperative pharyngeal bleeding after tonsillectomies in which the usual hemostatic measures, including surgical intervention, were often unsuccessful. Accordingly, the most commonly affected vessels are the internal maxillary artery in the pterygopalatine fossa (midfacial fracture) and the lingual and facial arteries after tonsillectomy.[194,195]

The treatment of external carotid artery aneurysms, like their etiology, is fundamentally different from the endovascular therapy of intracranial aneurysms. Because of their pathogenesis, extracranial aneurysms often have a broad connection with the parent vessel based on a tear in the vessel wall, similar to a pseudoaneurysm. Because the external carotid artery vessels communicate closely with one another in the transverse, horizontal, and vertical directions, every isolated aneurysm occlusion is prone to revascularization. It is best, therefore, to obliterate both the saccular protrusion and the parent vessel itself. Usually this can be done in the facial region without adverse functional consequences for the patient. Medium-sized PVA particles are the embolic material of first choice in these situations for producing secure and permanent occlusion of the parent vessel without jeopardizing integrity of the skin and underlying mucosa. More complex measures for endovascular aneurysm occlusion in the intracranial region or of extracranial portions of intra-cranial vessels (electrolytic detachable coils, covered or bare stents, temporary stents, and temporary balloons [remodeling technique]) are usually not necessary in the territory of the external carotid artery. This point should always be kept in mind, because PVA particles have proven to be a highly effective and economical solution. This is true as long as the parent vessel does not need to be preserved. But if it is necessary to preserve the main-taining vessel, the same principles and strategies apply as for the endovascular therapy of intracranial aneurysms.

Summary

Endovascular therapy is an established treatment modal-ity for many vascular diseases in the face and neck region. A major application is the preoperative embolization of hypervascular tumors (such as paragangliomas and JNAs) to enable a more complete resection; thus, lowering their recurrence rate. Endovascular therapy can also be used as a standalone palliative or even curative treatment for vascular malformations and recurrent bleeding. The spe-cial hemodynamic conditions in the skull base and face and neck regions, which are characterized by numerous interconnections among different vascular territories, require a therapeutic approach that is optimally tailored to those conditions. This includes placing a vascular occlusion as close to the actual lesion as possible. With refinements in catheter systems and the use of various embolic agents, interventional neuroradiology has access to tools that can effectively treat most of the vascular pathologies.

Endovascular interventions are suitable not only for elective treatments but also for emergency situations, especially in patients with life-threatening bleeding.

The source of the bleeding can be located and elimi-nated in one endovascular session. The principle of the progressive occlusion of bleeding vessels, proceeding in a distal-to-proximal direction with retrograde technique, offers a high success rate with effective protection from recurrent bleeds.[195]

Given the interdisciplinary approach to the treatment of many vascular lesions in the skull base and face and neck regions, it is essential to foster effective communica-tion between interventional and surgical colleagues and to develop coordinated treatment strategies. Moreover, peri-interventional care of the patient before, during, and after the procedure in immediate and intensive care units is crucial to the successful management of patients with complex vascular diseases.

References

[1] Schuknecht B, Simmen D. Importance of radiological imaging of the sinuses [in German]. Laryngorhinootologie 2002; 81: 126–146

[2] Konen E, Faibel M, Kleinbaum Y et al. State of the Art. Diagnostic imaging of paranasal sinus diseases [in German]. Clin Radiol 2000; 55: 856–860

[3] Simmen D, Jones N. Manual of Endoscopic Sinus Surgery: and Extended Applications. Stuttgart: Thieme; 2005

[4] Yousem DM, Gad K, Tufano RP. Resectability issues with head and neck cancer. AJNR Am J Neuroradiol 2006; 27: 2024–2036

[5] Holzmann D, Hegyi I, Rajan GP, Harder-Ruckstuhl M. Management of benign inverted sinonasal papilloma avoiding external approaches. J Laryngol Otol 2007; 121: 548–554

[6] Brors D, Draf W. The treatment of inverted papilloma Curr Opin Otolaryngol Head Neck Surg 1999; 7: 33–38

[7] Loevner LA, Sonners AI. Imaging of neoplasms of the paranasal sinuses. Magn Reson Imaging Clin N Am 2002; 10: 467–493

[8] Bockmuehl U. Malignant tumours of the paranasal sinuses and the anterior skull base. In: Anniko A, Bernal-Sprekelsen B, Bonkowsky V, Bradley PJ, Iurato S, eds. Otorhinolaryngology, Head and Neck Surgery (European Manual of Medicine). Berlin: Springer 2010:301–309

[9] Citardi MJ, Batra PS. Intraoperative surgical navigation for endoscopic sinus surgery: rationale and indications. Curr Opin Otolaryngol Head Neck Surg 2007; 15: 23–27

[10] Cohen NA, Kennedy DW. Endoscopic sinus surgery: where we are- and where we're going. Curr Opin Otolaryngol Head Neck Surg 2005; 13: 32–38

[11] Minovi A, Kollert M, Draf W, Bockmühl U. Inverted papilloma: feasi-bility of endonasal surgery and long-term results of 87 cases. Rhinol-ogy 2006; 44: 205–210

[12] Lee DK, Chung SK, Dhong HJ, Kim HY, Kim HJ, Bok KH. Focal hyperos-tosis on CT of sinonasal inverted papilloma as a predictor of tumor origin. AJNR Am J Neuroradiol 2007; 28: 618–621

[13] Dammann F, Pereira P, Laniado M, Plinkert P, Löwenheim H, Claussen CD. Inverted papilloma of the nasal cavity and the paranasal sinuses: using CT for primary diagnosis and follow-up. AJR Am J Roentgenol 1999; 172: 543–548

[14] Krouse JH. Endoscopic treatment of inverted papilloma: safety and efficacy. Am J Otolaryngol 2001; 22: 87–99

[15] Maroldi R, Farina D, Palvarini L, Lombardi D, Tomenzoli D, Nicolai P. Magnetic resonance imaging findings of inverted papilloma: differ-ential diagnosis with malignant sinonasal tumors. Am J Rhinol 2004; 18: 305–310

[16] Ojiri H. Potentially distinctive features of sinonasal inverted papil-loma on MR imaging. AJR Am J Roentgenol 2000; 175: 465–468

[17] Jeon TY, Kim HJ, Chung SK et al. Sinonasal inverted papilloma: value of convoluted cerebriform pattern on MR imaging. AJNR Am J Neuro-radiol 2008; 29: 1556–1560

[18] Som PM, Lawson W, Lidov MW. Simulated aggressive skull base ero-sion in response to benign sinonasal disease. Radiology 1991; 180: 755–759

[19] Unlu HH, Songu M, Ovali GY, Nese N. Inverted papilloma with new bone formation: report of three cases. Am J Rhinol 2007; 21: 607–610

[20] Karkos PD, Khoo LC, Leong SC, Lewis-Jones H, Swift AC. Computed tomography and/or magnetic resonance imaging for pre-operative planning for inverted nasal papilloma: review of evidence. J Laryngol Otol 2009; 123: 705–709

[21] Earwaker J. Paranasal sinus osteomas: a review of 46 cases. Skeletal Radiol 1993; 22: 417–423

[22] Schick B, Steigerwald C, el Rahman el Tahan A, Draf W. The role of endonasal surgery in the management of frontoethmoidal osteomas. Rhinology 2001; 39: 66–70

[23] Nabeshima K, Marutsuka K, Shimao Y, Uehara H, Kodama T. Osteoma of the frontal sinus complicated by intracranial mucocele. Pathol Int 2003; 53: 227–230

[24] Shady JA, Bland LI, Kazee AM, Pilcher WH. Osteoma of the front-oethmoidal sinus with secondary brain abscess and intracranial mucocele: case report. Neurosurgery 1994; 34: 920–923; discussion 923

[25] Gutenberg A, Larsen J, Rohde V. Frontal sinus osteoma complicated by extended intracranial mucocele and cerebral abscess: neuro-surgical strategy of a rare clinical entity. Cent Eur Neurosurg 2009; 70: 95–97

[26] Johnson D, Tan L. Intraparenchymal tension pneumatocele complicating frontal sinus osteoma: case report. Neurosurgery 2002; 50: 878–879; discussion 880

[27] Brunori A, de Santis S, Bruni P, Delitala A, Giuffre R, Chiappetta F. Life threatening intracranial complications of frontal sinus osteomas: report of two cases. Acta Neurochir (Wien) 1996; 138: 1426–1430

[28] Park MC, Goldman MA, Donahue JE, Tung GA, Goel R, Sampath P. Endonasal ethmoidectomy and bifrontal craniotomy with craniofacial approach for resection of frontoethmoidal osteoma causing tension pneumocephalus. Skull Base 2008; 18: 67–72

[29] Naraghi M, Kashfi A. Endonasal endoscopic resection of ethmoido-orbital osteoma compressing the optic nerve. Am J Otolaryngol 2003; 24: 408–412

[30] Castelnuovo P, Valentini V, Giovannetti F, Bignami M, Cassoni A. Iannetti G. Osteomas of the maxillofacial district: endoscopic surgery versus open surgery. J Craniofac Surg 2008; 19: 1446–1452

[31] Casselman JW, De Jonge I, Neyt L, De Clercq C, D'Hont G. MRI in craniofacial fibrous dysplasia. Neuroradiology 1993; 35: 234–237

[32] Chen YR, Wong FH, Hsueh C, Lo LJ. Computed tomography characteristics of non-syndromic craniofacial fibrous dysplasia. Chang Gung Med J 2002; 25: 1–8(engl.)

[33] Lustig LR, Holliday MJ, McCarthy EF, Nager GT. Fibrous dysplasia involving the skull base and temporal bone. Arch Otolaryngol Head Neck Surg 2001; 127: 1239–1247

[34] Parmar H, Gujar S, Shah G, Mukherji SK. Imaging of the anterior skull base. Neuroimaging Clin N Am 2009; 19: 427–439

[35] Jee W-H, Choi KH, Choe BY, Park JM, Shinn KS. Fibrous dysplasia: MR imaging characteristics with radiopathologic correlation. AJR Am J Roentgenol 1996; 167: 1523–1527

[36] Som PM, Schatz CJ, Flaum EG, Lanman TH. Aneurysmal bone cyst of the paranasal sinuses associated with fibrous dysplasia: CT and MR findings. J Comput Assist Tomogr 1991; 15: 513–515

[37] Han MH, Chang KH, Lee CH, Seo JW, Han MC, Kim CW. Sinonasal psammomatoid ossifying fibromas: CT and MR manifestations. AJNR Am J Neuroradiol 1991; 12: 25–30

[38] Nakagawa K, Takasato Y, Ito Y, Yamada K. Ossifying fibroma involving the paranasal sinuses, orbit, and anterior cranial fossa: case report. Neurosurgery 1995; 36: 1192–1195

[39] Sterling KM, Stollman A, Sacher M, Som PM. Ossifying fibroma of sphenoid bone with coexistent mucocele: CT and MRI. J Comput Assist Tomogr 1993; 17: 492–494

[40] Kendi ATK, Kara S, Altinok D, Keskil S. Sinonasal ossifying fibroma with fluid-fluid levels on MR images. AJNR Am J Neuroradiol 2003; 24: 1639–1641

[41] El-Saggan A, Olofsson J, Krossnes B. Sinonasal schwannoma: two case reports and review of literature. Int Congr Ser 2003; 1240: 503–507

[42] Yu E, Mikulis D, Nag S. CT and MR imaging findings in sinonasal schwannoma. AJNR Am J Neuroradiol 2006; 27: 929–930

[43] Sharma R, Tyagi I, Banerjee D, Pandey R. Nasoethmoid schwannoma with intracranial extension. Case report and review of literature. Neurosurg Rev 1998; 21: 58–61

[44] Murakami M, Tsukahara T, Hatano T, Nakakuki T, Ogino E, Aoyama T. Olfactory groove schwannoma—case report. Neurol Med Chir (Tokyo) 2004; 44: 191–194

[45] Ulu EMK, Cakmak O, Dönmez FY et al. Sinonasal schwannoma of the middle turbinate. Diagn Interv Radiol 2010; 16: 129–131

[46] Shinohara K, Hashimoto K, Yamashita M, Omori K. Schwannoma of the nasal septum removed with endoscopic surgery. Otolaryngol Head Neck Surg 2005; 132: 963–964

[47] Mannan AASR, Singh MK, Bahadur S, Hatimota P, Sharma MC. Solitary malignant schwannoma of the nasal cavity and paranasal sinuses: report of two rare cases. Ear Nose Throat J 2003; 82: 634–636, 638, 640

[48] Sanchez-Mejia RO, Pham DN, Prados M et al. Management of a sporadic malignant subfrontal peripheral nerve sheath tumor. J Neuro-oncol 2006; 76: 165–169

[49] Schick B, Kahle G. Radiological findings in angiofibroma. Acta Radiol 2000; 41: 585–593

[50] Sennes LU, Butugan O, Sanchez TG, Bento RF, Tsuji DH. Juvenile nasopharyngeal angiofibroma: the routes of invasion. Rhinology 2003; 41: 235–240

[51] Snyderman CH, Pant H, Carrau RL, Gardner P. A new endoscopic staging system for angiofibromas. Arch Otolaryngol Head Neck Surg 2010; 136: 588–594

[52] Sessions RB, Bryan RN, Naclerio RM, Alford BR. Radiographic staging of juvenile angiofibroma. Head Neck Surg 1981; 3: 279–283

[53] Fisch U. The infratemporal fossa approach for nasopharyngeal tumors. Laryngoscope 1983; 93: 36–44

[54] Radkowski D, McGill T, Healy GB, Ohlms L, Jones DT. Angiofibroma. Changes in staging and treatment. Arch Otolaryngol Head Neck Surg 1996; 122: 122–129

[55] Andrews JC, Fisch U, Valavanis A, Aeppli U, Makek MS. The surgical management of extensive nasopharyngeal angiofibromas with the infratemporal fossa approach. Laryngoscope 1989; 99: 429–437

[56] Bremer JW, Neel HB, III, DeSanto LW, Jones GC. Angiofibroma: treatment trends in 150 patients during 40 years. Laryngoscope 1986; 96: 1321–1329

[57] Onerci M, Oğretmenoğlu O, Yücel T. Juvenile nasopharyngeal angiofibroma: a revised staging system. Rhinology 2006; 44: 39–45

[58] Lloyd G, Howard D, Lund VJ, Savy L. Imaging for juvenile angiofibroma. J Laryngol Otol 2000; 114: 727–730

[59] Bleier BS, Kennedy DW, Palmer JN, Chiu AG, Bloom JD, O'Malley BW, Jr. Current management of juvenile nasopharyngeal angiofibroma: a tertiary center experience 1999–2007. Am J Rhinol Allergy 2009; 23: 328–330

[60] Sartor K, Karnaze MG, Winthrop JD, Gado M, Hodges FJ, III. MR imaging in infra-, para- and retrosellar mass lesions. Neuroradiology 1987; 29: 19–29

[61] Donovan JL, Nesbit GM. Distinction of masses involving the sella and suprasellar space: specificity of imaging features. AJR Am J Roentgenol 1996; 167: 597–603

[62] Naganuma H, Satoh E, Nukui H. Technical considerations of transsphenoidal removal of fibrous pituitary adenomas and evaluation of collagen content and subtype in the adenomas. Neurol Med Chir (Tokyo) 2002; 42: 202–212, discussion 213

[63] Pierallini A, Caramia F, Falcone C et al. Pituitary macroadenomas: preoperative evaluation of consistency with diffusion-weighted MR imaging—initial experience. Radiology 2006; 239: 223–231

[64] Stadlbauer A, Buchfelder M, Nimsky C et al. Proton magnetic resonance spectroscopy in pituitary macroadenomas: preliminary results. J Neurosurg 2008; 109: 306–312

[65] Sartoretti-Schefer S, Wichmann W, Aguzzi A, Valavanis A. MR differentiation of adamantinous and squamous-papillary craniopharyngiomas. AJNR Am J Neuroradiol 1997; 18: 77–87

[66] Freeman MP, Kessler RM, Allen JH, Price AC. Craniopharyngioma: CT and MR imaging in nine cases. J Comput Assist Tomogr 1987; 11: 810–814

[67] Davies MJ, King TT, Metcalfe KA, Monson JP. Intraventricular craniopharyngioma: a long-term follow-up of six cases. Br J Neurosurg 1997; 11: 533–541

[68] Pigeau I, Sigal R, Halimi P, Comoy J, Doyon D. MRI features of craniopharyngiomas at 1.5 Tesla. A series of 13 cases. J Neuroradiol 1988; 15: 276–287

[69] Samii M, Tatagiba M. Surgical management of craniopharyngiomas: a review. Neurol Med Chir (Tokyo) 1997; 37: 141–149

[70] Arndt S, Wiech T, Mader I, Aschendorff A, Maier W. Rare extracranial localization of primary intracranial neoplasm. Diagn Pathol 2008; 3: 14–19

[71] Pusey E, Kortman KE, Flannigan BD, Tsuruda J, Bradley WG. MR of craniopharyngiomas: tumor delineation and characterization. AJR Am J Roentgenol 1987; 149: 383–388

[72] Hald JK, Eldevik OP, Quint DJ, Chandler WF, Kollevold T. Pre- and postoperative MR imaging of craniopharyngiomas. Acta Radiol 1996; 37: 806–812

[73] Petrulionis M, Valeviciene N, Paulauskiene I, Bruzaite J. Primary extracranial meningioma of the sinonasal tract. Acta Radiol 2005; 46: 415–418

[74] Casselman JW. The skull base: tumoral lesions. Eur Radiol 2005; 15: 534–542

[75] Pieper DR, Al-Mefty O, Hanada Y, Buechner D. Hyperostosis associated with meningioma of the cranial base: secondary changes or tumor invasion. Neurosurgery 1999; 44: 742–746, discussion 746–747

[76] Taylor SL, Barakos JA, Harsh GR, IV, Wilson CB. Magnetic resonance imaging of tuberculum sellae meningiomas: preventing preoperative misdiagnosis as pituitary macroadenoma. Neurosurgery 1992; 31: 621–627, discussion 627

[77] Schick U, Hassler W. Surgical management of tuberculum sellae meningiomas: involvement of the optic canal and visual outcome. J Neurol Neurosurg Psychiatry 2005; 76: 977–983

[78] Kaplan RD, Coons S, Drayer BP, Bird CR, Johnson PC. MR characteristics of meningioma subtypes at 1.5 tesla. J Comput Assist Tomogr 1992; 16: 366–371

[79] Nagar VA, Ye JR, Ng WH et al. Diffusion-weighted MR imaging: diagnosing atypical or malignant meningiomas and detecting tumor dedifferentiation. AJNR Am J Neuroradiol 2008; 29: 1147–1152

[80] Obeid F, Al-Mefty O. Recurrence of olfactory groove meningiomas. Neurosurgery 2003; 53: 534–542, discussion 542–543

[81] Chirico G, Pergolizzi S, Mazziotti S, Santacaterina A, Ascenti G. Primary sphenoid esthesioneuroblastoma studied with MR. Clin Imaging 2003; 27: 38–40

[82] Hurst RW, Erickson S, Cail WS et al. Computed tomographic features of esthesioneuroblastoma. Neuroradiology 1989; 31: 253–257

[83] Pickuth D, Heywang-Köbrunner SH, Spielmann RP. Computed tomography and magnetic resonance imaging features of olfactory neuroblastoma: an analysis of 22 cases. Clin Otolaryngol Allied Sci 1999; 24: 457–461

[84] Laforest C, Selva D, Crompton J, Leibovitch I. Orbital invasion by esthesioneuroblastoma. Ophthal Plast Reconstr Surg 2005; 21: 435–440

[85] Regenbogen VS, Zinreich SJ, Kim KS et al. Hyperostotic esthesioneuroblastoma: CT and MR findings. J Comput Assist Tomogr 1988; 12: 52–56

[86] Schiro BJ, Escott EJ, McHugh JB, Carrau RL. Bone invasion by an esthesioneuroblastoma mimicking fibrous dysplasia. Eur J Radiol Extra 2008; 65: 69–72

[87] Schuster JJ, Phillips CD, Levine PA. MR of esthesioneuroblastoma (olfactory neuroblastoma) and appearance after craniofacial resection. AJNR Am J Neuroradiol 1994; 15: 1169–1177

[88] Som PM, Lidov M, Brandwein M, Catalano P, Biller HF. Sinonasal esthesioneuroblastoma with intracranial extension: marginal tumor cysts as a diagnostic MR finding. AJNR Am J Neuroradiol 1994; 15: 1259–1262

[89] Borges A. Imaging of the central skull base. Neuroimaging Clin N Am 2009; 19: 669–696

[90] Yu T, Xu YK, Li L et al. Esthesioneuroblastoma methods of intracranial extension: CT and MR imaging findings. Neuroradiology 2009; 51: 841–850

[91] Nguyen BD, Roarke MC, Nelson KD, Chong BW. F-18 FDG PET/CT staging and posttherapeutic assessment of esthesioneuroblastoma. Clin Nucl Med 2006; 31: 172–174

[92] Pickuth D, Heywang-Köbrunner SH. Imaging of recurrent esthesioneuroblastoma. Br J Radiol 1999; 72: 1052–1057

[93] Capelle L, Krawitz H. Esthesioneuroblastoma: a case report of diffuse subdural recurrence and review of recently published studies. J Med Imaging Radiat Oncol 2008; 52: 85–90

[94] Zollinger LV, Wiggins RH, III, Cornelius RS, Phillips CD. Retropharyngeal lymph node metastasis from esthesioneuroblastoma: a review of the therapeutic and prognostic implications. AJNR Am J Neuroradiol 2008; 29: 1561–1563

[95] Erdem E, Angtuaco EC, Van Hemert R, Park JS, Al-Mefty O. Comprehensive review of intracranial chordoma. Radiographics 2003; 23: 995–1009

[96] Ginsberg LE. Neoplastic diseases affecting the central skull base: CT and MR imaging. AJR Am J Roentgenol 1992; 159: 581–589

[97] Weber AL, Liebsch NJ, Sanchez R, Sweriduk ST, Jr. Chordomas of the skull base. Radiologic and clinical evaluation. Neuroimaging Clin N Am 1994; 4: 515–527

[98] Lee YY, Van Tassel P. Craniofacial chondrosarcomas: imaging findings in 15 untreated cases. AJNR Am J Neuroradiol 1989; 10: 165–170

[99] Oot RF, Melville GE, New PF et al. The role of MR and CT in evaluating clival chordomas and chondrosarcomas. AJR Am J Roentgenol 1988; 151: 567–575

[100] Sze G, Uichanco LS, III, Brant-Zawadzki MN et al. Chordomas: MR imaging. Radiology 1988; 166: 187–191

[101] Tashiro T, Fukuda T, Inoue Y et al. Intradural chordoma: case report and review of the literature. Neuroradiology 1994; 36: 313–315

[102] Meyer SP et al. Chordomas of the skull base. MR Features. AJNR Am J Neuroradiol 1992; 13: 16–36

[103] Asano S, Kawahara N, Kirino T. Intradural spinal seeding of a clival chordoma. Acta Neurochir (Wien) 2003; 145: 599–603, discussion 603

[104] Hermans R, De Vuysere S, Marchal G. Squamous cell carcinoma of the sinonasal cavities. Semin Ultrasound CT MR 1999; 20: 150–161

[105] Hunink MG, de Slegte RG, Gerritsen GJ, Speelman H. CT and MR assessment of tumors of the nose and paranasal sinuses, the nasopharynx and the parapharyngeal space using ROC methodology. Neuroradiology 1990;32(3):220–225

[106] Lloyd G, Lund VJ, Howard D, Savy L. Optimum imaging for sinonasal malignancy. J Laryngol Otol 2000; 114: 557–562

[107] Valencia MP, Castillo M. Congenital and acquired lesions of the nasal septum: a practical guide for differential diagnosis. Radiographics 2008; 28: 205–224, quiz 326

[108] Tiwari R, Hardillo JA, Mehta D et al. Squamous cell carcinoma of maxillary sinus. Head Neck 2000; 22: 164–169

[109] Som PM, Costantino PD, Silvers AR. Imaging central skull base neural tumor spread from paranasal sinus malignancies: a critical factor in treatment planning. Skull Base Surg 1999; 9: 15–21

[110] Bimbi G, Saraceno MS, Riccio S, Gatta G, Licitra L, Cantù G. Adenocarcinoma of ethmoid sinus: an occupational disease. Acta Otorhinolaryngol Ital 2004; 24: 199–203

[111] Orvidas LJ, Lewis JE, Weaver AL, Bagniewski SM, Olsen KD. Adenocarcinoma of the nose and paranasal sinuses: a retrospective study of diagnosis, histologic characteristics, and outcomes in 24 patients. Head Neck 2005; 27: 370–375

[112] Sklar EM, Pizarro JA. Sinonasal intestinal-type adenocarcinoma involvement of the paranasal sinuses. AJNR Am J Neuroradiol 2003; 24: 1152–1155

[113] Bradley PJ. Adenoid cystic carcinoma of the head and neck: a review. Curr Opin Otolaryngol Head Neck Surg 2004; 12: 127–132

[114] Rapidis AD, Givalos N, Gakiopoulou H et al. Adenoid cystic carcinoma of the head and neck. Clinicopathological analysis of 23 patients and review of the literature. Oral Oncol 2005; 41: 328–335

[115] Caldemeyer KS, Mathews VP, Righi PD, Smith RR. Imaging features and clinical significance of perineural spread or extension of head and neck tumors. Radiographics 1998; 18: 97–110, quiz 147

[116] Laine FJ, Braun IF, Jensen ME, Nadel L, Som PM. Perineural tumor extension through the foramen ovale: evaluation with MR imaging. Radiology 1990; 174: 65–71

[117] Sigal R, Monnet O, de Baere T et al. Adenoid cystic carcinoma of the head and neck: evaluation with MR imaging and clinical-pathologic correlation in 27 patients. Radiology 1992; 184: 95–101

[118] Hermans R. Neoplasm of the sinonasal cavity. In Hermans R, ed. Head and Neck Cancer Imaging. Berlin: Springer; 2008:191–217

[119] Phillips CD, Futterer SF, Lipper MH, Levine PA. Sinonasal undifferentiated carcinoma: CT and MR imaging of an uncommon neoplasm of the nasal cavity. Radiology 1997; 202: 477–480

[120] Musy PY, Reibel JF, Levine PA. Sinonasal undifferentiated carcinoma: the search for a better outcome. Laryngoscope 2002; 112: 1450–1455

[121] Wallace S, Pilon A, Kwok P, Messner LV, Hitchcock Y. Ophthalmic manifestations of an undifferentiated sinonasal carcinoma. Optom Vis Sci 2008; 85: 226–229

[122] Rischin D, Porceddu S, Peters L, Martin J, Corry J, Weih L. Promising results with chemoradiation in patients with sinonasal undifferentiated carcinoma. Head Neck 2004; 26: 435–441

[123] Enepekides DJ. Sinonasal undifferentiated carcinoma: an update. Curr Opin Otolaryngol Head Neck Surg 2005; 13: 222–225

[124] Ghosh S, Weiss M, Streeter O, Sinha U, Commins D, Chen TC. Drop metastasis from sinonasal undifferentiated carcinoma: clinical implications. Spine 2001; 26: 1486–1491

[125] Rosenthal DI, Barker JL, Jr, El-Naggar AK et al. Sinonasal malignancies with neuroendocrine differentiation: patterns of failure according to histologic presentation. Cancer 2004; 101: 2567–2573

[126] Babin E, Rouleau V, Vedrine PO et al. Small cell neuroendocrine carcinoma of the nasal cavity and paranasal sinuses. J Laryngol Otol 2006; 120: 289–297

[127] Esposito F, Kelly DF, Vinters HV, DeSalles AA, Sercarz J, Gorgulhos AA. Primary sphenoid sinus neoplasms: a report of four cases with common clinical presentation treated with transsphenoidal surgery and adjuvant therapies. J Neurooncol 2006; 76: 299–306

[128] Kanamalla US, Kesava PP, McGuff HS. Imaging of nonlaryngeal neuroendocrine carcinoma. AJNR Am J Neuroradiol 2000; 21: 775–778

[129] Roth TN, Gengler C, Huber GF, Holzmann D. Outcome of sinonasal melanoma: clinical experience and review of the literature. Head Neck 2010; 32: 1385–1392

[130] Batra K, Chhabra A, Rampure J, Tang S, Koenigsberg R, Gonzales C. CT and MRI appearances of primary sphenoid melanoma: a rare case. AJNR Am J Neuroradiol 2005; 26: 2642–2644

[131] Yousem DM, Li C, Montone KT et al. Primary malignant melanoma of the sinonasal cavity: MR imaging evaluation. Radiographics 1996; 16: 1101–1110

[132] Kim SS, Han MH, Kim JE et al. Malignant melanoma of the sinonasal cavity: explanation of magnetic resonance signal intensities with histopathologic characteristics. Am J Otolaryngol 2000; 21: 366–378

[133] Borges A, Fink J, Villablanca P, Eversole R, Lufkin R. Midline destructive lesions of the sinonasal tract: simplified terminology based on histopathologic criteria. AJNR Am J Neuroradiol 2000; 21: 331–336

[134] Kim GE, Koom WS, Yang WI et al. Clinical relevance of three subtypes of primary sinonasal lymphoma characterized by immunophenotypic analysis. Head Neck 2004; 26: 584–593

[135] Weber AL, Rahemtullah A, Ferry JA. Hodgkin and non-Hodgkin lymphoma of the head and neck: clinical, pathologic, and imaging evaluation. Neuroimaging Clin N Am 2003; 13: 371–392

[136] Quraishi MS, Bessell EM, Clark D, Jones NS, Bradley PJ. Non-Hodgkin's lymphoma of the sinonasal tract. Laryngoscope 2000; 110: 1489–1492

[137] Vedrine PO, Thariat J, Merrot O et al. Primary cancer of the sphenoid sinus—a GETTEC study. Head Neck 2009; 31: 388–397

[138] Aiken AH, Glastonbury C. Imaging Hodgkin and non-Hodgkin lymphoma in the head and neck. Radiol Clin North Am 2008; 46: 363–378, ix–x

[139] Ooi GC, Chim CS, Liang R, Tsang KW, Kwong YL. Nasal T-cell/natural killer cell lymphoma: CT and MR imaging features of a new clinicopathologic entity. AJR Am J Roentgenol 2000; 174: 1141–1145

[140] Yasumoto M, Taura S, Shibuya H, Honda M. Primary malignant lymphoma of the maxillary sinus: CT and MRI. Neuroradiology 2000; 42: 285–289

[141] Marsot-Dupuch K, Cabane J, Raveau V, Aoun N, Tubiana JM. Lethal midline granuloma: impact of imaging studies on the investigation and management of destructive mid facial disease in 13 patients. Neuroradiology 1992; 34: 155–161

[142] Karantanis D, Subramaniam RM, Peller PJ et al. The value of [(18)F] fluorodeoxyglucose positron emission tomography/computed tomography in extranodal natural killer/T-cell lymphoma. Clin Lymphoma Myeloma 2008; 8: 94–99

[143] Laigle-Donadey F, Taillibert S, Martin-Duverneuil N, Hildebrand J, Delattre JY. Skull-base metastases. J Neurooncol 2005; 75: 63–69

[144] Branstetter BF, IV, Weissman JL. Role of MR and CT in the paranasal sinuses. Otolaryngol Clin North Am 2005; 38: 1279–1299, x

[145] Tanaka K. A case of metastases to the paranasal sinus from rectal mucinous adenocarcinoma. Int J Clin Oncol 2006; 11: 64–65

[146] Simoens WA, van den Hauwe L, Van Hedent E et al. Amyloidoma of the skull base. AJNR Am J Neuroradiol 2000; 21: 1559–1562

[147] Park SB, Lee JH, Weon YC. Imaging findings of head and neck inflammatory pseudotumor. AJR Am J Roentgenol 2009; 193: 1180–1186

[148] Tomura N, Hirano H, Sashi R et al. Comparison of MR imaging and CT in discriminating tumor infiltration of bone and bone marrow in the skull base. Comput Med Imaging Graph 1998; 22: 41–51

[149] Lasjaunias P, Berenstein A. Ter Brugge Surgical Neuroangiography. 2nd ed. Vol 1–3. Berlin, Springer-Verlag; 2001, 2004, 2006

[150] Connors JJ, III, Wojak JC. Interventional neuroradiology: strategies and practical techniques. Philadelphia, PA: WB Saunders Company; 1999

[151] Harrigan MR, Deveikis JP. Handbook of Cerebrovascular Disease and Neurointerventional Technique. 2nd ed. Berlin: Springer-Verlag; 2013

[152] Djindjian R, Merland JJ. Super-Selective Arteriography of the External Carotid Artery. Berlin: Springer-Verlag; 1978

[153] Dawbarn RHM. The starvation operation for malignancy in the external carotid area. J Am Med Assoc 1904; 17: 792–795

[154] Tarkan Ö, Sürmelioğlu O, Tuncer U, Akgül E. Face skin necrosis following embolization for arteriovenous malformations: a case report. Oral Maxillofac Surg 2010; 14: 49–52

[155] Köti E, Frazzini VI, Kagetsu NJ. Epistaxis: vascular anatomy, origins, and endovascular treatment. AJR Am J Roentgenol 2000; 174: 845–851

[156] Laurent A, Beaujeux R, Wassef M, Rüfenacht D, Boschetti E, Merland JJ. Trisacryl gelatin microspheres for therapeutic embolization, I: development and in vitro evaluation. AJNR Am J Neuroradiol 1996; 17: 533–540

[157] Beaujeux R, Laurent A, Wassef M et al. Trisacryl gelatin microspheres for therapeutic embolization, II: preliminary clinical evaluation in tumors and arteriovenous malformations. AJNR Am J Neuroradiol 1996; 17: 541–548

[158] Sluzewski M, van Rooij WJ, Lohle PN, Beute GN, Peluso JP. Embolization of meningiomas: comparison of safety between calibrated microspheres and polyvinyl-alcohol particles as embolic agents. AJNR Am J Neuroradiol 2013; 34: 727–729

[159] Morse SS, Clark RA, Puffenbarger A. Platinum microcoils for therapeutic embolization: nonneuroradiologic applications. AJR Am J Roentgenol 1990; 155: 401–403

[160] Bank WO, Kerber CW. Gelfoam embolization: a simplified technique. AJR Am J Roentgenol 1979; 132: 299–301

[161] Berenstein A, Russell E. Gelatin sponge in therapeutic neuroradiology: a subject review. Radiology 1981; 141: 105–112

[162] Brothers MF, Kaufmann JC, Fox AJ, Deveikis JP. n-Butyl 2-cyanoacrylate—substitute for IBCA in interventional neuroradiology: histopathologic and polymerization time studies. AJNR Am J Neuroradiol 1989; 10: 777–786

[163] Kerber C. Letter: Intracranial cyanoacrylate: a new catheter therapy for arteriovenous malformation. Invest Radiol 1975; 10: 536–538

[164] Siekmann R. Basics and principles in the application of Onyx LD liquid embolic system in the endovascular treatment of cerebral arteriovenous malformations. Interv Neuroradiol 2005; 11 Suppl 1: 131–140

[165] Winn HR, Richardson AE, Jane JA. Late morbidity and mortality of common carotid ligation for posterior communicating aneurysms. A comparison to conservative treatment. J Neurosurg 1977; 47: 727–736

[166] Kato K, Tomura N, Takahashi S et al. Balloon occlusion test of the internal carotid artery: correlation with stump pressure and 99mTc-HMPAO SPECT. Acta Radiol 2006; 47: 1073–1078

[167] Tomura N, Omachi K, Takahashi S et al. Comparison of technetium Tc 99 m hexamethylpropyleneamine oxime single-photon emission tomograph with stump pressure during the balloon occlusion test of the internal carotid artery. AJNR Am J Neuroradiol 2005; 26: 1937–1942

[168] Palestro CJ, Sen C, Muzinic M, Afriyie M, Goldsmith SJ. Assessing collateral cerebral perfusion with technetium-99m-HMPAO SPECT during temporary internal carotid artery occlusion. J Nucl Med 1993; 34: 1235–1238

[169] Sugawara Y, Kikuchi T, Ueda T et al. Usefulness of brain SPECT to evaluate brain tolerance and hemodynamic changes during temporary balloon occlusion test and after permanent carotid occlusion. J Nucl Med 2002; 43: 1616–1623

[170] Standard SC, Ahuja A, Guterman LR et al. Balloon test occlusion of the internal carotid artery with hypotensive challenge. AJNR Am J Neuroradiol 1995; 16: 1453–1458

[171] Mathis JM, Barr JD, Jungreis CA et al. Temporary balloon test occlusion of the internal carotid artery: experience in 500 cases. AJNR Am J Neuroradiol 1995; 16: 749–754

[172] Houdart E, Saint-Maurice JP, Boissonnet H, Bonnin P. Clinical and hemodynamic responses to balloon test occlusion of the straight sinus: technical case report. Neurosurgery 2002; 51: 254–256; discussion 256–257

[173] Ernemann U, Löwenheim H, Freudenstein D, Koerbel A, Heininger A, Tatagiba M. Hemodynamic evaluation during balloon test occlusion of the sigmoid sinus: clinical and technical considerations. AJNR Am J Neuroradiol 2005; 26: 179–182

[174] Valavanis A, Christoforidis G. Applications of interventional neuroradiology in the head and neck. Semin Roentgenol 2000; 35: 72–83

[175] Small M, Murray JA, Maran AG. A study of patients with epistaxis requiring admission to hospital. Health Bull (Edinb) 1982; 40: 20–29

[176] Kucik CJ, Clenney T. Management of epistaxis. Am Fam Physician 2005; 71: 305–311

[177] Bertrand B, Eloy P, Rombaux P, Lamarque C, Watelet JB, Collet S. Guidelines to the management of epistaxis. B-ENT 2005 Suppl 1: 27–41, quiz 42–43

[178] Lasjaunias P, Marsot-Dupuch K, Doyon D. The radio-anatomical basis of arterial embolisation for epistaxis. J Neuroradiol 1979; 6: 45–53

[179] Willems PWA, Farb RI, Agid R. Endovascular treatment of epistaxis. AJNR Am J Neuroradiol 2009; 30: 1637–1645

[180] Pope LE, Hobbs CGL. Epistaxis: an update on current management. Postgrad Med J 2005; 81: 309–314

[181] Gottumukkala R, Kadkhodayan Y, Moran CJ, Cross WT, III, Derdeyn CP. Impact of vessel choice on outcomes of polyvinyl alcohol embolization for intractable idiopathic epistaxis. J Vasc Interv Radiol 2013; 24: 234–239

[182] Borden NM, Dungan D, Dean BL, Flom RA. Posttraumatic epistaxis from injury to the pterygovaginal artery. Am J Neuroradiol 1996; 17: 1148–1150

[183] Sharathkumar AA, Shapiro A. Hereditary haemorrhagic telangiectasia. Haemophilia 2008; 14: 1269–1280

[184] Layton KF, Kallmes DF, Gray LA, Cloft HJ. Endovascular treatment of epistaxis in patients with hereditary hemorrhagic telangiectasia. AJNR Am J Neuroradiol 2007; 28: 885–888

[185] Hofmann E, Arps H, Schwager K. Paragangliome der Kopf-Hals-Region. Radiologie Up2Date 2009;9(4): 337–353

[186] Shin SH, Piazza P, De Donato G et al. Management of vagal paragangliomas including application of internal carotid artery stenting. Audiol Neurootol 2012; 17: 39–53

[187] Abud DG, Mounayer C, Benndorf G et al. Intratumoral injection of cyanoacrylate glue in head and neck paragangliomas. AJNR Am J Neuroradiol 2004; 25: 1457–1462

[188] Wanke I, Jäckel MC, Goericke S, Panagiotopoulos V, Dietrich U, Forsting M. Percutaneous embolization of carotid paragangliomas using solely Onyx. AJNR Am J Neuroradiol 2009; 30: 1594–1597

[189] Gemmete JJ, Chaudhary N, Pandey A et al. Usefulness of percutaneously injected ethylene-vinyl alcohol copolymer in conjunction with standard endovascular embolization techniques for preoperative devascularization of hypervascular head and neck tumors: technique, initial experience, and correlation with surgical observations. AJNR Am J Neuroradiol 2010; 31: 961–966

[190] Quadros RS, Gallas S, Delcourt C, Dehoux E, Scherperel B, Pierot L. Preoperative embolization of a cervicodorsal paraganglioma by direct percutaneous injection of onyx and endovascular delivery of particles. AJNR Am J Neuroradiol 2006; 27: 1907–1909

[191] Pradhan B, Thapa N. Juvenile angiofibroma and its management. Nepal Med Coll J 2009; 11: 186–188

[192] Thiex R, Wu I, Mulliken JB, Greene AK, Rahbar R, Orbach DB. Safety and clinical efficacy of Onyx for embolization of extracranial head and neck vascular anomalies. AJNR Am J Neuroradiol 2011; 32: 1082–1086

[193] Benndorf G. Dural Cavernous Sinus Fistulas – Diagnosis and Endovascular Therapy. Berlin: Springer Verlag; 2010

[194] Cox MW, Whittaker DR, Martinez C, Fox CJ, Feuerstein IM, Gillespie DL. Traumatic pseudoaneurysms of the head and neck: early endovascular intervention. J Vasc Surg 2007; 46: 1227–1233

[195] Nadig S, Barnwell S, Wax MK. Pseudoaneurysm of the external carotid artery—review of literature. Head Neck 2009; 31: 136–139

Chapter 5

Management of the Internal Carotid Artery in Skull Base Tumor Surgery

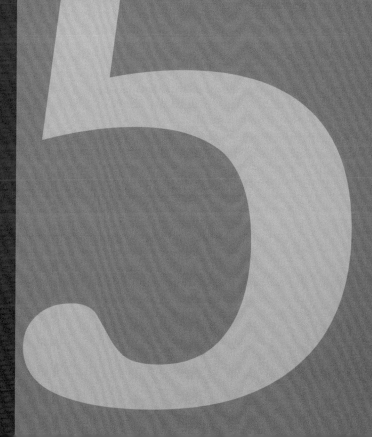

5 Management of the Internal Carotid Artery in Skull Base Tumor Surgery

Dietmar Frey, Peter Vajkoczy

5.1 Introduction

Skull base tumor surgery involving the internal carotid artery (ICA) has evolved significantly over the past years. Tumor involvement of the ICA endangers the blood supply to the brain, a major factor for mortality and morbidity in skull base surgery; thus, several approaches have been developed to overcome this problem.

Generally speaking, tumors that occur along the course of the ICA can be classified according to the respective segment they compromise. Head and neck tumors, such as squamous cell carcinoma, can often be approached easily. However, they are high-grade malignancies that mandate a complete resection. Incomplete resection results in a high rate of local recurrence. Therefore, despite the development of multimodal therapy for head and neck cancer and advancing nonsurgical options, in select patients the only chance for a curative approach consists of complete resection of the tumor and all involved tissue including the ICA. If resection of the ICA is indicated, the adequacy of the brain blood supply after exclusion of the involved vessel has to be evaluated preoperatively. Various algorithms have been proposed to ascertain the need for surgical revascularization. Thus, the need for clear and consistent guidelines regarding diagnosis and therapy for the treatment of malignancies of the head and neck region is obvious.

Lateral skull base tumors in the petrous segment of the ICA pose additional challenges with regard to preservation of nerves and vessels. Management of the ICA in the petrous segment came into focus after the development of facial nerve rerouting procedures. Tumors in this region are mostly benign; nevertheless, encasement of the ICA presents significant risk for intraoperative arterial rupture. Therefore, bypass procedures also have to be considered in these cases.

Tumors within the cavernous sinus may encase, stenose, or occlude the ICA. Meningiomas, pituitary adenomas, and other lesions can compromise the ICA in this segment. Parasellar meningiomas involve the ICA and its branches; therefore, these vessels are at high risk of being injured when complete resection is the goal.

This chapter addresses the management of the ICA in skull base tumor surgery, provides criteria for patient selection, gives an overview of preoperative diagnostic measures, outlines surgical indications, describes neurovascular procedures and operative techniques, and provides information about the postoperative management from a neurosurgeon's perspective.

5.2 Patient Selection

Patient selection for skull base tumor surgery and its potential disruption of neurovascular structures has to consider the individual patient with respect to oncological, neurological, and anatomical criteria. The question what patient group benefits from which surgery has to be answered with respect to location of the tumor, its known or suspected entity, its clinical consequence, its relation to vessels, and the patient's characteristics such as age and overall neurological and general status. The ICA may be affected by skull base tumors along its entire course resulting in encasement, stenosis, or occlusion with or without hemodynamic compromise. With respect to skull base tumor surgery it is practical to divide the ICA into four segments: cervical, petrous, cavernous, and intracranial segments (▶ Fig. 5.1).

5.2.1 Tumors Involving the Internal Carotid Artery

Head and Neck Tumors Involving the Internal Carotid Artery Cervical Segment

Head and neck cancers are mostly of epithelial origin, arising at the mucosa in the head and neck area, and thus consisting of squamous cells. Most tumors of the paranasal sinus, the oral cavity, and the nasopharynx, oropharynx, hypopharynx, and larynx fall into this category. The latter three may involve the ICA by direct extension; however, it is most commonly affected by metastatic lymphadenopathy. The annual worldwide incidence of these tumors is about half a million cases, accounting for 2 to 5% of adult malignancies.

Known risk factors for squamous cell tumors are tobacco and alcohol use, occupational hazards in woodworking, and exposure to textile fibers and nickel. Furthermore, Epstein-Barr virus is associated with the occurrence of nasopharyngeal cancer. Gene and chromosome analyses found deletions and mutations in chromosomes 3p, 9p, 13q, 17p, p53, as well as overexpression of epidermal growth factor receptor (EGFR). EGFR is reported to predict poor outcome and serves as a target molecule for antibody treatment.

Squamous cell tumors and other lesions such as malignant fibrous histiocytoma can compromise the cervical segment of the ICA (▶ Fig. 5.1).[1] If engulfment or complete encasement of the ICA is found, surgical treatment for complete resection is difficult since bleeding off the

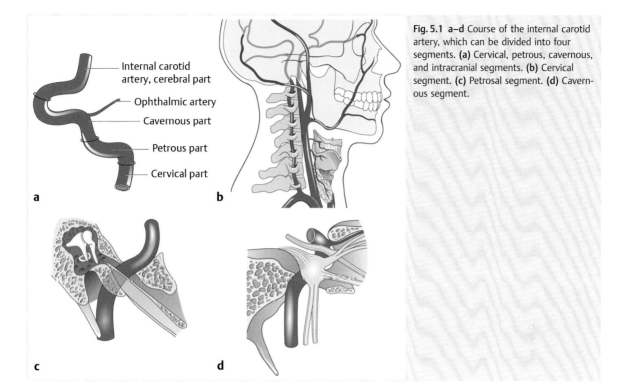

Fig. 5.1 a–d Course of the internal carotid artery, which can be divided into four segments. **(a)** Cervical, petrous, cavernous, and intracranial segments. **(b)** Cervical segment. **(c)** Petrosal segment. **(d)** Cavernous segment.

In figure labels:
- Internal carotid artery, cerebral part
- Ophthalmic artery
- Cavernous part
- Petrous part
- Cervical part

vessel endangers cerebral circulation and can lead to stroke. Nevertheless, aggressive surgical treatment and complete tumor removal are of prognostic relevance and provide the basis for adjuvant radiation therapy and chemotherapy. Incomplete resection can result in local recurrence rates of about 50%.[2]

Any tumor of the head and neck can compromise the ICA in the cervical segment. Complete tumor resection should be the primary goal; necessitating creative strategies to preserve sufficient blood flow to the brain. Therefore, any invasion of the ICA by a head and neck cancer and the need for complete tumor resection represents a challenge for the surgeon.

Salivary Gland Tumors

Salivary gland tumors differ in etiology, histopathology, and therapy. Tumors arising from the parotid, submandibular, sublingual, and minor salivary glands have no known specific risk factors. The majority of parotid tumors are benign, whereas about 50% of submandibular and sublingual lesions and most minor salivary gland tumors are malignant mucoepidermoid, adenoid cystic, and adenocarcinomas. Patients with benign salivary gland tumors generally undergo surgical excision of the lesion and, in case of invasion, radiation therapy such as neutron radiation. Adenoid cystic carcinoma can recur along neural structures many years after initial diagnosis even after complete resection.

Thyroid Cancer

Thyroid cancer as the most common malignancy of the endocrine system has an incidence of approximately 10/100,000 per year and can be classified according to its respective cellular origin into papillary or follicular, anaplastic, and medullary thyroid cancer. Treatment options include surgical resection, radioiodine treatment and ablation, and thyroid-stimulating hormone suppression therapy. In case of malignant disease as anaplastic thyroid cancer or medullary thyroid cancer, treatment primarily consists of surgical resection.

Carotid Body Tumors

Carotid body tumors arise from the paraganglion cells and are slow growing and mostly benign. They can affect cranial nerves including the vagus and hypoglossus nerves and can lead to transitory ischemic attacks or strokes due to stenosis or occlusion of the ICA. Their resection is associated with high complication rates including stroke morbidity and even mortality.

Lateral Skull Base Tumors with Possible Involvement of the Petrous Segment

Lateral skull base tumors such as glomus tympanicum and glomus jugulare paragangliomas, although rare, can affect the integrity of the ICA in the petrous segment (▶ Fig. 5.1). Surgical approaches to the intrapetrous ICA include the subtemporal and transcochlear approaches (and their multiple modifications). Glomus jugulare tumors arise from glomus body cells mostly originating from the jugular bulb. They are vascularized by branches of the external carotid artery as well as the ICAs. Cell proliferation occurs mainly along the vessels of origin and can be invasive. Due to invasion of either the acoustic canal or the labyrinth, hypoacusis and vertigo are major clinical symptoms.

Formerly, a major obstacle to approach the jugular foramen was the location of the facial nerve (i.e., the need to avoid its injury). Development of the infratemporal fossa approach, to tumors of the temporal bone and base of the skull, allowed the rerouting of the facial nerve; however, the ICA remained as an obstacle to access the jugular foramen.[3] Therefore, involvement of the ICA by tumors of the central and lateral skull base is the main factor precluding a total resection.

A glomus tympanicum tumor may involve the ICA starting at its site of origin, adjacent to jugular bulb (posterolateral aspect of the ICA vertical segment). Dissection of the vessel presents a high risk of rupture and catastrophic hemorrhage that correlates with the degree and complexity of involvement of the artery. Complex and aggressive tumors that endanger the vessel integrity of the petrous segment may lead to an incomplete removal. Therefore, sacrifice of the carotid artery may be considered in individual complex cases to achieve a complete tumor removal.

Tumors Involving the Cavernous Segment of the Internal Carotid Artery

Tumors that may affect the cavernous segment (▶ Fig. 5.1) of the ICA include meningiomas, schwannomas, chordomas, angiomas, pituitary adenomas, and others. Meningiomas are extra-axial tumors arising from mesodermal arachnoidal cells and are found anywhere in the cranium. Histopathology usually shows a benign pattern; however, about 2% are malignant and fast growing. Meningiomas represent one of the most common tumors of the central nervous system and account for up to 20% of primary intracranial neoplasms. Their incidence in autopsy studies is as high as 3% in patients older than 60 years. Of special interest with regard to involvement of the ICA are cavernous sinus meningiomas and variants of the medial sphenoid wing meningiomas, which can compress or encase the ICA or the middle cerebral artery and cause neurological deficits (i.e., transitory ischemic attacks or stroke). Meningiomas in this region tend to be supplied by branches of the ICA in contrast to the usual supply from external carotid branches. Taken together, in these patients assessment of cerebral blood flow and, if necessary, preparation for revascularization procedures prior surgery of the lesion itself are mandatory. Total resection is curative; however, depending on the location,

size, and relationship with neighboring structures, a complete removal may be impossible. This holds true especially when the tumor affects the cavernous segment of the ICA.

Most frequent symptoms include facial dysesthesia and numbness, facial pain, and paresis of ocular muscles. Diagnostic tests should include computed tomography (CT)/magnetic resonance (MR) imaging and, in suspected involvement of the ICA, though rare, CT or MR angiography. Treatment options are surgery, radiosurgery, and external beam radiation therapy. Surgery is favored in large symptomatic tumors, potentially in conjunction with adjuvant stereotactic radiosurgery. These tumors rarely mandate a brain revascularization procedure since they can be comfortably separated from the content of the cavernous sinus via an extradural transcavernous approach.

Chordomas and chondrosarcomas are rare low-grade malignancies most commonly located around the clivus and the sacral region. They do not respond to primary radiation therapy and due to their tendency for recurrence, they often require extensive total resection. In patients with clival chordomas, the ICA is often affected; therefore, a thorough preoperative evaluation with respect to the need for flow replacement is critical. This holds especially true in recurrent chordomas and when aiming for a radical curative resection.

Pituitary adenomas account for about 10% of intracranial neoplasms. The origin of cell proliferation is located in the anterior part of the pituitary gland, the adenohypophysis. At autopsy, around 25% of all examined pituitary glands showed microadenomas; and in radiographic series, 10% of patients had small tumors without any associated endocrine or neurological signs. In addition, hormonal dysfunction vision impairment, such as the classically described bitemporal hemianopsia, can be found if the optic chiasm is compressed. Extension into the cavernous sinus region, which happens in about 6 to 10% of cases, may exert pressure on the cranial nerves III, IV, V, and VI, resulting in oculomotor dysfunction, ptosis, trigeminal neuralgia, or diplopia. Clinical signs are mostly absent in tumors that involve the ICA; even complete encasement of the vessel does not necessarily result in functional flow impairment or neurological deficits.

Compression of neural or vascular structures in the cavernous sinus renders these tumors "invasive." Encasement of the ICA is an important predictor of perioperative morbidity and mortality. In case of invasion of the cavernous sinus and potential injury to the ICA, we recommend an assessment of the relation between tumor and vessels by MR imaging and CT or MR angiography; and if necessary, which is rare, by conventional angiography. If surgery is indicated, a transsphenoidal or transcranial approach may be performed according to the location, size, and morphology of the tumor and patient's individual needs. A transcranial approach can provide superior vascular control and may be preferable if a large-to-giant fibrous tumor. However, other algorithms of treatment should be considered including partial resection followed by observation or radiotherapy (external or stereotactic).

Any tumor in the cavernous sinus with the potential to affect the integrity of the ICA, and consequently endangering the blood supply to the brain, should undergo evaluation in terms of the feasibility for tumor resection and the subsequent perfusion of the brain, as well as the need for its revascularization. Outcomes regarding anatomy and functionality should be optimized. Similarly, complete resection of tumors that involve the ICA requires a thorough evaluation since sacrifice of the ICA, incidentally or intentionally, carries an unacceptable risk of neurological deficits.

5.2.2 Preoperative Diagnostic Procedures

Assessment of the extracranial and intracranial vascular status is crucial in patients with involvement of the ICA by tumor infiltration or compression. All the evaluations aim to ascertain: (1) the collateral blood flow to the vascular territory which is supplied by the affected carotid artery, to address the acute stroke risk following potential vessel sacrifice; (2) the cerebral vascular reserve in case of initial tolerance of vessel sacrifice (i.e., long-term delayed stroke risk); and (3) the availability of potential extracranial donor vessels for revascularization strategies.

Diagnostic imaging of the tumor and the vessels, mainly the ICAs, is performed by means of MR imaging, CT, angiography, and, if available, functional cerebral perfusion studies. The goals of diagnostic procedures include tumor localization, and assessment of its extent

and invasiveness. In some patients, especially those with head and neck cancer, the histological diagnoses can be obtained by biopsies. Furthermore, the relation of the ICA to the tumor has to be defined.

It is pivotal to note that depending on the collateralization of the affected ICA segment, sacrifice of the ICA may result in cerebral hypoperfusion and concomitant stroke. Extent of the collateral blood flow via the circle of Willis and leptomeningeal collaterals vary significantly; therefore, it is mandatory to identify high-risk patients. Those who do not tolerate vessel occlusion will need revascularization. Thus, angiographic studies should include occlusion testing of the affected segment.

Digital Subtraction Angiography and Balloon Test Occlusion

Conventional digital subtraction angiography (DSA) consists of a six-vessel angiography and selective injections according to the disease. Addition of a balloon test occlusion (BTO) assesses the tolerance to vessel sacrifice (► Fig. 5.2).

A balloon catheter is navigated into the ICA under fluoroscopic control, just proximal to the ICA segment to be sacrificed. A test occlusion of the common carotid artery is indicated in patients with head and neck tumors affecting the proximal cervical region. After inflation of the balloon, complete occlusion is verified by proximal injection of the contrast agent. For a hemodynamic analysis a separate catheter is placed into the contralateral ICA. Symmetry of the arterial, capillary, and venous filling can be evaluated after injection of contrast agent into the nonaffected ICA. Collateralization from the ICA to the contralateral cerebral hemisphere via the anterior communicating artery can thus be analyzed.

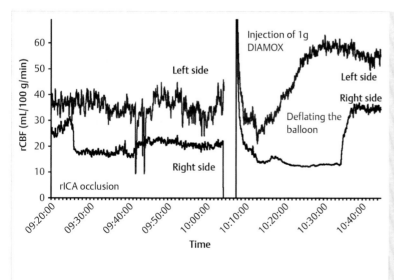

Fig. 5.2 Regional cerebral blood flow (rCBF) monitoring during balloon test occlusion (BTO) of right-affected internal carotid artery (rICA). rCBF probes were placed in the middle cerebral artery (MCA) territory of the affected hemisphere, and in the contralateral MCA territory. At 09:26:00, BTO of the right ICA is performed and a rCBF decrease of 40% in the respective MCA territory is recorded. On the contralateral hemisphere no significant changes can be seen at this point. After occlusion for 40 minutes, azetazolamide (Diamox) is administered and rCBF is shortly increased to 70 mL/100 g/min before reaching baseline values and lower in both hemispheres. After de-occlusion of ICA at 10:36:00, a compensatory increase to 35 mL/100 g/min is recorded. No neurological deficits were recorded during BTO.

After completion of the contralateral injection, the catheter is inserted into one vertebral artery (preferably the dominant one) and collateralization of the anterior territories via the posterior circulation can be ascertained. This provides an estimate of the capacity of the circle of Willis for collateral compensation after vessel sacrifice. Lack of filling of the middle cerebral artery territory via the anterior communication artery or delay of filling of the transverse sinus on the occluded side of more than 1 second (compared with the other transverse sinus) are considered as signs of inadequate collateralization (i.e., intolerance to vessel sacrifice).[4]

Currently, an angiographic assessment of the balloon test occlusion alone is considered insufficient to reliably identify patients that are at increased risk for stroke, and therefore need revascularization prior to sacrifice of the ICA. This is primarily due to a false-negative rate of the test of 10 to 15%. Consequently, additional direct or indirect monitoring of cerebral perfusion has been suggested.

Monitoring of Cerebral Perfusion during Balloon Test Occlusion

Sacrifice of one of the ICAs carries a high risk of provoking cerebral hypoperfusion and, thus, can ultimately lead to stroke. In addition, vessel sacrifice might be initially tolerated but may result in a loss of cerebrovascular reserve capacity due to a maximum dilation of precapillary arterioles. Loss of cerebrovascular reserve capacity results in a long-term increase in stroke risk of up to 30 to 45% in 2 years. Therefore, a thorough assessment of the cerebral hemodynamic status during BTO is an important supplement to the clinical and angiographic protocols.

To achieve this, various tests have been proposed and introduced including neurological/clinical evaluation, transcranial Doppler sonography, xenon-enhanced CT imaging, single-photon emission computed tomography, electroencephalography or monitoring of cerebral blood flow by implantation of a microprobe.

Clinical/Neurological Monitoring

Patients are under close surveillance during the DSA and BTO. Usual occlusion time ranges between 15 and 30 minutes and the patient undergoes repeated neurological examinations during this time. Simple motor and language tasks provide indirect evidence of adequate perfusion of eloquent areas (▶ Fig. 5.3). This approach requires a patient that is cooperative and able to understand and perform tasks; thus, the patient cannot be under general anesthesia. However, the sensitivity of the neurological examination alone is relatively low, and does not identify the loss of the cerebrovascular reserve capacity. Furthermore, a BTO of the ICA with clinical and angiographic monitoring alone is not able to significantly reduce the 10 to 15% false-negative rate.[5]

Transcranial Doppler Sonography

Transcranial Doppler sonography (TCD) has been introduced over recent years to predict hemodynamic intolerance in BTO procedures.[6,7] Usually, patients undergo TCD to assess baseline cerebral hemodynamics prior to DSA and BTO. Ideally the patient uses a custommade headset to decrease intertest variability. During the angiography session baseline values are obtained again before the test occlusion.

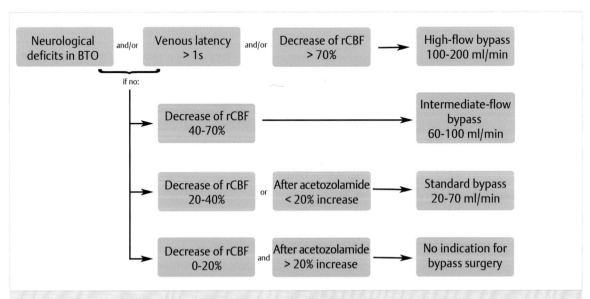

Fig. 5.3 Algorithm for decision making in revascularization surgery for carotid artery sacrifice. CBF, cerebral blood flow; STA-MCA, superficial temporal artery to middle cerebral artery.

Mean blood flow velocity and pulsatility index are generally recorded as surrogate parameters for indirectly assessing cerebral perfusion. TCD is performed on the middle cerebral artery of the affected side. Threshold values for critical reduction of the MBFV are set to 30, 35, or 40%, depending on the examiner. Patients with a reduction of less than 30 to 40% are deemed able to tolerate permanent occlusion of the respective vessel. A decrease below 50% of the baseline value seems to be a predictive factor for the development of ischemic symptoms. However, according to Sorteberg et al,[6] a decrease to 55% or less of the baseline value indicates the need for revascularization surgery, whereas a value of 65% or greater of baseline indicates tolerance of a permanent vessel occlusion. When the drop from baseline is between 55 and 65%, an additional parameter, the blood velocity pulsatility index should be considered. This value detects impaired autoregulation, which suggests hemodynamic intolerance. However, TCD also carries significant drawbacks: cerebral perfusion is assessed solely by indirect means, leptomeningeal collateralization is not addressed, a significant number of patients lack an adequate bone window for transcranial sonography, and the results are characterized by a high level of interexaminer variability. Therefore, techniques that assess cerebral perfusion directly and more objectively are superior to TCD.

Single-Photon Emission Computed Tomography

Single-photon emission computed tomography (SPECT) is a noninvasive method of cerebral blood flow measurement. It is well tolerated; however, its main disadvantage is the inability to generate absolute values and quantify cerebral blood flow. Cerebral blood flow measurement by SPECT is semiquantitative and records only relative changes during balloon occlusion testing and asymmetrical filling of the hemispheres. High intertest variability and low specificity has led to the search of other methods for quantification of cerebral blood flow in the setting of BTO.

Stable Xenon-Enhanced Computed Tomography

Stable xenon-enhanced CT (Xenon-CT) has been proposed for the quantification of cerebral perfusion to define thresholds of hemodynamic intolerance and, therefore, guide the surgical decision making.[8] This method is based on the principle that the rate of uptake and the rate of clearance of an inert substance in tissue are in proportion to the blood flow. In a first step, a DSA with test occlusion is initiated. After completion of a six-vessel angiography, an occlusion balloon catheter is introduced and inflated just proximal to the relevant segment. After 15 minutes, the balloon is deflated but kept in place. Any neurological

deficit mandates an immediate deflation of the balloon and interruption of the BTO. If the patient tolerates the test occlusion clinically, the examination proceeds to a Xenon-CT. In the scanner, the balloon is inflated again, and the cerebral perfusion is measured. The examination provides quantitative perfusion values for the cerebral hemisphere or individual regions of interest. Collateralization following vessel occlusion is assessed by the decrease of regional cerebral blood flow.

Cerebrovascular reserve capacity may be assessed by a hypotensive challenge or stimulation with acetazolamide. Acetazolamide is a potent vasodilator that is injected intravenously, and the subsequent increase in cerebral blood flow is monitored. A compromise of the cerebrovascular reserve capacity can be assumed when cerebral blood flow increases less than 10% following acetazolamide stimulation. Classification of patients according to their decrease in baseline perfusion and cerebrovascular reserve capacity enables us to tailor the revascularization procedure to the needs of the individual patient.

In current BTO protocols including Xenon-CT, a high risk of postocclusion cerebral infarction is ascribed if the patient does not tolerate the BTO clinically (i.e., develops neurological symptoms). A moderate risk of postocclusion neurological deficits is assigned when the Xenon-CT cerebral blood flow decreases below 30 mL/100 g/min during the test occlusion. If CBF, as measured by Xenon-CT during test occlusion, remains above 30 mL/100 g/min, patients are considered to be at low risk for developing a stroke.

Quantitative Cerebral Blood Flow Measurement by Xenon-Washout Procedure

Cortical cerebral blood flow measurements represent an alternative to Xenon-CT measurements.[9] During this test, xenon is injected via a distal lumen in the balloon catheter during occlusion. Two cadmium telluride scintillation detectors located over the frontal and occipital cortex ipsilateral to the balloon occlusion measure its washout. Cerebral blood flow is calculated using the tracer washout curve. Similar to the Xenon-CT technique, the absolute cerebral blood flow, the established threshold for hemodynamic intolerance, is 30 mL/100 g/min. Alternatively, in patients with low baseline values, intolerance is defined as a relative decrease by more than 30%.

Electroencephalography

Electroencephalography for monitoring during BTO for the identification of high-risk patients prior to surgery was previously used as an adjunct instrument. However, it has largely been abandoned in favor for other monitoring methods due to its poor specificity and its inability to generate quantitative results.

Measurement of Cerebral Blood Flow by Thermal Diffusion Flowmetry

In the last few years, we have introduced the measurement of cerebral blood flow by thermal diffusion flowmetry into our clinical practice. This technique allows for a continuous and real-time measurement of cerebral blood flow; as opposed to the previously mentioned imaging techniques that just provide a snapshot of cerebral perfusion. Technically, the microprobe is inserted through a 3.2 mm coronal burr hole over the hemisphere ipsilateral to the affected vessel in a standardized fashion. It is placed subcortically in the white matter at a depth of 20 mm below the dura according to the vascular region of interest (typically 6 cm lateral to midline).

Thermodilution involves the continuous measurement of temperature at two small gold plates fixed to the tip of the probe. One of the plates radiates heat; thus, the cerebral blood flow can be calculated from the difference in temperature between the two plates. High blood flow decreases the difference, whereas low blood flow increases the temperature difference. This method provides continuous and quantitative real-time data, which has been validated by Xenon-CT.[10] The microprobe provides absolute values for tissue perfusion in milliliters per 100 g per minute. Typical baseline values for a subcortical measurement range between 25 and 40 mL/100 g/min. Following 20 minutes of cerebral blood flow recording during BTO an acetazolamide challenge is performed. An impaired cerebrovascular reserve capacity is assumed if the cerebral blood flow increase is less than 10% than baseline.

Assessment of cerebral perfusion by the thermal diffusion probe has proven to be an excellent method during BTO. Patients with compromised cerebrovascular reserve capacity can be identified and according to cerebral blood flow change the patients can be stratified according to their stroke risk. Consequently, it serves to indicate the need for bypass surgery and to decide on the type of bypass. However, thermal diffusion flowmetry also carries some disadvantages. Its measurements are very focal and cannot be extrapolated to indicate the functional status of the complete territory at risk. In addition, it is invasive, as it requires insertion of a microprobe into the parenchyma. It should be noted, however, that in our experience no bleeding or infection has occurred with the implantation of the thermal diffusion probe. Finally, thermal diffusion measurements are strictly dependent on cerebral thermal stability; thus, rendering the cerebral blood flow measurements sometimes unstable.

Overall, there is no consensus regarding which BTO protocol to apply. All methods discussed herein contribute to the decision making. However, it would be inappropriate to base a decision of whether the ICA can be occluded with no risk of stroke or whether a bypass is indicated on BTO results alone, even when combined with complementary tests. The decision to perform a bypass surgery should be founded on the experience of the neurosurgeon, the evaluation of imaging findings, and the overall needs of the individual patient. Due to the remaining risk of a false-negative result, a more generalized approach to revascularization of patients scheduled for carotid artery sacrifice is justified in individual cases.

5.2.3 Patient Selection for Bypass Surgery

When considering carotid artery sacrifice, either intentionally or following accidental injury, it is desirable to precede the procedure with a thorough assessment of the patient's hemodynamic situation and compensatory potential. This is indispensable to decide whether the patient needs revascularization and to tailor the bypass type. The first step should be the general decision of whether or not the patient needs flow replacement or augmentation. This decision has to be based primarily on the angioarchitecture of the cerebrovascular system and the extent of collateral pathways in the event of carotid artery sacrifice. As previously described, multiple preoperative diagnostic tools have been developed and introduced into clinical practice to categorize the patients into different risk and treatment subgroups and to indicate the need for bypass surgery.

Our approach is that every patient undergoing surgery for a cervical or skull base tumor, where resection of the carotid artery is envisaged, or a significant accidental injury is possible, will undergo a thorough cerebrovascular evaluation with a six-vessel angiography and BTO applying radiological, clinical, and functional perfusion criteria. Recently, we have developed a BTO decision-making algorithm for carotid artery sacrifice, primarily based on clinical signs and the angiographic collateralization, as well as the results of cerebral blood flow analysis. Patients undergoing BTO who exhibit neurological deficits or demonstrate an asynchronous filling of the transverse sinus > 1 second, will definitely need revascularization with a large-caliber graft to replace carotid artery flow in the event of carotid artery sacrifice (i.e., sphenoid vein graft). Patients who do not exhibit these clinical and angiographic deficits may still need revascularization according to the cerebral blood flow studies. Patients demonstrating > 50% decrease in baseline perfusion also will qualify for revascularization with a medium- to large-caliber graft (i.e., a radial artery graft). For patients demonstrating a cerebral blood flow decrease of 30 to 50% we suggest a small-caliber bypass, which might mature over time and protect the patient during the perioperative period and at long term; that is, a superficial temporal artery to middle cerebral artery bypass. Finally, if baseline cerebral blood flow is reduced by < 30% an assessment of cerebrovascular reserve capacity becomes important. For patients with an impaired increase of cerebral blood flow upon acetazolamide stimulation we recommend a small caliber bypass to prevent a development of chronic hemodynamic insufficiency with an increased long-term stroke risk.

In addition to these principles, younger patients with a long life expectancy may require different treatment. Another important factor warrants consideration in younger patients with sufficient collateralization but facing the possibility of sacrificing one ICA. Following sacrifice of one ICA, the blood flow to the anterior circulation is mainly directed to the second ICA resulting in considerably higher flow velocities and shear stress rates in the remaining vessel. Theoretically, this vessel would consequently sustain a blood flow of up to 200 to 300 cm/s, which implies an increased risk of de novo aneurysm formation along the circle of Willis. Avoidance of this long-term complication in patients with a life expectancy of more than 20 years involves the augmentation of cerebral blood flow with a bypass, even when the cerebrovascular reserve capacity is not compromised.

5.3 Technique of Extracranial–Intracranial Bypass Surgery

Impairment of hemodynamics determines specific indications for bypass surgery. Bypass surgery in this context aims at replacing the difference in blood flow resulting from sacrifice of the carotid artery and endogenous collateral flow. Currently, we can choose among a panel of different types of bypass allowing us to tailor flow replacement to the individual needs of the patients and optimizing the risk/benefit ratio of the procedure.

5.3.1 Superficial Temporal Artery to Middle Cerebral Artery Bypass

In this classic technique, first described by Professor Yasargil, the frontal or parietal branch of the superficial temporal artery is anastomosed to a cortical branch of the middle cerebral artery in the perisylvian region (▶ Fig. 5.4). This is achieved with a minimally invasive keyhole approach where a 3 cm craniotomy is performed

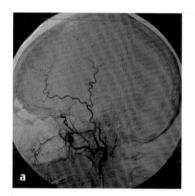
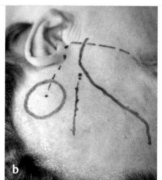
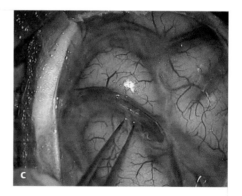
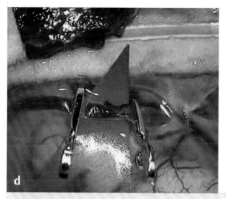
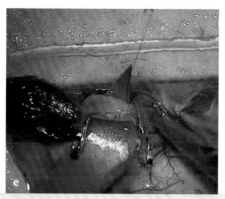
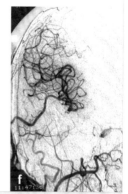

Fig. 5.4 a–f Standard superficial temporal artery to middle cerebral artery (STA-MCA) bypass procedure. **(a)** Lateral view of an angiogram of the external carotid artery on the right side depicting suitable frontal and parietal branches. If both branches are suitable we tend to use the frontal branch. **(b)** Projected end of the Sylvian fissure 6 cm above the external auditory canal (green circle), and course of the superficial temporal artery, with its frontal and parietal branches (red). **(c)** M3 segment of the middle cerebral artery as the recipient vessel is prepared for the anastomoses. **(d)** Temporary clips are placed on the recipient vessel. **(e)** Completed anastomosis with 10-0 interrupted sutures. **(f)** Postoperative angiogram demonstrating filling of middle cerebral artery territory via STA-MCA bypass.

at the end of the Sylvian fissure. The anastomosis can be performed using 10–0 interrupted or running sutures. Temporary occlusion time ranges between 15 and 25 minutes. Recently, we have shown that this temporary occlusion time is well tolerated and does not result in cerebral ischemia as evidenced by the lack of post-operative diffusion changes in the dependent vascular territory. Using our minimal invasive approach to superficial temporal artery to middle cerebral artery (STA-MCA) bypass surgery the mean surgical time has been reduced to 90 to 120 minutes with minimal invasiveness. In parallel, the complication rate could be significantly reduced to < 5%. The standard flow STA-MCA bypass provides a blood flow of about 20 to 70 mL/min and has an excellent 5-year patency rate of around 95%.

5.3.2 Intermediate-Flow Bypass with Radial Artery Graft Interposition

Radial artery interposition grafts deliver a blood flow of 60 to 100 mL/min with a 5-year patency rate of around 90 to 95%. The lumen of the radial artery is similar to the lumen of the M2 segment of the middle cerebral artery and serves as a physiological conduit for arterial blood. Technically, a bypass with radial artery interposition can be sequenced into three parts, the first, is the harvesting of the radial artery. One should ascertain that the area supplied by the radial artery is well collateralized by the ulnar artery. A second step includes a craniotomy and the exposure of the recipient vessel. Finally, the radial artery is anastomosed between the external carotid artery and the respective middle cerebral artery (▶ Fig. 5.5).

For radial artery harvesting the nondominant forearm is generally used. Allen testing confirms the patency of the palmar arch and sufficient blood supply to the hand via the ulnar artery. During surgery, the entire forearm is prepared and the radial artery is identified at the wrist by palpation or Doppler sonography. Then, a curvilinear skin incision is made running from the radial aspect of the wrist to the antecubital fossa, where the artery usually originates from the brachial artery. Dissection to the deep fascia is performed and the artery is prepared in a retrograde fashion beginning distally. Distally, the radial artery is covered by deep fascia, whereas in the middle forearm it is found between the brachioradial and the flexor carpi ulnaris muscles. According to the required length the artery is exposed and branches are coagulated by bipolar cautery or ligated at least 1 mm from the artery. Harvesting of the radial artery is performed just before graft insertion; thus, until then, the artery is left in situ and covered with papaverin-soaked sponges. Several techniques to prevent spasm of the artery after extraction have been developed, as the radial artery has a tendency for vasospasm. Any obstruction to blood flow, in specific vasospasm of the bypass graft, has to be prevented. A

pressure distension technique to prevent vasospasm of the arterial graft has been developed for this reason.[11] After extraction, the radial artery graft is flushed with heparin saline solution. A blunt cannula is introduced into the arterial graft at one end and saline solution is injected under pressure to distend the artery for a length of about 4 cm. In most cases the artery suddenly expands due to elevated pressure, and vasospasm is released in this part of the artery. This procedure is replicated segment after segment of the graft until extension has been achieved over the entire length and it is repeated from the other end in the same manner. In addition to preventing vasospasm, unsecured branches of the graft become visible due to leakage of the solution

Simultaneous to the bypass graft harvesting, a cervical skin incision is performed and the bifurcation of the common carotid artery is exposed. Usually, the proximal segment of the external carotid artery serves as the proximal anastomosis site. Then, a pterional craniotomy is performed and the recipient vessel is identified and exposed. This is done by splitting the Sylvian fissure and dissecting the most suitable M2 branch in terms of size and mobility. Due to the presence of perforating arteries, which can be subject to injury, the M1 segment of the middle cerebral artery is generally not used. To expose the carotid bifurcation, a skin incision is made at the level of the hyoid bone and the carotid sheath is opened. For an end-to-side anastomosis the external carotid artery has to be prepared 2 cm from the bifurcation. After tunneling of the radial artery graft it is connected to the M2 segment of the middle cerebral artery under temporary occlusion. Subsequently, an end-to-side anastomosis of the proximal site is performed.

5.3.3 High-Flow Bypass with Saphenous Vein Graft Interposition

High-flow bypass with a saphenous vein interposition graft affords maximal blood flow replacement (100 to 200 mL/min). Therefore, a saphenous vein graft is suitable if the carotid artery has to be fully bypassed due to the lack of collateral blood flow.[12] In terms of surgical technique, a venous bypass is between the proximal external carotid artery and an M2 segment of the middle cerebral artery. First, the saphenous vein is harvested.

The saphenous vein runs from the anteromedial malleolus to the medial epicondyle of the femur bone (▶ Fig. 5.6a). It joins the femoral vein after coursing the anterior surface of the thigh. It is of major importance to preoperatively exclude varicosis. For this reason and to facilitate harvesting, an ultrasonography is performed preoperatively and the course of the vein is marked on the skin. Exposure of the saphenous vein starts distally and dissection runs upward to expose and mobilize 25 to 30 cm of the vein. The ideal diameter of the graft is 2 to

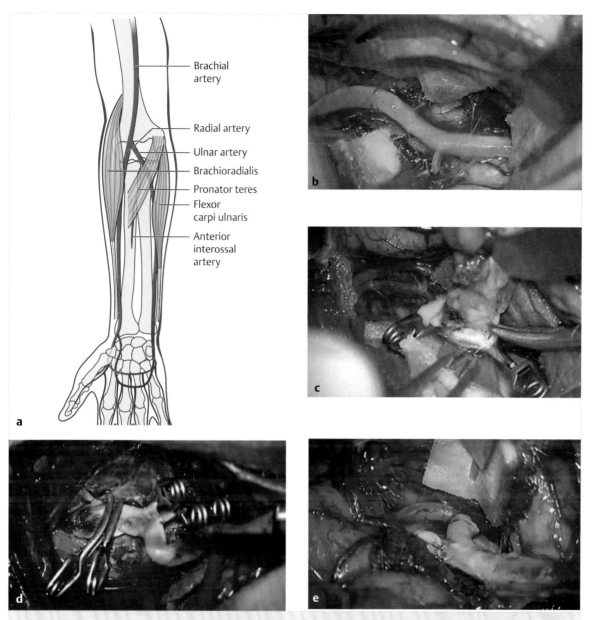

Fig. 5.5 a–e Intermediate-flow bypass using a radial artery graft. (a) Course of the radial artery in the forearm. (b) M2 segment of the middle cerebral artery as the recipient vessel following wide dissection of the Sylvian fissure. (c) Suturing of the end-to-side anastomosis using a radial artery graft with 8–0 running sutures. Temporary clips are applied to the M2 branch. (d) End-to-side anastomosis to the external carotid artery with the radial artery graft with 7–0 running sutured. Temporary clips are applied to the proximal and distal external carotid artery and to the superior thyroid artery. (e) Bypass filling of middle cerebral artery territory at the end of the procedure.

3 mm. Therefore, Doppler sonography should also localize the segment of optimal diameter to optimize the harvesting procedure(▸ Fig. 5.6b). Side branches are ligated or coagulated by bipolar cautery.

During preparation of the graft it is crucial to prevent leakage from the graft, which potentially could lead to postoperative bleeding, and to ensure laminar blood flow within the vessel by ligating and coagulating beyond the level of the vessel wall. After mobilization and preparation of the graft, it is left in situ until it is required.

Cervical and cranial exposures are performed as described above (▸ Fig. 5.5). In brief, a transverse incision is made at the level of the hyoid bone and the carotid bifurcation is identified and prepared as previously described (2 cm distal to the bifurcation). Subsequently, a pterional craniotomy is performed and the recipient

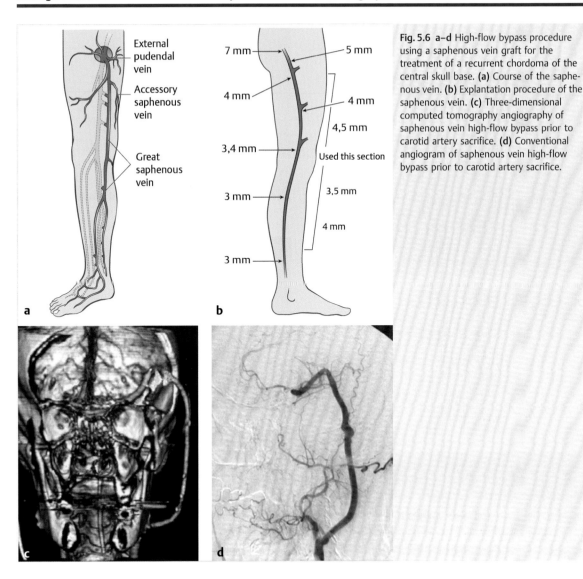

Fig. 5.6 a–d High-flow bypass procedure using a saphenous vein graft for the treatment of a recurrent chordoma of the central skull base. **(a)** Course of the saphenous vein. **(b)** Explantation procedure of the saphenous vein. **(c)** Three-dimensional computed tomography angiography of saphenous vein high-flow bypass prior to carotid artery sacrifice. **(d)** Conventional angiogram of saphenous vein high-flow bypass prior to carotid artery sacrifice.

vessel, usually the M2 segment of the middle cerebral artery, is prepared.

As soon as the anastomosis sites have fully been exposed, the saphenous vein graft is extracted and flushed with a heparin solution to extract any clots and check patency and lack of leaks of the graft. In addition, the graft is distended by controlled hydrostatic pressure. The ends of the graft are stripped of connective tissue and adventitia to maximize suture control. Care has to be taken to ensure the correct flow direction or to destroy the valves if flow direction ought to be reversed (▶ Fig. 5.6c, d).

After tunneling from the cervical to the cranial opening, the graft is pulled through and its patency is tested again. Anastomosis of the distal end is accomplished first. The distal end of the graft is anastomosed to an M2 segment of the middle cerebral artery. When using a saphenous vein graft this anastomosis is more challenging due to the size mismatch of the vessels. After the distal

anastomosis has been performed, the graft is connected to the external carotid artery with an end-to-side anastomosis technique.

5.3.4 Excimer Laser-Assisted Nonocclusive Anastomosis

Excimer laser-assisted nonocclusive anastomosis (ELANA) enables an extracranial–intracranial or intracranial–intracranial bypass without the need to temporarily occlude the recipient artery (▶ Fig. 5.7). Thus, the risk of causing cerebral infarction neurological deficits due to temporary occlusion can be reduced. This rather new technique was developed over the past 15 years by Professor Tulleken (Utrecht) and has been used in numerous neurovascular surgeries mainly to establish the distal anastomosis.[13,14] By allowing the proximal anastomoses

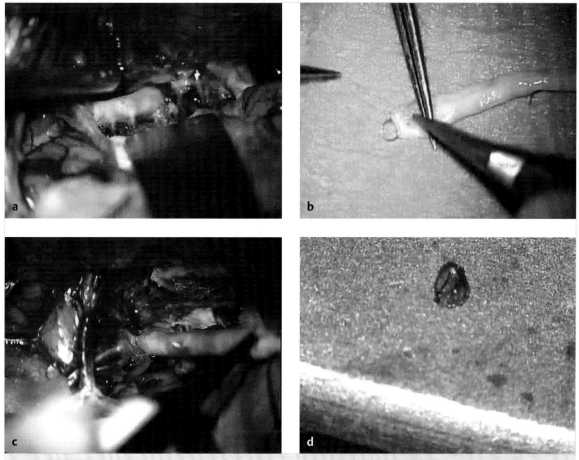

Fig. 5.7 a–d Excimer laser-assisted nonocclusive anastomosis (ELANA) technique for extracranial–intracranial bypass establishment. **(a)** The proximal intracranial recipient vessel: the proximal M1 segment of the middle cerebral artery. **(b)** A 2.6 mm or 2.8 mm platinum ring is sutured into the distal end of the saphenous vein graft using 8–0 interrupted sutures. **(c)** A laser catheter is introduced into the bypass graft and placed within the platinum ring in direct contact with the recipient vessel wall. **(d)** Vessel flap after 360° laser arteriotomy and extraction.

of high-flow bypasses without the need for temporary occlusion, it overcomes perioperative ischemia. Instead of having to occlude the recipient vessel for the arteriotomy and suturing, the anastomosis is created by a laser device.

As a first step, the graft previously attached to an anastomosis ring is sewn onto the recipient artery following conventional microsurgical protocols. Subsequently, the laser catheter device, consisting of an outer circular fiberoptic array ("laser knife") and a central suction, is introduced into the bypass graft, usually by a side branch up to the recipient's vessel wall. Then, the vessel wall inside the ring is fixed to the catheter by applying suction and the laser is activated in order to create the 360° anastomosis. The laser catheter is then retrieved and the vessel flap is secured.

The major advantage of the ELANA technique is the opportunity to create a vascular anastomosis without compromising the blood flow through the vessel. It can be reasoned that without the need for temporary

occlusion, temporary clips on the recipient or donor vessel are not needed and, consequently, vessel exposure and brain retraction can be minimized. Conversely, it has to be pointed out that the ELANA technique is reserved for a small subset of bypass procedures needing a proximal anastomosis in the light of little tolerance to temporary clipping. Therefore, the majority of bypasses are created using conventional microsurgical techniques, leaving the ELANA technique as an elegant supplement to our bypass armamentarium.

5.3.5 Intraoperative Assessment of Bypass Function

Patients with complex tumors that require vessel sacrifice and have demonstrated intolerance to vessel occlusion by BTO require a thorough intraoperative validation of adequate bypass function as a key to a safe and successful carotid artery sacrifice and radical tumor removal.

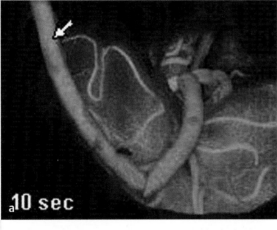

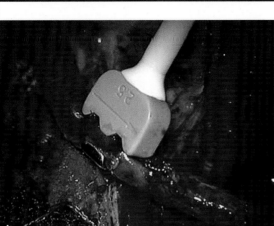

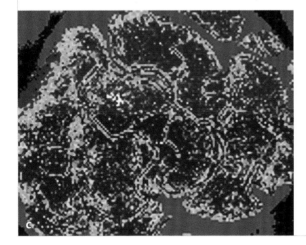

Fig. 5.8 **a–d** Intraoperative monitoring techniques for patient surveillance during intraoperative carotid artery sacrifice following extracranial–intracranial bypass surgery. **(a)** Intraoperative fluorescence angiography using indocyanine green (ICG) to assess patency of the anastomoses and bypass graft. **(b)** Doppler sonography provides quantitative information about blood flow (mL/min) within the bypass graft. **(c)** Laser speckle contrast analysis (LASCA) monitoring provides a false-color-coded image of the cortical perfusion. **(d)** Neurophysiological monitoring with motor-evoked potentials during temporary occlusion of the internal carotid artery. Note the loss of amplitude following clip application and its immediate recovery after clip removal.

Reasons for intraoperative graft failure include vasospasm, thrombosis, or technical shortcomings at the anastomotic site. Over the past years, different strategies have been devised to reliably assess graft patency and function intraoperatively (▶ Fig. 5.8). Obviously, intraoperative angiography is the gold standard for this task. However, invasiveness, personnel demands, and exposure to radiation argue against the routine use of intraoperative angiography.

Indocyanine Green Videoangiography

Recently, indocyanine green (ICG) videoangiography was introduced to aneurysm and neurovascular bypass surgery.[15,16] During this test, the fluorescent dye ICG is injected intravenously after completion of the bypass to visualize the filling of the bypass and its distal circulation using a near-infrared light integrated into the microscope. In our experience this novel method is ideal to check bypass patency intraoperatively. If occlusion or inadequate flow characteristics are encountered, the surgeon has the opportunity to immediately intervene. In addition, intraoperative ICG videoangiography not only shows failure of bypass patency but also directs the surgeon to the site of bypass failure and, thus, enables fast and precise revision. Using this technique, an early postoperative bypass patency rate near 100% seems feasible. However, additional monitoring is necessary to assess bypass function and blood delivery in more detail.

Neurophysiological Monitoring

Neurophysiological monitoring was introduced into neurosurgical practice decades ago. It represents a method of functional analysis and reflects the endpoint of the motor cortex activation and its subcortical pathways. In case of bypass surgery it enables the surgeon to validate adequate bypass function and sufficient perfusion of the downstream cerebral territory. In the event that the bypass is not delivering adequate flow rate, the surgeon will be warned to readdress the bypass intraoperatively. In our experience, intraoperative surveillance of motor function has advanced to be the single most important monitoring technique in decision making regarding sacrifice of a carotid artery.

Intraoperative Cerebral Blood Flow Monitoring by Thermal Diffusion Probe

Cerebral thermal diffusion flowmetry can evaluate cerebral perfusion intraoperatively. Preoperative assessment of cerebral perfusion by the thermal diffusion flowmetry as an excellent diagnostic instrument has been already discussed. Similar to neurophysiological monitoring, cerebral blood flow monitoring can provide important information about the patency and functioning of the bypass at the level of microcirculation. One has to consider, however, that data generated by the cerebral blood flow probe is by its nature calculated at a rather small region of the brain; therefore, it cannot guarantee anatomical and functional integrity of the complete territory at risk. It has been shown, however, that when placed in the region of interest the probe values are representative of the territory.[17] We have experienced no complications in terms of insertion and handling of the probe. The only technical drawback is that the probe depends on thermal stability, which cannot always be realized in the setting of an open skull.

Laser Speckle Contrast Analysis

Our group recently introduced laser speckle contrast analysis (LASCA) as a complementary diagnostic tool during neurovascular surgery.[18] It maps cortical blood flow intraoperatively and provides live imaging of relative changes of cerebral cortical blood flow. Developed as an advancement of laser Doppler flowmetry, it allows qualitative and semiquantitative measurement of tissue perfusion over a variable scan area. This new monitoring tool offers real-time measurements of cerebral perfusion with a good temporal and spatial resolution but cannot quantify tissue vascularization.

5.3.6 Antiaggregation and Anticoagulation Regimes

Preoperative administration of antiplatelet aggregation medications is recommended for the prevention of thrombosis and preservation of bypass. The standard regimen includes the administration of 100 mg/day acetyl salicylic acid. However, a significant number of patients show do not respond to this strategy; therefore, we suggest preoperative platelet function analysis for every patient. This allows the optimization of antiaggregation therapy by increasing the dose or changing to a more potent drug. In addition to antiplatelet aggregation therapy, an intraoperative heparin bolus of 3,000 IU might be administered prior to initiating perfusion in the newly created bypass graft.

5.4 Management of Internal Carotid Artery

Once the bypass surgery has been performed and a suitable flow replacement has been established, questions remain as to when to occlude the internal carotid artery when to proceed with tumor resection. In general, there are two possibilities: immediate intraoperative occlusion of the internal carotid artery by clipping, or delayed postoperative occlusion of the internal carotid artery by endovascular means. Since tumor resection is usually planned to follow carotid artery sacrifice an intraoperative occlusion of the internal carotid artery is the preferred strategy. Safe permanent vessel occlusion, however, can only be guaranteed if bypass patency and bypass function are reliably assessed intraoperatively. The usefulness of ICG videoangiography, bypass graft flow measurements, and monitoring of cerebral perfusion, as well as surveillance of adequate neurophysiological function, has been outlined above. Thus, given sufficient and reliable intraoperative monitoring we consider that immediate intraoperative occlusion is generally a safe and reasonable procedure, which can be followed by tumor resection without further delay.

5.5 Management of Tumor

Timing of the tumor resection with respect to bypass surgery is dependent on which vascularization procedure was indicated and performed. The greater the complexity, time consuming, and demanding the bypass procedure is, the more likely the resection of the tumor is planned as second surgery. Location of the tumor and its complexity, especially with regard to its involvement to the ICA, are also taken into account. In principle, if two different surgical approaches have to be used, one for the bypass and another for the tumor resection, it is prudent to proceed in two stages. Once the vessel is secured and has been sacrificed, the resection of the tumor can be performed in a separate session. We believe that two separate sessions are prudent since both the flow replacement procedure by bypass creation and the tumor resection are inherently complex and demanding procedures.

5.6 Combined Endovascular and Surgical Approach as an Alternative for Bypass Surgery

Recently, several approaches combining endovascular with surgical therapies have been developed for tumors involving the ICA or those that are liable to infiltrate it. In the treatment of head and neck cancer involving the ICA, several treatment options are available including radiotherapy and surgery with and without sacrifice of the ICA. When infiltration of the ICA is encountered, a novel combined approach allows radical tumor removal without compromising hemodynamics through the inflicted vessel. This alternative involves implantation of a stent covering the entire length of the ICA artery encased by the tumor. Surgery is performed 1 month later, and the carotid artery wall may be completely dissected from the stent and removed en bloc with the tumor. No deficits, either with regard to clinical signs or in terms of radiological findings, have been observed.[1] This approach seems to be superior to simply stripping or peeling the tumor off the vessel wall since the latter approach accepts a subtotal resection and leads to high recurrence rates due to microinvasion of the vessel wall.

A combined endovascular and surgical approach in the treatment of complex tympanojugular paragangliomas has also been proposed.[19] Infiltration of the tumor is one of the main factors with regard to operability, probability to resect the tumor totally and, hence, to positively influence patient's outcome. Involvement of the ICA by tympanojugular paragangliomas may be limited and surgery alone may allow a complete resection with no or minimal danger to the internal carotid artery. However, in patients with infiltrating and aggressive tympanojugular paragangliomas (especially in young patients), resection is prone to injury to the ICA, and complete resection of the tumor without sacrificing the vessel is virtually impossible. Some surgeons favor limiting the surgical intervention and only partially resect the tumor when ICA involvement occurs.[20]

In case of infiltrating tumor growth in young patients, partial resection is a poor option. A combined endovascular and surgical procedure approach is superior. As a first step, stenting of the cervical and petrous segment of the internal carotid is performed. Subsequently, patients undergo surgery with removal of the tumor. The rationale of this procedure is to define a plane of dissection and remove the tumor totally while having the vessel at risk secured by the stent. This procedure provides an elegant and intriguing approach to decrease the intraoperative risk of bleeding from the ICA as well as from its petrous and cavernous branches. It is not probable that, in patients presenting major encasement of the vessel wall, we could achieve a complete resection of the tumor without including the infiltrated vessel as well. It is intuitive that only en bloc resection of both tumor and vessel can provide complete removal of all tumor cells and prevent a local recurrence. Nevertheless, long-term results remain undefined.

Re-endothelialization of the stent poses an immediate risk for spreading of tumor cells. In addition, interventional complications of stenting such as bleeding, spasm, ischemic events, and rupture of the vessel wall, especially in patients who previously have been subject to radiotherapy, have to be weighed against the long-term benefits, which remain unclear. Unfortunately, there are no sufficient data regarding long-term outcomes with respect to in-stent restenosis after stent placement for this indication. This also applies to medial sphenoid wing meningiomas that can undergo endovascular stenting prior to surgery.

In one patient a meningioma extending into the cavernous sinus led to hemiparesis due to encasement and stenosis of the intracavernous internal carotid artery and subsequent cerebral hypoperfusion. Since the tumor produced ischemic symptoms, a vessel sacrifice could not be performed without risking permanent neurological deficits. Instead, percutaneous placement of a stent restored sufficient blood flow. In this case, other comorbidities preclude an extirpative surgery.[21]

In summary, stenting and subsequent surgery in cases of tumors exerting mass effects on the internal carotid artery and, thus, compromising the blood flow to the brain is a feasible alternative to a revascularization procedure followed by en bloc resection of the tumor. Nevertheless, it remains unclear whether complete tumor removal can be achieved and what is the ideal time lag between stenting and surgery.

We have developed an algorithm for indication of bypass surgery according to the results of the cerebral blood flow analysis. If the patient tolerates the acetazolamide challenge without exhibiting neurological deficits, but cerebral blood flow are increasing less than 30% of baseline value, an impairment of cerebrovascular reserve capacity is highly probable and the creation of a standard STA-MCA bypass is indicated. Without showing neurological deficits and with an increase of more than 30% of baseline value reserve capacity is intact and it is sound to refrain from bypass surgery. In this case no flow augmentation by way of bypass surgery is indicated and the respective internal carotid can be sacrificed without reasonably endangering perfusion of the brain. If hemodynamic insufficiency is not clinically apparent but can be found by a decrease of up to 30% in baseline measurements without hemodynamic challenge by acetazolamide, the establishment of an intermediate-flow radial artery graft bypass prior to tumor-related vessel sacrifice is indicated. In case of a drop of cerebral blood flow values of more than 30% in relationship to the baseline, the creation of a high-flow saphenous vein bypass is advocated. Finally, if neurological deficits can be observed during BTO we consider it best for the patient to be treated with high-flow bypass.

5.6.1 Cerebral Perfusion and Hemodynamics

For analysis of cerebral perfusion and hemodynamics patients undergo DSA. The synchronous opacification of hemispheric cortical veins is an important factor for evaluation of the cerebral blood flow characteristics and resulting hemodynamic tolerance. Additionally, collateralization from the ICA to the contralateral hemisphere via the anterior communicating artery can be evaluated. Furthermore arterial and venous filling of the territory of interest can be achieved via the vertebrobasilar circulation and assessed by injection of contrast agent into the dominant vertebral artery. Lateral vertebral angiography demonstrates if collateral circulation exists via the posterior communicating artery. The functioning of the circle of Willis can be evaluated. Threshold values with regard to delayed venous filling are from 0.5 to 1 second depending on the protocol used.[4] If opacification of the cortical veins in the territory originally supplied by the occluded vessel is delayed by more than 0.5 seconds compared with the contralateral hemisphere it is considered to be asynchronous and represents hemodynamic insufficiency.

Depending on supply of the collateral flow, either being via the anterior communicating artery of the contralateral ICA or through the posterior communicating artery of the vertebrobasilar circulation, the comparison of filling delay has to be based on the symmetry of the hemispheres or, in the case of posterior collateralization, the synchronicity between anterior and posterior filling. In patients with tumors involving the ICA, the main collateralization flow is directed via the anterior communicating artery. In summary, asymetrical or asynchronous filling suggests hemodynamic intolerance and is a predictor of developing stroke after unprotected permanent internal carotid artery occlusion. Studies have shown that about 50 to 75% of patients undergoing BTO show findings consistent with hemodynamic tolerance dependent on the respective protocol and patient population, and thus would not need protective bypass surgery. However, angiographic assessment alone cannot be considered sufficient for indication of bypass surgery in patients with tumors involving the ICA. A significant number of patients with latent hemodynamic insufficiency will be missed due to the comparably low sensitivity of angiographic findings alone. Therefore it is of major importance to rely also on diagnostic measures with the ability to quantify grades of vascularization.

Pearls and Pitfalls

When considering sacrifice of the ICA, either electively because of tumor involvement or as an emergency following an accidental injury, the adequacy of the brain blood supply after exclusion of the artery has to be assured before the sacrifice.

In such clinical scenarios the patient should undergo a six-vessel angiography with BTO applying radiological, clinical, and functional perfusion criteria to evaluate the cerebrovascular system.

If a patient does not tolerate vessel occlusion, generally there are two ways to maintain brain blood supply: revascularization by a bypass or stenting of the ICA.

BTO decision-making algorithm to indicate extracranial–intracranial bypass surgery:
a) Patients who exhibit neurological deficits or demonstrate an asynchronous filling of the transverse sinus > 1 second will need revascularization with a large-caliber graft.
b) Patients demonstrating > 50% decrease in baseline perfusion will qualify for a medium or large caliber graft.
c) Patients with 30 to 50% decrease in baseline perfusion will need a small caliber bypass.
d) In patients with < 30% reduced baseline perfusion, the cerebrovascular reserve capacity should be assessed by acetazolamide stimulation. If the increase is impaired, a small caliber bypass is recommended.

Types of extracranial–intracranial bypass:
a) STA-MCA bypass: the frontal or parietal branch of the superficial temporal artery is anastomosed to a cortical branch of the middle cerebral artery (blood flow 20–70 mL/min).
b) Radial graft artery interposition between external carotid artery and the middle cerebral artery (blood flow 60–100 mL/min).
c) Saphenous vein graft interposition between external carotid artery and the middle cerebral artery (blood flow 100–200 mL/min = high-flow bypass).

Intraoperative assessment of bypass function should be verified by ICG videoangiography, neurophysiological monitoring, thermal diffusion probe, and LASCA.

Bypass surgery or stenting and subsequent tumor surgery should be performed as a two-staged procedure: once the blood flow to the brain is secured the tumor can be removed in a separate session.

References

[1] Nussbaum ES, Levine SC, Hamlar D, Madison MT. Carotid stenting and "extarterectomy" in the management of head and neck cancer involving the internal carotid artery: technical case report. Neurosurgery 2000; 47: 981–984

[2] Sessa CN, Morasch MD, Berguer R, Kline RA, Jacobs JR, Arden RL. Carotid resection and replacement with autogenous arterial graft during operation for neck malignancy. Ann Vasc Surg 1998; 12: 229–235

[3] Fisch U. Infratemporal fossa approach to tumours of the temporal bone and base of the skull. J Laryngol Otol 1978; 92: 949–967

[4] van Rooij WJ, Sluzewski M, Slob MJ, Rinkel GJ. Predictive value of angiographic testing for tolerance to therapeutic occlusion of the carotid artery. AJNR Am J Neuroradiol 2005; 26: 175–178

[5] McIvor NP, Willinsky RA, TerBrugge KG, Rutka JA, Freeman JL. Validity of test occlusion studies prior to internal carotid artery sacrifice. Head Neck 1994; 16: 11–16

[6] Sorteberg A, Bakke SJ, Boysen M, Sorteberg W. Angiographic balloon test occlusion and therapeutic sacrifice of major arteries to the brain. Neurosurgery 2008; 63: 651–660, discussion 660–661

[7] Eckert B, Thie A, Carvajal M, Groden C, Zeumer H. Predicting hemodynamic ischemia by transcranial Doppler monitoring during therapeutic balloon occlusion of the internal carotid artery. AJNR Am J Neuroradiol 1998; 19: 577–582

[8] Field M, Jungreis CA, Chengelis N, Kromer H, Kirby L, Yonas H. Symptomatic cavernous sinus aneurysms: management and outcome after carotid occlusion and selective cerebral revascularization. AJNR Am J Neuroradiol 2003; 24: 1200–1207

[9] Marshall RS, Lazar RM, Young WL et al. Clinical utility of quantitative cerebral blood flow measurements during internal carotid artery test occlusions. Neurosurgery 2002; 50: 996–1004; discussion 1004–1005

[10] Vajkoczy P, Roth H, Horn P et al. Continuous monitoring of regional cerebral blood flow: experimental and clinical validation of a novel thermal diffusion microprobe. J Neurosurg 2000; 93: 265–274

[11] Sekhar LN, Duff JM, Kalavakonda C, Olding M. Cerebral revascularization using radial artery grafts for the treatment of complex intra-cranial aneurysms: techniques and outcomes for 17 patients. Neurosurgery 2001; 49: 646–658; discussion 658–659

[12] Friedman JA, Piepgras DG. Current neurosurgical indications for saphenous vein graft bypass. Neurosurg Focus 2003; 14: e1

[13] Langer DJ, Van Der Zwan A, Vajkoczy P, Kivipelto L, Van Doormaal TP, Tulleken CA. Excimer laser-assisted nonocclusive anastomosis. An emerging technology for use in the creation of intracranial-intracranial and extracranial-intracranial cerebral bypass. Neurosurg Focus 2008; 24: E6

[14] Bremmer JP, Verweij BH, Klijn CJM, van der Zwan A, Kappelle LJ, Tulleken CA. Predictors of patency of excimer laser-assisted nonocclusive extracranial-to-intracranial bypasses. J Neurosurg 2009; 110: 887–895

[15] Raabe A, Nakaji P, Beck J et al. Prospective evaluation of surgical microscope-integrated intraoperative near-infrared indocyanine green videoangiography during aneurysm surgery. J Neurosurg 2005; 103: 982–989

[16] Woitzik J, Horn P, Vajkoczy P, Schmiedek P. Intraoperative control of extracranial-intracranial bypass patency by near-infrared indocyanine green videoangiography. J Neurosurg 2005; 102: 692–698

[17] Horn P, Vajkoczy P, Thomé C, Muench E, Schilling L, Schmiedek P. Xenon-induced flow activation in patients with cerebral insult who undergo xenon-enhanced CT blood flow studies. AJNR Am J Neuroradiol 2001; 22: 1543–1549

[18] Hecht N, Woitzik J, Dreier JP, Vajkoczy P. Intraoperative monitoring of cerebral blood flow by laser speckle contrast analysis. Neurosurg Focus 2009; 27: E11

[19] Sanna M, Piazza P, De Donato G, Menozzi R, Falcioni M. Combined endovascular-surgical management of the internal carotid artery in complex tympanojugular paragangliomas. Skull Base 2009; 19: 26–42

[20] Witiak DG, Pensak ML. Limitations to mobilizing the intrapetrous carotid artery. Ann Otol Rhinol Laryngol 2002; 111: 343–348

[21] Heye S, Maleux G, Van Loon J, Wilms G. Symptomatic stenosis of the cavernous portion of the internal carotid artery due to an irresectable medial sphenoid wing meningioma: treatment by endovascular stent placement. AJNR Am J Neuroradiol 2006; 27: 1532–1534

Chapter 6

Multidisciplinary Endoscopic Skull Base Centers: Delivering Integrated Care

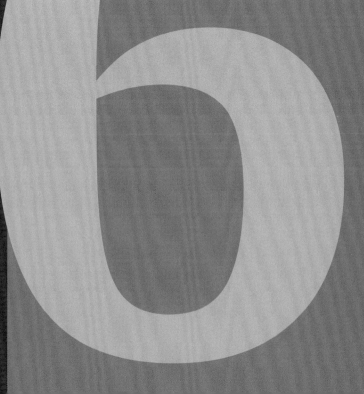

6 Multidisciplinary Endoscopic Skull Base Centers: Delivering Integrated Care

Nancy McLaughlin, Ricardo L. Carrau, Amin B. Kassam, Daniel M. Prevedello, Wolfgang Deinsberger, Ulrike Bockmühl

6.1 Introduction

During the past two decades there has been an increased use of endoscopic endonasal surgery for a variety of sinonasal and skull base pathologies. Thanks to the surgical expertise acquired by leading centers from around the world, endoscopic endonasal approaches have enabled a safe approach to deeply seated lesions.[1,2,3,4,5,6] Such approaches are currently recognized as a critical tool in the armamentarium of sinonasal and skull base surgeons as they provide access to the anterior, middle, and posterior cranial fossa. The favorable outcome is on one hand due to the satisfactory surgical results, and on the other due to the collaborative efforts of multiple caregivers. Effective health care requires a team of diverse health professionals to address the patient's specific needs throughout the care episode. Therefore, the multidisciplinary team approach is omnipresent in the outpatient preoperative, inpatient perioperative, and outpatient postoperative phases of care.

In this chapter, we review key elements assuring the progression and success of a multidisciplinary team approach and present how this concept has been implemented in dedicated endoscopic skull base centers.

6.2 Key Features of the Multidisciplinary Team Approach

Although physicians have traditionally been viewed as providers of clinical care, they should also be responsible for improving the quality of services delivered, not only during the acute phase of surgical care but also throughout the long-term follow-up as is mandated by most pituitary and skull base lesions. With today's medical system, which encourages specialization in specific fields of interest such as sinonasal and skull base endoscopic surgery, it is realistically impossible for one single physician to provide holistic care. Therefore, teamwork is recommended to pool together team members' skills, experience, and knowledge, and ultimately achieve the best overall outcome for patients.[7,8] Multidisciplinary practice is being recognized by many health care systems as central to improve patient care and outcomes, and to enhance patient safety.[8]

6.2.1 Formats of Teamwork

The process of teamwork is both complex and diverse.[8,9,10] Multiple terms are used in the literature to describe different structures of teamwork, namely multidisciplinary, interdisciplinary, and transdisciplinary team.[11] These three formats of teamwork describe a spectrum of collaborative work. In a multidisciplinary team different professions or different specialties in the same profession individually work to achieve their personal goals and meet to discuss their progress.[11] In interdisciplinary teams, the team first agrees upon the goals set forth (by the team). The members of an interdisciplinary team coordinate their efforts to the common treatment plan.[11] In transdisciplinary teams, the members not only share the goals but also the skills. This type of teamwork assures greater flexibility and interchangeability between members, enabling best use of resources.[11] In the context of sinonasal and skull base lesions, an interdisciplinary approach assures that all members share a common goal: improving quality of care delivered to patients afflicted with such pathologies. Within this overall interdisciplinary concept, the surgical team is in itself an interdisciplinary team, where all surgeons work together to obtain the best surgical result, each responsible for different parts of the surgery given their background. However, after numerous years of collaborative work, following the example of our team, neurosurgeons and head and neck surgeons may become interchangeable for every step of the procedure, creating a true transdisciplinary team. Various formats of teamwork may prevail at different moments throughout the episode of care, emphasizing that teamwork per se is much more important than the specific format it takes[12] (▶ Fig. 6.1).

6.2.2 Concepts of Teamwork

Multidisciplinary teamwork seeks an efficient and productive way to achieve the common goals set forth.[7] However, several barriers may prevent its potential to be fully exploited.[10] Xyrichis and colleagues reviewed important factors that can either inhibit or facilitate teamwork.

Team Structure

Having a structure is critical to a multidisciplinary team's success.[10] Team composition and overall size is dictated by the diversity of medical professionals required by the patient's care throughout the entire episode of care (▶ Fig. 6.2). Teams with multiple team members from the same specialty may not be as effective. Information exchange, communication between members, and personal familiarity is facilitated by geographic proximity.[13,14] Most importantly, the multidisciplinary team should have a skilled leader, able to channel the team's energy,

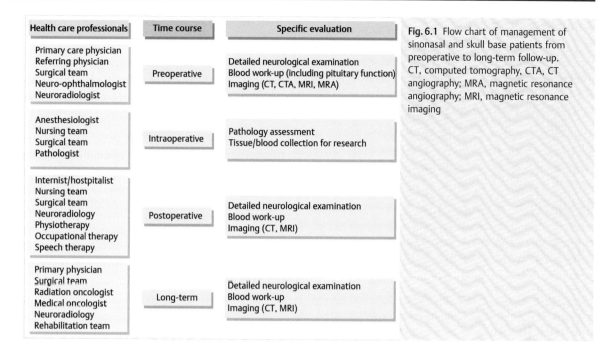

Health care professionals	Time course	Specific evaluation
Primary care physician Referring physician Surgical team Neuro-ophthalmologist Neuroradiologist	Preoperative	Detailed neurological examination Blood work-up (including pituitary function) Imaging (CT, CTA, MRI, MRA)
Anesthesiologist Nursing team Surgical team Pathologist	Intraoperative	Pathology assessment Tissue/blood collection for research
Internist/hostpitalist Nursing team Surgical team Neuroradiology Physiotherapy Occupational therapy Speech therapy	Postoperative	Detailed neurological examination Blood work-up Imaging (CT, MRI)
Primary physician Surgical team Radiation oncologist Medical oncologist Neuroradiology Rehabilitation team	Long-term	Detailed neurological examination Blood work-up Imaging (CT, MRI)

Fig. 6.1 Flow chart of management of sinonasal and skull base patients from preoperative to long-term follow-up. CT, computed tomography, CTA, CT angiography; MRA, magnetic resonance angiography; MRI, magnetic resonance imaging

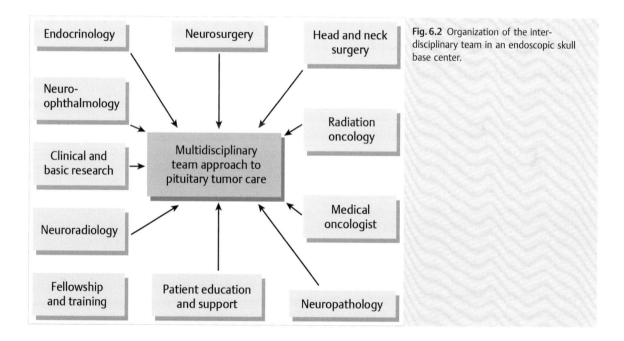

Fig. 6.2 Organization of the interdisciplinary team in an endoscopic skull base center.

maintain team momentum, and guide decision making.[15] Absence of leadership predicted lower levels of team effectiveness and was associated with poor quality teamworking.[1] In the context of sinonasal and skull base lesions, the leader should be a member of the surgical team, representing a team member involved in the patient's care throughout all phases of care: preoperative, perioperative, and postoperative. Beyond a specific team's structure, the health organization should have a common vision of multidisciplinary work. Organizational support is important for progressive development and continuous maturation of a multidisciplinary teamwork within the health organization. Disease or condition specific multidisciplinary teams should align their goals with those of their organization, share framework and tools, as well as resources. Health organizations should encourage innovations such as multidisciplinary collaborations, seeking to improve patient care.[10]

Team Processes

A well-established procedural organization is important for the effective working of the group.[10] Recurrent team meetings enable members to follow-up on their deliverables from previous meetings, set future goals, and clarify care processes, roles, and responsibilities.[16] All members, including verbal or written contacts with other members, must know means of communication within the multidisciplinary team. Communication within multidisciplinary teams supports collegial learning, expression of opinions on divergent views, development of new working relationships, and improvement in patient welfare.[7] Not only should teams have established processes on when to meet, how to communicate, what is to be discussed during the meetings, they should also have a procedural plan to evaluate their performance. Regular audits should be established with resultant effective and constructive feedback. Process measures and measurement of the impact of multidisciplinary care should be planned. At the end of an audit, members should participate in the development of new tools to optimize their efficiency and their impact on patient care.

6.3 Implementation of a Multidisciplinary Approach to Sinonasal and Skull Base Pathologies

Multiple groups around the world have developed excellence centers for the treatment of sinonasal and skull base pathologies using endoscopic endonasal approaches. This patient population requires specific care throughout the entire care episode, inspiring the elaboration of dedicated multidisciplinary teams to coordinate their care. The following is an overview of how various medical professionals can engage in a multidisciplinary approach, breaking down specialty silos and coordinating optimal delivery of care.

6.3.1 Preoperative Care

The primary care physician is a central player in the preoperative care of most patients. They are often the first medical specialists that are consulted by the patient for various symptoms, some more specific than others. Primary care physicians coordinate initial investigation including endocrine work-up and imaging. When the investigation is suggestive of a sinonasal or skull base lesion, a decision must be made to refer the patient to a team of specialists with extensive experience in such type of pathologies. Communication between the referring physician and the referred specialist is key.[8,10] The referred surgical team should clearly communicate the treatment plan to the referring physician to keep everyone implicated in the patients' care in the loop and to prevent disutility of resources and delay of care.

To offer a rigorous assessment, the patient should be evaluated by a team of surgeons able to advise and offer the complete spectrum of management options (including in some cases conservative treatment with serial imaging) and treatment modalities for sinonasal and skull base lesions, including oncological, radiation, and surgical aspects. The surgical team should be versatile in all approaches as well as reconstructive techniques to tailor the best surgical option for the patient. Together, the surgical team, composed of surgeons experienced in conventional transcranial and transfacial approaches, keyhole procedures, as well as in expanded endoscopic approaches, aims to achieve the most complete removal with preservation of the patient's neurological status. Thus, the first visit with the surgical team is important in many regards. It is the occasion to get a detailed medical history from the patient and perform a complete neurological examination with special emphasis on cranial nerves, sensorimotor, and cerebellar functions. In the presence of a clival, petroclival, or foramen magnum lesion, a detailed evaluation of the lower cranial nerve function is essential to document any subclinical dysfunction.

Furthermore, consultation with a speech therapist may help identify and/or quantify vocal cord and swallowing preoperative dysfunctions.

An endoscopic assessment of the nasal cavity should be performed prior to surgery to document sinus infection, septal integrity, septal deviations, and any other particular anatomical findings. Images should be reviewed with the patient as this helps them process the information and understand the following steps. If complementary imaging is required such as pituitary magnetic resonance imaging (MRI), magnetic resonance angiography (MRA), computed tomography angiography (CTA), or digital subtraction angiography (DSA), it should be explained to the patient and discussed with the neuroradiologist to obtain the most information out of the additional images.

If possible, a nurse practitioner should be implicated in the initial visit and serve as a reference person for any questions the patient may have and to clarify all the expectations related to the postoperative period. Centers dedicated at treating sinonasal and skull base pathologies should have educational material to help patients understand their pathology, their options, and preview the proposed treatment modality or combined treatment plan. The nurse practitioner can also help coordinate consultations with other members of the team.

Neuro-ophthalmologists are essential to evaluate preoperatively the visual acuity, presence of papilledema, presence of anisocoria and/or ptosis, and visual fields.

Endocrinologists are essential for assessing the patient's pituitary function prior to surgery by dosing specific hormones and performing precise stimulation tests. This evaluation is important since appropriate medical therapy for specific functional pituitary adenomas may decrease perioperative morbidities.[17]

Once surgery is recommended as a treatment plan, the primary physician should be informed and should coordinate the preoperative clearance. Prior to surgery, the surgical team must have responded all the patient's questions. In institutions where a research facility exists, participation to a tissue and/or blood bank should be offered on a voluntary basis to each patient prior to surgery.

6.3.2 Intraoperative Care

Perioperatively, the anesthesiologist is probably the most important member of the care team. For some patients with sinonasal, florid acromegaly, and skull base lesions, securing the airways may be a challenge and may require special intubation techniques. The surgical team and the anesthesiologist must discuss this possibility prior to intubation.

A dedicated surgical team performs the surgery. Given the collaborative efforts of skull base neurosurgeons, head and neck surgeons, neuro-otologist, and ophthalmologist, each part of the surgery is performed by the surgeon best acquainted with that specific part of the intervention. In some situations, as occurs during endoscopic endonasal approaches to the skull base, a head and neck surgeon and neurosurgeon perform the main part of the procedure simultaneously, demonstrating the concept of intraoperative multidisciplinary teamwork. This approach has been studied in the setting of acoustic neuroma surgery performed by a neurosurgeon and a neuro-otologist and was found to deliver optimal surgical results.[18] Combining expertise on a regular basis optimizes the surgical team's success in comparison with casual interaction.

Histopathology evaluation often confirms the presumed preoperative diagnosis representing another important member of the team. Detailed analysis of the histological characteristics and molecular signature are important for the adjuvant treatments recommended after surgery.

6.3.3 Postoperative Care

Following an expanded endonasal approach in which an intradural dissection was performed, close surveillance in an intensive care unit is required for the initial 24 hours. The patient's premorbid medical condition may also warrant this precaution. The surgical team must inform the intensivist/neurointensivist about the clinical history, preoperative neurological status, intervention performed, any intraoperative complication that might have occurred, and total blood loss. Informing the intensivist as well as the primary care physician assures optimal postoperative care for the patient. In cases of functional pituitary tumors or surgical procedures that might have altered the pituitary gland or pituitary stalk, the endocrinologist

should be invited to jointly follow the patient. During the first postoperative days, nurses at bedside, nurse practitioners, physiotherapists, occupational therapists, and the speech pathologists all contribute to the patient's recovery. These complementary disciplines' perspectives are essential to meet the needs of the patient and his/her family.

The patient's family is an important element is the patient's postoperative care. Given that they are at bedside most of the time, it is crucial that they understand what is to be expected in the postoperative period. It is important to inform them on symptoms and signs to look for, so they can inform the nursing staff. The family members also play a key role in the patient's recovery as they can stimulate progressive diet and mobilization. Their cooperation should be recognized and encouraged. The patient's discharge is organized only when the entire team believes this is safe. The patient's family or immediate caregiver should always be implicated in this decision since they will be looking after the patient at home. Common instructions must be given to the patient, preventing confusion and misunderstanding.

In the name of the sinonasal and skull base team, the nurse practitioner coordinates the discharge and follow-up instructions. The patient is seen in clinic 7 to 10 days after the surgery by the surgical team. At the same time, the head and neck surgeon may want to assess the sinonasal cavities. The definitive pathology is announced to the patient. If adjuvant treatment is required, the nurse practitioner coordinates the integration of medical oncologist and radio-oncologist to the team. It is important that the treatment plan be forwarded to the patient's primary physician to maintain all caregivers informed.

6.3.4 Long-term Follow-up

In the first year postoperative, clinical follow-ups every 3 to 6 months are important since they allow the patient to keep in contact with his surgical team. At all times, the nurse practitioner should be available to answer the patient's questions. A postoperative MRI should be performed at 3 months or earlier if the radiation or medical oncologists have specific concerns. This should be discussed between members of the medical team. For patients with preoperative visual deficits or new postoperative visual deficits, a follow-up should be organized within 4 to 6 weeks of surgery to re-evaluate the patient's vision.

In the presence of preoperative endocrinopathy or new postoperative hypopituitarism or diabetes insipidus, the patient should follow-up with his/her endocrinologist for fine-tuning of hormonal replacement and postoperative pituitary function assessment. In dedicated endoscopic skull base centers, organizing a patient support group integrates previous patients to the care team. In many institutions, the support group is a forum where new patients can meet and ask their questions directly to other patients afflicted with a pituitary pathology.

Members of the sinonasal and skull base interdisciplinary team should actively participate in the education of patients through presentations at the support group.

6.4 Trends for a Multidisciplinary Team at Endoscopic Skull Base Centers

Efforts to break down the silos between different professions and specialties to optimize patient care have been deployed at various degrees in different institutions. Tumor boards and virtual case review sessions, multidisciplinary clinics, multidisciplinary surgeries, multidisciplinary rounds, and care coordination meetings are examples of teamwork occurring throughout the entire phase of care. A review of the literature of these venues is beyond the scope of this chapter.[12] Importantly, many health care organizations are recognizing multidisciplinary team activities such as case reviews, tumor boards, and multidisciplinary rounds as central to improve patient safety, care, and outcomes.[19]

In addition, multidisciplinary teamwork may serve to achieve a greater resource efficiency by reducing duplication of investigations, sealing potential gaps in care management, minimizing variability in care delivery with the use of care protocols and care pathways, and minimizing the occurrence of errors. Implementation of multidisciplinary teams and reorganization of services may also result in centralization of various service lines, with potential advantages in value-based delivery of care (best outcome for the least cost).[8,20,21] Institutions recognizing these advantages will understand the importance of their support in the growth and maturation of multidisciplinary teams at skull base centers.

Various opportunities need to be created for health professionals to learn together. On an interpersonal level, members of the team should be encouraged to participate in communication and teamwork seminars.[10] Investment in team training is important since teamwork is not necessarily taught during medical training. Social activities should be coordinated to favor interpersonal ties between members and to facilitate a sense of belonging to the team. Although members currently possibly attend to their yearly specialty meeting, a common symposium on treatment of sinonasal and skull base pathologies should be organized yearly in every skull base center. This yearly local multidisciplinary meeting stimulates members to show their achievement within the last year and to propose new care programs. It is a forum where all disciplines are recognized as an active part of the patient's care. In the near future, international multidisciplinary meetings specific to a subspecialty will become the key element to improving holistic care for patients with sinonasal and skull base pathologies. These meetings should also implicate researchers working on various projects either clinical or basic science. Exchange of knowledge among specialists that have at heart the care of a specific group of pathologies will fuel research ideas and opportunities.

6.5 Conclusion

Multidisciplinary teamwork is critical for optimal care of patients afflicted with sinonasal and skull base pathologies. It drives quality improvement and overall improvement of patient outcomes. In whatever format (multidisciplinary, interdisciplinary, transdisciplinary), it is tightly interwoven in patient care from preoperative, perioperative, and postoperative phases of care. The multidisciplinary approach positions and keeps the patient at the center of the team's efforts throughout all his treatment, from beginning to end. Such collaborations are essential to help fully integrate clinical care, basic and translational research, and clinical trials.

References

[1] Cappabianca P, Cavallo LM, Esposito F, De Divitiis O, Messina A, De Divitiis E. Extended endoscopic endonasal approach to the midline skull base: the evolving role of transsphenoidal surgery. Adv Tech Stand Neurosurg 2008; 33: 151–199

[2] de Divitiis E, Esposito F, Cappabianca P, Cavallo LM, de Divitiis O, Esposito I. Endoscopic transnasal resection of anterior cranial fossa meningiomas. Neurosurg Focus 2008; 25: E8

[3] Fatemi N, Dusick JR, de Paiva Neto MA, Kelly DF. The endonasal microscopic approach for pituitary adenomas and other parasellar tumors: a 10-year experience. Neurosurgery 2008; 63 Suppl 2: 244–256; discussion 256

[4] Gardner PA, Kassam AB, Thomas A et al. Endoscopic endonasal resection of anterior cranial base meningiomas. Neurosurgery 2008; 63: 36–52; discussion 52–54

[5] Laufer I, Anand VK, Schwartz TH. Endoscopic, endonasal extended transsphenoidal, transplanum transtuberculum approach for resection of suprasellar lesions. J Neurosurg 2007; 106: 400–406

[6] Zada G, Kelly DF, Cohan P, Wang C, Swerdloff R. Endonasal transsphenoidal approach for pituitary adenomas and other sellar lesions: an assessment of efficacy, safety, and patient impressions. J Neurosurg 2003; 98: 350–358

[7] McCallin A. Interprofessional practice: learning how to collaborate. Contemp Nurse 2005; 20: 28–37

[8] Sargeant J, Loney E, Murphy G. Effective interprofessional teams: "contact is not enough" to build a team. J Contin Educ Health Prof 2008; 28: 228–234

[9] Delva D, Jamieson M, Lemieux M. Team effectiveness in academic primary health care teams. J Interprof Care 2008; 22: 598–611

[10] Xyrichis A, Lowton K. What fosters or prevents interprofessional teamworking in primary and community care? A literature review. Int J Nurs Stud 2008; 45: 140–153

[11] Young CA. Building a care and research team. J Neurol Sci 1998; 160 Suppl 1: S137–S140

[12] McLaughlin N, Carrau RL, Kelly DF, Prevedello DM, Kassam AB. Teamwork in skull base surgery: An avenue for improvement in patient care. Surg Neurol Int 2013; 4: 36

[13] Cook G, Gerrish K, Clarke C. Decision-making in teams: issues arising from two UK evaluations. J Interprof Care 2001; 15: 141–151

[14] Molyneux J. Interprofessional teamworking: what makes teams work well? J Interprof Care 2001; 15: 29–35

[15] Field R, West M. Teamwork in primary health care: 2. Perspectives from practices. J Interprof Care 1995; 9: 123–130

[16] Rutherford J, McArthur M. A qualitative account of the factors affecting team-learning in primary care. Education for Primary Care 2004; 15: 352–360

[17] Feelders RA, Hofland LJ, van Aken MO et al. Medical therapy of acromegaly: efficacy and safety of somatostatin analogues. Drugs 2009; 69: 2207–2226

[18] Tonn JC, Schlake HP, Goldbrunner R, Milewski C, Helms J, Roosen K. Acoustic neuroma surgery as an interdisciplinary approach: a neurosurgical series of 508 patients. J Neurol Neurosurg Psychiatry 2000; 69: 161–166

[19] Borrill C, West M, Shapiro D, Rees A. Team working and effectiveness in health care. British Journal of Health Care Management 2000; 6: 364–371

[20] Olofsson J. Multidisciplinary team a prerequisite in endoscopic endonasal skull base surgery. Eur Arch Otorhinolaryngol 2010; 267: 647

[21] Westin T, Stalfors J. Tumour boards/multidisciplinary head and neck cancer meetings: are they of value to patients, treating staff or a political additional drain on healthcare resources? Curr Opin Otolaryngol Head Neck Surg 2008; 16: 103–107

Chapter 7

360° Access to the Skull Base

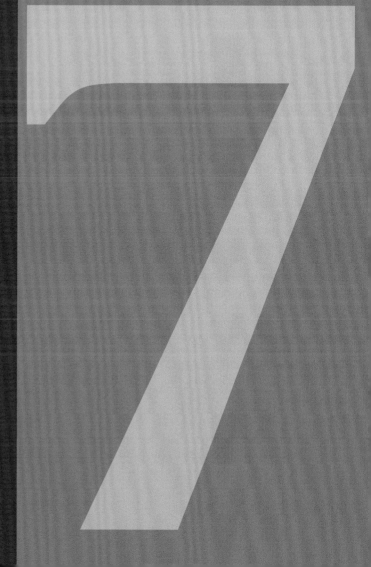

7 360° Access to the Skull Base

Nancy McLaughlin, Daniel M. Prevedello, Juan C. Fernandez-Miranda, Ricardo L. Carrau, Amin B. Kassam

7.1 Introduction

In general there are four primary approaches or trajectories to access the skull base: anterolateral, anteromedial, lateral, and posterolateral. Each of these can be further subdivided into:

- The external corridor (from the skin to the dura)
- The internal corridor (the dura to the lesion)
- The "precision zone" (the neurovascular structures, and in particular the cranial nerves, at the apex of the corridor)

The position of the tumor relative to the cranial nerves usually guides the decision as to which specific approach and trajectory is selected, with an overarching principle of avoiding crossing the plane of the cranial nerve when feasible.

When selecting the specific corridor there has been an increasing tendency to minimize the external and internal corridors and thereby reduce tissue and access-related trauma. This has led to the evolution of minimally invasive approaches in the external/internal corridors; for example, the transition from lateral rhinotomy external approach for anterior medial access to the ventral skull base to an endonasal approach to reach the same internal anterior medial structures. In the case of lateral and anterolateral trajectories this led to the evolution of "keyhole approaches" as pioneered by Axel Perneczky; posterolateral corridors evolved to retromastoid approaches championed by Peter Jannetta and Madjid Samii; and the evolution of the expanded endonasal approaches (EEAs) represented the transition of the anteromedial corridor to minimally invasive approaches.

EEAs have proven to provide safe anteromedial access along the sagittal and coronal planes to the anterior, middle, and posterior cranial fossa.[1,2,3,4] This has diversified the armamentarium of skull base approaches; however, the surgeon should be able to recognize when a transcranial lateral trajectory, endonasal anteromedial trajectory, or a combination of such approaches is better suited for the patient.[5,6,7] We refer to these circumferential trajectories to the skull base as "360° approaches" to the skull base.

This chapter reviews our decision algorithm in selecting the approach that will provide the most direct and least destructive route or combination of routes to facilitate the most complete resection with the least morbidity possible. It should be noted that while there is value in determining the morbidity of the external corridor (skin to dura), the primary long-term morbidity affecting the quality of life is most likely determined by the deeper corridor and the precision zone (working space between the cranial nerves and vasculature). In general the cranial nerves appear to be more sensitive to manipulation and thereby become a greater determinant of long-term morbidity; as a result, whenever possible, the primary driver in selecting the corridor is the avoidance of crossing the plane of the pertinent cranial nerve.

7.2 Skull Base Surgery: An Evolving Discipline

Skull base surgery has always been considered a challenging field given the deep location of pathologies and their proximity to eloquent neurovascular structures. Depending on the trajectory of the approach, skull base procedures may require extensive disruption of soft tissues and bone (external corridor), brain retraction (internal corridor), and neurovascular manipulation (precision zone) to gain access to the pathology. Earlier series underemphasized the access-related postoperative morbidities (temporary and sometimes permanent) that occur in patients undergoing extensive skull base approaches.[8] However, over recent decades, the outcome of patients with skull base lesions has significantly improved.

Significant advances in surgical technique and technology have contributed to reduce perioperative morbidity and mortality rates. From the surgeon's perspective, improved knowledge of skull base anatomy and mastering conventional skull base approaches and reconstructive techniques have contributed to render these procedures safer; therefore, reducing the risk of life-threatening complications.[9,10,11,12,13] The introduction of a multidisciplinary team to treat these pathologies has fueled the development of a variety of surgical strategies, techniques, and approaches. In addition, the refinement of reconstructive techniques has allowed surgeons to pursue more extensive approaches with the objective of complete tumor resection after open and endonasal procedures.[11,12] Advances in the surgical reconstruction of skull base defects have played a key role in the management of complex skull base lesions. Development of new reconstructive modalities and in particular vascularized reconstruction has led the way to extensive transcranial approaches.[11] By assuring sealing of the intracranial and extracranial compartments, reliable reconstructions have reduced serious and life-threatening complications. Meticulous reconstructive techniques have also contributed to improve postoperative quality of life by maximizing function preservation and optimizing cosmetic results. Concurrently, from a technological stand point, intraoperative frameless surgical navigation, improved optics, microinstrumentation, and high-speed drills have been invaluable in improving outcomes.

Despite these refinements in transcranial skull base surgery, some approaches have an inherently elevated risk for complications based on the trajectory selected and the relationship of neurovascular structures with the lesion and the surgical corridor.[8,14,15,16,17,18,19] As part of the natural evolution, the last decade focused on advances in the anteromedial corridor to provide anatomically driven approaches to the skull base. Over this time period, various skull base centers adopted the philosophy of more directed anatomically driven approaches in an attempt to minimize surgical morbidity.[9,10,13] Preservation of life is no longer the only goal; improving or maintaining quality of life is the overarching principle. It is self evident that the surgeon should aim to perform the most complete tumor resection while maintaining quality of life by preserving neurological function, psychological well being, and cosmesis.[13,20] Essentially, the first goal (degree of tumor resection) should not be achieved at the expense of the others, especially in patients with low-grade tumors where prolonged survival is expected. This philosophy marks a new era in the discipline of cranial base surgery, and has redirected its main aim from technical advances to improving overall patient outcome.

This modern trend applies to all skull base approaches. Specifically, keyhole surgeries, including the supraorbital (anterolateral) and retromastoid (posterolateral) approaches, have been increasingly used to address many different skull base pathologies of the anterior, middle, and posterior cranial fossae.[6,21,22,23] Explicitly, the keyhole concept advocated by Perneczky implies that a tailored anatomic corridor can provide access to a deep-seated lesion since the surgical field widens as the distance from the craniotomy increases, obviating the need for large craniotomies (external corridor), brain retraction (internal corridor), and unnecessary tissue exposure.[23] Importantly, such minimally invasive approaches should eliminate or reduce brain manipulation without sacrificing exposure or outcome. In addition, some have expanded the viewing angles afforded by these approaches by integrating the endoscope into these procedures.[24,25,26] Therefore, endoscope-assisted surgery via keyhole approaches for skull base lesions has evolved in the philosophy of maximum efficiency, maximum safety, and minimal invasiveness.

In an analogous manner, over the last two decades, the introduction of EEAs has provided a safe and effective method of reducing the corridor and providing a direct anterior medial trajectory for lesions located along the ventral skull base with cranial nerves along the dorsal perimeter.[1,2,3,4] EEAs are divided into two planes: (a) Median approaches (between the carotid arteries) are oriented rostrocaudally along the sagittal plane from the frontal sinus to the second cervical vertebra; therefore, enabling the treatment of pathologies in the anterior, middle, and posterior cranial fossa.[1,2,3,4] (b) Paramedian approaches (lateral to the carotid arteries) are divided into three different depths: anterior, middle, and posterior, each corresponding respectively to the anterior, middle, and posterior cranial fossa.[3] An EEA offers a direct median exposure through its direct ventral corridor; thus, enabling the removal of a lesion with the least destructive external and internal corridors (paranasal sinuses), and decreased brain and neurovascular structure (precision zone) manipulation. When indicated, its anterior and ventral trajectory allows prompt decompression of the visual apparatus and achieves early tumor devascularization.[5,6,27] Since the EEA has resulted in similar oncological results to those obtained with traditional open approaches for sinonasal, sellar, and skull base lesions, it is considered by many centers the preferred route for carefully selected lesions. As is the case in transcranial approaches, skull base reconstruction is paramount in the management of large skull base tumors. The development of skull base reconstructive techniques using vascularized flaps for large dural defects has significantly reduced the incidence of postoperative cerebrospinal fluid leaks, supporting its widespread use.[28,29,30] Recognition of the value of an EEA is in concert with the evolving philosophy of skull base surgery, aiming to accomplish tumor removal through less invasive routes, offering better overall outcome to patients.

7.3 The 360° Vision

Conceptually, the 360° paradigm is based on a detailed preoperative assessment of the lesion to determine the least destructive surgical corridor, or combination of corridors, that allow the most complete resection while associated with the least potential for complications and best overall outcome. This implies that the surgical team should be capable of performing the entire realm of skull base surgery, including traditional transcranial and minimal-access keyhole approaches, as well as endoscopic endonasal approaches to assess and offer the optimal surgical option for each individual patient (▶ Fig. 7.1**a**). In addition, the surgical team should be comfortable with the various reconstructive techniques to match the various surgical routes.[11,12,28,29,30] Some lesions may be completely addressed through either a transcranial (lateral) or an expanded endonasal (medial) approach; but this will be primarily dictated by the relative position of the cranial nerves involved. However, a single surgical approach may not allow complete exposure of the lesion.[9,31,32]

Applying the 360° paradigm we can categorize the skull base approaches into anteromedial, anterolateral, lateral, and posterolateral corridors (▶ Fig. 7.1**b**). There is a continuum between all approaches and in some cases a combination of two or more of the corridors might be more applicable to the patient's tumor. The possibility of combining transcranial lateral microsurgical approaches or proceeding to a multistage intervention has been

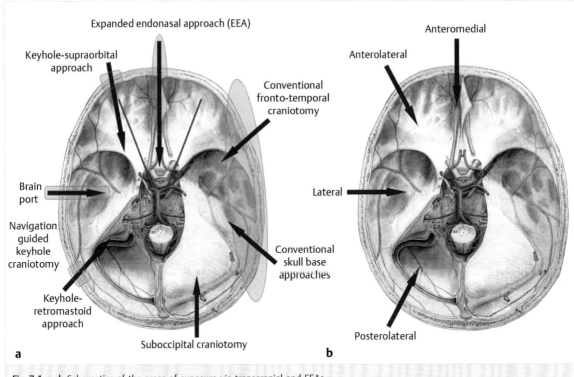

Fig. 7.1 a, b Schematics of the areas of exposure via transcranial and EEAs.

reported by many authors for the management of extensive cranial base lesions.[9,15,17,33,34] The risk of additional surgical morbidity attributable to a second surgical stage must be weighed against the risks of a more extensive and potentially more morbid single surgery requiring the manipulation or transposition of a cranial nerve to gain access to the tumor.[33] Recently, the combination of a medial EEA along with a lateral microsurgical approach has been described.[16,31]

7.3.1 Overview of Skull Base Approaches

The choice of a specific surgical corridor to treat a skull base lesion must take into consideration numerous factors related to the tumor and the patient's comorbidities.[5,6,7,14,35] With regard to the tumor's characteristics: its nature, location, size, consistency, and relation to surrounding vessels and nerves or their encasement are all important in the decision making.[6,18,35,36] In some circumstances, prior surgeries might also dictate the choice of approach in the case of a recurrence.[37] However, the most important consideration for any lesion involving the skull base is clearly its relationship to critical neurovascular structures. Preoperative cranial nerve function, their relationship with the lesion, and the potential risks for postoperative deficits must be carefully assessed preoperatively.

In the early era of skull base surgery vascular complications were the most feared and morbid events; however, as technique and technology have improved, the incidence of vascular complications has profoundly been reduced and their management when they rarely occur has been increasingly more effective. Postoperative morbidity related to cranial nerve deficits has become one of the primary determinants of the quality of life the patient is likely to enjoy, and, therefore, the primary determinant of the trajectory of the approach selected. As such, the anteromedial corridor via endonasal approaches along either the median or the paramedian plane are ideal for lesions in which nerves and vessels are located on the perimeter of the tumor.

Given the expanding armamentarium of skull base approaches, surgeons should recognize when a transcranial, endonasal, or a combination of such approaches is best suited to treat a lesion. The illustrated cases demonstrate how endonasal and transcranial approaches may be complementary, either simultaneously or sequentially, to treat complex skull base lesions.

7.3.2 Overview of Approaches to the Anterior Cranial Fossa

The anterior ventral cranial base is formed by the ethmoid, sphenoid, and frontal bones.[38] Its median osseous framework is formed anteriorly by the crista galli and the cribriform plate of the ethmoid bone, and posteriorly by the planum of the sphenoid body. These bony components cover the upper nasal cavity and the sphenoid sinus. The lateral part of the anterior skull base is formed by the frontal bone and the lesser wing of the sphenoid bone, which cover the orbits and optic canals respectively.[38]

Various transcranial anterior and anterolateral trajectories have been described for anterior skull base lesions. In general the anterolateral and lateral approaches rely on an external corridor that is a variant of a bicoronal or hemicoronal skin flap and accompanying craniotomy. The internal corridor (i.e., from the dura to the target) includes the subfrontal, the interhemispheric, and the pterional corridors. The anteromedial trajectory to this region relied heavily on using the transfacial and the craniofacial external corridors. This was done to provide a more direct route to the lesion using the paranasal sinuses as the internal corridor to avoid the effects of brain manipulation associated with the anterolateral corridors to reach the same ventral targets (precision zone). These risks related to the subfrontal and interhemispheric corridors should not be minimized and are related to the need for frontal lobe retraction, possible need to sacrifice the superior sagittal sinus, and damage to the olfactory tracts. The frontotemporal (pterional) craniotomy with the addition of an orbitotomy to the subfrontal and pterional approaches requires disarticulating the osseous framework to create an internal corridor with a more basal access, thus reducing the need for brain retraction and shortening the distance to the lesion. In particular the pterional craniotomy has the added advantage in that it can potentially use the cisternal space as an internal corridor; however, there still is a need for a certain degree of brain retraction and manipulation. The pterional approach is an essential tool in the skull base surgeon's armamentarium since it can be combined with other lateral and posterolateral corridors to gain access to the middle and posterior fossa respectively. While this lateral approach allows early identification of the ipsilateral carotid artery and optic nerves within the precision zone it is still tethered in circumstances in which the target lesion is located ventral and medial to the optic nerve. In such cases the nerve must be manipulated as it is in the trajectory of the dissection. This is best illustrated by craniopharyngiomas located in the subchiasmatic/retrochiasmatic space and interpeduncular fossa (▶ Fig. 7.2). Despite aggressive removal of bone along the external/internal corridors, when using a lateral trajectory the final working window becomes a small cone-shaped corridor crossing the oculomotor nerve, optic tract, internal carotid artery (ICA), and posterior communicating artery, with all of the associated perforators. In essence the nerve is located between the surgeon and the target; whereas in an anterior medial (EEA) trajectory, the target is located between the surgeon and the nerve.

Using this principle of keeping the target between the surgeon and the nerve, lesions of the median anterior skull base may be approached through a median EEA route[1] (▶ Table 7.1). The transcribriform, transplanum/transtuberculum, and transsellar approaches can be used independently or in combination depending on the tumor's rostrocaudal extension. A golden rule of the expanded endonasal approaches states that the plane of the cranial nerves should not be crossed (if possible) during the exposure or dissection. The lateral boundaries of the transcribriform approach are the laminae papyracea, which can be augmented by an endonasal medial supraorbital approach. Once the orbital soft tissue is lateralized, the meridian of the orbit can be reached in the anterior fossa, with the intraconal optic nerve representing the most lateral limit of the approach. Regarding the transplanum/transtuberculum approach, the optic nerves represent the lateral limit and must therefore be identified early during the exposure. For the paramedian approaches to the anterior cranial fossa, the transorbital approach implies removal of the lamina papyracea or the medial optic nerve canals. Intraconal dissection can be performed between the inferior and medial rectus muscle for pathologies medial to the optic nerve.

7.3.3 Overview of Approaches to the Middle Cranial Fossa

The ventral aspect of the middle cranial fossa is formed by the sphenoid and temporal bones. Its medial part is formed by the sphenoid bone body including the tuberculum sellae, pituitary fossa, middle and posterior clinoid processes, the carotid sulcus, and dorsum sellae. Laterally, it is formed by the lesser and greater sphenoid wings, as well as the squama and petrous bone.[38]

The middle cranial fossa can be accessed transcranially through various lateral approaches (▶ Fig. 7.2). A pterional craniotomy gives access to the middle cranial fossa as well as the supra and parasellar regions. A supraorbital approach also enables access to the suprasellar, parasellar, and cavernous sinus regions.[23,24] The temporozygomatic approach exposes the anterior part of the middle fossa. The posterior temporal floor can be exposed through a lateral corridor via a middle cranial fossa approach (subtemporal craniotomy strategically located above the external auditory canal), a posterolateral corridor through a posterior petrosectomy (combined approach), or a retromastoid suprameatal approach. Risks related to the transcranial middle cranial fossa approaches include temporal lobe retraction, injury to the vein of Labbe, and manipulation of the greater petrosal nerve with resultant facial nerve dysfunction. Recently, some have used the endoscopic-assisted keyhole supraorbital approach for resection of middle cranial fossa tumors to eliminate the need for excessive surgical manipulation.[24] Tumors within the infratemporal fossa may be approached through a preauricular–subtemporal–infratemporal fossa approach. However, independent of the external and

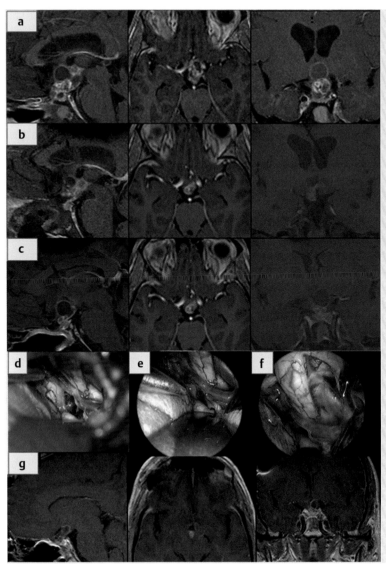

Fig. 7.2 a–g A 50-year-old man was referred to us after initial management at another institution. He was diagnosed in 2002 with a sellar and suprasellar cranio-pharyngioma composed of solid but mostly cystic components for which an EEA was performed (**a**). Given tumor recurrence, the patient underwent multiple endonasal surgical procedures, each time to remove the recurrent tumor and drain the cystic portions. The last EEA intervention was performed in March 2009 (**b, c**). Recently, the patient noticed a decrease in visual acuity of the right eye. Brain MRI showed mostly suprasellar cystic tumor recurrence. Surgical treatment of the recurrent cranio-pharyngioma was proposed through a supraorbital approach given that the majority of the cystic recurrence was located above the optic chiasm (**d f**). This route was chosen given the suprasellar and suprachiasmatic cyst location, the simplified closure, and to avoid mobilizing the previously placed and irradiated nasoseptal flap. Postoperatively the patient's vision improved progressively. Follow-up MRI showed satisfactory decompression of the optic chiasm (**g**).

internal corridors, in the end all lateral approaches are restricted by the position of the cranial nerves at the apex or precision zone.

Lesions in the median aspect of the middle cranial fossa may be treated by endonasal approaches[3] (▶ Fig. 7.3). The cavernous sinus and the cavernous ICA limit the endonasal transsellar approach laterally. Indeed, the cavernous ICA, which represents the meridian of the cavernous sinus, represents the lateral boundary of the transsellar approach. It is critical that the surgeon remains medial to the meridian of the cavernous ICA when using the transsellar corridor to avoid crossing the plane of cranial nerves III, IV, V1, and VI.

The transpterygoid approach is a basic component of most of the anterior median and paramedian trajectories to the middle fossa. It provides access to the medial component of the temporal fossa. The medial petrous apex approach enables treatment of medial petrous apex lesions. The petrous (horizontal) and paraclival (vertical) segments of the ICA are the lateral boundary of these two approaches. Meckel cave may be accessed through a suprapetrous-quadrangular space approach.[39] The limits of this approach are the petrous ICA inferiorly, the paraclival ICA medially, and cranial nerve VI superiorly, as it courses through the cavernous sinus and the maxillary division of the trigeminal nerve (V_2) laterally, referred to as the "quadrangular space." Pathologies within the superior cavernous sinus can be reached through a similar exposure with subsequent opening of the dura over the superior lateral portion of the cavernous sinus. This approach is usually reserved for cases with already established cranial nerve deficits (III, IV, VI) or for tumors refractory to adjuvant therapies.[3] Residual tumors inside the cavernous sinus in patients who have intact ocular

Table 7.1 Summary of conventional and expanded endonasal approaches to the anterior fossa

Expanded endonasal approach		Open approaches (most frequently used)		Cistern exposed	Accessed regions			Common pathologies
Approach	Bone removed	Keyhole approach	Conventional approach		Brain	Cranial nerve	Vessel	
Median approaches								
Transcribriform	Cribriform plate, crista galli	Supraorbital: unilateral frontal mini-craniotomy ± orbital osteotomy	Anterior: Subfrontal: unilateral or bilateral frontal craniotomy ± orbital osteotomy Interhemispheric: bilateral frontal craniotomy Transfacial approaches: (including transmandibular, transmaxillary, extended maxillectomy) Craniofacial approaches (including transbasal) Anterolateral: Pterional: frontotemporal craniotomy ± orbital osteotomy	Interhemispheric fissure	Gyrus rectus, orbitofrontal gyrus	Olfactory	A2, frontopolar, orbital frontal arteries	Olfactory groove meningioma, esthesioneuroblastoma, encephalocele, cerebrospinal fluid leak, sinonasal tumor
Transplanum/transtuberculum	Planum sphenoidale, tuberculum sellae, middle clinoid	Supraorbital: unilateral minifrontal craniotomy ± orbital osteotomy	Anterior: Subfrontal: unilateral or bilateral frontal craniotomy ± orbital osteotomy Anterolateral: Pterional: frontotemporal craniotomy ± orbital osteotomy	Suprasellar cistern, prechiasmatic cistern	Gyrus rectus, orbitofrontal gyrus	Optic nerve, optic chiasm	Internal carotid arteries, superior hypophyseal arteries, anterior communicating artery, A2s	Planum meningioma, suprasellar pituitary macroadenoma, craniopharyngioma, optic nerve glioma, suprasellar Rathke cleft cyst, germ cell tumor
Transsellar	Sphenoid, sellar floor and face	Supraorbital: unilateral frontal mini-craniotomy ± orbital osteotomy (especially for lesions with important suprasellar extension)	Anterior: Subfrontal: bilateral frontal craniotomy ± orbital and zygomatic osteotomies Craniofacial approaches: transbasal with frontal bar Anterolateral: Pterional: frontotemporal craniotomy ± orbital osteotomies	Sellar fossa, suprasellar cistern (suprasellar extension cases)	(Pituitary gland and diaphragma sellae)	Optic nerve, optic chiasm	Cavernous internal carotid artery, superior and inferior hypophyseal arteries	Micro and macroadenoma, craniopharyngioma, Rathke cleft cyst
Paramedian approaches								
Transorbital	Lamina papyracea, medial optic canal	Transconjunctival approach, Lynch approach, lateral orbitotomy	Anterior: Orbitofrontal: small frontal bone flap with superior orbital rim removal Lateral orbitotomy	No cistern Orbital contents	Extraocular muscles Orbital contents	Optic nerve	Anterior and posterior ethmoidal arteries, ophthalmic artery with its central retina artery branch	Sinonasal malignancy, schwannoma, cavernoma, meningioma, hemangioma

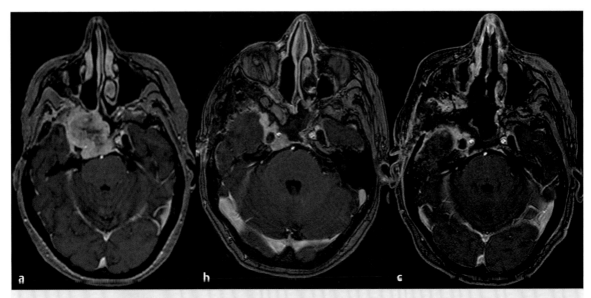

Fig. 7.3 a–c A 66-year-old woman presented with diplopia and new right abducens palsy. She had been operated 3.5 years ago for an infratemporal fossa hemangiopericytoma via a transcranial approach and subsequently irradiated. Imaging documented a recurrent mass in the primary tumoral site. Detailed analysis of the preoperative imaging suggested that the cisternal part of VI cranial nerve passed through the lesion toward its intradural component (**a**). To avoid transgressing the plane of the VI cranial nerve, tumor removal proceeded through a pterional approach with an additional orbitotomy, allowing resection of the tumor extending lateral to the plane of the VI cranial nerve (**b**). In a second stage, the tumor medial to the abducens was removed through the anteromedial corridor via an expanded endonasal approach (**c**). The patient had an uneventful postoperative course and completely recuperated from her VI cranial nerve palsy.

function are approached in very select circumstances to avoid unnecessary morbidity.[40]

7.3.4 Overview of Approaches to the Posterior Cranial Fossa

The ventral part of the posterior cranial fossa is formed by the sphenoid, temporal, and occipital bones. Its medial part is formed by the dorsum sellae, clivus, and foramen magnum of the occipital bone.[41] Its upper third includes the dorsum sella and posterior clinoids down to the level of the Dorello canal. The middle third extends from Dorello canal down to the jugular foramen. The lower third extends from jugular foramen through the cervicomedullary junction and foramen magnum. The lateral part is formed by the posterior surface of the temporal and occipital bones. The petro-occipital fissure and the jugular foramen lie between the occipital and temporal bones.

The posterior cranial fossa can be reached through a variety of lateral and posterolateral and posterior trajectories[9] (▶ Table 7.3). The transpetrosal approaches access the posterior cranial fossa through the middle fossa through an anterior petrosectomy (Kawase) or a posterolateral corridor and include the retrolabyrinthine presigmoid, partial labyrinthectomy, translabyrinthectomy, and transcochlear approaches. The transpetrosal approaches enable access to lesions located between the tentorium and cranial nerves IX and X (jugular foramina). Risks related to the transpetrosal approaches include hearing loss (depending on the amount of drilling on the labyrinth). The retrosigmoid craniotomy is a standard neurosurgical procedure that exposes the posterolateral posterior fossa, notably the cerebellopontine angle. Potential complications related to this approach include cranial nerve lesion (III through to XII) and cerebellar retraction. Posterior corridors, such as the suboccipital craniotomy, offer a direct access to the posterior fossa in a median axis. If a viewing angle is required across the front of the brainstem, the far lateral/transcondylar or the extreme lateral approach may be performed. These approaches offer a better exposure of the lower brainstem and lower vascular complex.[17] However, these procedures risk injury to the vertebral artery and dysfunction of cranial nerves IX to XII. Once again, independent of the lateral and posterior lateral trajectory selected, the apex becomes restricted by the position of the cranial nerves. In accessing this region this issue is even further exaggerated due the compact location of the cranial nerves in situations in which the tumor is ventral when coming from a lateral approach, often requiring the surgeon to work between them and or mobilizing the pertinent cranial nerve.

In these circumstances, an anteromedial trajectory provides a good alternative, keeping the tumor between the surgeon and the pertinent cranial nerve. The part of

Table 7.2 Summary of conventional and expanded endonasal approaches to the middle cranial fossa

| EEA | | Open approaches (most frequently used) | | Cistern exposed | Accessed regions | | | Common pathologies |
Approach	Bone removed	Keyhole approach	Conventional approach		Brain	Cranial nerve	Vessel	
Medial petrous apex approach	Maxillary antrostomy, pterygoid base; Middle clivus; petrous apex	Subtemporal keyhole approach with anterior petrosectomy	Lateral: Middle fossa approach with anterior petrosectomy Transmastoid approach with posterior petrosectomy	Ambient cistern, prepontine cistern	Midbrain, pons	VI (at Dorello canal)	Internal carotid artery and lateral clival artery	Cholesterol granuloma, chondrosarcoma, chordoma, osteomyelitis, benign inflammatory lesions
Inferior cavernous sinus/quadrangular space	Posterior maxillary antrostomy extending laterally to expose V2, pterygoid base (wedge)	Subtemporal keyhole approach	Lateral: Middle fossa approach Infratemporal approach	Prepontine cistern Meckel cave	Temporal lobe	V1, V2, and V3; VI (in the cavernous sinus – superior boundary)	Internal carotid artery (paraclival-medial, petrous – inferior); infero-lateral trunk	Meckel cave region including invasive adenoid cystic carcinomas, juvenile nasal angiofibroma, meningioma, schwannoma, invasive pituitary adenoma
Superior cavernous sinus	Posterior maxillary antrostomy extending laterally to expose V2, pterygoid base (wedge) Medial superior orbital fissure (SOF), face of cavernous sinus	Pterional mini-craniotomy with modified orbito-zygomatic (OZY) osteotomies and cavernous sinus peeling	Anterolateral: Pterional: frontotemporal craniotomy ± orbital osteotomy Orbitozygomatic: frontotemporal craniotomy + orbitotomy + zygomatic osteotomies with middle fossa peeling	III Cranial nerve cistern	Temporal lobe	III, IV, V1, V2, VI (in the cavernous sinus) *sympathetic fibers around internal carotid artery	Internal carotid artery cavernous segment and its inferolateral trunk; and meningohypophyseal trunk	Tumors refractory to medical treatment or radiosurgery, established cranial nerve deficit, apoplectic or functional invasive macroadenoma or refractory meningiomas that invade the cavernous sinus with resultant cavernous sinus syndrome
Temporal/infratemporal approach	Posterior maxillary antrostomy; base, medial and lateral pterygoid plate Middle fossa	Subtemporal keyhole approach	Lateral: Subtemporal/infratemporal craniotomy (preauricular transzygomatic)	Temporal and infra-temporal fossa (no real cistern)	Temporal lobe	III, IV, V1, VI in superior orbital fissure; V2, V3 and its branches	Internal carotid artery; maxillary artery and its branches	Trigeminal schwannoma; nasopharyngeal carcinoma, encephalocele and cerebrospinal fluid leak of the middle cranial fossa

Table 7.3 Summary of conventional and expanded endonasal approaches to the posterior fossa

Expanded endonasal approach		Open approaches (most frequently used)		Cistern exposed	Accessed region			Common pathologies
Approach	Bone removed	Keyhole approach	Conventional approach		Brain	Cranial nerve	Vessel	
Median approaches								
Posterior clinoid (trans/subsellar approaches) Pituitary transposition	Upper third of clivus, posterior clinoids, dorsum sellae	Retrosigmoid approach	Anterior: Interhemispheric: bilateral frontal craniotomy Anterolateral: Pterional: frontotemporal craniotomy ± orbital osteotomy Frontotemporal transcavernous approach frontotemporal craniotomy + orbitotomy + zygomatic complex osteotomies Lateral middle fossa approach with anterior petrosectomy Posterior RMC Presigmoid with posterior petrosectomy	Suprasellar cistern, anterior recess of third ventricle, basilar cistern, interpeduncular cistern	Uncus, hypo-thalamus, infundibulum, mammillary body, midbrain, cerebral peduncles	II, III, VI	Basilar apex P1, posterior communicating artery, P2, perforators, superior cerebellar artery	Retrosellar craniopharyngioma, pituitary macroadenoma, petroclival meningioma
Transclival	Middle third of clivus, petrous apex, Dorello canal	Retrosigmoid keyhole approach	Anterior: Craniofacial transbasal Posterolateral: Posterior transpetrosal retrolabyrinthine approach Combined petrosal (combination of a retrolabyrinthine approach with an extended middle fossa and anterior petrosectomy) Complete petrosectomy Retrosigmoid	Prepontine cistern, pontomedullary cistern	Ventral pons, upper medulla	V, VI, VII, VIII	Midbasilar, anterior inferior cerebellar artery, vertebrobasilar junction	Petroclival meningioma, chordoma, chondrosarcoma, sinonasal tumor
Craniovertebral junction	Inferior third of clivus; foramen magnum	Retrosigmoid keyhole approach	Posterolateral: Lateral suboccipital approach: occipital bone and posterior ring of foramen magnum Extreme lateral approach Transcondylar/far lateral approach	Premedullary; pontomedullary cistern	Lower medulla, cervicomedul-lary junction	IX, X, XI, XII	VBJ, medullary perforators, vertebral artery, posterior inferior cerebellar arteries	Foramen magnum meningioma, chordoma, X schwannomas

Table 7.3 continued

	Expanded endonasal approach	Open approaches (most frequently used)		Cistern exposed	Accessed regions			Common pathologies
Transodontoid	Foramen magnum, ring of C1, odontoid, upper body of C2	Transcervical	Anterior: Transoral (including transpharyngeal and transpalatine) approaches: splitting of soft palate and removal of hard palate Transfacial approaches (including transmandibular, transmaxillary, extended maxillectomy) Craniofacial approaches (including transbasal)	Caudal extension of pontomedullary cistern	Cervicomedullary junction, ventral cervical spinal cord at C1 and C2	XII, C1	Vertebral artery at intradural insertion, anterior spinal arteries	Rheumatoid arthritis/basilar invagination, foramen magnum meningioma
Paramedian approaches								
Infrapetrous	Posterior maxillary antrostomy, medial and lateral pterygoid plate	Subtemporal/infratemporal keyhole approach, anterior petrosectomy	Lateral: Subtemporal/infratemporal craniotomy (preauricular transzygomatic) Anterior petrosectomy Transmastoid Infracochlear	Paramedian section of the prepontine cistern Cerebellar-pontine angle and cistern	Temporal lobe; pons	V_2, V_3 and its branches; VI cranial nerve posteriorly; VII and VIII laterally	Internal carotid artery (vertical paraclival segment, anterior genu and horizontal petrous segment)	Chondrosarcoma, chordoma, cholesterol granulomas that do not protrude medially, petroclival meningioma (as a complementary corridor)
Condylar/hypoglossal canal (inferior third extension of the infrapetrous) (lateral extension of an inferior third transclival approach)	Transpterygoid; clivus (inferior third Medial condylectomy	RMC	Posterior: Transcondylar/far lateral approach	Premedullary cistern; cerebellar–medullary cistern	Lower medulla, cervicomedullary junction	XII	Internal carotid artery (petrous and parapharyngeal segments), vertebral artery, medullary perforators	Invasive carcinoma, paraganglioma, schwannoma, skull base meningioma, chordoma
Jugular foramen (lateral extension of the condylar/hypoglossal approach)	Medial and anterior maxillectomy; endoscopic Denker approach (Sturman-Canfield)	RMC	Posterolateral: Extreme lateral approach Posterior: Transcondylar/far lateral approach	Premedullary cistern	Lower medulla, cervicomedullary junction	X, XI, XII	Internal carotid artery (petrous and parapharyngeal segments), jugular vein, vertebral artery, medullary perforators	Invasive carcinoma, paraganglioma, schwannoma, skull base meningioma, chordoma

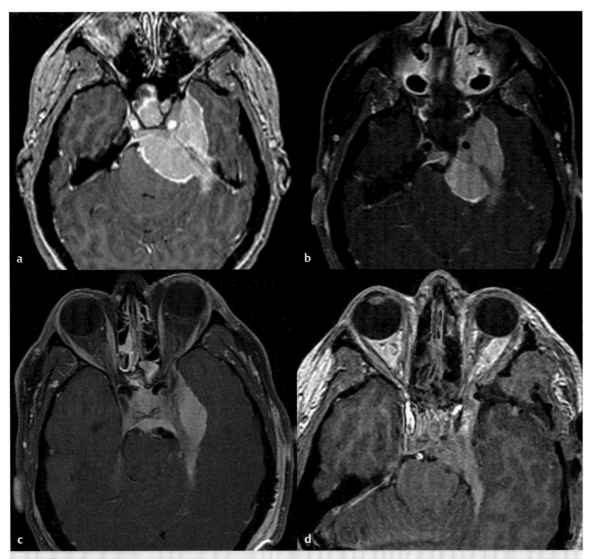

Fig. 7.4 a–d A 38-year-old woman was diagnosed with a petroclival meningioma extending into the sella and middle fossa. This lesion was found incidentally during investigation for an unrelated reason (**a**). At the time of consultation, the patient was intact neurologically. Tumor removal was staged, beginning with an expanded endonasal approach to decompress her optic apparatus through an anteromedial corridor (**b**); followed by a retromastoid approach to decompress her brainstem (**c**); and finally by an orbitozymatic route to complete tumor removal (**d**). The pathology confirmed the diagnosis of a benign meningioma and the patient remains intact neurologically.

the posterior cranial fossa that can be reached through an EEA extends rostrocaudally from the dorsum sellae to the foramen magnum and laterolaterally between the jugular foramina, hypoglossal canals, occipital condyles, and parapharyngeal spaces[2,4] (▶ Fig. 7.4). A transclival approach gives access to the ventral pons and upper medulla. Cranial nerves II and III are the lateral limits for the upper third of clivus. In addition, cranial nerves V through X are part of the lateral boundaries during a panclival approach. A transodontoid and foramen magnum/craniovertebral approach may supplement a transclival approach, allowing access to the foramen magnum,

anterior aspect of the ring of C1, odontoid, and upper body of C2.[4] Its exposure and dissection remains medial to the lower cranial nerves. Among the paramedian EEAs to the posterior fossa, the petroclival approach is used to access lesions that are deep along the midportion of the petrous bone, as it adds to the medial petrous apex exposure. This latter approach is limited laterally by the middle cranial fossa and the ICA. The infrapetrous approach builds on the infratemporal approach and is usually used to access tumors below the petrous ICA into the petrous apex. This approach is limited laterally by the VII and VIII cranial nerves and inferolaterally by the XII cranial nerve.

The plane of the XII cranial nerve limits the jugular foramen/hypoglossal canal approach laterally. It may provide access to the same region as the far lateral but from a median corridor; therefore, we named it the far medial exposure.[42]

7.4 Principles of the 360° Philosophy

The key principles that guide the 360° skull base approach are:

- The primary goal should be most complete tumor resection through the least destructive route and minimizing morbidity; thus, preserving neurological function, cosmesis, and quality of life.
- The skull base team should be familiar with multiple transcranial approaches, keyhole craniotomies, endoscopic endonasal approaches, and reconstructive techniques in order to offer the approach or combination of approaches that are best suited to treat the individual patient based on anatomy, rather than personal preferences.
- The most important factor influencing the choice of a specific route is the relationship to critical neurovascular structures; particularly, transgressing the plane of cranial nerves and dissecting between small windows between them should be fundamentally avoided. Specifically, keep the tumor between the surgeon and the nerve!
- Meticulous skull base reconstruction (vascular when feasible) is key to both transcranial and expanded endonasal approaches, as it prevents life-threatening complications, maximizes postoperative function (vision, mastication, speech, sinonasal physiology), and restores optimal cosmesis.
- Skull base surgery requires a multidisciplinary approach, putting the patient at the center of the team's efforts. A multidisciplinary surgical team composed of skull base neurosurgeons, otolaryngologist–head and neck surgeons, neuro-otologists, plastic surgeons, and ophthalmologists offers a combined expertise that allows the best surgical approach and reconstruction. The close collaboration of neuroanesthesiologist, neurointensivist, neuroradiologist, radio-oncologist, and oncologist assures optimal treatment throughout the treatment regimen.

Currently, each patient should be evaluated with a 360° approach, where a devoted team seeks the best and least destructive corridor to treat a specific lesion or decides which combination of approaches should be performed to ultimately obtain the best overall outcome. Clinical outcome should be the primary determinant in deciding upon particular treatment for an individual patient.[13] The risks of radical surgery, including increased morbidity and mortality, should be weighed against the risk of rapid or delayed recurrence following subtotal removal.[20,30] When facing malignancies and subtotal resection of benign lesions, adjuvant treatments including radiation, chemotherapy, and immunotherapy may help achieve local tumor control and survival with preservation of quality of life.

References

[1] Kassam A, Snyderman CH, Mintz A, Gardner P, Carrau RL. Expanded endonasal approach: the rostrocaudal axis. Part I. Crista galli to the sella turcica. Neurosurg Focus 2005; 19: E3

[2] Kassam A, Snyderman CH, Mintz A, Gardner P, Carrau RL. Expanded endonasal approach: the rostrocaudal axis. Part II. Posterior clinoids to the foramen magnum. Neurosurg Focus 2005; 19: E4

[3] Kassam AB, Gardner P, Snyderman C, Mintz A, Carrau R. Expanded endonasal approach: fully endoscopic, completely transnasal approach to the middle third of the clivus, petrous bone, middle cranial fossa, and infratemporal fossa. Neurosurg Focus 2005; 19: E6

[4] Kassam AB, Snyderman C, Gardner P, Carrau R, Spiro R. The expanded endonasal approach: a fully endoscopic transnasal approach and resection of the odontoid process: technical case report. Neurosurgery 2005; 57 Suppl: E213; discussion E213

[5] de Divitiis E, Esposito F, Cappabianca P, Cavallo LM, de Divitiis O. Tuberculum sellae meningiomas: high route or low route? A series of 51 consecutive cases. Neurosurgery 2008; 62: 556–563, discussion 556–563

[6] Fatemi N, Dusick JR, de Paiva Neto MA, Malkasian D, Kelly DF. Endonasal versus supraorbital keyhole removal of craniopharyngiomas and tuberculum sellae meningiomas. Neurosurgery 2009; 64 Suppl 2: 269–284, discussion 284–286

[7] Zimmer LA, Theodosopoulos PV. Anterior skull base surgery: open versus endoscopic. Curr Opin Otolaryngol Head Neck Surg 2009; 17: 75–78

[8] Sekhar LN, Wright DC, Richardson R, Monacci W. Petroclival and foramen magnum meningiomas: surgical approaches and pitfalls. J Neurooncol 1996; 29: 249–259

[9] Bambakidis NC, Gonzalez LF, Amin-Hanjani S et al. Combined skull base approaches to the posterior fossa. Technical note. Neurosurg Focus 2005; 19: E8

[10] Bambakidis NC, Kakarla UK, Kim LJ et al. Evolution of surgical approaches in the treatment of petroclival meningiomas: a retrospective review. Neurosurgery 2007; 61 Suppl 2: 202–209, discussion 209–211

[11] Imola MJ, Sciarretta V, Schramm VL. Skull base reconstruction. Curr Opin Otolaryngol Head Neck Surg 2003; 11: 282–290

[12] Moyer JS, Chepeha DB, Teknos TN. Contemporary skull base reconstruction. Curr Opin Otolaryngol Head Neck Surg 2004; 12: 294–299

[13] Neil-Dwyer G, Lang DA, Davis A. Outcome from complex neurosurgery: an evidence based approach. Acta Neurochir (Wien) 2000; 142: 367–371

[14] Erkmen K, Pravdenkova S, Al-Mefty O. Surgical management of petroclival meningiomas: factors determining the choice of approach. Neurosurg Focus 2005; 19: E7

[15] Javed T, Sekhar LN. Surgical management of clival meningiomas. Acta Neurochir Suppl (Wien) 1991; 53: 171–182

[16] Pirris SM, Pollack IF, Snyderman CH et al. Corridor surgery: the current paradigm for skull base surgery. Childs Nerv Syst 2007; 23: 377–384

[17] Safavi-Abbasi S, de Oliveira JG, Deshmukh P et al. The craniocaudal extension of posterolateral approaches and their combination: a quantitative anatomic and clinical analysis. Neurosurgery 2010; 66 Suppl Operative: 54–64

[18] Bricolo AP, Turazzi S, Talacchi A, Cristofori L. Microsurgical removal of petroclival meningiomas: a report of 33 patients. Neurosurgery 1992; 31: 813–828, discussion 828

[19] Siwanuwatn R, Deshmukh P, Figueiredo EG, Crawford NR, Spetzler RF, Preul MC. Quantitative analysis of the working area and angle of attack for the retrosigmoid, combined petrosal, and transcochlear approaches to the petroclival region. J Neurosurg 2006; 104: 137–142

[20] Ausman JI. A revolution in skull base surgery: the quality of life matters! Surg Neurol 2006; 65: 635–636

[21] Li Z, Lan Q. Retrosigmoid keyhole approach to the posterior cranial fossa: an anatomical and clinical study. Eur Surg Res 2010; 44: 56–63

[22] Mostafa BE, El Sharnoubi M, Youssef AM. The keyhole retrosigmoid approach to the cerebello-pontine angle: indications, technical modifications, and results. Skull Base 2008; 18: 371–376

[23] Reisch R, Perneczky A. Ten-year experience with the supraorbital subfrontal approach through an eyebrow skin incision. Neurosurgery 2005; 57 Suppl: 242–255, discussion 242–255

[24] Kabil MS, Shahinian HK. The endoscopic supraorbital approach to tumors of the middle cranial base. Surg Neurol 2006; 66: 396–401; discussion 401

[25] Perneczky A, Fries G. Endoscope-assisted brain surgery: part 1—evolution, basic concept, and current technique. Neurosurgery 1998; 42: 219–224; discussion 224–225

[26] Zheng X, Liu W, Yang X et al. Endoscope-assisted supraorbital keyhole approach for the resection of benign tumors of the sellar region. Minim Invasive Ther Allied Technol 2007; 16: 363–366

[27] Gardner PA, Kassam AB, Thomas A et al. Endoscopic endonasal resection of anterior cranial base meningiomas. Neurosurgery 2008; 63: 36–52, discussion 52–54

[28] Hadad G, Bassagasteguy L, Carrau RL et al. A novel reconstructive technique after endoscopic expanded endonasal approaches: vascular pedicle nasoseptal flap. Laryngoscope 2006; 116: 1882–1886

[29] Kassam A, Carrau RL, Snyderman CH, Gardner P, Mintz A. Evolution of reconstructive techniques following endoscopic expanded endonasal approaches. Neurosurg Focus 2005; 19: E8

[30] Kassam AB, Thomas A, Carrau RL et al. Endoscopic reconstruction of the cranial base using a pedicled nasoseptal flap. Neurosurgery 2008; 63 Suppl 1: ONS44–ONS52; discussion ONS52–ONS53

[31] de Notaris M, Cavallo LM, Prats-Galino A et al. Endoscopic endonasal transclival approach and retrosigmoid approach to the clival and petroclival regions. Neurosurgery 2009; 65 Suppl: 42–50; discussion 50–52

[32] Kabil MS, Jarrahy R, Shahinian HK. The application of craniofacial techniques and intracranial endoscopy to pituitary surgery. J Craniofac Surg 2005; 16: 812–818

[33] Chang SW, Wu A, Gore P et al. Quantitative comparison of Kawase's approach versus the retrosigmoid approach: implications for tumors involving both middle and posterior fossae. Neurosurgery 2009; 64 Suppl: ons44–ons51; discussion ons51–ons52

[34] Nakase H, Ohnishi H, Matsuyama T, Morimoto T, Sakaki T. Two-stage skull base surgery for tumours extending to the sub- and epidural spaces. Acta Neurochir (Wien) 1998; 140: 891–898

[35] Carrabba G, Dehdashti AR, Gentili F. Surgery for clival lesions: open resection versus the expanded endoscopic endonasal approach. Neurosurg Focus 2008; 25: E7

[36] Dehdashti AR, Ganna A, Witterick I, Gentili F. Expanded endoscopic endonasal approach for anterior cranial base and suprasellar lesions: indications and limitations. Neurosurgery 2009; 64: 677–687; discussion 687–689

[37] Cavallo LM, Prevedello DM, Solari D et al. Extended endoscopic endonasal transsphenoidal approach for residual or recurrent craniopharyngiomas. J Neurosurg 2009; 111: 578–589

[38] Rhoton AL, Jr. The anterior and middle cranial base. Neurosurgery 2002; 51 Suppl: S273–S302

[39] Kassam AB, Prevedello DM, Carrau RL et al. The front door to Meckel's cave: an anteromedial corridor via expanded endoscopic endonasal approach- technical considerations and clinical series. Neurosurgery 2009; 64 Suppl: ons71–ons82; discussion ons82–ons83

[40] Walsh MT, Couldwell WT. Management options for cavernous sinus meningiomas. J Neurooncol 2009; 92: 307–316

[41] Rhoton AL, Jr. The foramen magnum. Neurosurgery 2000; 47 Suppl: S155–S193

[42] Morera VA, Fernandez-Miranda JC, Prevedello DM et al. "Far-medial" expanded endonasal approach to the inferior third of the clivus: the transcondylar and transjugular tubercle approaches. Neurosurgery 2010; 66 Suppl Operative: 211–219; discussion 219–220

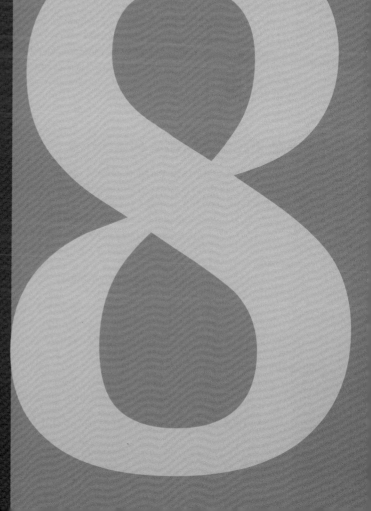

Chapter 8

The Sinonasal Corridor

8 The Sinonasal Corridor

Ulrike Bockmühl, Ricardo L. Carrau, Bradley A. Otto, Daniel M. Prevedello, Amin B. Kassam

8.1 Introduction

In general, an ideal surgical approach to the skull base should provide adequate access to facilitate the resection, debulking and/or repair of the target lesion, and allow the possibility to extend the resection margins and the identification and protection of important neurovascular structures. It should produce minimal facial scarring, no deformity, and should preserve the neurological and masticatory functions. In addition, the approach should facilitate the reconstruction of the surgical defect.

The endoscopic endonasal approach offers many if not all these characteristics. It presents the advantage of using pre-existent air spaces that facilitate reaching various areas of the skull base, while avoiding external incisions/scars, and obviating the need for the translocation of maxillofacial skeleton. While advantageous in these and other respects, the sinonasal corridor should be optimized to adequately access the skull base, avoiding sinonasal complications and minimizing sequelae.[1] Two concepts are critical for the endoscopic endonasal exposure: bilateral nasal access to allow for a two-surgeon, four-hand technique, and maximum removal of bone at the skull base to create a wide surgical corridor. In addition, the planning and execution of the sinonasal corridor must take into consideration the anticipated reconstructive needs and technique, incorporating the elevation of pedicle or rotation flaps or sparing the intended pedicle to preserve the potential of employing the flap if needed. Olfactory and ciliary function must be preserved as much as possible. Ideally, at the end of the procedure the entire sinonasal cavity should be completely lined by mucosa (original, graft, or flap).

8.2 Preoperative Planning

Each patient undergoes a detailed patient examination comprising functional testing of all cranial nerves and basic cognitive function. As appropriate for each individual patient, standard metabolic and endocrine tests, preoperative visual assessment tests including visual acuity, and, if possible, baseline standardized visual fields are performed.

Preoperative imaging customarily includes high-resolution computed tomography (CT) and/or magnetic resonance imaging (MRI) which must be reviewed in detail with special attention to sinus anatomy and the relationship of the tumor and planned corridor to neurovascular structures.[2] In patients with tumor in close relationship to major vasculature (internal carotid artery, circle of Willis, cavernous sinus) we prefer CT angiography (CTA) in lieu of a CT scan, as it provides the best demonstration of critical vessels and exquisite bone definition.

8.3 Intraoperative Preparation and Other General Considerations

To avoid surgical errors and miscommunications we use a modification of the surgical safety checklist proposed by the World Health Organization (▶ Fig. 8.1). It is imperative that the entire surgical staff is engaged during the performance of the checklist. These safeguards have diminished surgical errors worldwide.

Intraoperatively, we monitor cranial nerves III, IV, VI, VII, and IX to XII (i.e., electromyography [EMG]), as well as brain and brainstem functions (i.e., somatosensory evoked potentials and brainstem auditory evoked responses, respectively) according to the extension of the tumor and the surgical approach.[3,4,5] The digital dataset of a contrasted CT or CTA and/or MRI are fused for intraoperative navigation. Similarly, we use an acoustic Doppler sonography probe to complement the intraoperative navigation. The Doppler provides real-time information regarding the position of important vessels and blood flow. If a significant blood loss is anticipated the patient is typed and crossed for packed red blood cells (according to institutional logistics, this can be done preoperatively). To complete our intraoperative preparation, we administer a prophylactic perioperative antibiotic regimen, most commonly a third-generation cephalosporin with cerebrospinal fluid (CSF) penetration. In addition, we administer corticosteroids when manipulation of the cranial nerves is anticipated but avoid their use in functional pituitary tumor surgery, as it interferes with the monitoring of cortisol levels. Vasoconstriction and decongestion of the nasal cavity are achieved by spraying or packing cottonoids soaked in oxymetazoline 0.05% (or epinephrine 1/20,000). Injecting the lateral nasal wall (agger nasi) and septum with a solution of lidocaine 1% with epinephrine 1/100,000 enhances hemostasis.

Surgery proceeds under general endotracheal anesthesia with the patient in supine position, neck slightly flexed, tilted to the left, and turned to the right, and the head on a three-pin fixation system similar to a microscopic surgery position (▶ Fig. 8.2). This better aligns the nasal passage with the wrists of the surgeon. Greater extension of the neck is advisable if the lesion extends anterior to the cribriform plate or if a frontal sinusotomy is necessary, as this provides a better angle for the visualization of the most anterior skull base and frontal sinus. Flexion of the neck is

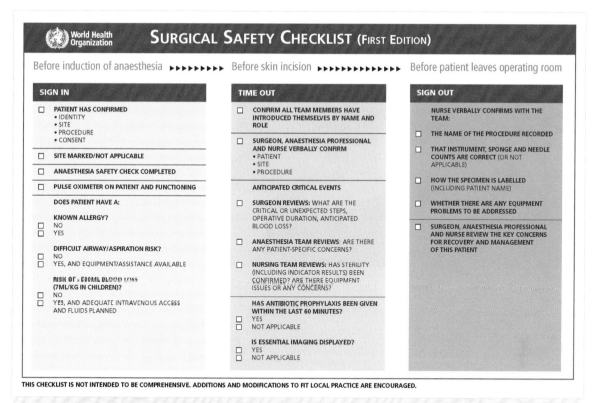

Fig. 8.1 World Health Organization surgical safety checklist. (Image provided courtesy of the World Health Organization.)

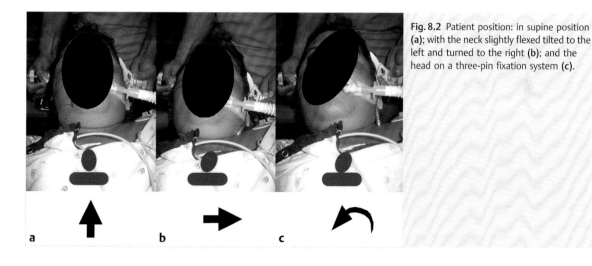

Fig. 8.2 Patient position: in supine position **(a)**; with the neck slightly flexed tilted to the left and turned to the right **(b)**; and the head on a three-pin fixation system **(c)**.

helpful for low endonasal approaches to the upper cervical spine. These positioning suggestions help the surgeon to position him or herself in a manner that avoids strain and fatigue of the surgeon's back, neck, and hands. Similarly, to avoid undue strain of the surgeon's neck, the display monitors should be facing the surgeons at eye level. Alternatively, the head could be resting on a conforming pillow or a gel horseshoe head-holder to allow freedom of movement during the surgery. We prefer to fix the head, however, when drilling over critical structures is anticipated, when we anticipate a prolonged surgery (avoid decubitus ulcers), and when EMG monitoring is necessary (precludes the use of paralytics).

We favor an optical surgical navigation system using a facemask for registration (Stryker Navigation; Stryker, Kalamazoo, Michigan, United States); however, other navigation systems may be equally suitable. The camera is placed at the head of the operating table and its tracker is

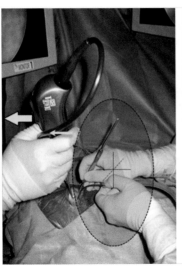
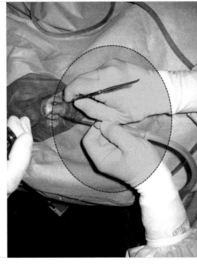

Fig. 8.3 Three- or four-hand dissection technique.

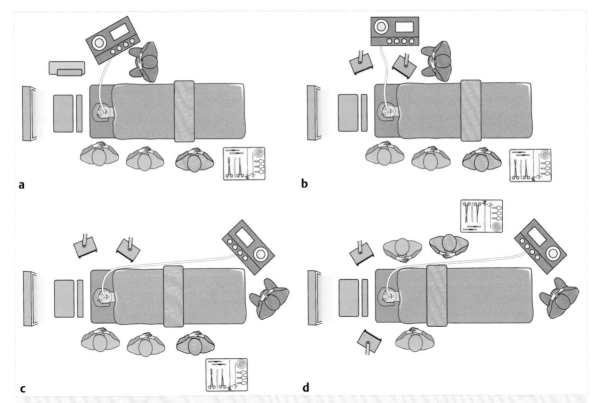

Fig. 8.4 a–d Different configurations for the operating suite setup. Blue, patient; green, surgeons; gray, nurse; orange, navigation and monitors; pink, anesthesia team.

fixed to the three-pin fixation system. For their placement one needs to consider the position of the surgeons and video monitors to avoid problems with the line of sight of the camera.

Our surgical team is composed of two surgeons who will perform a three- or four-hand dissection technique (▶ Fig. 8.3). This brings some important considerations regarding positioning of surgeons, patient, anesthesia staff, and equipment, as well as the position of other paraphernalia and flow of personnel. There is an infinite number of ways to set up the operating suite. ▶ Fig. 8.4 shows our most common setups. Our current configuration is that the anesthesia team is positioned toward the feet of the patient and the surgical team to the right side. The surgical

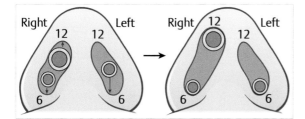

Fig. 8.5 Endonasal position of the instruments. The endoscope is at the 12 o'clock position of the right nostril retracting the nasal vestibule superiorly to increase the available space for other instruments. The suction tube is introduced at the 6 o'clock position on the ipsilateral side. The dissection instruments are usually introduced through the left nasal cavity.

technician or nurse is positioned toward the left of the bed (▶ Fig. 8.4c). When we have a left-handed surgeon, that surgeon goes to the patient's left side (▶ Fig. 8.4d). However, the ideal arrangement varies according to individual preferences, equipment, and size and geometry of the operating suite; thus, every team has to ascertain what works best under their circumstances.

Most of the surgery proceeds using a 0° rod-lens endoscope, although endoscopes with angled lenses (30°, 45°, and 70°) are used as needed. The endoscope is introduced at the 12 o'clock position of the right nostril and is used to retract the nasal vestibule superiorly, increasing the available space for other instruments (▶ Fig. 8.5). A suction tip is introduced at the 6 o'clock position on the ipsilateral side. Although the primary dissection instruments or powered instrumentation are usually introduced through the left nasal cavity, they may be freely exchanged throughout the case, taking advantage of the best angle of approach.

8.4 Surgical Technique

8.4.1 Basic Sinonasal Corridor

We begin our approach with the preparation and expansion of the sinonasal corridor and, if needed, incorporate the harvesting of the Hadad-Bassagaisteguy nasoseptal flap (HBF)[5] into the approach. The location of the HBF pedicle over the rostrum of the sphenoid places the pedicle at risk during dissection along the anterior face of the sphenoid or the posterior septum.[6,7] Other pedicled flaps, such as the anterior and posterior lateral nasal wall flaps[8,9], and pericranial,[10,11] and temporoparietal flaps,[12] may be harvested after completion of the extirpative surgery. Expansion of the natural nasal corridor usually includes bilateral inferior turbinate lateralization, a right middle-turbinectomy, a posterior septectomy, bilateral wide sphenoidotomies, and removal of the anterior floor of the sphenoid sinuses (▶ Fig. 8.6).

The inferior turbinates are in-fractured and then out-fractured to achieve optimal lateralization. This maneuver expands the lower nasal corridor providing more space for instrumentation and better visualization of the posterior choana. The middle and superior turbinates are carefully lateralized, avoiding mucosal tears and avoiding a fracture of the superior insertion of the middle turbinate as it inserts into the vertical lamella of the cribriform plate. Fractures in this area may produce a CSF leak and tear the olfactory filaments; thus, potentially leading to olfactory dysfunction. We, however, prefer a right partial middle turbinectomy (i.e., lower half), as this provides more space for the endoscope and allows the surgeon to place it away from the dissecting instruments (▶ Fig. 8.7). This also improves postoperative access to the sphenoid sinus for débridement and surveillance (▶ Fig. 8.8). Preservation of the superior half is desirable, as this spares the olfactory epithelium. The resected middle turbinate is kept sterile, as it can be the source of mucoperiosteum for free grafting.

All instruments tend to converge at the median area of the posterior nose. A middle turbinectomy prevents convergence of the scope (it remains at a lateral position, parallel to the lateral wall); therefore, avoiding the soiling of the lens and the criss-crossing with the dissecting instruments. The superior turbinates may be partially resected to provide direct visualization of the optic apices and subsequently the optic nerve canals. Occasionally, anterior and/or a posterior ethmoidectomies are needed

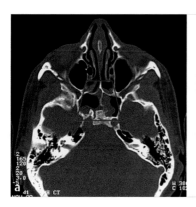
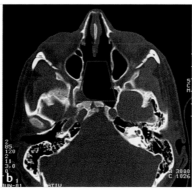

Fig. 8.6 a, b Basic sinonasal corridor.
(a) Axial CT scan of a squamous cell carcinoma of the sphenoid sinus.
(b) Postoperative axial CT scan showing the sinonasal corridor marked by the red trapezoid box.

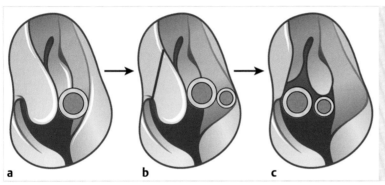

Fig. 8.7 a–c Importance of partial middle turbinectomy (lower half). **(a)** Right nasal cavity with endoscope alone. **(b)** Right nasal cavity with endoscope and suction. **(c)** Right nasal cavity after partial middle turbinectomy with endoscope and suction.

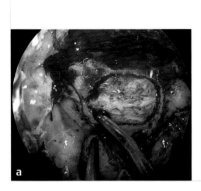

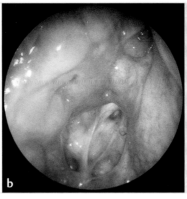

Fig. 8.8 a, b Endoscopy pictures of the basic sinonasal corridor at surgery **(a)** and postoperatively after wound healing is complete **(b)**.

to provide space for the endoscope and dissecting instruments. In our experience, this is more common in children where the space of the developing nasal cavity is limited.

Hadad-Bassagaisteguy Flap

The HBF, a pedicled nasoseptal flap based on the posterior septal arteries, is harvested from the widest nasal cavity (▶ Fig. 8.9). This is commonly the right side, as this is the side of the middle turbinectomy. However, a septal spur, or tumor involvement of the sphenoid rostrum, posterior septum, or pterygopalatine fossa may dictate harvesting the HBF from the contralateral septal mucoperiosteum. This is also true for the need of a transpterygoid approach.[13,14] The HBF is used for the reconstruction of the surgical defect separating the sinonasal tract from the cranial cavity and/or protecting neurovascular structures. Its pedicle is posterior; thus, its harvesting is one of the first steps of the surgery, as our surgical approach usually requires a posterior septectomy and bilateral wide sphenoidotomies, which would destroy its pedicle.

Once the flap has been elevated, the posterior bony septum is removed, while preserving the contralateral mucosa. The contralateral mucosa is then elevated from the sphenoid sinus and incised in a horizontal plane, superiorly 2 cm below the olfactory sulcus, and inferiorly 4 to 5 mm above the junction of septum and floor of the nose. A third incision is made vertically at the level of the rostrum of the sphenoid. This creates an anteriorly based mucoperiosteal flap that is then rotated to the contralateral anterior septum to cover the HBF donor site (Caicedo reverse septal flap). The flap is then sutured with transseptal quilting stitches using an absorbable suture. This completes the posterior septectomy; thus, facilitating bilateral instrumentation without displacing the septum into the path of the endoscope, and increases the lateral angulation and range of motion of instruments. The remaining mucosa above the level of the maxillary crest is incised anteriorly and posteriorly to rotate over the denuded bone at this area.

The HBF is stored in the nasopharynx until the extirpative part of the surgery is completed (▶ Fig. 8.9). However, in those patients who require surgery that involves the lower clivus, nasopharynx, or craniocervical junction, the HBF is stored in the ipsilateral antrum. This requires a large nasomaxillary window. Alternatively, a stitch may be placed in the anterior aspect of the flap then retracted outside of the nose by the weight of a hemostat. This allows the flap to assume a position that is parallel and against the length of the lateral nasal wall, keeping it out of the plane of dissection. This maneuver also decreases congestion or contraction of the flap during the procedure.

In cases where the HBF is not needed, the pedicle may be preserved by dissecting the strip of mucosa containing its blood supply and then removing the bony rostrum.

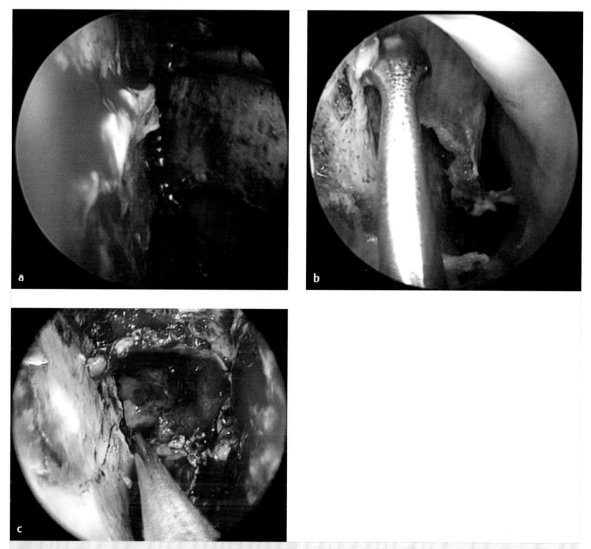

Fig. 8.9 a–c Endoscopy picture of the Hadad-Bassagaisteguy flap (HBF). Elevation of the anterior **(a)** and inferior aspects of the HBF. The flap is placed apposing the denuded bony walls and pushed into the nasopharynx for protection during surgery **(c)**.

The posterior septectomy is limited to that portion that is required to provide a bilateral approach. This is best accomplished by performing the posterior aspect of the HBF incisions including those at the posterior choanae, rostrum of the sphenoid, and posterosuperior septum. The mucosa is the elevated and displaced to expose the rostrum and the posterior septum, which can then be removed sparing the strips of mucosa that constitute the pedicles.

Sphenoidotomy

A sphenoidotomy is initiated by enlarging the natural ostium of the sphenoid sinus or by entering the sphenoid at the junction of the nasal septum and the rostrum of the sphenoid sinus. Removal of the bony rostrum is com-

pleted using Kerrison rongeurs and/or a surgical drill. We use a "Total Performance System" drill (TPS; Stryker) with an angled hand-piece and 3 to 4 mm rough diamond (hybrid) short and long burrs. The sphenoidotomies are extended laterally to the level of the medial pterygoid plates and lateral wall of the sphenoid sinus, superiorly to the level of the planum sphenoidale, and inferiorly to the floor of the sphenoid sinus. Wide bilateral sphenoidotomies and a posterior septectomy provide bilateral access and visualization of key anatomical structures such as optic nerves and internal carotid arteries (▶ Fig. 8.10). Any intersinus or intrasinus septations with the potential to displace the instruments medially are drilled down to be in-plane with the walls of the sphenoid sinus. Care is taken as most septations insert in the internal carotid artery and optic nerve canals.

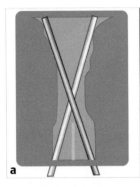
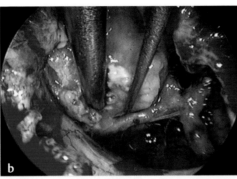

Fig. 8.10 a, b Sphenoidotomy. (a) Bilateral access and visualization after wide bilateral sphenoidotomies and a posterior septectomy. (b) Optimal endoscopy view of key anatomical structures as nerves and arteries.

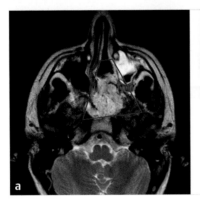
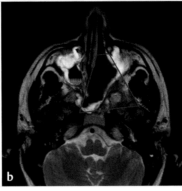

Fig. 8.11 a, b Lateral expansion of the sinonasal corridor. (a) Axial MRI scan of a left-side juvenile angiofibroma. (b) Axial MRI scan after tumor removal. The resulting sinonasal corridor is marked by the red trapezoid box.

8.4.2 Expanded Sinonasal Corridor

Lateral Exposure

Exposure of tumors that involve a transpterygoid approach requires expansion of the corridor in a lateral direction. This usually implies an endoscopic medial maxillectomy including a wide nasomaxillary window, an inferior turbinectomy, and removal of the medial maxillary wall (lateral wall of the nose) ipsilateral to the tumor. This exposes the entire posterior wall of the antrum and, upon its removal, the entire pterygopalatine fossa (▶ Fig. 8.11 and ▶ Fig. 8.12). Nonetheless, an endoscopic medial maxillectomy is limited anteriorly by the nasolacrimal duct, which becomes both the fulcrum for the rod-lens endoscope and an impediment to move the scope laterally. An endoscopic Denker approach eliminates this obstacle by removing the most anterior aspect of the medial maxilla including the piriform aperture. This can be extended laterally removing the medial aspect of the anterior wall of the maxilla; therefore expanding the lateral angle of exposure.

An initial step to complete an endoscopic Denker approach is to carry a vertical incision on the mucosa that covers the edge of the piriform aperture (just anterior to the anterior head of the inferior turbinate). The incision is carried through periosteum to facilitate a subperiosteal dissection that exposes the anterior aspect of the maxilla. The most anterior aspect of the medial maxillary wall is removed using a backbiting rongeurs or a high-speed drill. We can usually spare the lacrimal duct opening, resecting just that area inferior to it. If needed, the nasolacrimal duct and its canal can be divided sharply. Bone removal is extended anteriorly to remove the piriform aperture and laterally to remove the anterior wall of the maxillary sinus. These steps create a single cavity that connects the antrum, nasal cavity, ethmoid and sphenoid sinuses, and nasopharynx (▶ Fig. 8.13).[15,16]

Anterosuperior Exposure

An anterosuperior extension of the sinonasal corridor is needed for the transcribriform and transplanum approaches or to remove lesions in the ethmoidal cells and frontal sinus (▶ Fig. 8.14).

First, complete ethmoidectomies are performed, exposing the medial orbital walls, (i.e., lamina papyracea or periorbita and the anterior skull base). One must identify the ethmoidal arteries (in most cases only the anterior ethmoidal artery is prominently displayed) and the frontal recess. Adjacent bony partitions are fractured and teased out resulting in an opening that corresponds to a simple drainage or type I drainage according to Draf's classification.[17] The frontal sinus drainage is then extended achieving a type II drainage by resecting the floor of the frontal sinus between the lamina papyracea and the middle turbinate anterior to the ventral margin of the olfactory fossa (type IIa) or extending the resection medially to the nasal septum (type IIb).[17] This is usually done with a high-speed or curved drill.

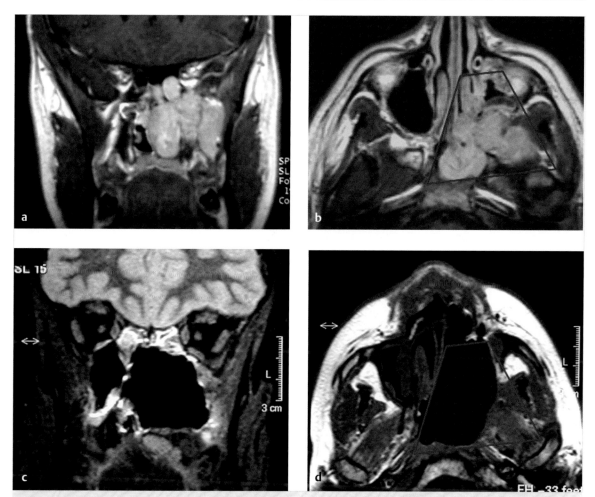

Fig. 8.12 a–d Far lateral expansion of the sinonasal corridor. Coronal (a) and axial (c) MRI scans of a left-side juvenile angiofibroma extending into the infratemporal fossa. Axial (b) and coronal (d) MRI scans after tumor removal. The resulting sinonasal corridor is marked by the red trapezoid box.

If there is a unilateral lesion we try to preserve the contralateral skull base in order save the olfactory filaments but only if possible from the oncological point of view (▶ Fig. 8.15). If the complete anterior skull base has to be exposed, we start by drilling out a Draf type III drainage (also known as median drainage, modified endoscopic Lothrop procedure, or bilateral frontal sinus drill-out procedure ▶ Fig. 8.16). Typically, we start by identifying the first olfactory fibers (bilaterally): the middle turbinate is cut from anterior to posterior along its origin at the skull base. Around 10 to 15 mm posterior to the anterior attachment of the middle turbinate one can find a small artery coming out of the lamina cribrosa; the first olfactory fiber is just posterior to it. We follow with the drilling out of the remaining frontal sinus floor and the lower part of intersinus septa. This will finally result in the so-called "Frontal T"[17] (▶ Fig. 8.17). The posterior border of the resected perpendicular nasal septum represents its long crus, and the posterior margins of the frontal sinus

floor resection provide the shorter wings. Drilling the cribriform plate rostrocaudally will follow the coagulation of soft tissue and olfactory filaments, as well as the anterior and posterior ethmoidal arteries. After bilateral removal of the cribriform plate, the crista galli is drilled eggshell thin, fractured and then taken out. ▶ Fig. 8.18 shows an intraoperative endoscopic view of the exposed frontal lobes. The intradural resection is described in the next chapter. Select sinonasal or anterior skull base pathologies may require additional lateral exposure; thus, the anterosuperior corridor can be complemented with a lateral expansion, a transpterygoid corridor, or a transorbital module.

A criticism of the endoscopic endonasal approach is the "impossibility" of obtaining en bloc resection. This is often achieved in smaller lesions. When it is not possible, we perform a sequential multilayer tumor removal. Radical extirpation of the disease does not depend on en bloc resection as shown by our long-term results of

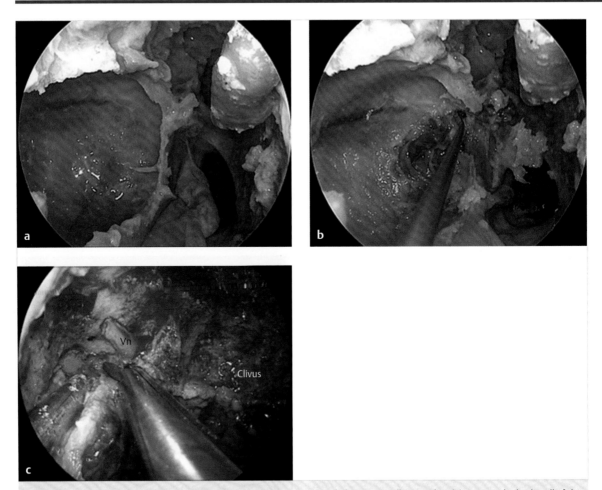

Fig. 8.13 a–c Endoscopy views of lateral expanded exposure. A right expanded anteromaxillary window **(a)** exposes the back wall of the antrum. The latter is removed following the anterior vascular compartment from medial to lateral, exposing the maxillary artery **(b)**. Thus facilitates the identificationand dissection of the neural compartment.
Vn, vidian nerve.

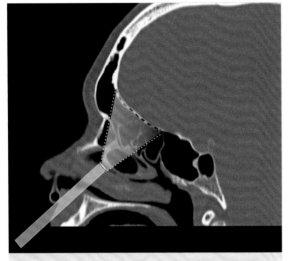

Fig. 8.14 Anterosuperior expansion of the sinonasal corridor marked by the red dashed line.

inverted papilloma and malignant tumors.[18,19] Instead, the primary purpose is to identify and widely remove the tumor origin as well as the infiltrated structures (i.e., anterior skull base, dura, or lamina papyracea). Therefore, it is acceptable to resect larger tumors segmentally.[18,20,21,22,23,24,25]

8.5 Complications

Avoidance of complications in endoscopic endonasal surgery is based among other factors on the anticipation of potential pitfalls and understanding of their mechanism. Several risk factors that may increase the possibility of complications include previous sinus surgery leading to the absence of anatomical landmarks, bleeding, infection, extensive disease, and inexperience of the surgeon.

Complications can be classified according to severity as *minor* and *major* and according to the time of appearance as *intraoperative* or *postoperative*.

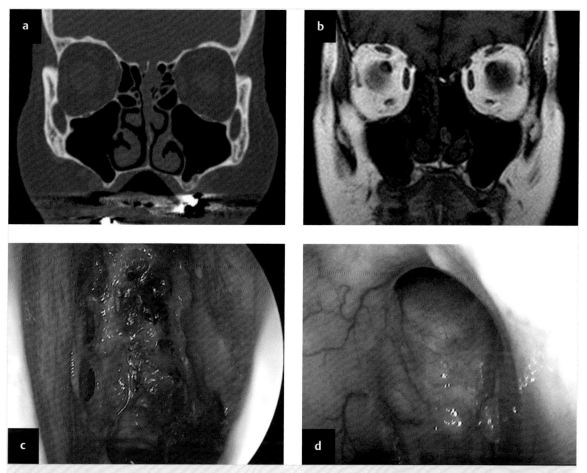

Fig. 8.15 a–d Left-sided anterosuperior expansion of the sinonasal corridor. (a) Coronal CT scan presenting a circumscribed sinonasal carcinoma at the left anterior skull base. (b) Coronal MRI scan after tumor removal. (c) Endoscopy view 4 weeks postoperative showing the anterior skull base with crusting that can remain for up to 1 year. (d) Endoscopy view of the type II frontal sinus drainage according to Draf.[17]

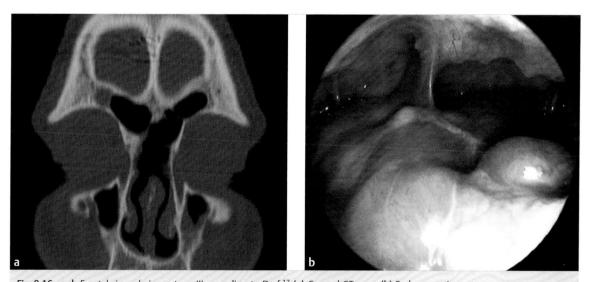

Fig. 8.16 a, b Frontal sinus drainage type III according to Draf.[17] (a) Coronal CT scan. (b) Endoscopy view.

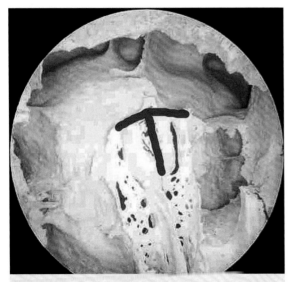

Fig. 8.17 "Frontal T" according to Draf.

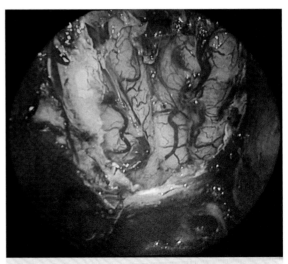

Fig. 8.18 Endoscopy view of the complete exposed anterior skull base (i.e., after removal of the dura).

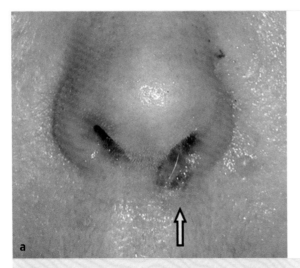

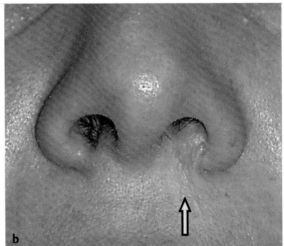

Fig. 8.19 a, b Alar sill injury after endoscopic endonasal surgery. This is often considered a "minor" complication but it can have a severe impact on a patient's cosmetic appearance. (a) 5 days postoperative. (b) 1 year postoperative.

8.5.1 Minor Complications

Minor complications are those that cause little morbidity and do not compromise the life of the patient. In patients who undergo endonasal sinus surgery they occur in between 2 and 21%[26,27,28,29] and include synechiae, crusting, minor bleeding, nasal septal perforation, headache, facial pain, alteration of dental sensitivity, edema, local infection, periorbital ecchymosis, palpebral edema, subcutaneous emphysema or paraffin granuloma due to ointment packages and alar sill injuries (▶ Fig. 8.19), postoperative sinusitis, epiphora, and hyposmia.

8.5.2 Major Complications

Major complications present significant morbidity and a possibility of mortality. They comprise orbital injuries (i.e., damage of the optical nerve or the extraocular muscles), intracranial damage (i.e., CSF leak, intracranial hemorrhage and hematoma, damage to the brain itself, meningitis, cerebral abscess, damage to the cranial nerves, pneumocephalus or stroke and bleeding due to injury of the internal carotid artery, the anterior cerebral arteries and their fronto-orbital or frontopolar branches, the vertebral artery as well as the cavernous sinus). The incidence of major complications due to endonasal sinus surgery has been reported to vary between 0.75 and 8%.[26,30]

8.5.3 Immediate Complications

The most frequent immediate complications are intraoperative bleeding, and orbital or nerve injuries. Kassam et al[7,25,31] described 0.9% vascular and 1.8% neural injuries of 800 patients who underwent expanded endoscopic surgeries.

8.5.4 Delayed Complications

Delayed complications included CSF leak, meningitis, progressive loss of vision or smell, bleeding, synechia, and infection. Kassam et al[7,25,31] reported an incidence of infections in 1.9% and < 5% CSF leaks in a cohort undergoing endoscopic skull base surgeries. Castelnuovo et al[32] reported a success rate for the first dural repair attempt with 93% (7% failure). Komotar et al[33] determined a rate of successful repair of about 90% for both endoscopic and open cohorts. They found, however, significantly lower complications in patients undergoing endoscopic endonasal surgery compared with those undergoing open approaches (e.g., meningitis [1.1 versus 3.9%], abscess/wound infection [0.7 versus 6.8%], sepsis [0 versus 3.8%], and perioperative mortality [0 versus 1.4%]).

8.6 Postoperative Care

We advocate a noncontrasted CT scan immediately after surgery for all patients in whom the dura has been transgressed. Similarly, we usually perform a contrasted MRI within 24 hours of surgery in patients undergoing an oncologic resection (e.g., esthesioneuroblastoma, adenocarcinoma, chondrosarcoma, or chordoma). This confirms the adequacy of the resection and, secondarily, the adequacy of reconstruction and vascularity and positioning of the reconstructive flap.

There are differences between European and American postoperative hygiene regimens.

8.6.1 Kassel Hospital (Germany)

All patients with anterior skull base resection (both cribriform plates and crista galli) and duraplasty or dura strengthening as all cases with a large common nasal cavity are packed by an ointment tamponade on a silicone sheet that is placed directly on the duraplasty. The silicon film helps re-epithelialization creating a moisture chamber. If the tumor can be resected by a unilateral operation the nose is packed with rubber finger stalls (Rhinotamp; Vostra, Aachen, Germany). These are removed 3 to 7 days postoperatively. In all expanded endonasal resections the silicone film and the ointment tamponade will be taken out after 7 days. Usually, the patients are hospitalized for 3 days (simple cases) or up to 10 days (severe cases). During the time of nasal packing the patients are given antibiotics (usually a third-generation cephalosporin). After removal of the nasal packing the patients have to nurse their noses (i.e., using ointment several times a day). They get weekly or bi-weekly gentle débridement and suctioning at an outpatient clinic.

Follow-up consists of endoscopic examination of the nasal cavity and MRI (▶ Fig. 8.20). In all malignant tumors we perform regular clinical controls quarterly in the first and second year after operation, semi-yearly in the third year, and yearly thereafter. Three months after surgery patients undergo MRI of the paranasal sinuses including the skull base and the brain, as well as of the neck to exclude lymph node metastases. Afterwards MRI is

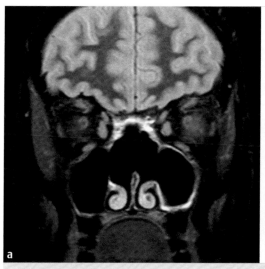
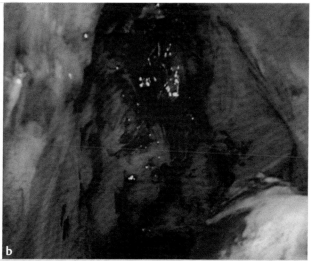

Fig. 8.20 a, b Follow-up after anterior skull base tumor removal. **(a)** Coronal MRI scan presenting the expanded sinonasal corridor without any sign of tumor recurrence. **(b)** Endoscopic examination of the nasal cavity showing some remaining granulation 6 months postoperatively.

repeated yearly. Importantly, preoperative staging includes thoracic CT, which is also repeated yearly post-operatively, since solitary metastases are resectable.

8.6.2 Ohio State University

Patients with transdural resection undergo reconstruction a vascularized flap, which is bolstered by a temporary packing consisting of Nasopore (Stryker) followed by expandable sponges. Silicone splints commonly cover the nasal septum. In those patients whose surgery does not involve communication with the subarachnoid space (i.e., CSF), we use only Nasopore, which degrades into a suction-able paste. Barring any systemic or endocrinological abnormality the latter patients may be discharged after an overnight observation. Those with transdural surgeries typically remain in the hospital for 3 days.

Patients are prescribed normal saline sprays and decongestants sprays immediately after surgery. Outpatient care is initiated 5 to 7 days after surgery with removal of packing and silicone splints followed by gentle suctioning and débridement of the nasal passages. Manipulation of the flap or defect is avoided until 4 weeks after surgery. After this initial débridement the patient is asked to start a regimen of nasal irrigations with normal saline solution (3–4 times per day). Débridement and suctioning is performed on a weekly or bi-weekly basis.

8.7 Conclusion

By exploiting the natural sinonasal corridor, the entire ventral and central skull base can be approached to successfully treat benign and malignant lesions. Its access can be adapted and enlarged as necessary while obviating some of the morbidity associated with an open procedure.

Pearls and Pitfalls

- An appropriate sinonasal corridor is fundamental for successful endonasal surgery.
- Ideally, the surgery is carried by two surgeons, an oto-laryngologist–head and neck surgeon and a neuro-surgeon, working simultaneously with a three- or four-hand technique.
- Bilateral nasal access, and a posterior septectomy, bilateral wide sphenoidomies, and removal of the anterior floor of the sphenoid sinuses are essential to provide optimal space for instrumentation.
- Surgeons must anticipate the reconstructive needs as the expansion of the corridor may destroy or interfere with the harvesting of the nasoseptal and lateral wall flaps. In addition one must consider alternative methods of reconstruction.
- As much as possible, the entire sinonasal cavity should be lined by mucosa (original, graft, or flap) at the end of the surgical procedure.

References

[1] Bayram M, Sirikci A, Bayazit YA. Important anatomic variations of the sinonasal anatomy in light of endoscopic surgery: a pictorial review. Eur Radiol 2001; 11: 1991–1997

[2] Barges-Coll J, Fernandez-Miranda JC, Prevedello DM et al. Avoiding injury to the abducens nerve during expanded endonasal endoscopic surgery: anatomic and clinical case studies. Neurosurgery 2010; 67: 144–154; discussion 154

[3] Thirumala PD, Mohanraj SK, Habeych M et al. Value of free-run electromyographic monitoring of extraocular cranial nerves during expanded endonasal surgery (EES) of the skull base. J Neurol Surg Rep 2013; 74: 43–50

[4] Thirumala PD, Kodavatiganti HS, Habeych M et al. Value of multimodality monitoring using brainstem auditory evoked potentials and somatosensory evoked potentials in endoscopic endonasal surgery. Neurol Res 2013; 35: 622–630

[5] Hadad G, Bassagasteguy L, Carrau RL et al. A novel reconstructive technique after endoscopic expanded endonasal approaches: vascular pedicle nasoseptal flap. Laryngoscope 2006; 116: 1882–1886

[6] Shah RN, Surowitz JD, Patel MR et al. Endoscopic pedicled nasoseptal flap reconstruction for pediatric skull base defects. Laryngoscope 2009; 119: 1067–1075

[7] Zanation AM, Carrau RL, Snyderman CH et al. Nasoseptal flap reconstruction of high flow intraoperative cerebral spinal fluid leaks during endoscopic skull base surgery. Am J Rhinol Allergy 2009; 23: 518–521

[8] Fortes FS, Carrau RL, Snyderman CH et al. The posterior pedicle inferior turbinate flap: a new vascularized flap for skull base reconstruction. Laryngoscope 2007; 117: 1329–1332

[9] Prevedello DM, Barges-Coll J, Fernandez-Miranda JC et al. Middle turbinate flap for skull base reconstruction: cadaveric feasibility study. Laryngoscope 2009; 119: 2094–2098

[10] Patel MR, Shah RN, Snyderman CH et al. Pericranial flap for endoscopic anterior skull-base reconstruction: clinical outcomes and radioanatomic analysis of preoperative planning. Neurosurgery 2010; 66: 506–512; discussion 512

[11] Zanation AM, Snyderman CH, Carrau RL, Kassam AB, Gardner PA, Prevedello DM. Minimally invasive endoscopic pericranial flap: a new method for endonasal skull base reconstruction. Laryngoscope 2009; 119: 13–18

[12] Fortes FS, Carrau RL, Snyderman CH et al. Transpterygoid transposition of a temporoparietal fascia flap: a new method for skull base reconstruction after endoscopic expanded endonasal approaches. Laryngoscope 2007; 117: 970–976

[13] Fortes FS, Sennes LU, Carrau RL et al. Endoscopic anatomy of the pterygopalatine fossa and the transpterygoid approach: development of a surgical instruction model. Laryngoscope 2008; 118: 44–49

[14] Kassam AB, Vescan AD, Carrau RL et al. Expanded endonasal approach: vidian canal as a landmark to the petrous internal carotid artery. J Neurosurg 2008; 108: 177–183

[15] Chen MK, Lai JC, Chang CC, Liu MT. Minimally invasive endoscopic nasopharyngectomy in the treatment of recurrent T1–2a nasopharyngeal carcinoma. Laryngoscope 2007; 117: 894–896

[16] Yoshizaki T, Wakisaka N, Murono S, Shimizu Y, Furukawa M. Endoscopic nasopharyngectomy for patients with recurrent nasopharyngeal carcinoma at the primary site. Laryngoscope 2005; 115: 1517–1519

[17] Draf W. Endonasal frontal sinus drainage type I–III according to Draf. In: Kountakis S, Senior B, Draf W, eds. The Frontal Sinus. Berlin Heidelberg New York: Springer; 2005:219–232

[18] Bockmühl U, Minovi A, Kratzsch B, Hendus J, Draf W. Stellenwert der endonasalen mikro-endoskopischen Tumorchirurgie. Laryngo Rhino Otol (Stuttg) 2005; 84: 884–891

[19] Minovi A, Kollert M, Draf W, Bockmühl U. Inverted papilloma: feasibility of endonasal surgery and long-term results of 87 cases. Rhinology 2006; 44: 205–210

[20] Kraft M, Simmen D, Kaufmann T, Holzmann D. Long-term results of endonasal sinus surgery in sinonasal papillomas. Laryngoscope 2003; 113: 1541–1547

[21] Nicolai P, Castelnuovo P, Bolzoni Villaret A. Endoscopic resection of sinonasal malignancies. Curr Oncol Rep 2011; 13: 138–144

[22] Nicolai P, Castelnuovo P, Lombardi D et al. Role of endoscopic surgery in the management of selected malignant epithelial neoplasms of the naso-ethmoidal complex. Head Neck 2007; 29: 1075–1082

[23] Nicolai P, Villaret AB, Bottazzoli M, Rossi E, Valsecchi MG. Ethmoid adenocarcinoma—from craniofacial to endoscopic resections: a single-institution experience over 25 years. Otolaryngol Head Neck Surg 2011; 145: 330–337

[24] Castelnuovo PG, Belli E, Bignami M, Battaglia P, Sberze F, Tomei G. Endoscopic nasal and anterior craniotomy resection for malignant nasoethmoid tumors involving the anterior skull base. Skull Base 2006; 16: 15–18

[25] Kassam AB, Prevedello DM, Carrau RL et al. Endoscopic endonasal skull base surgery: analysis of complications in the authors' initial 800 patients. J Neurosurg 2011; 114: 1544–1568

[26] Keerl R, Stankiewicz J, Weber R, Hosemann W, Draf W. Surgical experience and complications during endonasal sinus surgery. Laryngoscope 1999; 109: 546–550

[27] Stankiewicz JA. Complications of endoscopic sinus surgery. Otolaryngol Clin North Am 1989; 22: 749–758

[28] Stankiewicz JA. Complications in endoscopic intranasal ethmoidectomy: an update. Laryngoscope 1989; 99: 686–690

[29] Stankiewicz JA. Cerebrospinal fluid fistula and endoscopic sinus surgery. Laryngoscope 1991; 101: 250–256

[30] Stamm AC. Complications of micro-endoscopic sinus surgery. In: Stamm AC, Draf W, eds. Micro-endoscopic Surgery of the Paranasal Sinuses and the Skull Base. Berlin Heidelberg New York: Springer; 2000:581–593

[31] Kassam AB, Thomas A, Carrau RL et al. Endoscopic reconstruction of the cranial base using a pedicled nasoseptal flap. Neurosurgery 2008; 63 Suppl 1: ONS44–ONS52; discussion ONS52–ONS53

[32] Castelnuovo PG, Delú G, Locatelli D et al. Endonasal endoscopic duraplasty: our experience. Skull Base 2006; 16: 19–24

[33] Komotar RJ, Starke RM, Raper DM, Anand VK, Schwartz TH. Endoscopic endonasal versus open repair of anterior skull base CSF leak, meningocele, and encephalocele: a systematic review of outcomes. J Neurol Surg A Cent Eur Neurosurg 2013; 74: 239–250

Chapter 9

Expanded Endoscopic Endonasal Approaches

9

9 Expanded Endoscopic Endonasal Approaches

Nancy McLaughlin, Daniel M. Prevedello, Daniel F. Kelly, Ricardo L. Carrau, Amin B. Kassam

9.1 Introduction

Endoscopic endonasal skull base surgery has burgeoned during the past two decades. In early 1990s, some reported the use of the endoscope as the sole visualizing tool during surgery for pituitary lesions.[1] Numerous centers around the world followed the lead and adopted a pure endoscopic approach to the sella.[1,2]

Detailed anatomical studies have contributed greatly to the understanding of skull base anatomy from the endoscopic perspective. This, along with improvements in intraoperative image guidance, acoustic Doppler ultrasound, and electrophysiologic monitoring, has enabled surgeons to approach skull base lesions beyond the sella turcica. By 1997, the entire ventral cranial base had been systematically approached using endoscopic endonasal techniques. Numerous anatomical and clinical studies have documented the feasibility and safety of extended endoscopic approaches along the sagittal and coronal planes.[3,4,5,6,7,8,9,10,11,12,13] Expanded endonasal approaches (EEAs) are considered important tools for skull base surgery, as they provide access to the anterior, middle, and posterior cranial fossa in appropriately selected cases.[14,15,16,17]

When compared with traditional transcranial approaches, an EEA has numerous advantages. Through its direct ventral corridors, an EEA offers a more direct median exposure, enabling the removal of a lesion with minimal brain and neurovascular manipulation. It allows prompt decompression of the visual apparatus, when indicated, and devascularizes tumors arising at the skull base early during the procedure; therefore, facilitating their removal.[2,6,7,12] Significantly, these surgical advantages may decrease operative time, length of hospitalization, and morbidity. Furthermore, EEAs may increase patient comfort and are not associated with surgical cosmetic defects.

This chapter reviews general concepts of expanded endoscopic endonasal surgery and describes specific techniques for EEAs along the sagittal and coronal planes.

9.2 Indications and Preoperative Work-up

EEAs are used to treat a wide variety of pathologies (▶ Table 9.1) that require access to the entire ventral skull base, including the anterior, middle, and posterior fossae. Unlike other surgical approaches, EEAs avoid brain manipulation and/or retraction; therefore, EEAs are useful to treat lesions in the skull base or between the skull base and the brain. Median lesions that have displaced critical neurovascular structures to the perimeter are ideal for EEA.

Table 9.1 Classification of pathologies treated via the expanded endonasal approach

Category	Example
Inflammatory sinus disease	Mucocele Allergic fungal sinusitis
Infection	Epidural abscess Osteomyelitis
Trauma	Cerebrospinal fluid leak Optic nerve decompression
Benign neoplasm	Pituitary adenoma Craniopharyngioma Meningioma Fibro-osseous lesions Angiofibroma
Malignant neoplasm	Sinonasal malignancies Esthesioneuroblastoma Chordoma Chondrosarcoma Metastases
Miscellaneous	Rathke cleft cyst Dermoid cyst Epidermoid cyst Vascular pathologies (aneurysm, arteriovenous malformation)

Preoperative high-resolution computed tomography (CT) angiography (CTA) is obtained for most skull base pathologies (except for routine pituitary adenomas or other sellar lesions), as it simultaneously displays osseous, vascular, and soft-tissue anatomy. A magnetic resonance image (MRI) is also obtained to assess tumor location and extension and to document its relation to critical soft tissues. CTA and MRI are fused for intraoperative navigation using both bony and parenchymal algorithms ("windows"). Image fusion is used to confirm the visual impression of the surgical anatomy, notably critical neurovascular structures, thereby facilitating a targeted resection. Intraoperative CT scanning can be performed, if necessary, to update the image-guidance system.

Serology and endocrine laboratory tests are performed as appropriate prior to surgery. Depending on the lesion's pathology, location, and extension, the presence of cranial neuropathies should be addressed preoperatively by a neuro-ophthalmologist and/or otolaryngologist–head and neck surgeon (ORL-HNS).

Under general anesthesia, the patient is positioned supine with the head fixed in a Mayfield head-holder. Head fixation reduces intraoperative movement of the head, especially during drilling and neurovascular dissection and secures the head in those patients in whom paralytic agents cannot be administered due to the need for cranial nerve monitoring (electromyography [EMG]).

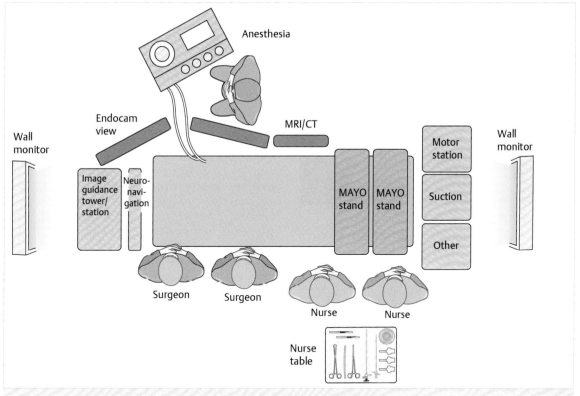

Fig. 9.1 Floor plan of the operating room during an expanded endonasal approach.

Patients who need limited surgery and no EMG monitoring can be positioned on a Mayfield horseshoe headholder. In all cases, the vertex is tilted slightly to the left with the face turned to the right by 15 to 20°. Depending on the location on the sagittal axis, the head may be extended or flexed to gain a more ventral or caudal access. We routinely use frameless stereotactic image guidance.

We advocate neurophysiological monitoring, including cortical function (somatosensory evoked potentials) with or without brainstem function (brainstem evoked responses), for cases that will require intradural surgery or dissection near the circle of Willis or internal carotid arteries. When dissection of cranial nerves is predicted based on tumor anatomy, cranial nerve EMG is also performed.

In our operating suite the anesthesia team is positioned toward the feet of the patient and the surgical team to the right side. The surgical technician or nurse can be positioned on either side of the bed. Other configurations are appropriate according to the geometry and dimensions of the operating suite, surgeon's handedness, body habitus, or surgeon's preference. The surgical team is ideally composed of a neurosurgeon and an ORL-HNS; both knowledgeable in ventral skull base endoscopic anatomy and experienced in conventional skull base surgery and expanded endoscopic surgery

(or at least have additional members of their team that are facile with open techniques). A surgical navigation device, monitor, and camera are positioned at the head of the patient (▶ Fig. 9.1). After optimal positioning, the skin of the external nose and nasal vestibule as well as the abdomen (fat graft donor site) is prepped with an antiseptic solution. The intranasal space and mucosa are not prepped. Perioperative broad-spectrum antibiotic prophylaxis is administered.

9.3 Surgical Technique

9.3.1 General Concepts for Endoscopic Endonasal Skull Base Surgery

Successful endoscopic endonasal skull base surgery procedures require bilateral nasal access for a two-surgeon, three-/four-hand technique. They also require removal of enough bone at the skull base to create a wide surgical corridor that exposes key anatomical landmarks (▶ Fig. 9.2). Bilateral access through a wide corridor prevents crisscrossing of instruments, minimizes soiling of the endoscope lens, allows dynamic movement of the scope, helps maintain an unobstructed view of the surgical field, and

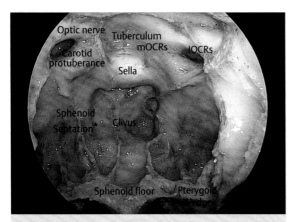

Fig. 9.2 Key anatomic landmarks for the transsphenoidal expanded endonasal approach.
lOCRs, lateral opticocarotid recesses; mOCRs, medial opticocarotid recesses.

increases lateral angulation. Bimanual dissection is especially important for managing significant bleeding, as it allows visualization while controlling the hemorrhage; thus, avoiding injury to adjacent structures.[18]

Endoscopic endonasal tumor resection uses the same intracranial dissection techniques and principles as microneurosurgery. Specifically, capsular bipolar coagulation, capsular mobilization, extracapsular dissection of neurovascular structures, and coagulation and removal of the capsule are sequentially performed. Depending on the consistency of the tumor, debulking may rely on bimanual suctioning, ultrasonic aspiration and/or piecemeal removal with cutting instruments. Grasping and pulling must be avoided.

9.3.2 Transsellar Approach to Complement an Expanded Endonasal Approach[14]

Although the transsellar approach is not considered an "expanded approach," it may be part of the corridor for the removal of extrasellar lesions such as extensive pituitary adenomas and craniopharyngiomas (▶ Fig. 9.3). For example, a transsellar approach might be combined with transplanum and/or transclival EEA to access intradural disease.

During the transsellar approach, the anterior wall of the sphenoid (rostrum) is removed to expose the lateral recesses (i.e., pterygoid recess), the planum–tuberculum junction and opticocarotid recesses (OCRs). The floor of the sphenoid is drilled back to be in-plane with the level of the clivus, giving a greater rostrocaudal trajectory into the suprasellar space. In addition to the wide bilateral sphenoidotomies, the posterior nasal septum is resected with backbiting forceps or microdebrider. These steps provide bilateral access, facilitate bilateral instrument

maneuverability, increase lateral angulation, and optimize visualization of anatomical structures. These are key components of a transsellar exposure, as they were initiated by our group a decade ago, and constitute the foundation of subsequent expanded endoscopic endonasal approaches to the skull base.[14,15]

Intrasphenoidal septations are drilled down carefully, since most often they lead directly to the internal carotid artery (ICA) and/or optic nerve canals. After the sphenoid mucosa is removed, the posterior wall of the sphenoid sinus is completely exposed. A series of key anatomical landmarks can be identified: the sellar prominence in the center, the bone strut covering the superior intercavernous sinus (SIS) above, the clival recess below, the carotid prominences lateral to the sella, and more superiorly the optic nerves, with the associated medial and lateral OCRs. Bone removal over the sellar face should extend laterally beyond the medial portions of the cavernous sinus to expose the superior and inferior intercavernous sinuses. The medial OCR does not need to be opened unless the lesion has suprasellar and lateral extensions toward the opticocarotid cistern.

The cavernous sinuses and the ICAs limit the transsellar approach laterally.

9.3.3 Expanded Endonasal Approaches: Anatomical Modules

The ventral skull base may be divided in modules based on anatomical corridors (▶ Table 9.2).[14,15,16,19] As described below, these modules are oriented between the carotid arteries (sagittal or median plane) or lateral to the carotid arteries (coronal or paramedian plane).

Sagittal Plane

Median approaches (between the carotid arteries) are oriented rostrocaudally along the sagittal plane from the frontal sinus to the second cervical vertebra, enabling access through the crista galli, cribiform plate, planum, tuberculum, dorsum sella, and clivus (▶ Fig. 9.4, ▶ Fig. 9.5).[14,15,17,20]

Transtuberculum/Transplanum Approach

The transtuberculum/transplanum approach[14] is indicated for craniopharyngiomas, tuberculum sellae meningiomas, epidermoid tumors, and other lesions involving both the posterior aspect of the anterior skull base and suprasellar space (▶ Fig. 9.6). The bony exposure of this approach frequently builds on the transsellar approach. It includes removal of the planum sphenoidale and tuberculum sellae. Importantly, the optic canals must be identified in the orbital apex early in the exposure, as they represent the lateral limit of the transplanum approach. Bilateral posterior ethmoidectomies are performed to extend the bony

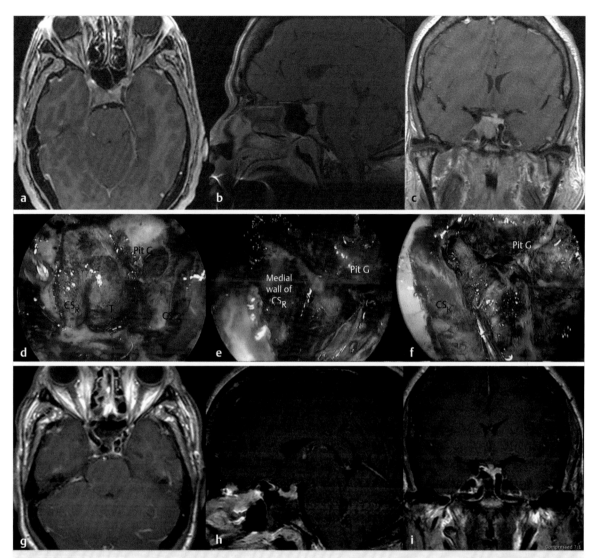

Fig. 9.3 a–i Illustrative case of a transsphenoidal approach for a functional pituitary macroadenoma. **(a–c)** Preoperative imaging. **(d–f)** Intraoperative findings. **(g–i)** Postoperative imaging.
CSL, left cavernous sinus; CSR, right cavernous sinus; Pit G, pituitary gland; T, tumor.

resection rostrally. Ethmoidal septations are drilled flush with the anterior cranial base and the lamina papyracea bilaterally. To preserve olfactory function, the resection should not extend anterior to the posterior ethmoidal arteries (PEAs), and the most rostral margin of the nasal septum is left attached to the skull base. If the dissection is pursued anterior to the PEA, the cribriform plate and olfactory fibers will be injured, potentially compromising olfaction. The planum sphenoidale is drilled eggshell-thin from a rostral-to-caudal direction. After removal of both medial OCRs and the tuberculum sellae, the SIS is exposed, cauterized, and mobilized or divided. This enables access to suprasellar extensions of tumors in the prechiasmatic cisterns. The paraclinoid carotid canals can also be opened using Kerrison rongeurs. Arterial feeders arising from the distal portion of the paraclinoid carotid artery at the level of the medial OCR as well as from the PEAs may be identified and coagulated.

The most important structures related to this approach are the optic nerves, which mark the lateral limits of the transplanum approach, the ICAs, and the anterior cerebral arteries (A1 artery, recurrent artery of Heubner, anterior communicating artery [AcoA], and perforator arteries). Care to avoid damage to the AcoA and the recurrent artery of Heubner is necessary when dissecting superior surface of an intradural tumor. Similar efforts are required to preserve the subchiasmatic perforating vessels during subchiasmatic extracapsular dissection.

Table 9.2 Modular classification of the expanded endonasal approaches

Sagittal plane (midline)	Coronal plane (paramedian)
Transfrontal	Anterior coronal plane
Transcribriform	• Supraorbital
Transtuberculum/transplanum	• Transorbital
Transselar	Middle coronal plane
Transclival	• Medial petrous apex (zone 1)

• Superior third
  ○ Transdorsum sellae (intradural)
  ○ Subsellar (extradural)
	• Inferior cavernous sinus/ quadrangular space (zone 3)
	• Superior cavernous sinus (zone 4)

• Middle third	• Infratemporal approach (zone 5)
• Inferior third	
• Panclival	Posterior coronal plane
Transodontoid and foramen magnum/craniovertebral junction approach	• Petroclival approach (zone 2)

	• Infrapetrous
	  ○ Transcondylar
	  ○ Transhypoglossal

	• Parapharyngeal space
	  ○ Medial (jugular foramen)
	  ○ Lateral

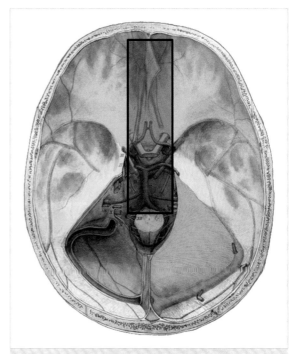

Fig. 9.4 Sagittal plane. Red bar, all modules oriented between the carotid arteries; blue, anterior cranial fossa; yellow, middle cranial fossa; green, posterior cranial fossa.

Transcribriform Approach

A transcribriform approach[14] is most frequently combined with a transplanum approach to remove large anterior fossa meningiomas, esthesioneuroblastomas, or other invasive sinonasal malignancies (▶ Fig. 9.7). It requires extending the rostral aspect of the transplanum approach to the level of the crista galli or even the frontal sinus. Boundaries of this module are the laminae papyraceae laterally, the frontal sinus anteriorly, and the transition with the planum sphenoidale posteriorly at the level of the PEA.

The attachment of the anterior portion of the nasal septum to the skull base is resected since olfaction is most likely already compromised. Complete ethmoidectomies expose the medial orbital walls. Drilling of the skull base begins at the frontoethmoidal recess in a rostrocaudal direction. The anterior and posterior ethmoidal arteries are identified, coagulated, and transected medially, contributing to tumor devascularization; failure to coagulate or clip the ethmoidal arteries may lead to a postoperative retrobulbar hematoma. The lamina papyracea can be removed to gain lateral exposure, taking care not to disrupt the periorbita. Prior to drilling the cribriform plate, the soft tissues including mucosa, olfactory filaments, and branches of ethmoidal arteries must be coagulated, further contributing to tumor devascularization. After bilateral removal of the cribri-

form plate, the crista galli is drilled eggshell-thin and fractured.

The most important bounding structures are the orbits and the anterior cerebral arteries (A2) and their branches (fronto-orbital, frontopolar). For example, dissection over the superior pole of an anterior fossa meningioma proceeds along the interhemispheric fissure where the A2 and frontopolar arteries will be draped over the tumor surface. Extracapsular dissection may also proceed toward the parasellar cistern (inferior pole), enabling identification of the optic nerves and the AcoA. This provides proximal control of both A2 arteries during dissection along the interhemispheric fissure.

Transclival Approach

The transclival approach[15] is frequently used for resection of extradural and intradural diseases such as chordomas and chondrosarcomas (▶ Fig. 9.8). It is also used to access lesions anterior to the brainstem such as meningiomas and craniopharyngiomas.

A transclival approach can be used to selectively remove the upper, middle, or lower third of the clivus, or the entire clivus (panclivectomy). The upper third includes the dorsum sella in the midline and posterior clinoids in the paramedian region down to the level of the Dorello canal. The dorsum sellae and posterior clinoids may be removed either intradurally via a transsellar approach or extradur-

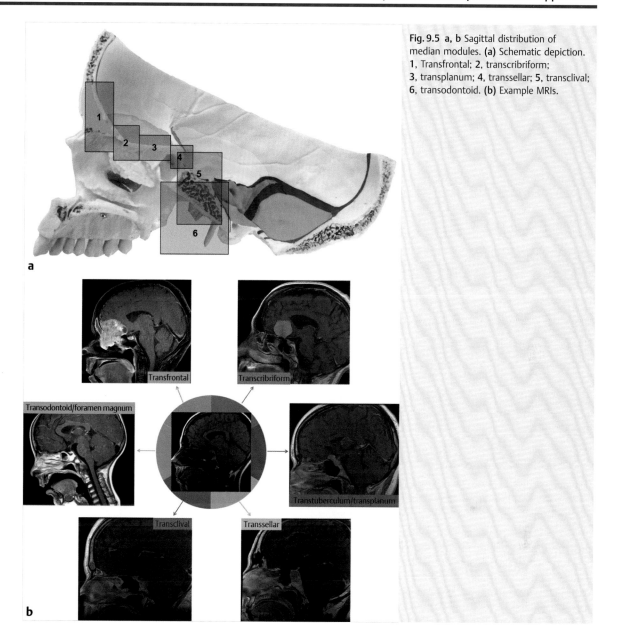

Fig. 9.5 a, b Sagittal distribution of median modules. **(a)** Schematic depiction. 1, Transfrontal; 2, transcribriform; 3, transplanum; 4, transsellar; 5, transclival; 6, transodontoid. **(b)** Example MRIs.

ally via a subsellar approach, elevating the contents of the pituitary fossa en bloc and allowing for access to the basilar artery and interpeduncular cistern. In some cases, a pituitary gland transposition may be required to obtain an unobstructed visualization of the posterior wall of the sella and gain access to the interpeduncular cistern.[20]

The middle third of the clivus extends from the Dorello canal down to the jugular foramen and can be directly accessed at the posterior aspect of the sphenoid sinus. Its resection is limited laterally by both ascending paraclival ICAs.

The lower third of the clivus extends from jugular foramen through the cervicomedullary junction and foramen magnum. If drilling is continued inferiorly from the mid-dle third of the clivus, removal of the lower third of the clivus is limited laterally by the fossa of Rosenmuller and the torus tubarius.

A panclival approach extends from the dorsum sellae and posterior clinoids to the anterior aspect of the foramen magnum. To gain such a caudal access, certain modifications must be brought to the initial bilateral sphenoid sinus exposure. The nasal septum should be completely detached from the sphenoid rostrum. Wide sphenoidotomies provide deeper positioning of the scope and a direct caudal view. After removing the basipharyngeal fascia from the floor of the sphenoid sinus and clivus face, the sphenoid floor is drilled until it is in-plane with the clivus. The vidian artery and its corresponding nerve

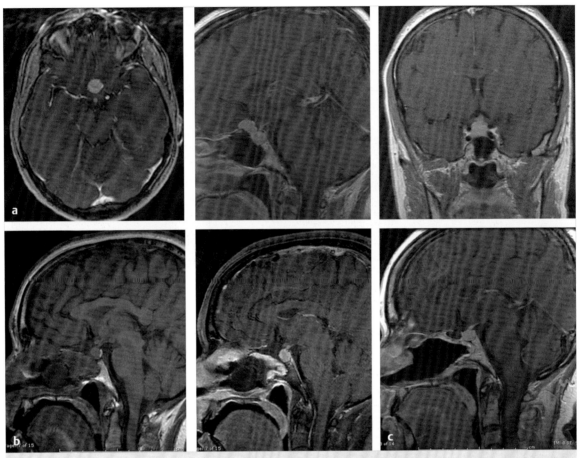

Fig. 9.6 a–c Illustrative case of a transplanum/transtuberculum sellae approach for a tuberculum sella meningioma. **(a)** Preoperative imaging. **(b)** immediate postoperative imaging. **(c)** MRI 3 months after surgery.

must be located before drilling the clivus since these structures travel in the vidian canal to join the anterior genu of the ICA.[21] If drilling is required inferior and lateral to the anterior genu of the ICA, the vidian canal is used as the superior limit.[22]

The dura is opened in short segments to ensure its meticulous coagulation as well as that of the basilar venous plexus. The dural incision is extended laterally under the horizontal petrous ICA toward the fossa of Rosenmuller, where the Eustachian tubes disappear obliquely into the skull base. Opening of the dura at the level of the ICA genu should be performed under direct visualization, as the abducens nerves enter the Dorello canal just medial, superior, and dorsal to the anterior ICA genu.

The most important neural structures related to the transclival approach are the brainstem and cranial nerves II and III for the upper third of clivus, cranial nerve VI for the middle clivus, and cranial nerves IX to XII for the lower clivus. Cranial nerves V, VII, and VIII are located lateral to this corridor and rarely come into consideration during a transclival approach. Vascular structures associated with a transclival approach include the vertebral

arteries, vertebrobasilar junction, basilar artery, superior cerebellar arteries, posterior cerebral arteries, and respective perforating arteries.

Transodontoid and Foramen Magnum/ Craniovertebral Approach

A transodontoid approach[17] implies the removal of the odontoid process off from the axis. It provides access the extradural craniocervical junction for resection of the odontoid process in degenerative or inflammatory disease (▶ Fig. 9.9). A transodontoid approach also can expose the ventral medulla and upper cervical spinal cord for access to related intradural pathologies. Although this approach is a caudal extension of the transclival approach, it may be performed independently; thus, not requiring sphenoidotomies. Foramen magnum meningiomas are the most frequent intradural lesions treated using this approach.

After removing the nasopharyngeal mucosa, the paraspinal muscles and the atlanto-occipital membrane are exposed and partially resected. At this point, the lower

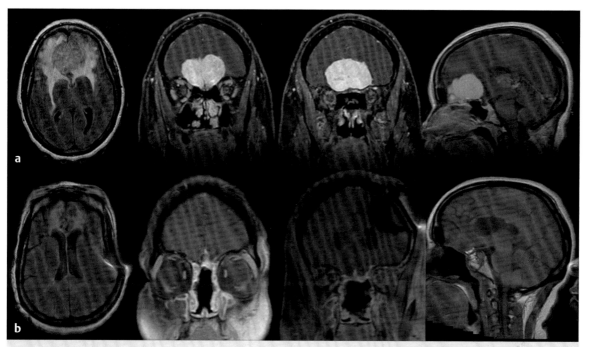

Fig. 9.7 a, b Illustrative case of a transcribriform approach for an olfactory groove meningioma. **(a)** Preoperative imaging. **(b)** Postoperative imaging.

clivus and the anterior arch of C1 are exposed. If the pathology requires a foramen magnum exposure, only the superior aspect of C1 ring is drilled to expose the tip of the odontoid. The medial aspects of the occipital condyles are removed without entering the joint capsule. However, if a transodontoid exposure is needed, the anterior arch of C1 is drilled and the odontoid process is exposed and drilled out to the posterior cortical shell, which is preferentially removed by sharp dissection. After removal of the dens, the normal dura covering the brainstem is exposed; however, in the setting of rheumatoid arthritis, the underlying pannus is exposed and removed. A posterior cervical fusion might be necessary if instability is produced. However, if one of the alar ligaments and occipital condyle-C1 articular facet capsules are preserved, stability can be maintained.

The most important neurovascular structures are the vertebral arteries, posterior inferior cerebellar arteries, brainstem, and lower cranial nerves. Since the ICAs can be positioned close to the midline in their parapharyngeal segment under the mucosa, they might also be at risk of injury. Therefore, a CTA performed prior to surgery is useful to rule out this midline location and potential disastrous situation.

Coronal Plane

Paramedian approaches (lateral to the carotid arteries) are divided into three different levels: anterior, middle, and posterior. The anterior coronal plane has an intimate relation with the anterior fossa and orbits, the middle coronal plane with the middle fossa and temporal lobe, and the posterior coronal plane with the posterior fossa (▶ Fig. 9.10).

Anterior Coronal Plane

Transorbital and supraorbital approaches are indicated for resection of sinonasal lesions that invade the posterior medial wall of the orbit (such as sinonasal malignancies), resection of intraconal lesions that are inferior and medial to the optic nerve (such as schwannomas, cavernomas, and meningiomas), and decompression of the optic nerves in the presence of unresectable intraconal pathologies. Both approaches require wide resection of the anterior and posterior ethmoid cells to expose the lateral wall of the sinonasal cavity.

Depending on the pathology, the transorbital approach may be performed unilaterally or bilaterally. Intraconal access is gained by removing the lamina papyracea and/ or the medial optic canals, opening the periorbita, and creating a corridor between the inferior and medial rectus muscle or superior oblique and medial rectus muscle. In the supraorbital approach, the medial wall of the orbit is removed and the orbital tissues are displaced laterally to visualize the orbital roof.

The optic nerves, the anterior and posterior ethmoidal arteries, and the ophthalmic artery with its central retina artery branch are the most important structures in the anterior coronal plane.

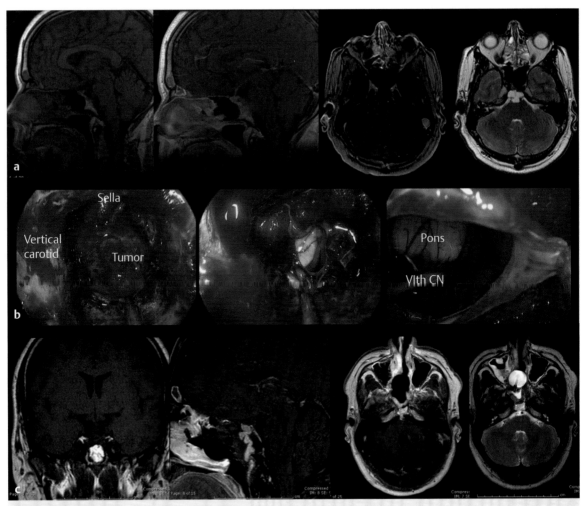

Fig. 9.8 a–c Illustrative case of a transclival approach for a clival chordoma. (a) Preoperative imaging. (b) Intraoperative findings. (c) Postoperative imaging.
CN, cranial nerve.

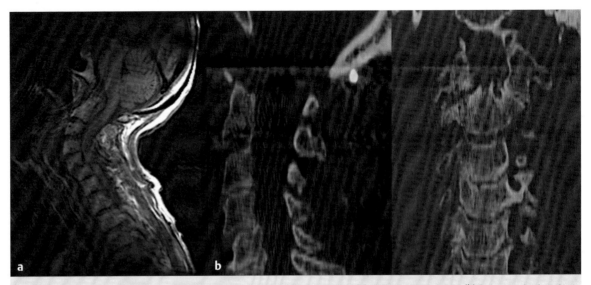

Fig. 9.9 a, b Illustrative case of a transodontoid approach for basilar invagination. (a) Preoperative imaging. (b) Postoperative imaging, sagittal and coronal views.

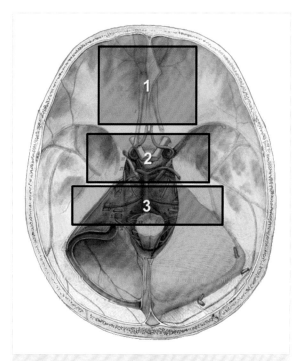

Fig. 9.10 Coronal plane. **1**, Anterior coronal plane; **2**, middle coronal plane; **3**, posterior coronal plane. Blue, anterior cranial fossa; yellow, middle cranial fossa; green, posterior cranial fossa.

Middle Coronal Plane

Approaches that access the middle coronal plane[16] are grouped on the basis of their relationship to the petrous carotid artery. Infrapetrous approaches give access to the medial petrous apex and the petroclival junction. Suprapetrous approaches give access to the inferior and superior cavernous sinus as well as the infratemporal/middle fossa.

Transpterygoid Approach

This exposure allows direct access to the medial cranial skull base (pterygoid recess) where spontaneous cerebrospinal fluid (CSF) leaks are frequently encountered. The transpterygoid approach[16] is to the middle and posterior coronal plane what the transsphenoidal approach is to the sagittal plane. The first step requires a wide midmeatal maxillary antrostomy or medial maxillectomy that provides access to the back wall of the maxillary sinus. The sphenopalatine and posterior nasal arteries should be identified and ligated. Next, the posterior wall of the maxillary sinus is removed, giving access to the pterygopalatine fossa.[23,24] The soft tissues of the pterygopalatine fossa are either elevated in a medial-to-lateral direction, or resected to expose the base of the pterygoid process.

The vidian canal and foramen rotundum are identified posteriorly in the sphenoid bone. The vidian canal must

be identified early in the exposure since this canal and the medial pterygoid plate are critical landmarks for endoscopic approaches to the petrous apex.[21,22] The vidian canal leads directly to the an area that corresponds to the anterior genu of the ICA, at a point where the petrous portion of the ICA angles superiorly to form the vertical paraclival ICA. The medial pterygoid plate is drilled medial and inferior to the vidian canal while following it posteriorly, toward the foramen lacerum. After identifying the anterior genu of the ICA, the lateral and superior part of the medial pterygoid plate can also be drilled. At this point, the lateral sphenoid recess is completely exposed.

Medial Petrous Apex[16]

This approach, which builds on the transpterygoid and transclival approaches, is indicated to access lesions in the medial petrous apex such as chondrosarcomas and cholesterol granulomas (▶ Fig. 9.11). However, if the pathology is located posterior to the ICA, without medial expansion or bony remodeling, this medial–lateral corridor is not recommended as it risks damage to the ICA. An infrapetrous approach (posterior coronal plane) may be safer for lesions behind the petrous ICA.

To access the petrous apex, removal of the bone covering the paraclival carotid may be required if the ICA needs to be mobilized laterally.[25] Access can be enhanced by drilling a portion of the lateral clivus at its junction with the petrous apex.

The most important structures related to this module are the ICAs and cranial nerve VI at the Dorello canal.

Inferior Cavernous Sinus/Quadrangular Space

This approach[26] also has been termed suprapetrous to indicate its orientation above the course of the horizontal segment of the ICA. It is indicated to access lesions in the Meckel cave or the quadrangular space (defined inferiorly by the petrous ICA, superiorly by the cranial nerve VI, medially by the paraclival ICA, and laterally by the gasserian ganglion). The Meckel cave is delimited inferiorly by the petrous ICA, medially by the ascending paraclival ICA, superiorly by the VI cranial nerve in the cavernous sinus, and laterally by the maxillary division of the trigeminal nerve (V_2). Pathologies commonly encountered in this region are invasive adenoid cystic carcinomas, meningiomas, schwannomas, and invasive pituitary adenomas (▶ Fig. 9.12).

A transpterygoid approach is initially performed and the vidian nerve is followed posteriorly up to the area of the foramen lacerum and the anterior genu of the ICA. Removal of the posterior wall of the maxillary antrum is extended laterally until the maxillary branch (V_2) of the trigeminal nerve is identified and followed to the foramen rotundum. The medial pterygoid plate is drilled inferior and medial to the vidian canal. Next, the bone

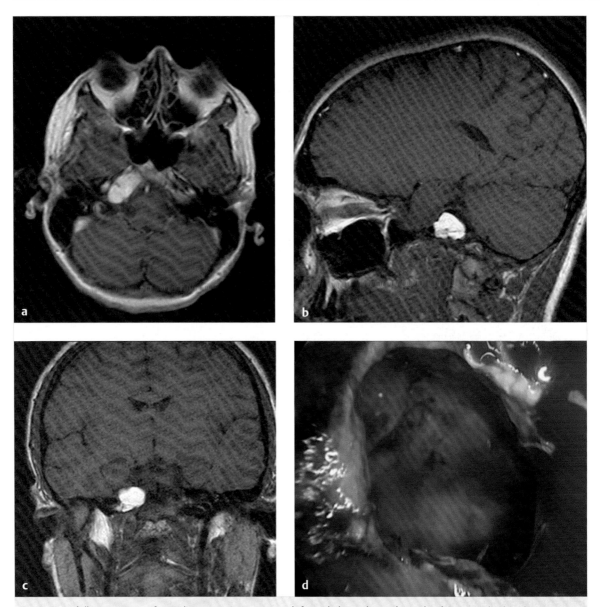

Fig. 9.11 a–d Illustrative case of a median petrous apex approach for a cholesterol granuloma. **(a–c)** Preoperative imaging. **(d)** Intraoperative imaging documenting complete drainage of the lesion.

between the vidian canal and V_2 is removed, taking into consideration that this bony corridor narrows progressively as it deepens. Removing this bone accesses the quadrangular space. If mobilization of the ICA is required to gain access to the lesion, the bone covering the horizontal petrous ICA, the anterior genu, and parasellar ICA may need to be removed. The inferior cavernous sinus is accessed by opening dura from the genu of the ICA (medial) toward the V_2 (lateral).

Structures at risk include those at the boundaries of the Meckel cave: the ICA and the trigeminal and abducens cranial nerves.

Superior Cavernous Sinus

This approach requires the same bone removal and ICA exposure as the inferior cavernous sinus/quadrangular approach. However, it is rarely indicated as it is associated with a high risk of cranial nerve injury. The superior cavernous sinus approach is usually reserved for cases with pre-existent cranial nerve deficits (III, IV, VI).[16,27]

The medial margin of the parasellar ICA should be clearly identified to protect it during the dural incision. The dura is then opened in a medial-to-lateral direction directly over the superior lateral portion of the cavernous sinus. If the cavernous sinus has been thrombosed by the

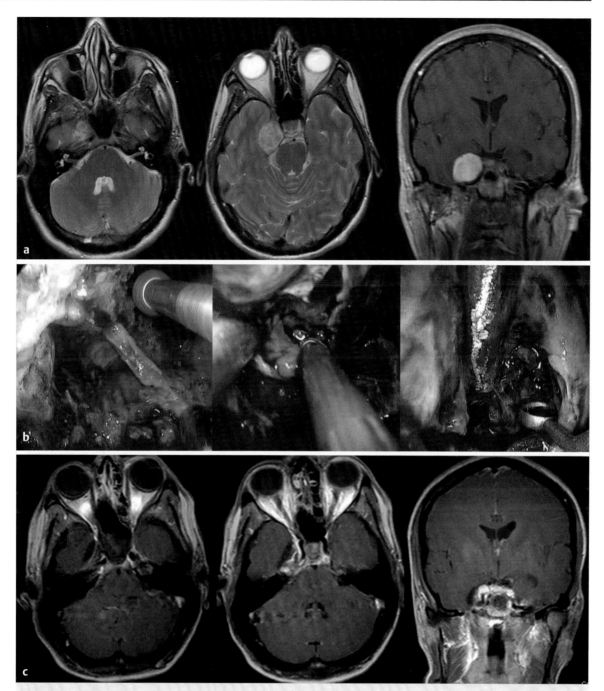

Fig. 9.12 a–c Illustrative case of a quadrangular approach for a trigeminal nerve schwannoma (V$_2$). **(a)** Preoperative imaging. **(b)** Intraoperative findings. **(c)** Postoperative imaging.

lesion, little venous bleeding occurs during initial opening. However, once the tumor is removed, significant bleeding may occur.

Important structures related to this approach include cranial nerves III, IV, V, and VI, as well as the ICAs with their accompanying sympathetic fibers.

Infratemporal Approach

Neoplasms can expand a corridor through the pterygomaxillary fissure, extending rostrally to the middle fossa and laterally into the infratemporal fossa, or they can arise within the fossa itself. Pathologies approached via

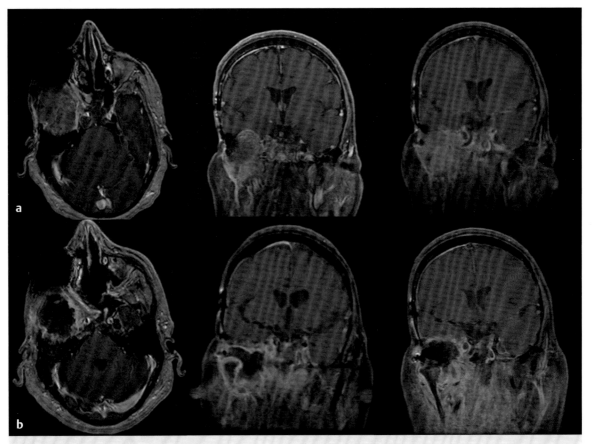

Fig. 9.13 a, b Illustrative case an infratemporal approach for a skull base chordoma. (**a**) Preoperative imaging. (**b**) Postoperative imaging.

this route include skull base juvenile angiofibromas, meningiomas, schwannomas, CSF leaks, and select sinonasal malignancies (▶ Fig. 9.13). The infratemporal approach[16] to these lesions begins after the medial pterygoid plate is isolated, the vidian canal is identified, and the maxillary antrostomy is completed.

The medial pterygoid plate is identified and removed flush with the middle cranial fossa and foramen rotundum. Tumor debulking only begins after identifying the anterior genu of the ICA and horizontal petrous segment of the ICA. During the lateral dissection, the internal maxillary artery and its branches must be isolated and ligated. The dissection is pursued laterally until the lateral pterygoid plate (LPP) is identified. The LPP is drilled rostrally until it is flush with the middle fossa and foramen ovale. Profuse venous bleeding from the pterygopalatine venous complex may require packing and staged resection to allow time for the venous complex to thrombose. Since the bony landmarks are often remodeled or eroded, and the soft tissues displaced, image guidance is required.

Relevant structures to this module are the internal maxillary artery and its branches, the vidian nerve, the trigeminal nerves (V_2 and V_3) and their branches, and the superior orbital fissure.

Posterior Coronal Plane

The posterior coronal plane extends rostrocaudally from the petroclival region to the foramen magnum and laterolaterally between the jugular foramina, hypoglossal canals, occipital condyles, and parapharyngeal spaces.

Petroclival

A petroclival approach is used to access deep-seated lesions along the midportion of the petrous bone. This approach begins as a medial petrous apex exposure. After identification of the vidian canal, just lateral to the junction of the sphenoid floor with the medial pterygoid plate, it is drilled circumferentially, following it back to the anterior genu of the ICA.[21,22] The anterior genu of the ICA is the most important landmark of this approach since it determines its lateral boundary. The petrous (horizontal), genu, and the paraclival (vertical) segments of the ICA are unroofed to allow for their lateral displacement. Once the anterior genu of the ICA has been well identified, the medial portion of the clivus can be drilled safely. The lateral portion of the clivus at the petroclival junction can be drilled laterally beneath the petrous ICA until the underlying dura of the posterior fossa and its accompanying venous plexus are identified. The horizontal segment of the petrous carotid and overlying cavernous sinus represent the superior boundary of this exposure; the middle fossa represents the superolateral boundary. The paramedian segment of the prepontine cistern can be accessed by opening the dura.

Important structures associated with this approach include the vidian nerves and the ICAs.

Infrapetrous

An infrapetrous approach[16] is based as an infratemporal approach and is usually indicated for chondrosarcomas and cholesterol granulomas arising in this region (▶ Fig. 9.14). After identifying V_2, the vidian canal and the anterior genu of the ICA, the medial pterygoid plate is drilled until is flush with the middle cranial fossa and the foramen rotundum. As the lateral pterygoid plate is drilled, V_3 is identified along its posterior edge and used to guide drilling toward the foramen ovale. The medial aspect of the cartilaginous segment of the Eustachian tube is resected. The inferior surface of the petrous apex is reached by drilling the bone and cartilage between the horizontal petrous segment of the ICA and the Eustachian

tube, medial to V_3. The horizontal petrous and vertical paraclival segment of ICA are identified and skeletonized. Finally, drilling and tumor dissection proceed under the petrous ICA into the petrous apex.

Vital structures related to the infrapetrous module are the inner ear with cranial nerves VII and VIII laterally, the petrous ICA superiorly, and cranial nerve XII inferolaterally.

Jugular Foramen/Hypoglossal Canal

This approach is most commonly indicated for the resection of chondrosarcomas, paragangliomas, schwannomas, and skull base meningiomas. The Eustachian tube must be identified in this approach since it determines the position of the parapharyngeal ICA (ascending segment) as it penetrates the carotid canal into the petrous bone. The fossa of Rosenmüller is followed laterally. The medial aspect of the occipital condyle is encountered lateral to the foramen magnum and followed laterally. The hypoglossal canal is rostrolateral to the condyle; its location should be confirmed with intraoperative image guidance and function of the nerve is followed by EMG monitoring. Once the ICA is localized, the jugular foramen is identified

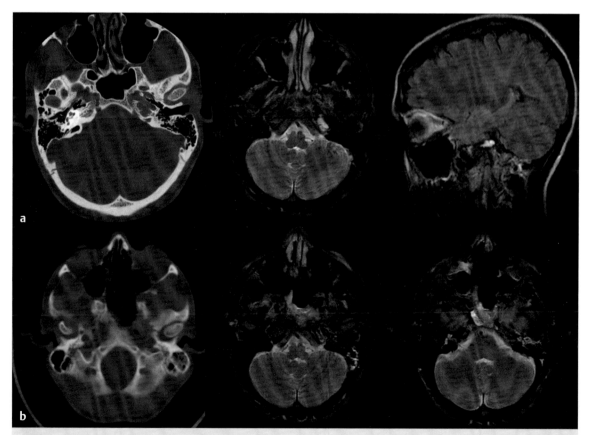

Fig. 9.14 a, b Illustrative case of an infrapetrous approach for a petrous apex cholesterol granuloma that was impossible to approach medially. (a) Preoperative imaging. (b) Postoperative imaging.

Table 9.3 Intraoperative complications during 800 cases of an expanded endonasal approach performed by the authors

Category	Consequence	Type of lesion and/or defect
Vascular	Death (0%)	None
	Transient deficit (0.1%)	P1 perforator
	Permanent deficit (0.4%)	Pontine bleed (quadriplegic) Imax laceration (hemiplegic) Frontopolar avulsion (right lower limb paresis)
	No deficit (0.4%)	Ophthalmic (already blind) (1 case) ICA lacerations (2 cases)
Neural injury	Permanent deficit (0.5%)	IX, X, XII (1 case) IX, X (1 case) VI (2 cases)
	Transient deficit (1.5%)	III nerve (2 cases) V3 motor (1 case) V1 nerve (4 cases) IX, X (1 case) Hemiparesis (4 cases)

Results based on a study of 800 cases using an expanded endonasal approach.
ICA, internal carotid artery; Imax, internal maxillary artery.

Table 9.4 Postoperative complications after 800 cases of an expanded endonasal approach performed by the authors

Category	Consequence	Type of complication
Infection (1.4%)	Death (0.1%)	Meningitis + status epilepticus (1 case)
	Successfully treated (1.1%)	Intradural abscess (1 case) Extradural abscess (1 case) Meningitis (7 cases)
	Deficit (0.1%)	Intradural abscess—incapacitated (1 case)
Systemic (2.8%)	Death (0.7%)	PE < 30 days (2 cases) PE > 30 days (2 cases) Pneumonia + MI < 30 days (1 case) Multiorgan failure > 30 days (1 case)
	Successfully treated (2.1%)	Acute renal failure—transfusion (1 case) Respiratory failure (7 cases) PE < 30 days (5 cases) MI (3 cases) Immediate postoperative asystole (1 case)
Delayed deficit (1.9%)	Permanent deficit (0.6%)	Visual deficit (perfusion) (2 cases) Visual deficit (late hypotension) (1 case) Visual deficit (hematoma) (1 case) Hemiplegia (postoperative apoplexy) (1 case)
	Transient deficit (1.3%)	Visual deficit (omphalocele) (1 case) Visual deficit (hematoma) (4 cases) Visual deficit (nasal balloon) (2 cases) III nerve (hematoma) (1 case) Proptosis (retrobulbar hematoma) (1 case) Ataxia (OG tube passed clivectomy) (1 case)

MI, myocardial infarction; OG, orogastric; PE, pulmonary embolism.

immediately lateral. Cranial nerves IX, X, and XI are located in between the jugular vein and the ICA.

Important structures related to this approach are the internal maxillary artery, the ICA (pharyngeal and petrous segments), the trigeminal nerve, the jugular foramen with the jugular vein and accompanying lower cranial nerves (IX, X, XI), and cranial nerve XII exiting the hypoglossal canal inferiorly.

9.4 Complications

Intraoperative and postoperative complications are minimal when an EEA is undertaken by an experienced surgical team that is familiar with endoscopic ventral skull base anatomy, using proper instrumentation, and adhering to endoscopic surgical principles. Complications in our first 800 expanded endoscopic surgeries have been compiled and categorized (▶ Table 9.3 and ▶ Table 9.4). The most significant risk is injury to the ICA. The anterior cerebral arteries, optic nerve, cranial nerves III and IV, pituitary gland, and orbits are at risk when the anterior fossa is approached. Similarly, the abducens cranial nerve and trigeminal branches are at risk during approaches to the middle fossa. When the posterior fossa is approached, the brainstem, basilar artery, and vertebral arteries and branches, as well as the cranial nerves, including IX, X, XI and XII, are at risk. Anytime the dura is opened, there is a risk of CSF leak and it should be reconstructed with vascularized tissue or similarly reliable technique.

9.5 Sequential Learning and Training for Expanded Endonasal Approaches

Endoscopic skull base surgery is complex; thus, it *must* be learned in a stepwise fashion.[19] Surgical learning could be categorized by complexity and technical difficulty into five increasing levels that are associated with an increasing risk of major complications (▶ Table 9.5). Each level must be fully mastered before proceeding to the next, since a higher level translates into increased anatomical

Table 9.5 Training program for endonasal cranial base surgery

Level	Procedures
Level I	Endoscopic sinonasal surgery Endoscopic sphenoethmoidectomy Sphenopalatine artery ligation Endoscopic frontal sinusotomy
Level II	Advanced sinus surgery Cerebrospinal fluid leaks Lateral recess sphenoid Sella/pituitary (intrasellar)
Level III (extradural)	Medial orbital decompression Optic nerve decompression Sella/pituitary (extrasellar) Petrous apex (medial expansion) Transclival approaches (extradural) Transodontoid approach (extradural)
Level IV (intradural)	Presences of cortical cuff
A	Transplanum approach
	Transcribriform approach
	Preinfundibular lesions
B	Absence of cortical cuff (direct vascular contact)
	Transplanum approach
	Transcribriform approach
	Infundibular lesions
	Retroinfundibular lesions
	Transclival approach
	Foramen magnum approach
C	Internal carotid artery dissection
Level V	Middle coronal plane (paramedian)
A	Suprapetrous carotid approaches
	Infrapetrous carotid approaches
	Transpterygoid approaches
	Infratemporal approach
B	Posterior coronal plane (paramedian)
C	Vascular surgery

complexity, technical difficulty, and potential risk of neurovascular injury.

- **Level I** includes endoscopic sinonasal surgeries such as endoscopic sphenoethmoidectomy, sphenopalatine artery ligation, orbital decompression, and endoscopic frontal sinusotomy. Since neurovascular structures are well protected under the bony skull base, the risk of a major complication during such procedures is considered low.
- **Level II** represents the initial step for endoscopic endonasal skull base surgery and includes repair of CSF leaks and intrasellar surgeries. These surgeries involve a connection with the intradural space; therefore the risk of complications increases from level I procedures.

- **Level III** includes extrasellar extradural dissections. This level encompass any endoscopic endonasal surgery that require drilling of the skull base to expose the periosteal layer of dura, such as for optic nerve decompression, exposure of petrous apex lesions with a medial expansion, and extradural transclival and transodontoid approaches. A critical understanding the endoscopic ventral skull base anatomy is required since a vast number of noble neurovascular structures are immediately beneath the dura.
- **Level IV** includes intradural surgery; therefore, encompassing any intervention in which the surgeon intentionally opens the dura to access either purely intradural pathologies or extradural lesions that have invaded the subdural space. Theoretically, the likelihood of complications increases significantly.
- **Level V** procedures represent cerebrovascular surgery including aneurysm and arteriovenous malformation treatment and resection of tumors that surround or invade major intracranial vessels or any segment of the ICA. Also, any endoscopic procedure that extends beyond the carotid in the midcoronal and posterior coronal plane is considered a level V procedure since it requires dissecting and transposing the ICAs with the use of angled scopes. This is a daunting maneuver that carries a risk of catastrophic complications.

Each specific surgical module and corresponding level of difficulty has an associated learning curve that each surgeon needs to experience before achieving ease and proficiency. Each step requires hands-on practice and insightful analysis to master the necessary skills. It is generally recognized that the learning curve is steepest and, therefore, the required hands-on time is longest for the paramedian approaches. The ideal number of cases that must be performed before a surgeon feels comfortable with a specific level depends on innate eye–hand coordination, previously acquired surgical skills, prior surgical experience with the specific pathology, and frequency of endoscopic endonasal surgeries. Mentoring, courses, and other means of insightful feedback can accelerate the learning process. For example, neurosurgeons who are versed in endoscopic-assisted keyhole supraorbital or retrosigmoid approaches have acquired skills working through these narrow corridors that are similar to those required for EEAs. In both approaches, the surgeon must work bimanually along a long, constricted corridor, manipulating custom surgical instruments through a small superficial opening. Neurosurgeons, who are used to microsurgical visualization through conventional open skull base approaches, will have to commit energy and time to overcome the barriers of the confined corridor and endoscopic visualization. Similarly, an ORL-HNS, who is trained and versed in endoscopic techniques, will find that the skills will be second nature after gaining experience with the skull base anatomy. Most have to attend courses and train to acquire endoscopic skills.

It is recommended that the endoscopic surgical team perform at least 30 to 50 pituitary procedures at each level before proceeding to the next level.[28,29,30,31] If the endoscopic surgical team chooses to perform high-level procedures (levels IV and V), each surgeon must commit to the team approach, assuring regular surgical activity with an adequate volume of cases. Whatever level of competence is achieved, it is important for surgeons to recognize their own limitations and not attempt procedures that are beyond their training and institutional capabilities.

In addition to the learning opportunities encountered in the operating theater with each specific case, participation in cadaveric dissection courses under the guidance of an experienced group may enhance the understanding of particular anatomical relationships that cannot be adequately explored in the operating room. Cadaveric dissection courses also give insight into more advanced levels IV and V.

9.6 Postoperative Care and Outcome

Close surveillance in an intensive care unit is recommended after an EEA if an intradural dissection was performed or if a premorbid medical condition warrants this precaution. Otherwise patients routinely go to a step-down unit. General principles of multilayer reconstruction and use of free tissue grafts and vascularized pedicled flaps are reviewed in a companion chapter. Lumbar drains are not routinely used prior to transsellar or EEAs but may be considered for a high-flow CSF leaks (opening of the ventricles or more than one cistern), extensive arachnoid dissection, or morbid obesity. Any sign of a CSF leak after surgery requires immediate reoperation for identification and repair.

Endocrine follow-up is indicated in the immediate postoperative period in cases of functional pituitary tumors or surgical procedures that might have altered the pituitary gland or pituitary stalk. Urinary output, specific urinary gravity, and serum sodium should be monitored closely. Antibiotics are administered while the patient has endonasal packing.

Numerous series have demonstrated equivalent oncologic results for endoscopic versus standard transcranial resection of sinonasal, sellar, and various skull base lesions when performed in dedicated centers.[2,3,7,10,11,13,32,33] Overall, endoscopic skull base surgery shares the same primary goal of oncological surgery as open procedures (i.e., to perform a complete tumor excision). Since EEAs have a ventral perspective that facilitates resection of bony and dural invasion, in select cases the resection of infiltrative skull base tumors may be more extensive with EEA than with traditional skull base approaches. In addition, the endoscopic panoramic view of the surgical field facilitates the planning of resection margins.[19] Furthermore, since more lateral areas can be visualized and dynamically magnified with the endoscope, the intraoperative assessment of the surgical field for tumor remnants is improved.

Although results of EEA for various skull base pathologies are promising, the collective experience is currently too small and too brief to describe long-term tumor control. Larger series and longer follow-up are required to determine in which circumstances the EEA is superior to standard open surgery.

9.7 Conclusion

Over the past two decades, endoscopic endonasal surgery has evolved significantly. In experienced hands, pathologies of the ventral skull base in which the neurovascular structures are located on the lesions perimeter can be safely and successfully accessed using endoscopic endonasal approaches. Importantly, these minimally invasive approaches have not yet reached their limits; therefore, their indications and contraindications have not yet matured. Tumor type, size, shape, fibrosity, vascularity, extradural locoregional extension, major vessel encasement, dural invasion, and intradural extension have not proven to be limiting factors to endoscopic endonasal surgery; although, they increase the complexity and difficulty of the surgery. These factors and the patient's comorbidities, as well as the skills and experience of the operating team, must be considered when choosing the best surgical route for a given patient. Each patient should be evaluated with a 360° strategy, using the surgical approach that will yield the best resection (possible and/or desirable), while using the least destructive route with the frequency and severity of complications. Modular approaches may and should be combined as mandated by the lesion and its location.[14,15,16] However, when a lesion cannot be completely removed through an EEA, an open route may be considered or a combination of endonasal and open approaches.[3,7,8]

To date, endonasal endoscopic surgery is still in evolution: the limits have not yet been reached. Greater familiarity with endoscopic ventral skull base anatomy and continued development of instrumentation will stimulate further advances in this field. The collective experience of EEA for the management of skull base lesions will need to be assessed on a large scale in the near future.

Pearls and Pitfalls

- EEAs are based on modular anatomic corridors that avoid crossing the plane of cranial nerves or major vascular structures.
- EEAs offer several advantages: (a) early tumor devascularization; (b) minimal pituitary gland, brain, and neurovascular manipulation; (c) direct access to the ventral osseous framework of the skull base such as the cribriform plate, clivus, and medial optic canal.
- The extent of the sinonasal corridor (i.e., exposure) is dictated by the pathology, its location, and skull base extension.
- An EEA is best as a binarial, bimanual access that allows for a two-surgeon, three-/four-hand technique.
- Endoscopic skull base surgery applies similar principles to microscopic skull base surgery. Excessive retraction, grasping, and avulsion of tissues must be avoided.
- Reconstruction of skull base defect is a critical phase of the surgery and, when faulty, a major cause of morbidity. Vascularized flaps provide the most reliable technique for reconstruction.
- EEAs are best performed by a team composed of a neurosurgeon and a head and neck surgeon, both with experience in conventional skull base surgery and expanded endoscopic surgery.
- Familiarity with the cranial base anatomy from the ventral endoscopic perspective is critical to performing endoscopic cranial base surgery.
- Endoscopic skull base surgery must be learned in an incremental and modular fashion by all skull base surgeons, irrespective of their specialty.

References

[1] Doglietto F, Prevedello DM, Jane JA, Jr, Han J, Laws ER, Jr. Brief history of endoscopic transsphenoidal surgery—from Philipp Bozzini to the First World Congress of Endoscopic Skull Base Surgery. Neurosurg Focus 2005; 19: E3

[2] O'Malley BW, Jr, Grady MS, Gabel BC et al. Comparison of endoscopic and microscopic removal of pituitary adenomas: single-surgeon experience and the learning curve. Neurosurg Focus 2008; 25: E10

[3] Carrabba G, Dehdashti AR, Gentili F. Surgery for clival lesions: open resection versus the expanded endoscopic endonasal approach. Neurosurg Focus 2008; 25: E7

[4] de Divitiis E, Cappabianca P, Cavallo LM, Esposito F, de Divitiis O, Messina A. Extended endoscopic transsphenoidal approach for extrasellar craniopharyngiomas. Neurosurgery 2007; 61 Suppl 2: 219–227; discussion 228

[5] de Divitiis E, Cavallo LM, Cappabianca P, Esposito F. Extended endoscopic endonasal transsphenoidal approach for the removal of suprasellar tumors: Part 2. Neurosurgery 2007; 60: 46–58; discussion 58–59

[6] de Divitiis E, Esposito F, Cappabianca P, Cavallo LM, de Divitiis O, Esposito I. Endoscopic transnasal resection of anterior cranial fossa meningiomas. Neurosurg Focus 2008; 25: E8

[7] Dehdashti AR, Ganna A, Witterick I, Gentili F. Expanded endoscopic endonasal approach for anterior cranial base and suprasellar lesions: indications and limitations. Neurosurgery 2009; 64: 677–687; discussion 687–689

[8] Fatemi N, Dusick JR, de Paiva Neto MA, Malkasian D, Kelly DF. Endonasal versus supraorbital keyhole removal of craniopharyngiomas and tuberculum sellae meningiomas. Neurosurgery 2009; 64 Suppl 2: 269–284; discussion 284–286

[9] Frank G, Pasquini E, Doglietto F et al. The endoscopic extended transsphenoidal approach for craniopharyngiomas. Neurosurgery 2006; 59 Suppl 1: ONS75–ONS83; discussion ONS75–ONS83

[10] Fraser JF, Nyquist GG, Moore N, Anand VK, Schwartz TH. Endoscopic endonasal transclival resection chordomas: operative technique, clinical outcome, and review of the literature. J Neurosurg 2010; 112: 1061–1069

[11] Gardner PA, Kassam AB, Snyderman CH et al. Outcomes following endoscopic, expanded endonasal resection of suprasellar craniopharyngiomas: a case series. J Neurosurg 2008; 109: 6–16

[12] Laufer I, Anand VK, Schwartz TH. Endoscopic, endonasal extended transsphenoidal, transplanum transtuberculum approach for resection of suprasellar lesions. J Neurosurg 2007; 106: 400–406

[13] Zada G, Kelly DF, Cohan P, Wang C, Swerdloff R. Endonasal transsphenoidal approach for pituitary adenomas and other sellar lesions: an assessment of efficacy, safety, and patient impressions. J Neurosurg 2003; 98: 350–358

[14] Kassam A, Snyderman CH, Mintz A, Gardner P, Carrau RL. Expanded endonasal approach: the rostrocaudal axis. Part I. Crista galli to the sella turcica. Neurosurg Focus 2005; 19: E3

[15] Kassam A, Snyderman CH, Mintz A, Gardner P, Carrau RL. Expanded endonasal approach: the rostrocaudal axis. Part II. Posterior clinoids to the foramen magnum. Neurosurg Focus 2005; 19: E4

[16] Kassam AB, Gardner P, Snyderman C, Mintz A, Carrau R. Expanded endonasal approach: fully endoscopic, completely transnasal approach to the middle third of the clivus, petrous bone, middle cranial fossa, and infratemporal fossa. Neurosurg Focus 2005; 19: E6

[17] Kassam AB, Snyderman C, Gardner P, Carrau R, Spiro R. The expanded endonasal approach: a fully endoscopic transnasal approach and resection of the odontoid process: technical case report. Neurosurgery 2005; 57 Suppl: E213; discussion E213

[18] Kassam A, Snyderman CH, Carrau RL, Gardner P, Mintz A. Endoneurosurgical hemostasis techniques: lessons learned from 400 cases. Neurosurg Focus 2005; 19: E7

[19] Snyderman CH, Carrau RL, Kassam AB et al. Endoscopic skull base surgery: principles of endonasal oncological surgery. J Surg Oncol 2008; 97: 658–664

[20] Kassam AB, Prevedello DM, Thomas A et al. Endoscopic endonasal pituitary transposition for a transdorsum sellae approach to the interpeduncular cistern. Neurosurgery 2008; 62 Suppl 1: 57–72; discussion 72–74

[21] Osawa S, Rhoton AL, Jr, Seker A, Shimizu S, Fujii K, Kassam AB. Microsurgical and endoscopic anatomy of the vidian canal. Neurosurgery 2009; 64 Suppl 2: 385–411; discussion 411–412

[22] Kassam AB, Vescan AD, Carrau RL et al. Expanded endonasal approach: vidian canal as a landmark to the petrous internal carotid artery. J Neurosurg 2008; 108: 177–183

[23] Cavallo LM, Messina A, Gardner P et al. Extended endoscopic endonasal approach to the pterygopalatine fossa: anatomical study and clinical considerations. Neurosurg Focus 2005; 19: E5

[24] Solari D, Magro F, Cappabianca P et al. Anatomical study of the pterygopalatine fossa using an endoscopic endonasal approach: spatial relations and distances between surgical landmarks. J Neurosurg 2007; 106: 157–163

[25] Zanation AM, Snyderman CH, Carrau RL, Gardner PA, Prevedello DM, Kassam AB. Endoscopic endonasal surgery for petrous apex lesions. Laryngoscope 2009; 119: 19–25

[26] Kassam AB, Prevedello DM, Carrau RL et al. The front door to Meckel's cave: an anteromedial corridor via expanded endoscopic endonasal approach- technical considerations and clinical series. Neurosurgery 2009; 64 Suppl: ons71–ons82; discussion ons82–ons83

[27] Walsh MT, Couldwell WT. Management options for cavernous sinus meningiomas. J Neurooncol 2009; 92: 307–316

[28] Cappabianca P, Cavallo LM, Colao A, de Divitiis E. Surgical complications associated with the endoscopic endonasal transsphenoidal approach for pituitary adenomas. J Neurosurg 2002; 97: 293–298

[29] Cavallo LM, Briganti F, Cappabianca P et al. Hemorrhagic vascular complications of endoscopic transsphenoidal surgery. Minim Invasive Neurosurg 2004; 47: 145–150

[30] Koc K, Anik I, Ozdamar D, Cabuk B, Keskin G, Ceylan S. The learning curve in endoscopic pituitary surgery and our experience. Neurosurg Rev 2006; 29: 298–305; discussion 305

[31] Snyderman C, Kassam A, Carrau R, Mintz A, Gardner P, Prevedello DM. Acquisition of surgical skills for endonasal skull base surgery: a training program. Laryngoscope 2007; 117: 699–705

[32] Gardner PA, Kassam AB, Thomas A et al. Endoscopic endonasal resection of anterior cranial base meningiomas. Neurosurgery 2008; 63: 36–52; discussion 52–54

[33] Tabaee A, Anand VK, Barrón Y et al. Endoscopic pituitary surgery: a systematic review and meta-analysis. J Neurosurg 2009; 111: 545–554

Chapter 10

Transpterygoid Approaches

10

10 Transpterygoid Approaches

Carlos Diogenes Pinheiro-Neto, Pornthep Kasemsiri, Ricardo L. Carrau, Daniel M. Prevedello, Amin B. Kassam

10.1 Introduction

Located centrally at the base of the skull, the sphenoid bone is divided in three main regions: greater wings, lesser wings, and pterygoid processes. The pterygoid processes project inferiorly from the body of the sphenoid bone and are situated behind the posterior wall of the maxillary sinus and soft tissues of the pterygopalatine fossa. The pterygoid process comprises two plates, medial and lateral, which are fused anteriorly. One can find two foramina at their base (attachment to the skull base): the foramen rotundum and the pterygoid or vidian canal, where the V_2 and vidian nerves respectively exit the skull base.[1,2]

Endoscopic endonasal approaches to the skull base are based on the principle of using anatomical corridors to access a region of interest.[3] We define a transpterygoid approach as one requiring the partial or complete removal of the pterygoid process. It should be noted that this requires access through the air space of the antrum, removal of the posterior and/or lateral antral wall, and control of the neurovascular contents of the pterygopalatine fossa, namely the internal maxillary artery and its terminal branches, the sphenopalatine ganglion and its associated nerves (vidian, greater palatine, and V_2). Endoscopic endonasal transpterygoid approaches (EETAs) include those that access the lateral recess of the sphenoid sinus,[4,5,6] the foramen lacerum or petrous internal carotid artery (ICA), the Meckel cave or cavernous sinus,

lateral nasopharynx (fossa of Rosenmüller), and infratemporal fossa.[7,8,9]

Considering the goals and anatomical intricacies of the transpterygoid route, EETAs can be divided in five main types (▶ Table 10.1).

- **Type A** involves the partial removal of the medial and/or lateral pterygoid plates, and may be indicated for the transposition of a temporoparietal fascia flap.[10]
- **Type B** involves the removal of the medial aspect of the base of the pterygoid process. It is usually indicated for lesions at the lateral recess of the sphenoid sinus above the level of the vidian canal, such as cerebrospinal fluid (CSF) leaks of the Sternberg canal.
- **Type C** involves dissecting the vidian canal removing the base of the pterygoid plates to reach the petrous apex (infrapetrous or retropetrous), the Meckel cave, or, rarely, the cavernous sinus (zones 1, 2, 3, and 4, respectively).
- **Type D** provides access to the infratemporal fossa (zone 5) and requires a variable removal of the plates.
- **Type E** involves the removal of the medial pterygoid plate or even the entire pterygoid process, and medial third of the Eustachian tube to provide exposure of the lateral nasopharynx (fossa of Rosenmüller) or the lateral aspect of the craniocervical junction.[11]

A safe and effective endoscopic endonasal transpterygoid approach requires an experienced surgeon who is familiarized with the complex endoscopic anatomy of the

Table 10.1 CPK classification of endonasal transpterygoid approaches

EETA type	Antral corridor	Extended resection of pterygoid bone	Region		Indications
			Vidian foramen	Foramen rotundum	
A		Partial removal of the pterygoid process	Superior	Medial Inferior	Extended pterygopalatine fossa approach to augment the corridor for a temporoparietal fascia flap
B	Nasoantral window	Anterior aspect of the base of the pterygoid process	Superior	Medial Inferior	Lesions at the lateral recess of the sphenoid sinus (e.g., CSF leak from the Sternberg canal)
C		Base of pterygoid process with dissection of vidian canal	Superior	Lateral Superior	Lesions of the petrous apex or the Meckel cave
D	Medial maxillectomy ± Denker approach	Partial or complete removal of the pterygoid plates with dissection of the petrous ICA (combined Type B + C)	Inferior	Lateral Inferior	Extensive lesion requiring access to the infratemporal fossa and control of the petrous ICA
E	Medial maxillectomy + Denker approach	Partial or complete removal of the pterygoid plates with dissection of the petrous ICA and removal of the Eustachian tube	Inferior and superior	Lateral Inferior and superior	Nasopharyngeal tumors, extensive tumors of the skull base (e.g., chordomas, chondrosarcomas)

EETA, endoscopic endonasal transpterygoid approach; CSF, cerebrospinal fluid; ICA, internal carotid artery.

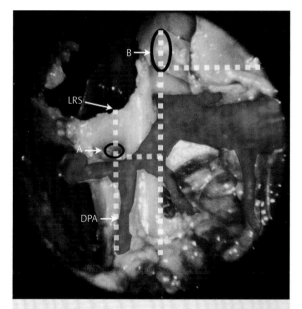

Fig. 10.1 Cadaveric dissection of the left pterygopalatine fossa demonstrating a sphenoidotomy extended toward the lateral recess (LRS) of the sphenoid sinus and dissection of the internal maxillary artery and its terminal branches. The descending palatine artery (DPA) is seen in front of the pterygoid plates. Vertical and horizontal dashed lines intersecting at the vidian (A) and rotundum (B) foramina help to estimate the extent of the approach. In general, lesions above the vidian foramen (A) and inferomedial or superolateral to the foramen rotundum (B) can be exposed with a wide nasoantral window and removal of the posterior wall of the antrum. Lesions below the vidian foramen (A) and inferolateral to the foramen rotundum (B) require a medial maxillectomy with or without a Denker approach and removal of the lateral wall of the maxillary sinus. If extensive lesions are located at the region above or below the vidian foramen (A) and lateral to the foramen rotundum (B), they require a medial maxillectomy with a Denker approach.

10.2 Preoperative Work-up and Indications

Planning includes the staging and histological diagnosis of the lesion. A high-resolution computerized tomography (CT) scan provides important information about the bone structure. If the lesion or approach are intimately associated to major vessels, the addition of CT angiography (CTA) provides a map of the vasculature around and within the surgical field. Magnetic resonance imaging (MRI) is fundamental to define the soft-tissue interfaces including the tumor extension. Interventional angiography is recommended for highly vascular lesions, but only if embolization, ICA sacrifice, or ICA stenting is being considered. In these cases, the diagnostic and interventional phases of the angiography are completed in the same procedure. A significant exception is a patient undergoing a balloon occlusion test of the ICA to ascertain the adequacy of collateral cerebral blood flow. Sacrifice or stenting of the ICA is usually planned as a separate procedure.

A thorough evaluation of the cranial nerves and ocular function is critical. Pre-existent and anticipated deficits should be addressed, especially those of lower cranial nerves, which may affect swallowing and possibly complicate the perioperative management. Similarly, hormonal and electrolyte balance should be optimized. Need for blood products should be anticipated based on the patient's preoperative hematocrit, and tumor vascularity, size and extent, and its relation to major vessels.

As previously stated, EETAs are indicated to access lesions that are situated deep in the skull base, including infratemporal fossa (ITF), nasopharynx, petrous apex, cavernous sinus, and the Meckel cave. There is an enormous variability of pathologies that can arise or extend in these areas. Lesions that can affect the petrous apex include cholesterol granuloma, petrous apicitis, congenital cholesteatoma, mucocele, chondrosarcoma, chordoma, and other rare tumors such as squamous cell carcinoma.[7] Lesions that can compromise the Meckel cave include meningioma, trigeminal schwannoma, pituitary adenoma, malignancies with a predisposition toward perineural spread (i.e., adenoid cystic carcinoma, melanoma, cutaneous squamous cell carcinoma), chondrosarcoma, chordoma, and other rare lesions.[8] Among others, the infratemporal fossa can be involved by juvenile nasopharyngeal angiofibromas, maxillary or mandibular nerve schwannomas, solitary fibrous tumors, meningoceles, adenoid cystic carcinomas lymphoma, and sarcomas. An endoscopic approach can provide adequate exposure for a complete resection, debulking of the lesion, or for tissue sampling (to establish a diagnosis before a definitive treatment).[12]

region (▶ Fig. 10.1 and ▶ Fig. 10.2). Critical landmarks for the approach need to be identified including the sphenopalatine foramen with the sphenopalatine and posterior nasal arteries, the greater palatine canal containing the descending palatine artery and the greater palatine nerve, as they travel from the pterygopalatine fossa to the greater palatine foramen, the vidian (i.e., pterygoid) and palatovaginal canals, V2 foramen, and the pterygomaxillary and inferior orbital fissures. In addition, the surgeon must have a deep anatomical understanding of the structures within the pterygopalatine fossa (pterygopalatine ganglion, maxillary artery, and maxillary division of the trigeminal nerve) and the anatomical relationships of structures adjacent to the pterygoid plates especially the ICA, Eustachian tube, pterygoid muscles, and mandibular division of the trigeminal nerve (▶ Fig. 10.1 and ▶ Fig. 10.2).

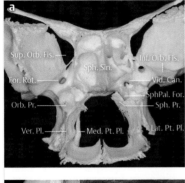
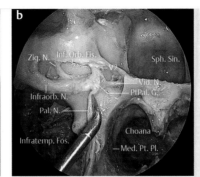
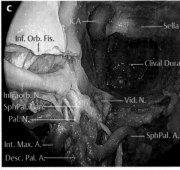
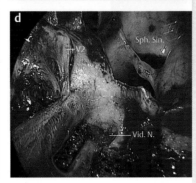
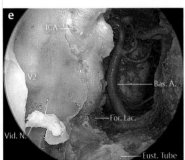
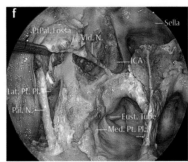

Fig. 10.2 a–f The complex anatomy of the pterygoid region needs to be recognized for a transpterygoid approach. The pterygoid process includes medial and lateral plates that project inferiorly from the body of the sphenoid bone (**a**). Important landmarks include the sphenopalatine foramen with the sphenopalatine and posterior nasal arteries, the greater palatine canal containing the descending palatine artery and the greater palatine nerve, the vidian canal, foramen rotundum, and the pterygomaxillary and inferior orbital fissures (**a–d**). Detailed anatomical illustration of the structures within the pterygopalatine fossa (pterygopalatine ganglion, internal maxillary artery, and maxillary division of the trigeminal nerve) (**c, d**); and the anatomical relationships of structures adjacent to the pterygoid plates, especially the ICA, Eustachian tube, pterygoid muscles, and mandibular division of the trigeminal nerve (**e**). When approaching the Meckel cave, the vidian nerve can be preserved with a transposition technique (**f**).

Bas. A., basilar artery; Desc. Pal. A., descending palatine artery; Eust. Tube, Eustachian tube; For. Lac., foramen lacerum; For. Rot., foramen rotundum; ICA, internal carotid artery; Inf. Orb. Fis, inferior orbital fissure; Infraorb. N., infraorbital nerve; Infratemp. Fos., infratemporal fossa; Int. Max. A., internal maxillary artery; Lat. Pt. Pl., lateral pterygoid plate; Med. Pt. Pl., medial pterygoid plate; Orb. Pr., orbital process; Pal. N., palatine nerve; PtPal. Fossa, pterygopalatine fossa; PtPal. G., pterygopalatine ganglion; Sph. Pr., sphenoid process; Sph. Sin., sphenoid sinus; SphPal. A., sphenopalatine artery; SphPal. For., sphenopalatine foramen; SphPal. Gan., sphenopalatine ganglion; Sup. Orb. Fis., superior orbital fissure; V2, maxillary division of the trigeminal nerve; Ver. Pl., vertical plate; Vid. Can., vidian canal; Vid. N., vidian nerve; Zig. N., zygomatic nerve.

10.3 Surgical Technique

10.3.1 Perioperative Preparation

Image guidance is a critical adjunct during any endoscopic endonasal transpterygoid approach; therefore, its use should be anticipated. We prefer to use CTA for intraoperative guidance during the resection of lesions requiring a transpterygoid approach, as it provides a map of the bony structures as well as the vasculature. In addition, a CTA can be fused with MRI to provide better definition of the soft-tissue interfaces (Stryker Navigation; Stryker, Kalamazoo, Michigan, United States). Electrophysiological monitoring of cranial nerves, somatosensory evoked

potentials and/or brain stem evoked responses is used according to the extent of the resection and the relationship to neurovascular structures. Perioperative broad-spectrum antibiotics, with adequate CSF penetration, are administered before the beginning of the surgery and are continued for 48 to 72 hours postoperatively.

After orotracheal intubation, the patient is placed in a three-pin head-holder with the neck tilted slightly to the left and turned slightly to the right. The nose is decongested with topical 0.05% oxymetazoline. A povidone solution is applied to the perinasal and periumbilical areas (in the event that an autologous fat-free graft is required for reconstruction). If the patient presents a high risk for ICA injury, the thigh is also prepped in case a muscle patch is needed. A solution of lidocaine 1% with epinephrine (1:100,000 to 1:200,000) is injected in the septum and middle meati.

10.3.2 Surgical Exposure

A 0° rod-lens endoscope (Karl Storz, Tuttlingen, Germany) provides visualization for most of the surgery. Angled lens endoscopes are advantageous to "look around the corner"; however, they are more difficult to use for instrumentation, as they provide a somewhat distorted view and require angled instruments to match the visual field. This presents the problem of being able to see more than what can be controlled; therefore, we prefer the use of the 0° rod-lens endoscope that can be used with straight instruments (a line of sight that matches to the geometry of the instruments). EETA types A, B, and C require a partial middle turbinectomy, a wide nasoantral window (NAW), and a wide ipsilateral sphenoidotomy. The NAW should be maximized extending anteroposteriorly from the nasolacrimal duct to the posterior antral wall, and cephalocaudally from orbit to the inferior turbinate.

In most cases, we perform bilateral wide sphenoidotomies (exposing the vidian foramen bilaterally) and a posterior septectomy to create a single cavity that facilitates visualization and bimanual instrumentation. In the contralateral side, a Hadad-Bassagaisteguy nasoseptal flap (HBF)[13] is harvested and transposed into the nasopharynx or into the ipsilateral antrum (for exposure of the nasopharynx). Transposition of the HBF into the antrum requires a large maxillary antrostomy similar to that described for the side of the ITF dissection. Alternatively, the HBF is placed against the lateral wall of the nose with a traction suture that is externalized through the ipsilateral nostril. A generous posterior septectomy is performed (preserving 2 to 3 cm of the anterior septum) to allow bimanual instrumentation through both sides of the nose. This extensive posterior septectomy allows the visualization of the entire posterior wall of the maxillary sinus using a 0° endoscope that crosses over from the contralateral side of the nose. The donor site of the HBF is relined using a mucoperiosteal-free graft (i.e., from the middle turbinate) or a Caicedo reverse flap.[14,15,16]

Conversely, EETA types D and E require a medial maxillectomy that occasionally needs to be extended anteriorly (endoscopic Denker approach). A medial maxillectomy provides a wide opening into the maxillary sinus extending from the inferior orbital wall to the floor of the nasal cavity and from the nasolacrimal duct to the posterior wall of the antrum. A NAW exposes the superior half of the posterior wall of the maxillary sinus; whereas, a medial maxillectomy exposes the entire height of the posterior wall (when using a 0° rod-lens endoscope; ▶ Fig. 10.2).

According to the need for exposure and the configuration and dimensions of the patient's sinonasal tract, the approach may also require anterior and posterior ethmoi-

dectomies. A detailed description of these basic steps can be found in other pertinent chapters.

Following a wide NAW or a medial maxillectomy, one must dissect the mucoperiosteum over the remaining posterolateral wall of the nasal cavity, corresponding to the level of the superior third of the posterior wall of the antrum (over the perpendicular plate of the palatine bone). This dissection yields the sphenopalatine foramen with the sphenopalatine and posterior nasal arteries. Using 1 to 2 mm Kerrison rongeurs, the anterior aspect of the sphenopalatine foramen can be removed to expose the pterygopalatine fossa. The periosteum of the posterior wall of the antrum is displaced and preserved so that its bone may be resected without injuring any of the vascular structures within the pterygopalatine fossa. Bone removal is extended inferiorly to reach the level of the superior aspect of the inferior turbinate (after a NAW) or the antral floor (after a medial maxillectomy), and laterally to reach the inferior orbital fissure.

The medial aspect of the posterior wall of the maxillary sinus deserves special attention, as the greater palatine canal is located at this area. This canal is formed by the oblique groove of the posteroinferior aspect of the maxillary bone and the greater palatine groove, which is deep to the lateral surface of the perpendicular plate of the palatine bone.[17,18] The descending palatine artery (▶ Fig. 10.2b, c, d, f) travels together with the greater palatine nerve through this bone canal. EETA types D and E require lateral expansion of this bone corridor removing the lateral wall of the maxillary sinus. As previously stated, this may require an endoscopic Denker approach.

After complete exposure of the anterior aspect of the pterygopalatine fossa (through NAW or medial maxillectomy) and identification of the infraorbital nerve as it enters the infraorbital canal, its medial aspect is dissected removing the orbital process and the perpendicular plate of the palatine bone. Inferiorly, the medial and anterior walls of the greater palatine canal are removed to expose and release the descending palatine artery and the greater palatine nerve. It is important to verify that the dissection extends inferiorly to the greater palatine foramen, as that will facilitate the lateral mobilization of the soft tissues of the pterygopalatine fossa (▶ Fig. 10.2b, d, f).

Subsequently, the sphenoid process of the palatine bone is removed to expose the vidian and palatovaginal canals.[19,20] The palatovaginal artery, a terminal branch of the internal maxillary artery (IMA), is sectioned to allow the lateralization pterygopalatine fossa and identification of the vidian foramen at the base of the pterygoid plates and the lateral aspect of the pterygoid wedge (junction of the sphenoid floor and superior aspect of the medial pterygoid plate). At this point the periosteum of the anterior aspect of the pterygoid plates may be dissected leaving the contents of the pterygopalatine fossa enclosed in a periosteal sac formed by the periosteum of the posterior maxilla and that of the pterygoid plates. For a type A approach, a partial removal of the pterygoid process enlarges the tunnel to allow the passage of a reconstructive flap (i.e., temporoparietal fascia flap, radial forearm free flap). Extent of this tunnel expansion and removal of the pterygoid plates is dictated by the geometry and dimensions of the pterygopalatine fossa, antrum, and soft-tissue flap. During a type B approach, the sphenoidotomy can be extended laterally, removing the anterior wall of the lateral recess (i.e., pneumatized base of the pterygoid process) above the level of the vidian canal. Occasionally, if the pneumatization of the pterygoid process extends to the greater wing of the sphenoid, the vidian neurovascular bundle needs to be sacrificed to allow further lateral mobilization of the soft tissues of the pterygopalatine fossa. It is usually adequate to remove the medial aspect of the pterygoid process base for a type C approach (petrous apex or Meckel cave approach).[7,8] During a type C approach, the floor of the sphenoid sinus is drilled until it is flush with the level of the clival recess. Subsequently, the vidian canal is dissected; initially drilling the canal from 3 to 9 o'clock. Once the ICA position is confirmed, the superior hemicircumference is drilled and removed. Lateral transposition of the vidian nerve may be enough to expose the base of pterygoid process while preserving the neurovascular bundle.[21] To preserve the integrity of the vidian nerve, following the identification of the anterior genu of the ICA, the vidian canal is drilled until eggshell thin. A dissector can be used to fracture the thin residual bone while preserving the periosteum of canal, as it protects the nerve during its manipulation. Once the vidian canal is unroofed, the vidian nerve can be released and transposed from its canal.[21] Finally, the vidian nerve, descending palatine artery, greater palatine nerve, and pterygopalatine fossa are transposed laterally "en bloc" (▶ Fig. 10.2f). With that mobilization, it is feasible to achieve sufficient exposure to completely remove the pterygoid plates. Once the bone removal is finished, the ITF can be approached preserving the pterygopalatine fossa. The trunk of the IMA, however, will need to be divided at the level of the pterygomaxillary fissure before entering the ITF.

As previously stated, to dissect the lateral aspect of the ITF (EETA types D and E) it is often, albeit not always, necessary to extend the medial maxillectomy anteriorly (endoscopic Denker); thus, achieving the necessary line of sight laterally. This modification includes the removal of the remaining inferior turbinate and anterior aspect of the inferior meatus with backbiting rongeurs, osteotomes, or drill. In select cases the removal may be confined to the area inferior to the nasolacrimal opening. For a full exposure, however, we remove the piriform aperture and ascending process of the maxilla dissecting the lacrimal duct and transecting it sharply. Exposure of the piriform aperture requires a vertical incision just anterior to the head of the inferior turbinate, right on the edge of the aperture. This edge can be palpated with a blunt dissector to optimize the placement of the incision, which is then carried through the periosteum down to bone. A subperiosteal lateral dissection exposes the anterior maxilla. The medial maxillectomy is then extended to remove the piriform aperture and sufficient anterior maxillary wall to expose the entire lateral wall of the antrum. This modification allows the placement of the endoscope and dissecting instruments in such a way that the line of sight extends laterally to encompass the most lateral aspect of the ITF.

To enter the ITF (EETA type D) the IMA is divided at the pterygomaxillary fissure and the vidian neurovascular bundle, and the branch of the sphenopalatine ganglion to V_2 is divided just distal to their respective foramina; thus, allowing the inferior and lateral displacement of soft tissue of the pterygopalatine fossa. This exposes the entire height of the pterygoid process. Before the removal of the lateral pterygoid plate, the lateral and medial pterygoid muscles are detached following a subperiosteal plane (avoids bleeding from the pterygoid plexus). The infratemporal fossa can be approached (EETA type D) after the pterygoid plates are removed. Several surgical landmarks are critical to approach the ITF. The V_3 and foramen ovale are identified just posterior to the base of the lateral pterygoid plate; the tensor veli palatini is medial to the lateral pterygoid plate (at the pterygoid fossa) and just anterior to the Eustachian tube. The petrous ICA is posterior to the foramen ovale (V_3) (▶ Fig. 10.2e). As previously implied the parapharyngeal ICA is posterior to the Eustachian tube. Removal of the Eustachian tube in a lateral and superior direction, including its bony canal, directs the surgeon to the carotid canal, which is just posterior. For an extensive lesion in the ITF, the type E approach is required. It involves the resection of the entire pterygoid process and the separation of the Eustachian tube from the cartilage of the foramen lacerum (to avoid injuring the petrous ICA) and preservation of the soft tissue posterior to the Eustachian tube (to avoid injuring the parapharyngeal ICA).[22]

10.3.3 Postoperative Care and Outcome

After the surgery, the patient is transferred to an intensive care unit for continuous monitoring and early detection of complications. Special attention should be given to the fluid and metabolic disturbances that can occur during the early postoperative period. The two more common disturbances are diabetes insipidus and the syndrome of inappropriate secretion of antidiuretic hormone. The physician should be alert to others major complications that can occur after skull base surgery, especially cerebral edema, stroke, air embolus, and seizures.

Patients who need an EETA for the resection of tumors situated in the infratemporal fossa frequently present with some degree of function impairment of the masticatory muscles. It is important to follow-up with physiotherapy. Rehabilitation is fundamental to achieve good outcomes and a better quality of life for the patients.

10.4 Complications

EETAs provide access to regions adjacent to critical neurovascular structures.[23] Dissection in such a complex area has a considerable potential risk for complications. Injury of the IMA in the pterygopalatine fossa may result in a significant intraoperative bleeding. Reduction of the lacrimation can be a concern in the postoperative period when an injury to the sphenopalatine ganglion or the vidian nerve occurs. This is especially true for patients with V_1 or dysfunction and/or facial paralysis, who cannot protect their cornea adequately. There is also a risk of injury to the maxillary and mandibular division of the trigeminal nerve (facial hypoesthesia arises). Trismus is common after dissection of the pterygoid muscles. Analgesics and stretching exercises should be started early in the postoperative period to avoid permanent and progressive scarring of the muscles that could lead to severe limitation of the oral opening.

Other complications can occur with the transpterygoid approach, especially when this approach is used to reach areas such as the infrapetrous region or Meckel cave. Injury to the ICA produces catastrophic bleeding and is potentially fatal. Other complications include sixth nerve palsy, CSF leak, central nervous system injury, and orbital injury.

Pearls and Pitfalls

- A transpterygoid approach implies the partial or complete removal of the pterygoid process.
- A transpterygoid approach is the preliminary step to accessing modules in the middle coronal plane (i.e., transcavernous, petrous apex, and suprapetrous approaches), and lateral posterior fossa.
- Key anatomical landmarks include the foramen ovale and V3, foramen rotundum and V2, the vidian foramen and nerve, the Eustachian tube and the petrous ICA.
- The transpterygoid approach gives access to pathologies of the lateral recess of the sphenoid sinus, foramen lacerum or petrous ICA, Meckel cave or cavernous sinus, lateral nasopharynx, and infratemporal fossa.
- Potential risks of surgery include injury of the ICA, second and third division of trigeminal nerve, the sixth cranial nerve, and the brainstem.

References

[1] Osawa S, Rhoton AL, Jr, Seker A, Shimizu S, Fujii K, Kassam AB. Microsurgical and endoscopic anatomy of the vidian canal. Neurosurgery 2009; 64 Suppl 2: 385–411; discussion 411–412

[2] Fortes FSG, Sennes LU, Carrau RL et al. Endoscopic anatomy of the pterygopalatine fossa and the transpterygoid approach: development of a surgical instruction model. Laryngoscope 2008; 118: 44–49

[3] Pirris SM, Pollack IF, Snyderman CH et al. Corridor surgery: the current paradigm for skull base surgery. Childs Nerv Syst 2007; 23: 377–384

[4] Bolger WE. Endoscopic transpterygoid approach to the lateral sphenoid recess: surgical approach and clinical experience. Otolaryngol Head Neck Surg 2005; 133: 20–26

[5] DelGaudio JM. Endoscopic transnasal approach to the pterygopalatine fossa. Arch Otolaryngol Head Neck Surg 2003; 129: 441–446

[6] Al-Nashar IS, Carrau RL, Herrera A, Snyderman CH. Endoscopic transnasal transpterygopalatine fossa approach to the lateral recess of the sphenoid sinus. Laryngoscope 2004; 114: 528–532

[7] Zanation AM, Snyderman CH, Carrau RL, Gardner PA, Prevedello DM, Kassam AB. Endoscopic endonasal surgery for petrous apex lesions. Laryngoscope 2009; 119: 19–25

[8] Kassam AB, Prevedello DM, Carrau RL et al. The front door to Meckel's cave: an anteromedial corridor via expanded endoscopic endonasal approach - technical considerations and clinical series. Neurosurgery 2009; 64 Suppl: ons71–ons82, discussion ons82–ons83

[9] Vescan AD, Snyderman CH, Carrau RL et al. Vidian canal: analysis and relationship to the internal carotid artery. Laryngoscope 2007; 117: 1338–1342

[10] Fortes FSG, Carrau RL, Snyderman CH et al. Transpterygoid transposition of a temporoparietal fascia flap: a new method for skull base reconstruction after endoscopic expanded endonasal approaches. Laryngoscope 2007; 117: 970–976

[11] Kasemsiri P, Carrau RL, Prevedello DM et al. How I do it: endoscopic endonasal transpterygoid approaches. Acta de Otorrinolaringología y Cirugía de Cabeza y Cuello. 2012 Supplement: 119–124

[12] Herzallah IR, Germani R, Casiano RR. Endoscopic transnasal study of the infratemporal fossa: a new orientation. Otolaryngol Head Neck Surg 2009; 140: 861–865

[13] Hadad G, Bassagasteguy L, Carrau RL et al. A novel reconstructive technique after endoscopic expanded endonasal approaches: vascular pedicle nasoseptal flap. Laryngoscope 2006; 116: 1882–1886

[14] Caicedo-Granados E, Carrau R, Snyderman CH et al. Reverse rotation flap for reconstruction of donor site after vascular pedicled nasoseptal flap in skull base surgery. Laryngoscope 2010; 120: 1550–1552

[15] Kimple AJ, Leight WD, Wheless SA, Zanation AM. Reducing nasal morbidity after skull base reconstruction with the nasoseptal flap: free middle turbinate mucosal grafts. Laryngoscope 2012; 122: 1920–1924

[16] Kasemsiri P, Carrau RL, Otto BA et al. Reconstruction of the pedicled nasoseptal flap donor site with a contralateral reverse rotation flap: technical modifications and outcomes. Laryngoscope 2013; 123: 2601–2604

[17] Daniels DL, Mark LP, Ulmer JL et al. Osseous anatomy of the pterygopalatine fossa. AJNR Am J Neuroradiol 1998; 19: 1423–1432

[18] Mellema JW, Tami TA. An endoscopic study of the greater palatine nerve. Am J Rhinol 2004; 18: 99–103

[19] Rumboldt Z, Castillo M, Smith JK. The palatovaginal canal: can it be identified on routine CT and MR imaging? AJR Am J Roentgenol 2002; 179: 267–272

[20] Borden NM, Dungan D, Dean BL, Flom RA. Posttraumatic epistaxis from injury to the pterygovaginal artery. AJNR Am J Neuroradiol 1996; 17: 1148–1150

[21] Prevedello DM, Pinheiro-Neto CD, Fernandez-Miranda JC et al. Vidian nerve transposition for endoscopic endonasal middle fossa approaches. Neurosurgery 2010; 67 Suppl Operative: 478–484

[22] Fortes FSG, Pinheiro-Neto CD, Carrau RL, Brito RV, Prevedello DM, Sennes LU. Endonasal endoscopic exposure of the internal carotid artery: an anatomical study. Laryngoscope 2012; 122: 445–451

[23] Kassam AB, Gardner P, Snyderman C, Mintz A, Carrau R. Expanded endonasal approach: fully endoscopic, completely transnasal approach to the middle third of the clivus, petrous bone, middle cranial fossa, and infratemporal fossa. Neurosurg Focus 2005; 19: E6

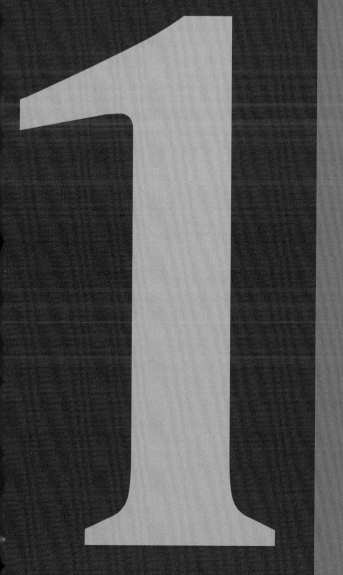

Chapter 11

Endoscopic Transsphenoidal Pituitary Surgery: Endoneurosurgery

11 Endoscopic Transsphenoidal Pituitary Surgery: Endoneurosurgery

Giorgio Frank, Ernesto Pasquini, Matteo Zoli, Diego Mazzatenta, Vittorio Sciarretta, Marco Faustini Fustini

11.1 Introduction

The transsphenoidal route is a direct and rapid extracerebral approach to the sellar region and, therefore, it is the most widely used technique for procedures involving this area. Since its introduction by Schloffer in 1907,[1] it has been refined, thanks to improvements in techniques and instrumentation. The technique has progressed with the aim of finding a less invasive approach; thus, evolving from the original sublabial[2] and transnasal[3] transseptal approaches to the direct endonasal approach in which the sphenoidotomy begins directly in the depth of the nasal cavity at the junction between the vomer and the septum.[4] The procedure was originally performed with the naked eye; however, in the 1960s, Hardy introduced the use of the microscope.[5] This instrument, combining the benefits of magnification and coaxial illumination, seemed, at the time, to have resolved the problems caused by the narrowness and depth of the operating field. In reality, the cone-shaped beam of illumination of the microscope and the rigidity of the working canal created by the surgical speculum persist in limiting vision and maneuverability of this approach.

The rod-lens endoscope is the latest innovation in the field of optical instrumentation; it allows the "surgeon's eye" to penetrate the depth of the operating field, and it provides a panoramic and/or angled view independent of the depth and width of the access route. It was Guiot in 1963[6] who first suggested its use in transsphenoidal surgery, but its real acceptance by neurosurgeons had to wait for it to be perfected and for further surgical technical advances. Jankowski[7] was the first to use endonasal endoscopy for the removal of pituitary adenomas, combining the use of the endoscope with the transethmoidal approach performed without a surgical speculum. The endonasal technique was subsequently perfected and popularized by the groups of Jho and Carrau, and Cappabianca and de Divitiis.[8,9,10] These pioneers first explored the feasibility of the procedure, focusing their attention on minimal postoperative discomfort, lower complication rate, quick postoperative recovery rate, and short hospital stay.

The above characteristics are well accepted as being representative of this type of surgery and attention has now shifted to its efficacy in the treatment of pituitary diseases.[11]

Transsphenoidal surgery began in Bologna in the 1930s[12] and evolved with the introduction of the operating microscope at the end of 1960s. In 1998, we replaced transsphenoidal microscopic surgery with endoscopic surgery. Close collaboration with ear, nose, and throat (ENT) surgeons, experienced in endoscopic sinonasal surgery, facilitated the changeover of technique. The change has been smooth and there has not been a single case in which there has been a return to a microsurgical approach after an endoscopic approach has been attempted.

In this chapter, we provide an update of our experience using endoscopic transsphenoidal pituitary surgery in the treatment of pituitary adenomas. We would like to discuss some changes, with respect to previous statements,[13] that have come about as a result of our increasing experience.

11.2 Indications

Indications for endoscopic transsphenoidal pituitary surgery are the same as for transsphenoidal microscopic surgery; for the most part, these include tumors growing from the sella and expanding in a symmetrical fashion in the suprasellar space. Due to its tolerability, endoscopic transsphenoidal pituitary surgery is the treatment of choice for elderly patients and for patients in poor condition. It is ideal in children, due to the narrowness of the surgical tunnel. Finally, endoscopic transsphenoidal pituitary surgery facilitates the approach in cases of relapse since transseptal dissection is unnecessary. Some of the "classic" contraindications to the transsphenoidal approach, such as some asymmetrical tumors, significant cavernous sinus growth, or supradiaphragmatic dumbbell-shaped tumors, are partially overcome by using "extended" endoscopic transsphenoidal approaches such as the ethmoido-pterygo-sphenoidal (EPSea), the supradiaphragmatic (SDPhea), the transsphenoidal-transclival (TTea), and the pterygomaxillary (PMea) approaches.[14,15,16,17]

11.3 Surgical Technique

11.3.1 Standard Technique

Instrumentation

Critical instrumentation for the endoscopic technique includes a xenon 300 W cold light fountain source, an endoscopic video camera, a video recorder, and 0 to 30° and 45° rod-lens endoscopes with a diameter of 4 mm and length of 18 mm. A cleaning system with pedal control is used to reduce the need to remove the endoscope from the nose. During the tumor removal phase, we use a mechanical holder for the endoscope and video camera to allow the surgeon to work with both hands (▶ Fig. 11.1).

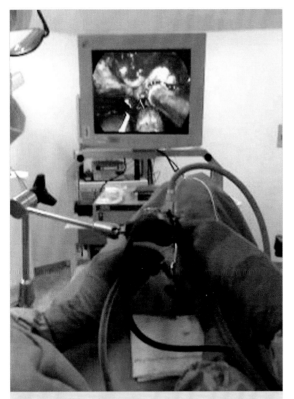

Fig. 11.1 Endoscope fixed on mechanic holder. During the tumor removal phase, we use a mechanical holder for the endoscope and video camera to allow the surgeon to work with both hands. The presence of three surgical instruments in the sphenoid sinus at the same time is shown on the screen.

The classic bayonet-shaped instruments have been replaced with straight, double-action, or pistol-handled instruments.

We use image-guided navigation, instead of fluoroscopy, in recurrent tumors, conchal or presellar pneumatization, and to localize vascular structures during the approach. In parasellar lesions, the acoustic Doppler is helpful, in addition to the neuronavigator, for localizing the internal carotid artery (ICA).

Median Transsphenoidal Endoscopic Approach

Surgery is performed under general anesthesia using orotracheal intubation; the patient is placed in a semisitting position with his head turned toward the surgeon and resting freely in the horseshoe head-holder. In cases in which image-guided navigation is required, the head is fixed in a three-pin holder (Mayfield). The oropharynx is packed with moist gauze to prevent blood and secretions from the operative site reaching the stomach. The nasal mucous membranes are decongested with oxymetazoline 0.5%. The periumbilical abdomen is routinely prepared for the harvesting of a free fat graft. In the case of an extended supradiaphragmatic approach, we prepare the lateral thigh for harvesting fascia lata.

The surgical procedure can be schematically divided into three stages: (1) exposure of the sellar wall; (2) adenomectomy; and (3) final exploration and closure of the surgical field.

Stage 1: Exposure of the Sellar Wall

The operation is performed through both nostrils. The lateral dislocation of the middle and upper turbinates allows the localization of the sphenoethmoidal recesses and the natural ostia of the sphenoid sinus (▶ Fig. 11.2**a, b ,c**).

The opening of the sphenoid sinuses starts with the enlargement of the natural ostia, using Kerrison rongeurs or a Stammberger punch. A semilunar incision is made in the posterior part of the septum to separate the mucoperiosteum from the bone of the perpendicular lamina of the ethmoidal bone and the natural ostia of the sphenoid sinus (▶ Fig. 11.2**d**). For cases in which it is difficult to expose the sphenoid ostia, the entry point to the sphenoid sinus may be obtained by means of direct perforation of the anterior wall at the junction of the keel of the sphenoid bone and the posterior nasal septum, approximately 1 cm above the rim of the choana and close to the septum.

Access to the sphenoid sinus should be wide, extending from the roof to the floor of the sphenoid vertically and expanding the sphenoid ostia laterally. In case of poor sphenoid pneumatization and/or a short distance between the posterior and the anterior wall of the sphenoid sinus, it is necessary to remove a posterior part of the septum (0.5–1 cm). This surgical step improves access to the deep surgical field through both nasal fossae thus allowing the surgeon to operate bimanually.

Intersinus septa, which reduce vision and limit maneuverability in front of the sella, are removed. It is not necessary to remove the sphenoid sinus mucosa, which may be simply laterally displaced. Preservation of the mucosa permits faster postoperative stabilization of the sphenoid cavity with less incidence of sphenoid sinus inflammation, and the opening of the natural ostia reduces the risk of postoperative mucoceles. The opening of the sellar floor should be as wide as possible, laterally, from one cavernous sinus to the other and vertically from the superior to the inferior intercavernous sinuses.

Stage 2: Adenomectomy

This stage begins with the incision of the sellar dura. A classic cruciform incision is made with a single blade curved microsciscors, or, if histological examination of the dura is required, a rectangular window is removed. Tumor is removed by suction or using a curette. It is mandatory to avoid any traction before mobilizing the tumor with a curette or dissector. To prevent a premature collapse of the supradiaphragmatic cistern, it is suggested

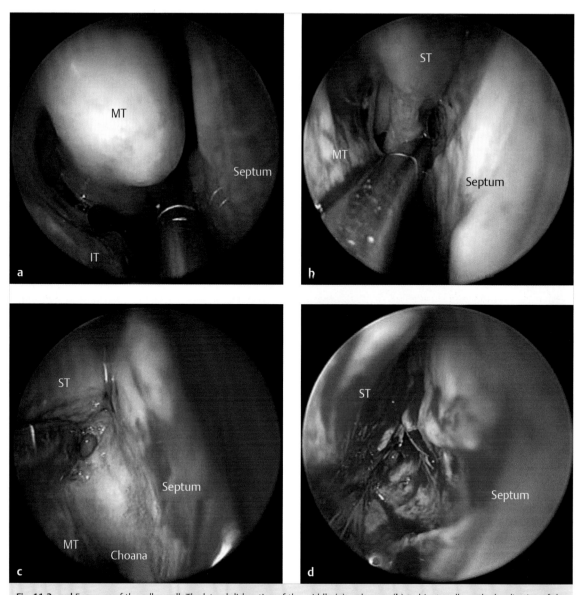

Fig. 11.2 a–d Exposure of the sellar wall. The lateral dislocation of the middle (**a**) and upper (**b**) turbinates allows the localization of the sphenoethmoidal recesses and the natural ostia of the sphenoid sinus (**c**). A semilunar incision is made in the posterior part of the septum to separate the mucoperiosteum from the bone of the perpendicular lamina of the ethmoidal bone and the natural ostia of the sphenoid sinus (**d**).
IT, inferior turbinate; MT, middle turbinate; ST, superior turbinate.

that the tumor be mobilized and removed first from its inferior and lateral portion and then from its posterior and superior portion.

Final Exploration and Closure of the Surgical Field

Hemostasis is obtained using cotton packing, and exploration of the surgical field using angled 30° and 45° endoscopes allows localization and removal of any remnant tumor. In the absence of cerebrospinal fluid (CSF) leaks, the surgical cavity is packed with gelatin sponge; otherwise, if a CSF leak is detected or suspected, autologous free fat is grafted in the sellar cavity and the dural gap is closed with a middle turbinate mucoperiosteal graft.[18]

The sphenoid sinus is gently packed with gelatin sponge and, finally, the middle turbinates are medially displaced to their normal position. Nasal packing is not routinely required except in cases where the middle turbinate has been resected.

11.3.2 Extended Approaches

Ethmoido-pterygo-sphenoidal Endoscopic Approach

The EPSea[15,16,17] is reserved for soft tumors involving the cavernous sinus that do not tend to infiltrate the vessel wall. This type of procedure permits the frontal exposure of the cavernous sinus with the possibility of direct control of its medial and lateral compartments.

The procedure is performed by means of a transethmoidal route, and a complete sphenoethmoidectomy with a wider meatotomy is required. The medial portion of the posterior wall of the maxillary sinus is resected and the sphenopalatine artery is cauterized with bipolar forceps or closed with titanium hemoclips. Partial resection of the pterygoid process is performed taking into account the degree of pneumatization of the lateral recess of the sphenoid sinus and the need for visualization of the lateral and inferior walls of the sphenoid sinus (▶ Fig. 11.3a).

With the exception of a tumor exclusively located in the lateral portion of the cavernous sinus, the dural opening is made in the sellar region and progressively enlarged following the tumor from its medial to its lateral portion (▶ Fig. 11.3b). Venous bleeding is usually negligible because the sinus is plugged by the tumor and the bleeding is generally well controlled with gelatin sponge, cotton packing, and/or Floseal (Baxter International, Deerfield, Illinois, United States). After tumor removal, progressive slow bleeding is possible.

Supradiaphragmatic Approach

Indications for a SDPhea are strictly median extra-arachnoidal tumors that are not accessible using a standard approach, as in the case of some adenomas, Rathke cleft cysts, craniopharyngiomas, and meningiomas.[14]

The nasal phase of the surgical procedure is the same as that of standard endoscopic transsphenoidal pituitary surgery except for a systematic unilateral middle turbi-

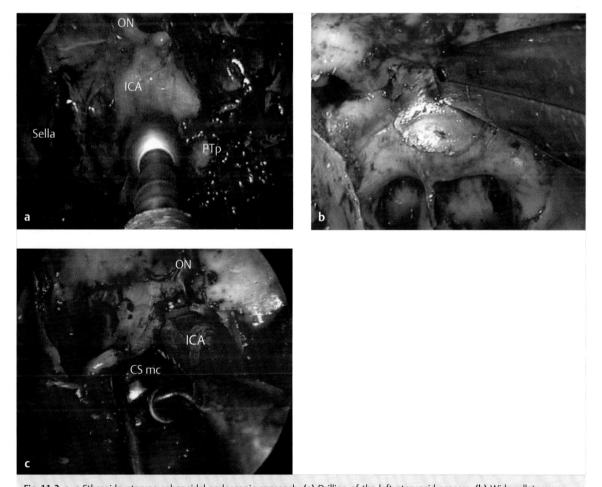

Fig. 11.3 a–c Ethmoido-pterygo-sphenoidal endoscopic approach. **(a)** Drilling of the left pterygoid process. **(b)** Wide sellotomy including the removal of the tuberculum sella. **(c)** Bimanual tumor removal from left cavernous sinus.
CS mc, cavernous sinus medial compartment; ICA, internal carotid artery; ON, optic nerve canal; PtP, pterygoid process.

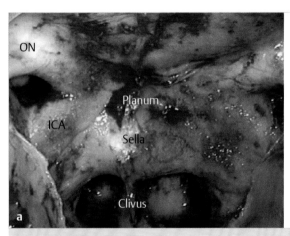
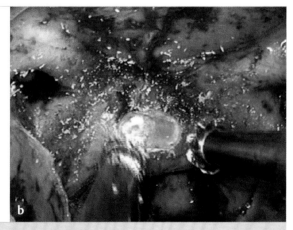

Fig. 11.4 a, b The bony removal starts at the level of the sella turcica (**a**), Close to the optic nerve and chiasm we prefer levering off the thin bone with the Kerrison rongeurs (**b**), to avoid potential tissue damage by the thermal injury caused by the burr. ICA, internal carotid artery; ON, optic nerve canal.

nectomy. The middle turbinectomy is performed to improve surgical maneuverability and to preserve the mucoperiosteum for plastic repair.

The approach to the planum sphenoidale is the same as that first described by Weiss.19

The bony removal starts at the level of the sella turcica (▶ Fig. 11.4b), and the degree of rostral extension to the tuberculum and planum sphenoidale is tailored to the size and location of the lesion. Having thinned down the skull base with the coarse diamond burr, we prefer levering off the thin bone with Kerrison rongeurs (▶ Fig. 11.4c). The optic nerves represent the lateral extent of this approach (▶ Fig. 11.5a). The medial part of the lateral opticocarotid recesses should be rongeured cautiously, but exposure lateral to the recesses risks damaging the optic nerves and carotid arteries, and, thus, must be avoided.

A durotomy is performed in a "horizontal-H" fashion, with the superior limb of the H being placed on the dura rostral to the superior intercavernous sinus, and the inferior limb placed on the sellar dura (▶ Fig. 11.5a). Following cauterization (▶ Fig. 11.5b), or placement of hemoclips on the superior intercavernous sinus, a short median vertical incision between the two horizontal limbs is performed. Similar to the extent of the bony removal, the size of the durotomy is also determined by the size and location of the lesion. Unnecessary extensions are avoided to minimize the extent of the durotomy to reduce the risk of postoperative CSF leaks.

The surgical route gives direct access to the region of the suprasellar cistern, chiasm, and pituitary stalk (▶ Fig. 11.5d). Generally, an expanding mass displaces the optic nerves laterally, the chiasm superiorly, and the pituitary stalk posteriorly, and pushes the vascular structures laterally. Whenever possible, we advocate preserving the arachnoid plane, which wraps the dome of the tumor, and performing a centrifugal removal of the tumor.

Other Approaches

The transsphenoidal-transclival and the pterygomaxillary approaches are rarely used for pituitary lesions, and are always combined with an EPSea. For this reason, they are not discussed and but they are included in cases treated by an EPSea.

11.4 Materials and Methods

Between May 1998 and December 2009 at the Center of Pituitary Tumor Surgery of the Neurosurgical Department of "Bellaria" Hospital in Bologna, Italy, 1,029 patients underwent endoscopic transsphenoidal pituitary surgery for tumors involving the sella and parasellar regions (▶ Table 11.1). In this chapter, we report our experience in the treatment of 851 cases of pituitary adenomas because they are the most representative and homogeneous group in sellar pathology, and the presence of well-defined remission criteria makes a comparative study between endoscopic and microscopic surgery easier. All other sellar and extrasellar pathologies were excluded from this report.

11.4.1 Preoperative and Postoperative Evaluation

All patients underwent preoperative endocrinological, neuroradiological, and neurophthalmological evaluation. After an overnight fast, plasma samples were collected for the measurement of cortisol, free thyroxine (FT4), thyrotropin (TSH), corticotropin (ACTH), prolactin (PRL), growth hormone (GH), luteinizing hormone, follicle-stimulating hormone, insulinlike grown factor-I (IGF-I), testosterone (in males), and estradiol (in females). A 24-hour urine collection was obtained for the measurement of urinary free cortisol.

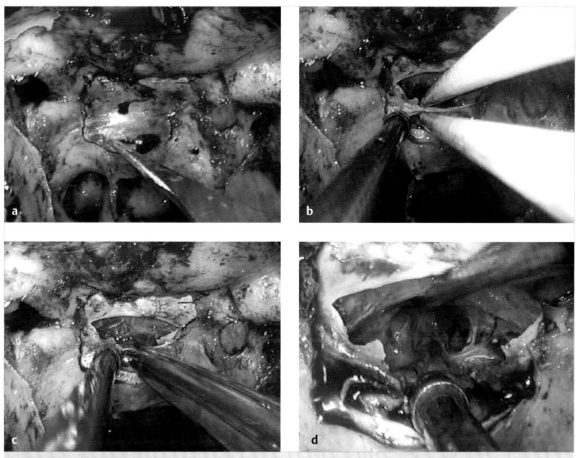

Fig. 11.5 a–d The lateral extent of a supradiaphragmatic approach is represented by the lateral opticocarotid recesses. The durotomy is performed in a "horizontal-H" fashion, with the superior limb of the H being placed on the dura rostral to the superior intercavernous sinus, and the inferior limb being placed on the sellar dura (**a, b**). Following cauterization (**b**) of on the superior intercavernous sinus, a midline vertical incision between the two horizontal limbs is performed (**c**). The surgical route gives direct access to the region of the suprasellar cistern, the chiasm, and the pituitary stalk (**d**).

Table 11.1 Number of expansive lesions treated from May 1998 to December 2009

Pathology	Number of lesions	Number of lesions treated by endoscopic approach			
		MTea	EPSea	SDPhea	PM
Pituitary adenoma	851	765	67	19	0
Rathke cleft cyst	56	55	0	1	0
Craniopharyngioma	45	6	0	39	0
Chordomas/chondrosarcoma	37	10	19	0	8
Meningioma	16	0	0	14	2
Metastasis	9	8	0	1	0
Astrocytoma	5	0	0	5	0
Pseudotumoral inflammation	2	2	0	0	0
Cholesterol apex granuloma	2	0	0	0	2
Trigeminal neuroma	2	0	0	0	2
Capillary hemangioma	2	0	2	0	0
Germinoma	2	0	0	2	0
Total number of lesions	1,029	846	88	81	14
Number of lesions (%)	0	82	9	8	1

EPSea, ethmoidal-pterygosphenoidal approach; MTea, median transsphenoidal approach (including the extension to the middle and lower clivus); PM, pterygomaxillary ± EPS; SDPhea, supradiaphragmatic approach.

All patients underwent radiological assessments by means of magnetic resonance imaging (MRI) and computed tomography (CT) scans. All patients received short-term prophylaxis with cefazolin 1 g intravenous (IV) during induction and 1 g IV after 6 hours. Clindamycin was used in patients allergic to penicillin. Patients with secondary hypoadrenalism received a loading dose infusion of 50 to 100 mg hydrocortisone.

Our postoperative protocol consisted of an endocrinological evaluation on the third postoperative day and again at 1, 3, and 6 months. Follow-up MRI was performed 3 months postoperatively and then yearly. Early neuroradiological examinations by MRI or CT were performed for specific indications. An endoscopic rhinologic evaluation was performed 1 month postoperatively to evaluate the normalization of the nasal and sphenoid cavities. A neuro-ophthalmological check-up was routinely performed 3 months after surgery, only in cases of preoperative dysfunction or postoperative referred visual disturbances.

11.4.2 Pituitary Adenoma Outcome Analysis

We analyzed 851 patients who underwent endoscopic transsphenoidal pituitary surgery for pituitary adenomas. Six hundred and ninety-four patients were surgically treated for the first time while 157 (47 from our center) had been previously treated with microscopic or endoscopic surgery, with or without radiotherapy.

Pituitary adenomas were clinically, histologically, and immunohistochemically investigated. They were classified as functioning (GH-, PRL-, ACTH-, or TSH-secreting adenomas) or nonfunctioning (NF) adenomas (▶ Table 11.2).

Patients' ages ranged from 7 to 89 years (mean 49 years, median 50 years). There was at least one 6-month follow-up (range 6–142 months, mean 34 months, median 26 months) (▶ Table 11.2).

We performed an intraoperative evaluation of invasiveness in every case, which was then classified as: 0, no invasiveness; 2, cavernous sinus invasion; 3, invasion of bone and/or neurological structures; 4, invasion of cavernous sinus plus bone and/or neurological structure invasion.

Tumors were classified into two groups according to consistency: tumors with soft consistency (easy removable using suction) and tumors with hard consistency (not removable using suction but excised en bloc or piece by piece using scissors). The proliferative index (Ki-67) was measured in all cases; p53 was not routinely measured and was therefore not included in the overall results.

Endocrinological cure was defined as follows. In GH-secreting adenomas, remission was defined by a normal sex- and age-adjusted IGF-I level (GH nadir < 1 ng/mL after oral glucose tolerance test[20]). In PRL-secreting adenomas, remission was defined as having normal serum PRL levels (< 30 ng/mL in females, < 15 ng/mL in males) at their latest check-up, without having had previous dopaminergic therapy for at least 2 months.[21] In ACTH-secreting adenomas, remission was defined as an early morning cortisol level < 50 nmol/L requiring substitutive therapy, and then as the normalization of 24 hour urinary free cortisol levels.[22] In TSH-secreting adenomas, remission was defined as normalization of the free triiodothyronine (FT3), FT4, and TSH levels.[23]

The results were evaluated for each surgical procedure at a 3-month follow-up, with respect to the entity of tumor removal by MRI, and to the evaluation of visual symptoms and/or endocrinological status. Overall results of the multimodal management of the individual patients were classified in the comprehensive evaluation comparing MRI and clinical data at a 6-month or longer follow-up.

Tumor removal was judged on the basis of MRI: 1, radical (no evidence of residual tumor); 2, subtotal (residual tumor < 20%); 3, partial (residual tumor < 50%); and 4, insufficient (residual tumor > 50%).

We defined the clinical (endocrinological and visual) parameters as follows: 1, unchanged (no modification of preoperative symptoms); 2, normalized (symptom resolution); 3, improved (symptom reduction without normalization); and 4, worsened (symptom deterioration or new functional and/or endocrinological symptoms).

Finally, the comprehensive evaluation was defined as: 1, cured (radical removal and clinical cure); 2, controlled (subtotal removal with symptom resolution, or radical removal with amelioration of symptoms without the need for subsequent postoperative therapy [normal for NF adenomas] or remission/control with other therapies [surgery and/or medical therapy and/or radiotherapy] [normal for functioning adenomas]); and 3, not cured (disease progression despite other therapy).

Table 11.2 Number of patients who underwent surgical procedures for functioning or NF adenomas, and the number and percentage of patients with intraoperative cavernous sinus invasion from 1998 to December 2009

Type of tumor	Sex, n (%)		Total, n (%)
	Male	Female	
GH	76 (41)	110 (59)	186 (22)
PRL	38 (36)	67 (64)	105 (12)
ACTH	40 (34)	77 (66)	117 (14)
TSH	8 (61.5)	5 (38.5)	13 (1.5)
NF	241 (56)	189 (44)	430 (50.5)
Total	402 (47)	448 (53)	851

ACTH, corticotropin-secreting adenoma; GH, growth-hormone-secreting adenoma; NF, nonfunctioning adenoma; PRL, prolactin-secreting adenoma; TSH, thyrotropin-secreting adenoma.

Table 11.3 Symptoms and type of pituitary adenoma

Type of tumor	Symptom, n					
	Incidental findings	Apoplexy	Recurrence/ residual/progression	Endocrinologic disturbances	Visual disturbances	Neurologic deficit
GH	8	2	34	135	1	2
PRL	7	6	13	72	6	
ACTH	5	7	28	77	3	1
TSH	1	3	3	7	1	1
NF	77	40	93	62	143	15
Total, n (%)	98 (11.5)	56 (6.5)	171 (20)	352 (41)	154 (18)	19 (2)

ACTH, corticotropin-secreting adenoma; GH, growth-hormone-secreting adenoma; NF, nonfunctioning adenoma; PRL, prolactin-secreting adenoma; TSH, thyrotropin-secreting adenoma.

In the statistical analysis, a contingency table was analyzed using the chi-square test for independence.

11.4.3 Results

Symptoms are shown in ▶ Table 11.3. The median transsphenoidal endoscopic approach was used in 765 patients, while in 67 patients the EPSea was used, and in 19 patients the SDPhea was used (▶ Table 11.4).

Median surgical time was 45 minutes (range 35–90 minutes) for the median transsphenoidal endoscopic approach, 90 minutes (range 60–180 minutes) for EPSea, and 120 minutes (range 90–200 minutes) for SDPhea.

There was no perioperative mortality. Patient hospital stay ranged from 2 to 91 days (median 4 days).

Surgical Results

The evaluation of the surgical results for individual procedures was made on the basis of gross tumor removal as shown by MRI and the resolution of clinical and/or biohumoral signs at 3 months.

Gross Tumor Removal

The 3-month follow-up MRI showed that macroscopic radical removal of the tumor was obtained in 707 (83%)

procedures, 124 (14.5%) were subtotal, 15 (2%) were partial, and only in 5 (0.5%) patients was the tumoral debulking deemed insufficient (▶ Table 11.5).

Short-term Endocrinological Results

▶ Table 11.6 shows the short-term (< 3 months) results for individual procedures. One hundred and thirty-five of 186 (72.5%) patients with acromegaly were in remission after surgery. Eighty-three of 105 (79%) PRL-secreting adenomas, operated due to resistance to medical therapy, achieved endocrinological remission. Eighty-four of 107 (78.5%) ACTH-secreting adenomas were cured and 11 of 13 (84.6%) TSH-secreting adenomas were in remission. Finally, 73 of 168 (43%) NF adenomas with preoperative endocrinological disturbance normalized. The majority complained of mild hyperprolactinemia (less than 120 ng/mL) and they showed a normal PRL level in the postoperative analysis.

Short-term Visual and Neurological Outcome

Different grades of visual disturbances and neurological deficits (▶ Table 11.7 and ▶ Table 11.8) were observed in 306 (36%) and 51 (6%) patients, respectively. Visual

Table 11.4 Type of pituitary adenoma and type of surgical approach

Type of tumor	Surgical approach, n		
	MTea	EPSea	SDPhea
GH	176	10	
PRL	91	10	4
ACTH	106	7	4
TSH	12		1
NF	380	40	10
Total, n (%)	765 (90)	67 (8)	19 (2)

EPSea, ethmoidal-pterygosphenoidal approach; MTea, median transsphenoidal (including the extension to the middle and lower clivus) approach; SDPhea, supradiaphragmatic approach.

Table 11.5 Surgical results: gross tumor removal related to the type of tumor

Type of tumor	Follow-up MRI at 3 months, n (%)			
	Radical	< 20%	< 50%	> 50%
GH	152 (82)	28 (15)	4 (2)	2 (1)
PRL	86 (82)	18 (17)	1 (1)	0
ACTH	105 (90)	11 (9)	1 (1)	0
TSH	11 (85)	2 (15)	0	0
NF	353 (82)	65 (15)	9 (2)	3 (1)
Total	707 (83)	124 (14.5)	15 (2)	5 (0.5)

Table 11.6 Surgical results: endocrinological results at the 3-month follow-up for a single procedure

Type of tumor	Endocrinology results at 3 months (number of patients)				
	Preoperative endocrinological disturbances	Unchanged	Normalized	Improved	Adjunctive temporary or permanent endocrinological disturbances
GH	186/186	17	133 + 2*	34	2
PRL	105/105	6 + 1*	77 + 6*	15	7
ACTH	107/107	25 + 1*	83 + 1*	4 + 3*	5
TSH	13/13	1	10 + 1*	1	1
NF	168/430	301	73	0	56
Total	851	350	376	54	71

ACTH, corticotropin-secreting adenoma; GH, growth-hormone-secreting adenoma; NF, nonfunctioning adenoma; PRL, prolactin-secreting adenoma; TSH, thyrotropin-secreting adenoma; *patients with adjunctive temporary or permanent endocrinological disturbances.

Table 11.7 Surgical results: visual disturbances results at the 3-month follow-up for a single procedure

Type of preoperative visual deficit	Visual disturbance results at 3 months(number of patients)				
	Unchanged	Normalized	Improved	Worsened	Total
PVD monolateral	1	35	2	0	38
PVD bilateral	21	131	75	1	228
SVD monolateral	2	2	20	0	24
SVD bilateral	0	1	10	0	11
PVD-SVD	1	0	4	0	5
Total, n (%)	25 (8)	169 (55)	111 (36)	1 (0.1)	306 (36)

PVD, partial visual deficit; SVD, severe visual deficit.

Table 11.8 Surgical results: neurological deficit results at the 3-month follow-up for a single procedure

Type of preoperative neurological deficit	Neurological deficit results at 3 months (number of patients)				
	Unchanged	Normalized	Improved	Worsened	Total
None	0	0	0	1	1
Ophthalmoplegia (CN III, IV, VI)	7	23	6	1	37
Trigeminal Neuralgia/ophthalmoplegia	1	4	1	0	6
Intracranial hypertension/hydrocephalus	1	0	1	0	2
Coma	0	1	1	0	2
Total	9 (19)	28 (58)	9 (19)	2/851 (0.2)	48 (5.6)

dysfunction resolved in 169 (55%) patients, improved in 111 (36%) patients, and was unchanged in 25 (8%) patients. In one patient, visual worsening occurred, due to overpacking of the surgical cavity, and it was only partially corrected by early surgical revision.

Preoperative neurological symptoms (▶ Table 11.8) resolved completely after surgery in 28 patients (58%), improved in 9 (19%), and were unchanged in 9 (19%). Two out of 851 (0.2%) patients complained of postoperative ophthalmoplegia, of whom one did not have preoperative neurological symptoms.

Comprehensive Evaluations

The parameters in ▶ Table 11.9 describe the overall results for individual patients (804 patients instead of 851 procedures) treated surgically with and without other postoperative therapy at a 6-month or longer follow-up (mean 31, median 24, range 6–102 months).

Statistical Analysis

A comprehensive evaluation for each type of tumor was made using the following parameters: sex, size, previous

Table 11.9 Comprehensive evaluations: results obtained for individual patients who underwent one surgical procedure (remission and controlled without other therapy) or other therapies (surgery and/or medical therapy and/or radiotherapy)

Tumor	Secondary treatment	Outcome (number of patients)			
		Cured	Controlled	Not cured	Total
GH	None	130	0	0	130
	Medical	0	34	5	39
	Radiotherapy	0	7	0	7
	Radiotherapy + surgery	0	1	0	1
GH, total (%)		130 (73.4)	42 (23.7)	5 (2.8)	177
PRL	None	75	3	0	78
	Medical	0	18	1	19
	Radiotherapy	0	3	1*	4
PRL, total (%)		75 (74.2)	24 (23.7)	2 (1.9)	101
ACTH	None	79	2	5	86
	Medical	0	1	2	3
	Craniotomy	0	2	0	2
	Radiotherapy	0	5	4 + 1*	10
	Radiotherapy + adrenalectomy	0	3	0	3
ACTH, total (%)		79 (75.9)	13 (12.5)	12 (11.5)	104
TSH	None	10	0	0	10
	Medical	0	1	0	1
	Radiotherapy	0	1	0	1
TSH, total (%)		10 (83.3)	2 (16.6)	0	12
NF	None	344	51	2 + 1*	398
	Medical	0	2	1	3
	Craniotomy	0	3	1*	4
	Radiotherapy	0	5	0	5
NF, total (%) l		344 (83.9)	61 (14.8)	5 (1.2)	410
Total (%)		638 (79.3)	142 (17.6)	24 (2.9)	804

*Died from disease.

ACTH, corticotropin-secreting adenoma; GH, growth-hormone-secreting adenoma; NF, nonfunctioning adenoma; PRL, prolactin-secreting adenoma; TSH, thyrotropin-secreting adenoma;

surgery, tumor consistency, intraoperative invasivity, and proliferative index (Ki-67).

Secreting Adenomas

GH-secreting Adenomas

We treated 177 patients, 65 of whom had microadenomas and 112 had macroadenomas. Their ages varied from 14 to 78 years (mean 47 years); 73 were male (41.2%) and 104 were female (58.82%). Two patients died from causes not related to the disease at 50 and 57 months postoperatively.

We performed 186 procedures on 177 patients; cure was obtained in 130 (73.4%) (▶ Table 11.10). The statistical analysis of all parameters showed significance or only previous surgery ($p = 0.0024$) and invasiveness ($p < 0.0001$) (▶ Table 11.10).

PRL-secreting Adenomas

We treated 101 patients, 46 of whom had microadenomas and 55 had macroadenomas. Their ages varied from 7 to 82 years (mean 38 years); 36 were male (35.6%) and 65 were female (64.4%). Two patients died from causes not related to the disease at 11 and 46 months, respectively. One patient developed multiple brain metastases 6 years after surgery; he underwent a retrosigmoid approach for removal of symptomatic clival lesions and died 1 year later from progression of the disease.

We performed 105 procedures on 101 patients; cure was obtained in 75 (74.2%) (▶ Table 11.11). The statistical analysis of all parameters showed significance for only previous surgery ($p = 0.0137$), size ($p = 0.0064$), and invasiveness ($p < 0.0001$) (▶ Table 11.11).

Table 11.10 Growth-hormone-secreting adenomas: comprehensive evaluation for each parameter

Statistical parameter		Number of patients	Outcome, number of patients (%)			Chi-square test for independence	
			Cured	Controlled	Not cured	p Value	Significant association
Sex	Male	73	58 (79.5)	12 (16.4)	3 (4.1)	0.1275	No
	Female	104	72 (69.2)	30 (28.8)	2 (1.9)		
Previous surgery	None	151	118 (78.1)	30 (19.9)	3 (2.0)	0.0024	Yes
	Yes	26	12 (46.2)	12 (46.2)	2 (7.7)		
Size	Micro	65	52 (80)	10 (15.4)	3 (4.6)	0.0916	No
	Macro	112	78 (69.6)	32 (28.6)	2 (1.8)		
Invasiveness	Invasive	36	16 (44.4)	17 (47.2)	3 (8.3)	<0.0001	Yes
	Not invasive	141	114 (80.9)	25 (17.7)	2 (1.4)		
Consistency	Soft	167	122 (73.1)	40 (24.0)	5 (3.0)	0.8092	No
	Hard	10	8 (80.0)	2 (20.0)	0 (0.0)		
Proliferative index	Ki-67 <3%	150	110 (73.3)	35 (23.3)	5 (3.3)	0.6168	No
	Ki-67 >3%	27	20 (74.1)	7 (25.9)	0 (0)		

Table 11.11 Prolactin-secreting adenoma: comprehensive evaluation for each parameter

Statistical parameter		Number of	Outcome, number of patients (%)			Chi-square test for independence	
			Cured	Controlled	Not cured	p Value	Significant association
Sex	Male	36	23 (63.9)	5 (13.9)	6 (16.7)	0.3182	No
	Female	65	56 (86.2)	8 (12.3)	6 (9.2)		
Previous Surgery	None	91	71 7.	19 20.9	1 1.1	0.0137	Yes
	Yes	10	4 40	5 50.0	1 10.0		
Size	Micro	46	41 89.1	5 10.9	0 0.0	0.0064	Yes
	Macro	55	34 61.8	19 34.5	2 3.6		
Invasiveness	Invasive	16	4 25.0	11 68.8	1 6.3	<0.0001	Yes
	Not invasive	85	71 (83.5)	13 (15.3)	1 (1.2)		
Consistency	Soft	94	71 (75.5)	21 (22.3)	2 (2.1)	0.4494	No
	Hard	7	4 (57.1)	3 (42.9)	0		
Proliferative index	Ki-67 <3%	80	63 (78.8)	17 (21.3)	0	0.0079	Yes
	Ki-67 >3%	21	12 (57.1)	7 (33.3)	2 (9.5)		

ACTH-secreting Adenomas

We treated 104 patients, 73 of whom had microadenomas and 31 had macroadenomas. Their ages varied from 14 to 80 years (mean 40 years); 34 were male (32.7%) and 70 were female (67.3%). Two patients died from causes not related to the disease at 4 and 28 months postoperatively. Two patients died from disease progression after 18 and 45 months postoperatively (one of them developed multiple metastases).

We performed 117 procedures on 104 patients; cure was obtained in 79 (75.9%) (▶ Table 11.12). Statistical analysis of all parameters showed significance for only previous surgery (p = 0.0081) and invasiveness (p = 0.0237) (▶ Table 11.12).

TSH-secreting Adenomas

We treated 12 patients with TSH-secreting adenomas, one of whom was an unusual case of an ectopic TSH-secreting pituitary adenoma arising from the vomerosphenoidal junction.[24] The ages of the patients varied from 14 to 72 years (mean 48 years; 7 were male [58.3%] and 5 were female [41.7%]). As yet, we have encountered no causes of death related or unrelated to the disease.

Table 11.12 Corticotropin-secreting adenomas: comprehensive evaluation for each parameter

Statistical parameters		Number of patients	Outcome, number of patients (%)			Chi-square test for independence	
			Cured	Controlled	Not cured	p Value	Significant association
Sex	Male	34	23 (67.6)	5 (14.7)	6 (17.6)	0.3182	No
	Female	70	56 (80.0)	8 (11.4)	6 (8.6)		
Previous surgery	None	81	67 (82.7)	8 (9.9)	6 (7.4)	0.0081	Yes
	Yes	23	12 (52.2)	5 (21.7)	6 (26.1)		
Size	Micro	73	57 (78.1)	8 (11.0)	8 (11.0)	0.7112	No
	Macro	31	22 (71.0)	5 (16.1)	4 (12.9)		
Invasiveness	Invasive	7	3 (42.9)	1 (14.3)	3 (42.9)	0.0237	Yes
	Not invasive	97	76 (78.4)	12 (12.4)	9 (9.2)		
Consistency	Soft	97	75 (77.3)	12 (12.4)	10 (10.3)	0.3237	No
	Hard	7	4 (57.1)	1 (14.3)	2 (28.6)		
Proliferative index	Ki-67 < 3%	86	68 (79.1)	10 (11.6)	8 (9.3)	0.2136	No
	K-i67 > 3%	18	11 (61.1)	3 (16.7)	4 (22.2)		

Table 11.13 Nonfunctioning adenomas: comprehensive evaluations for each parameter

Statistical parameter		Number of patients	Outcome, number of patients (%)			Chi-square Test for independence	
			Cured	Controlled	Not cured	p Value	Significant association
Sex	Male	231	192 (83.1)	36 (15.6)	3 (1.3)	0.8853	No
	Female	179	152 (84.9)	25 (14.0)	2 (1.1)		
Previous surgery	None	331	296 (89.4)	33 (10.0)	2 (0.6)	< 0.0001	Yes
	Yes	79	48 (60.8)	28 (35.4)	3 (3.8)		
Size	Micro	9	7 (77.8)	2 (22.2)	0 (0.0)	0.7839	No
	Macro	401	337 (84.0)	59 (14.7)	5 (1.2)		
Invasiveness	Invasive	81	55 (67.9)	25 (30.9)	1 (1.2)	< 0.0001	Yes
	Not invasive	329	289 (87.8)	36 (10.9)	4 (1.2)		
Consistency	Soft	358	305 (85.2)	52 (14.5)	1 (0.3)	< 0.0001	Yes
	Hard	52	39 (75.0)	9 (17.3)	4 (7.7)		
Proliferative index	Ki-67 < 3%	348	293 (84.2)	50 (14.4)	3 (0.9)	0.2605	No
	K-i67 > 3%	62	51 (82.3)	11 (17.7)	2 (3.2)		

We performed 13 procedures on 12 patients; cure was obtained in 10 (83.3%) (▶ Table 11.9). Due to the small number of cases treated, the statistical analysis was not significant.

Nonfunctioning Adenomas

All tumors, except nine, were macroadenomas. We treated 431 patients. Their ages varied from 15 to 89 years (median 56 years); 231 were male (56.3%) and 179 were female (43.7%). Two patients died from causes unrelated to the disease at 8 and 43 months postoperatively. Two patients died at 2 and 3 months after surgery due to tumoral progression; brain invasion was discovered at autopsy. Two patients died at 6 and 7 months from causes related to surgical complications.

We performed 430 procedures in 410 patients; cure was obtained in 344 (83.9%) (▶ Table 11.13). Statistical analysis of all the parameters showed significance for previous surgery ($p < 0.0001$), consistency ($p < 0.0001$) and invasiveness ($p < 0.0001$) (▶ Table 11.13).

11.5 Complications

Surgical and medical complications are summarized in ▶ Table 11.14 and ▶ Table 11.15. ▶ Table 11.14 shows the number and percentage of complications related to the

Table 11.14 Surgical complications and type of surgical procedure

Surgical complication	MiTea	EPSea	SDPhea	Total (%)
Epistaxis	12		1	13 (1.5)
Postoperative CSF leak	9	1	3	13 (1.5)
CN palsy	1		1	2 (0.1)
Neurological	2		1	3 (0.3)
Visual impairment	2	1	1	4 (0.5)
ICA injury		1		1 (0.1)
Hematoma/ ischemia	10	2	2	14 (1.6)
Total (%)	36/765 (4.7)	5/67 (7.4)	9/19 (47)	50 (5.9)

CN, cranial nerve; CSF, cerebrospinal fluid; EPSea, ethmoidal-pterygo-sphenoidal approach; ICA, internal carotid artery; MTea, median transsphenoidal approach (including the extension to the middle and lower clivus); SDPhea, supradiaphragmatic approach.

Table 11.15 Surgical and medical complications

Surgical complication	Number of patients (%)
Epistaxis	13 (1.5)
Postoperative CSF leak	13 (1.5)
Visual impairment	4 (0.4)
CN palsy	1 (0.2)
Neurological	3 (0.3)
ICA injury	1 (0.1)
Hematoma/ischemia	14 (1.6)
Intra-/perioperative death	0
Medical complication	
Temporary DI	26 (3.0)
Permanent DI	10 (2.3)
Partial hypopituitarism	45 (5.2)
Total hypopituitarism	5 (1.1)
SIADH	7 (0.8)
Meningitis	4 (0.4)
Cardiovascular	3 (0.3)
Pulmonary	1 (0.1)

CN, cranial nerve; CSF, cerebrospinal fluid; DI, diabetes insipidus; SIADH, syndrome of inappropriate antidiuretic hormone secretion.

surgical approach. We calculated the difference from the population with and without complications and the type of surgical approach (standard versus extended approaches). A two-sided p value of 0.0002 was considered extremely significant.

11.5.1 Rhinosinusal Complications

Thirteen (1.5%) cases of delayed (from few hours to 18 days after surgery) epistaxis were observed; nasal packing was required in the majority of the cases, and coagulation of the sphenopalatine artery in only five cases.

No cases of postoperative sinusitis or mucocele were observed. Patients with a history of chronic rhinosinusitis were treated pre- and postoperatively for their disease. All patients underwent frequent nasal cleaning with a hypotonic solution and a transnasal endoscopic examination 3 to 4 weeks after the surgical procedure.

11.5.2 Intrasellar Complications

In 139 (16.3%) cases there was intraoperative evidence of a CSF leak, which necessitated reconstruction with the use of abdominal fat or fascia lata together with the mucoperiosteum of the middle turbinate. Thirteen patients (1.5% overall, 10% of the intraoperative CSF leak group) experienced a postoperative CSF leak that required reintervention. Only the first five patients with intraoperative CSF leaks underwent lumbar drainage.

In four cases, a worsening of visual capacity was observed; it was related to the overpacking of the sella with the abdominal fat and it was corrected by early surgical revision. The correction was partial in one patient.

11.5.3 Suprasellar and Parasellar Complications

Vascular and neurological complications may be related to the approach phase and/or to vascular dissection during tumor resection, especially in cases where the tumor exceeded the sella limits.

Neurological complications may be the consequence of vascular damage or may be due to direct injury of the neural tissue (e.g., the curettes that pierce the diaphragma sellae and penetrate the neural tissue) and nerves.

A direct injury of a cranial nerve III palsy without a preoperative neurological deficit was observed in one patient. This damage was related to a blind surgical maneuver with a curette during the tumor removal from the superolateral compartment of the right cavernous sinus in a TSH-secreting adenoma with a hard consistency.

One female patient with invasive clivus and cavernous sinus NF adenoma suffered ICA injury. The rupture was due to an unrecognized bone dehiscence with erroneous clamping of the ICA wall during the sella approach. The bleeding was controlled intraoperatively with a tamponade. Angiography was performed immediately and the carotid artery was occluded by means of endovascular coils. The patient had no postoperative neurological sequelae.

Hematoma and ischemia were considered to be complications only if symptomatic; 14 patients complained of these complications. Six patients with intrasellar hematomas and mild symptoms recovered spontaneously a few days after surgery. Eight patients required reintervention (three with a median transsphenoidal endoscopic approach and five using a transcranial approach). Only six patients complained of neurological sequelae; three of them died 6 (two patients) and 7 months after surgery from related causes.

11.5.4 Medical Complications

Among the medical complications, there were 45 (5.2%) partial pituitary insufficiencies and 5 (1.1%) total pituitary insufficiencies, which required substitutive therapy, and 26 (3%) transient and 10 (2.3%) permanent cases of diabetes insipidus. Syndrome of inappropriate antidiuretic hormone secretion (SIADH) was observed in 32 (7%) patients and appeared from 3 to 10 days after surgery. We believe that it may be underestimated in our database because it more frequently occurs after discharge and is subclinical.

Quality of Nasal Function

To verify the tolerability of the surgical procedure for the nasal phase, we analyzed 40 patients with no anamnestic alteration of nasal function, no previous acute or chronic sinusitis, and no previous nasal surgery. In the preoperative evaluation, all patients underwent a specific subjective anamnestic test for nasal symptomatology, a nasal endoscopy, and a rhinomanometric test 1 and 3 months after surgery as well as the standard examinations (endocrinological, neuro-ophthalmological, and MRI). We performed another re-evaluation of all patients with nasal endoscopy, a nasal function test, and a rhinomanometric test. We did not find septum perforations, significant synechiae, or sinusitis. No patient complained of a deterioration of their nasal function; on the contrary, 13 patients with a simple alteration of the ostiomeatal complex that was corrected during the operation showed mild to significant improvement of subjective/objective nasal functionality.

11.6 Discussion

Currently, transsphenoidal surgery is considered the technique of choice for the treatment of an expansive lesion of the sellar region. Three main types of anterior approaches to the sella are currently in use: transseptal-transsphenoidal microsurgery, endonasal transsphenoidal microsurgery, and endoscopic endonasal transsphenoidal surgery.

The microscopic transeptal-transsphenoidal approaches evolved from the technique proposed by Cushing and Hirsh in 1910.[2,3] This technique requires a submucosal dissection, by means of an orogingival or septal incision to create a tunnel toward the posterior wall of the sphenoid sinus. In this approach, it is necessary to use a mechanical surgical speculum.

In 1987, Griffith[4] proposed an endonasal sphenoidotomy through a sphenoethmoidal recess. Here it is also necessary to use a surgical speculum. More recently, to overcome the difficulty of the lateral and superior vision

of the microscope, an angled endoscope is frequently used in the final exploration.

In 1992, Jankosky[7] first described an endoscopic transethmoidal approach to the sella for three pituitary tumors; in 1997, Jho and Carrau then[8] described an endonasal approach in 50 patients principally affected by pituitary adenomas. De Divitiis[10] and Cappabianca[9] popularized endoscopic endonasal pituitary surgery in Europe and perfected the technique, contributing to the development of proper instrumentation.

The endoscopic technique employs a rod-lens endoscope as a light source and optical instrument; it arrives at the sellar wall through a natural corridor (nasal cavity-natural ostium of the sphenoid sinus-sphenoid cavity) and does not use a surgical speculum.

Endoscopic transsphenoidal pituitary surgery represents the latest and most recent step in the evolution of the transsphenoidal approach, retaining expediency, good tolerance, effectiveness, and a low complication rate, characteristic of the original procedure.

We made a statement as the conclusion of a previous paper[13] and we would now like to verify, after our increased experience, whether the situation has changed. Comparing our first 314 cases (5.5 years) with the subsequent 537 cases (the last 5 years), we can state the following.

11.6.1 Expediency

The average time for an uncomplicated surgical procedure is still 40 minutes, which is the same as our pituitary surgical experience with microscopy.

11.6.2 Good Tolerance

Tolerance is difficult to estimate because it is composed of subjective and objective components. The first could be estimated by asking patients who had previously undergone a microsurgical transsphenoidal approach to express a tolerance comparison between the two experiences using a score between 0 (absolute comfort) and 10 (intolerability) for each procedure; in all cases, tolerance of the endoscopic approach improved at least three points with respect to the microsurgical transsphenoidal procedure. The second component of tolerance may be judged by the necessity of using analgesics, by the difficulties of nasal breathing, and by hospital stay/recovery time. After a median transsphenoidal endoscopic approach, postoperative pain was minimal and analgesics were rarely required. Conversely, headache, mainly due to pneumocephalus, was normally present in the early postoperative period after the supradiaphragmatic approach. It was controlled by analgesics and by maintaining a supine position for at least 24 to 48 hours. Nasal breathing contributes to a comfortable postoperative period. After a median transsphenoidal endoscopic approach, nasal packing was rarely required; conversely, after a supradiaphragmatic approach, where one middle turbinate is routinely sacrificed, nasal packing was regularly performed, at least ipsilaterally. Time of postoperative recovery may be very short, but we think that it is prudent not to consider discharge earlier than 3 to 4 days. This is, in our opinion, the minimum time required for endocrinological and water/electrolyte balance assessment. Other possible delayed complications, such as SIADH, may be detected and controlled by planning outpatient follow-ups. For this reason, patients were discharged after a minimum time of 3 days after a median transsphenoidal endoscopic approach; conversely, when using the supradiaphragmatic approach, the median hospital stay was 9 days, mainly depending on the need to verify the absence of a CSF leak. Therefore, the hospital stay for the median transsphenoidal endoscopic approach was unchanged with respect to our early experience and was the same as for the microscopy approach; conversely, the hospital stay for the supradiaphragmatic approach was three times longer and the lack of available data make comparison with a microscopy series impossible.

11.6.3 Effectiveness

A slight improvement in results emerges when comparing our recent series with the previous series. However, our final comment remains the same: in intrasellar adenomas, the overall effectiveness of an endoscopic transsphenoidal is comparable with that of the microscopy series, but in macroadenomas with extrasellar growth the endoscopic technique demonstrates a capacity for greater resection.[13]

In detail we can report that:

- In GH-secreting adenomas using modern remission criteria, the overall results were comparable to Kreutzer et al (69.2% versus 70%).[25] Conversely, in macroadenomas, we obtained slightly better results (69.6%) as compared with the percentages (46–64%) reported in the literature.[1,12,26,27,28]
- In PRL-secreting adenomas, the results also confirm a good remission rate in microadenomas (89.1%) but an improvement in remission rate in macroadenomas (61.8%) in comparison with the literature.[21,24,29,30]
- In ACTH-secreting adenomas, we obtained better results with microadenomas (78.1%) compared with macroadenomas (71.0%). In microadenomas, we included the 18 cases in which MRI did not identify any lesion. This circumstance is a well-documented poor prognostic factor.[31]

Our experience confirms the rarity of TSH-secreting adenomas. Despite a good percentage cure rate, the small number of patients with this type of tumor does not allow a significant evaluation of overall results.

Our results regarding NF adenomas indicate that tumor size does not influence the outcome as much as it does the real intraoperative invasiveness of the neoplasm and its consistency ($p < 0.0001$) (▶ Table 11.14). As a matter of fact, we obtained disease control in 97.5% of patients, with a low rate of medical and surgical complications, when adopting a single surgical procedure.

Statistical analysis showed a significant negative correlation in all types of tumors with intraoperative invasiveness and with patients who had previously been surgically treated. The other two variables with a negative prognostic correlation were the size of the tumor in PRL-secreting adenomas and the consistency in NF adenomas

11.6.4 Complications

Reports of endoscopy in the literature[10,11,32] indicate a lower complication rate when compared with microscopy surgery.[28,33,34] The comparison between our early and late series confirms the statement of Ciric[33]: "An unexpected increase in the complication rate may be observed with the acquisition of great confidence and it may be due to the assumption of increasingly risky procedures." Furthermore, the late series includes numerous extended approaches, which are associated with an obvious increase in complication rates.

Nasal complications are reduced because the endoscopic technique "skips" the nasal phase since it starts in the sphenoethmoidal recess. Moreover, we think that active and constant collaboration with an ENT surgeon is beneficial with respect to any nasal alterations that may result; this could improve nasal function, as we found in our study and which has been discussed previously.

We did not observe postoperative sinusitis in short-term or long-term follow-up. A 1-month postoperative ENT check-up may also play an active role. We did not experience postsurgical mucoceles, which could be explained by the fact that the median transsphenoidal endoscopic approach utilizes a natural cavity and, together with the enlargement of the natural ostia, can reduce the possibility of their closure postoperatively.

The main "nasal" complication consisted of postoperative epistaxis from the septal branch of the sphenopalatine artery; this occurred infrequently (1.5%). In the majority of cases, only ambulatory nasal packing was necessary; in five patients, cauterization of the vessel was necessary in the operating theater. This complication occurred in the first 14 days after surgery and was a very unpleasant experience for the patient.

CSF leak and meningitis are the main complications in transsphenoidal surgery. In our experience meningitis was rare (0.4%) and it occurred as a complication of a postoperative CSF leak. In our data, we did not consider a CSF leak as a complication if it had been detected and repaired intraoperatively. This type of CSF leak (▶ Table 11.1) observed in our series in 84 (18.2%) patients is a foreseeable and sometimes unavoidable event. We considered a postoperative CSF leak as a complication; we observed 12 (2.6%) postoperative CSF leaks. Although we performed early repairs by means of a transnasal endoscopic duraplasty, meningitis occurred in four (0.4%) patients, and this was resolved in all cases by means of medical therapy and without neurological consequences.

As far as hemorrhagic complications are concerned, these include direct injury of the ICA, a compressive hematoma in the surgical field, an extrasellar hemorrhage, and, finally, a hemorrhage from a residual tumor.[35] In this type of pathology, we had a single case of ICA bleeding; the paraclival ICA was lacerated during the resection from the sphenoidal sinus of an invasive adenoma. First, the hemorrhage was controlled by packing of the sphenoidal sinus; an emergency angiography showed a pseudoaneurysm and the vessel was occluded uneventfully using an endovascular technique.

Hemorrhage into the surgical field does not require treatment except for symptomatic cases. Revision endonasal surgery was necessary to remove the compressive hematoma in three cases. Extrasellar hemorrhages, due to damage to the intradural vessels (two patients) or due to bleeding or hemorrhagic infarction of a residual mass (three patients), were treated using a craniotomy.

We observed a single case of ophthalmoplegia, which was due to oculomotor nerve paresis as a result of injury from a right-angled curette that penetrated the subdural space. Visual worsening may be a consequence of direct trauma, compression, or ischemic damage of the optochiasmatic structures. Four patients experienced visual impairment due to overpacking. We performed early surgical revision: three patients were normalized and one patient was only partially corrected.

Endocrinological complications were pituitary insufficiency, diabetes insipidus, and SIADH. The first two complications are predictable and preventable with careful maneuvers during the dissection of the tumor. The experience of the surgeon in recognizing and sparing the normal pituitary tissue allows the preservation of pituitary functionality. We observed postoperative insufficiency in 16 (3.5%) patients.

SIADH is a complication that is predictable but not preventable. We observed it in 32 (7%) patients. Unrecognized SIADH may be a very dangerous systemic complication and its early detection and medical correction is very important. We therefore routinely plan outpatient electrolyte tests 10 days after surgery.

11.6.5 Final Remarks

During the last decade increased experience has been gained in endoscopic transphenoidal pituitary surgery, allowing us to make some observations regarding the state of the art of this technique. The median transsphenoidal endoscopic approach confirms the characteristics of expediency, good tolerability, safety, and effectiveness of transsphenoidal procedures. In particular, we confirm our previous statement that, in endosellar lesions, the results are not very different from the best microsurgical series, but when dealing with tumors that have an extra-

sellar extension, the resection ability afforded by the endoscopy technique seems superior to the microscopy technique. The complication rate related to the approach phase is reduced; however, complications related to tumor resection during the median transsphenoidal endoscopic approach remain similar to those reported in the literature for microsurgical techniques.

A confounding factor in the evaluation of the endoscopic transsphenoidal pituitary surgery may be that the median transsphenoidal endoscopic approach and the extended approaches (SDPhea and EPSea), which are increasingly being performed using an endoscopic technique, are considered by some to be one and the same. However, while the former can be rightly compared with the microsurgical transsphenoidal approach, the latter should be more correctly compared with transcranial approaches. The debate on the extended approaches is open and it should be centered mainly on the balance between the unquestionable advantages of these approaches, avoiding brain and nerve manipulation, and the increased risk of complications, which depends on the pathology to be treated.

Pearls and Pitfalls

- Pituitary gland tumors should be managed in a multidisciplinary setting, including endocrinologists and neuroradiologists, as well as neurosurgeons and head and neck surgeons.
- Compared with traditional transsphenoidal approaches, endoscopic approaches to the sella are associated with higher rates of complete tumor removal (macroadenomas).
- Surgery is the mainstay treatment for nonsecreting adenomas presenting with compressive symptoms, as well as for functional ACTH-secreting and GH-secreting adenomas.
- Patients with prolactinomas are primarily treated medically.
- A complete resection is the aim for all hormone-secreting (i.e., functional) tumors.
- Simple drainage is usually sufficient for Rathke cleft cysts.
- In nonsecreting adenomas, craniopharyngiomas, and meningiomas, complete tumor removal should be balanced against the expected associated morbidity.
- Avoid sharp dissection during tumor removal and remove the adenoma remaining in the extra-arachnoid plane to avoid CSF leakage.
- Remove the parasellar extension of the tumor under direct view and using dedicated blunt and sharp instruments combined with atraumatic suctioning to avoid ICA injury.
- Preservation of at least one-third of the normal pituitary gland in the sella prevents panhypopituitarism.

References

[1] Sciarretta V, Mazzatenta D, Ciarpaglini R, Pasquini E, Farneti G, Frank G. Surgical repair of persisting CSF leaks following standard or extended endoscopic transsphenoidal surgery for pituitary tumor. Minim Invasive Neurosurg 2010; 53: 55–59

[2] Cushing H. Surgical experience with pituitary disorders. JAMA 1914; 63: 1515–1525

[3] Hirsch O. Endonasal method of removal of hypophyseal tumors, with a report of two successful cases JAMA 1910; 55: 772–774

[4] Griffith HB, Veerapen R. A direct transnasal approach to the sphenoid sinus. Technical note. J Neurosurg 1987; 66: 140–142

[5] Hardy J. Surgery of the pituitary gland, using the trans-sphenoidal approach. Comparative study of 2 technical methods[in French] Union Med Can 1967; 96: 702–712

[6] Guiot G, Rougerie J, Fourestier A et al. Intracranial endoscopic explorations [in French]. Presse Med 1963; 71: 1225–1228

[7] Jankowski R, Auque J, Simon C, Marchal JC, Hepner H, Wayoff M. Endoscopic pituitary tumor surgery. Laryngoscope 1992; 102: 198–202

[8] Jho HD, Carrau RL. Endoscopic endonasal transsphenoidal surgery: experience with 50 patients. J Neurosurg 1997; 87: 44–51

[9] Cappabianca P, Alfieri A, de Divitiis E. Endoscopic endonasal transsphenoidal approach to the sella: towards functional endoscopic pituitary surgery (FEPS). Minim Invasive Neurosurg 1998; 41: 66–73

[10] de Divitiis E, Cappabianca P, Cavallo M. Endoscopic endonasal transsphenoidal approach to the sellar region. In: de Divitiis E, Cappabianca P, eds. Endoscopic Endonasal Transsphenoidal Surgery. Vienna NewYork: Springer; 2003:91–130

[11] Dehdashti AR, Ganna A, Karabatsou K, Gentili F. Pure endoscopic endonasal approach for pituitary adenomas: early surgical results in 200 patients and comparison with previous microsurgical series. Neurosurgery 2008; 62: 1006–1015; discussion 1015–1017

[12] Cavina C. Lo stato attuale della chirurgia ipofisaria. Riv Otoneurooftalmol 1932; 9: 205–370

[13] Frank G, Pasquini E, Farneti G et al. The endoscopic versus the traditional approach in pituitary surgery. Neuroendocrinology 2006; 83: 240–248

[14] Cappabianca P, Frank G, Pasquini E, de Divitiis O, Calbucci F. Extended endoscopic endonasal transsphenoidal approaches to the suprasellar region, planum sphenoidale and clivus. In: de Divitiis E, Cappabianca P, eds. Endoscopic Endonasal Transsphenoidal Surgery. Vienna NewYork: springer; 2003:176–187

[15] Frank G, Pasquini E. Approach to the cavernous sinus. In: de Divitiis E, Cappabianca P, eds. Endoscopic Endonasal Transsphenoidal Surgery. Vienna NewYork: Springer; 2003:159–175

[16] Pasquini E, Sciarretta V, Farneti G, Mazzatenta D, Modugno GC, Frank G. Endoscopic treatment of encephaloceles of the lateral wall of the sphenoid sinus. Minim Invasive Neurosurg 2004; 47: 209–213

[17] Pasquini E, Sciarretta V, Frank G et al. Endoscopic treatment of benign tumors of the nose and paranasal sinuses. Otolaryngol Head Neck Surg 2004; 131: 180–186

[18] Schloffer H. Erfolreiche Operation eines Hypophysentumors auf nasalem Wege. Wien Klin Wchnschr 1907; 20: 621–624

[19] Webb SM, Rigla M, Wägner A, Oliver B, Bartumeus F. Recovery of hypopituitarism after neurosurgical treatment of pituitary adenomas. J Clin Endocrinol Metab 1999; 84: 3696–3700

[20] Giustina A, Barkan A, Casanueva FF et al. Criteria for cure of acromegaly: a consensus statement. J Clin Endocrinol Metab 2000; 85: 526–529

[21] Losa M, Mortini P, Barzaghi R, Gioia L, Giovanelli M. Surgical treatment of prolactin-secreting pituitary adenomas: early results and long-term outcome. J Clin Endocrinol Metab 2002; 87: 3180–3186

[22] Gittoes NJL, Sheppard MC, Johnson AP, Stewart PM. Outcome of surgery for acromegaly—the experience of a dedicated pituitary surgeon. QJM 1999; 92: 741–745

[23] Losa M, Giovanelli M, Persani L, Mortini P, Faglia G, Beck-Peccoz P. Criteria of cure and follow-up of central hyperthyroidism due to thyrotropin-secreting pituitary adenomas. J Clin Endocrinol Metab 1996; 81: 3084–3090

[24] Mortini P, Losa M, Barzaghi R, Boari N, Giovanelli M. Results of transsphenoidal surgery in a large series of patients with pituitary adenoma. Neurosurgery 2005; 56: 1222–1233; discussion 1233

[25] Kreutzer J, Vance ML, Lopes MB, Laws ER, Jr. Surgical management of GH-secreting pituitary adenomas: an outcome study using modern remission criteria. J Clin Endocrinol Metab 2001; 86: 4072–4077

[26] Nishizawa S, Oki Y, Ohta S, Yokota N, Yokoyama T, Uemura K. What can predict postoperative "endocrinological cure" in Cushing's disease? Neurosurgery 1999; 45: 239–244

[27] Ahmed S, Elsheikh M, Stratton IM, Page RCL, Adams CBT, Wass JAH. Outcome of transphenoidal surgery for acromegaly and its relationship to surgical experience. Clin Endocrinol (Oxf) 1999; 50: 561–567

[28] Semple PL, Laws ER, Jr. Complications in a contemporary series of patients who underwent transsphenoidal surgery for Cushing's disease. J Neurosurg 1999; 91: 175–179

[29] Nomikos P, Buchfelder M, Fahlbusch R. Current management of prolactinomas. J Neurooncol 2001; 54: 139–150

[30] Tyrrell JB, Lamborn KR, Hannegan LT, Applebury CB, Wilson CB. Transsphenoidal microsurgical therapy of prolactinomas: initial outcomes and long-term results. Neurosurgery 1999; 44: 254–261; discussion 261–263

[31] Bochicchio D, Losa M, Buchfelder M. Factors influencing the immediate and late outcome of Cushing's disease treated by transsphenoidal surgery: a retrospective study by the European Cushing's Disease Survey Group. J Clin Endocrinol Metab 1995; 80: 3114–3120Review

[32] Jho HD. Endoscopic transsphenoidal surgery. J Neurooncol 2001; 54: 187–195

[33] Ciric I, Ragin A, Baumgartner C, Pierce DB. Complications of transsphenoidal surgery: results of a national survey, review of the literature, and personal experience. Neurosurgery 1997; 40: 225–236; discussion 236–237

[34] Weiss MH. Transnasal transsphenoidal approach. In: Apuzzo MLJ, ed. Surgery of the Third Ventricle. Baltimore: Williams & Wilkins; 1987:476

[35] Laws ER, Jr. Vascular complications of transsphenoidal surgery. Pituitary 1999; 2: 163–170

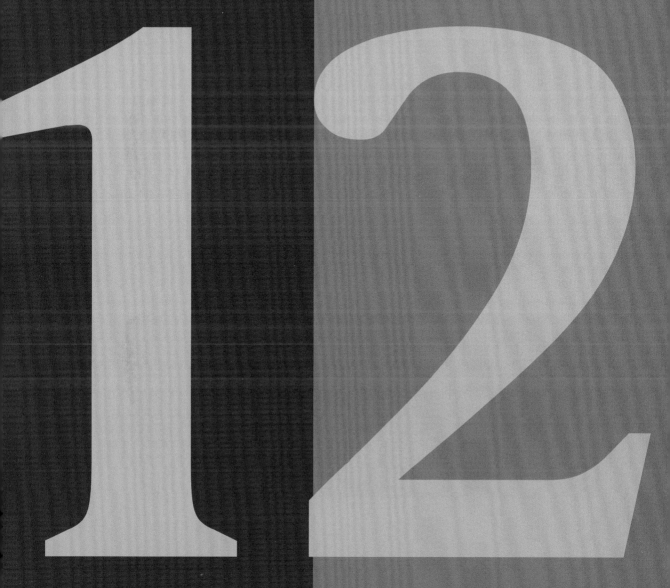

Chapter 12
Tumor-Specific Strategies

12 Tumor-Specific Strategies

12.1 Inverted Papilloma

Paolo Castelnuovo, Apostolos Karligkiotis, Paolo Battaglia, Federica Sberze, Davide Lombardi, Piero Nicolai

12.1.1 Introduction

An inverted papilloma is a primary benign epithelial tumor of the sinonasal region that may be locally aggressive invading adjacent paranasal sinuses, surrounding bone, and vital structures such as the orbit or the skull base. The two peculiar features that have dictated the standard methods of treatment are its high propensity toward recurrence and its possible transformation into malignant.[1]

Surgery is considered the mainstay in the treatment of an inverted papilloma. Until late 1960s, transnasal removal was routinely performed without microscopic or endoscopic assistance. In this period, the incidence of recurrence was as high as 78% due to incomplete removal of the tumor.[2] Following this, the recurrence rate was reduced to 0 to 29% when transfacial surgical procedures were largely used and lateral rhinotomy and midfacial degloving became the gold standard for the treatment of inverted papillomas.[3] External approaches including skin or mucosal incisions and maxillary osteotomies can be frequently associated with persistent or transitory complications such as epiphora, chronic dacryocystitis, cheek paresthesia, and temporary diplopia.[4]

In 1992, Waitz and Wigand first reported the treatment of inverted papillomas by a purely endoscopic approach.[5] Large series published in the last two decades have demonstrated how this technique seems to produce results that are comparable with external approaches while avoiding the major complications and facial scars associated with osteotomies and external incisions.[6,7,8] In 2006, a meta-analysis clearly showed that endoscopic surgery is a reliable alternative to traditional external techniques for the vast majority of lesions.[1]

The association of inverted papilloma with squamous cell carcinoma (SCC) has been overestimated, with incidences reported to be as high as 56%.[9] Recent data, coming from accurate reviews of the literature and data resulting from large series, clearly show that the incidence of malignant transformation in individual series of inverted papillomas ranges from 2 to 13%.[3,10,11,12,13,14] In a collective review reporting more than 2,000 inverted papillomas, there was an association with synchronous carcinoma in 7.1% of cases and metachronous carcinoma in 3.6%.[15]

An exclusive endoscopic approach may be contraindicated in the following situations: (1) massive involvement of the mucosa of the frontal sinus and/or within a large supraorbital cell; (2) the concomitant presence of a malignancy involving critical areas, such as the orbit or the facial skin; and (3) the presence of abundant scar tissue from previous surgery.[16]

It is mandatory to underline that recurrence occurs more often due to a surgical error rather than to some characteristic of the tumor itself; therefore, great care must be taken to achieve complete removal no matter which approach is used.[6,17] The extension of the tumor and its relationship with surrounding structures is very important for the surgical planning. It is best assessed preoperatively by magnetic resonance imaging (MRI) in which the cerebriform-columnar pattern is a valuable indicator to suggest inverted papilloma in the differential diagnosis[18] (▶ Fig. 12.1). Recent studies suggest that osteitis and focal hyperostosis on computed tomography (CT) can predict the site of attachment of the lesion.[19,20]

12.1.2 Technical Considerations

Endoscopic approaches cannot always obtain an en bloc resection. However, it is not the concept of an en bloc resection per se that has to be fulfilled to achieve complete removal. What really matters when dealing with benign tumors is the radicality of the resection obtained

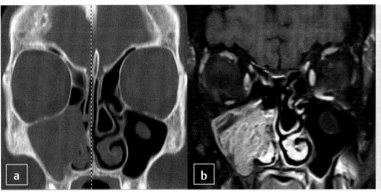

Fig. 12.1 a, b Preoperative imaging of inverted papilloma. **(a)** Coronal CT scan revealing complete opacification of the right maxillary sinus. The medial wall of the sinus is pushed medially and the bone partially reabsorbed. Note the characteristic shape resembling the "continent of Africa." **(b)** MRI: T1-weighted, fat-saturated, with gadolinium enhancement showing the typical cerebriform-columnar pattern of inverted papilloma.

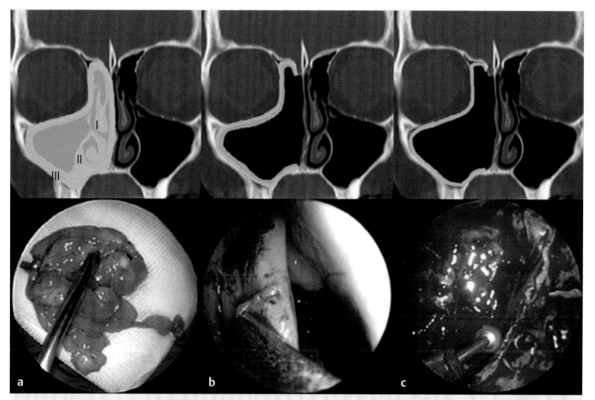

Fig. 12.2 a–c Sequential layer resection technique for inverted papilloma. **(a)** Schematic representation of the three layers to be removed. The first step of the technique is: debulking or piecemeal removal of the exophytic portion of the tumor (I, light blue). **(b)** Second step: subperiosteal dissection of the tissues (II, orange). **(c)** Third step: drilling of the underlying bone (III, green).

at the end of the procedure. It is crucial to achieve a complete resection of the lesion leaving the margins histologically free of disease.

Endoscopes provide a magnified view and the possibility to explore around corners thanks to their angled lenses. This facilitates the possibility of obtaining a radical resection using a "piecemeal" technique.[21] We remove inverted papillomas using a technique called "progressive multilayer resection" since the tumor is removed following consecutive anatomical layers (▶ Fig. 12.2). There are three important general principles to be respected to obtain oncological radicality.

The first step consists in debulking the vegetating portion of the mass in the sinonasal tract to reach its actual insertion. Through-cutting or powered instruments can be used to remove the lesion sufficiently to permit the identification of its attachment to the mucosa. Multiple frozen sections (biopsies) must be performed around the macroscopically healthy mucosa to define the margins of the lesion.

The second step consists in removing the mucosa on a subperiosteal plane and centripetal direction to reach the central residual lesion. The incisions must be performed around the tumor on seemingly healthy tissue. The tissues are then dissected subperiosteally towards the

center of the nasal cavity, achieving a "radical resection". The dissected tissue is then extracted through the vestibule or the oral cavity.

The third step consists in drilling out the bone underlying the pedicle of the neoplasm; this guarantees oncological radicality.[4] The latest endonasal drills (straight and curved) that are used for this step do not harm the skin or the mucosa around the vestibule.

The site of the lesion and the area of mucosa involved dictate the extent of the operation. Cases in which the origin of the lesion is clearly identifiable as being small can be managed with a very conservative approach[22] (▶ Fig. 12.3).

12.1.3 Surgical Technique

Surgery is performed with the patient placed under hypotensive general anesthesia and placed in supine reverse Trendelenburg position. The nasal cavities are packed with pledges soaked in 2% oxymetazoline, 1% oxybuprocaine, and epinephrine (1/100,000) solution for 10 minutes.

Rod-lens endoscopes of 4 mm diameter, with 0 and 45° lenses are used. An irrigation sheath connected to an irrigation pump can be useful for maintaining the endoscope lens clean during surgery. Straight, angled, and

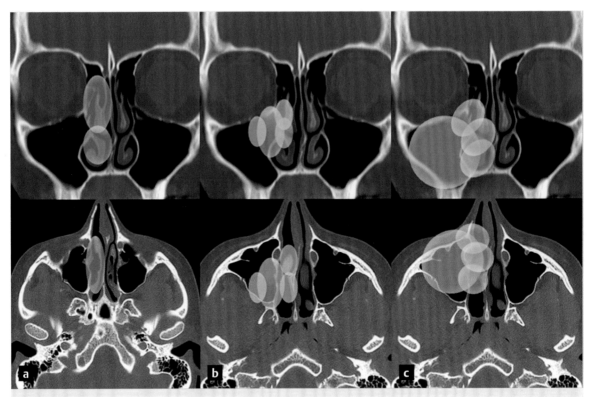

Fig. 12.3 **a–c** Different extensions of inverted papillomas toward the ethmoid and maxillary sinus. **(a)** Involvement of the nasal cavity, middle meatus, ethmoid and/or superior meatus (blue). **(b)** Involvement of the medial and posterior wall of the maxillary sinus with extension in the ethmoid and/or nasal cavity (green). **(c)** Involvement of the anterolateral wall or of the anteromedial angle of the maxillary sinus with ethmoidal and/or nasal extension (yellow).

double-ended instruments are needed to dissect the tissues both laterally and behind angles. A shaver is very useful during the first step of the procedure for debulking the exophytic portion of the tumor until the site of origin is identified. A suction trap, incorporated in the suction line, permits collecting the tumor, which is then sent for histological examination. A diode laser may help surgeons to perform bloodless incisions. The endonasal pen-style, compact, powerful, lightweight, high-performance microdrills equipped with extended handles are used with diamond or cutting burrs to remove the bone in the sinuses or the skull base without harming surrounding tissues. The recently introduced curved drills are very useful for reaching far lateral (maxillary sinus) and far superior (frontal sinus, supraorbital cell) sites (▶ Fig. 12.4).

The endoscopic approaches for removal of the tumor are classified as follows.

Type 1 Endoscopic Approach for Inverted Papilloma

Type 1 endoscopic resection (▶ Fig. 12.5a) can be performed for those inverted papillomas that involve the middle meatus, the ethmoid and/or the sphenoid sinuses, and the frontal infundibulum. Lesions protruding into the maxillary sinus that do not directly involve the mucosa can also be treated with this kind of procedure (▶ Fig. 12.3a). When the lesion occupies the whole nasal cavity, the operation starts with the debulking of the mass and exposure of the fundamental surgical landmarks, such as the maxillary line, the insertion of the middle turbinate, and the choana. The mucosal incision is performed along the maxillary line with a cold knife (blade) or diode laser, and the underlying bone is drilled with a diamond burr to obtain exposure of the infundibulum and identification of the lamina papyracea in a subperiosteal plane. The dissection continues in a centripetal way, laterally among the lamina papyracea as far as the posterior ethmoidal cells, and superiorly as far as the ethmoidal roof. The middle turbinate is usually resected at the insertion on the skull base and included in the surgical piece. The sphenopalatine artery and its branches must be cauterized using bipolar forceps. In endoscopic endonasal surgery, it is very important to use a bipolar electrocautery with a pistol-grip design, protected sheaths and small-angled microtips for easy insertion and maneuverability (360° rotation) inside the nasal cavity to avoid the instrument crossing with the endoscope. A second recommendation is the use of bipolar forceps since the monopolar type can cause optic nerve injuries

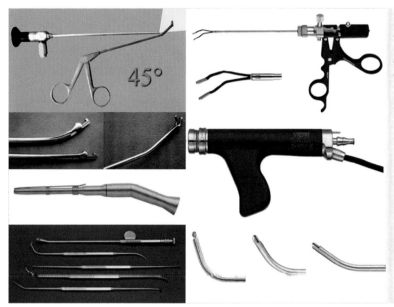

Fig. 12.4 Various microinstruments for endoscopic sinus surgery: 45° endoscopes, pen-style microdrill, angled double-curved dissectors and forceps, bipolar forceps, curved drills, and shavers.

by electrical diffusion through the blood. The superior turbinate is resected only when the inverted papilloma involves the posterior ethmoid. Dissection of the olfactory fissure is performed in rare cases of medial mucosal extension of the tumor. The olfactory fibers must be transected very carefully to avoid a cerebrospinal fluid (CSF) leak. In the case of an iatrogenic dural defect, the duraplasty is performed during surgery.

The mucosa lying on the anterior wall of the sphenoid sinus, from the skull base to the choana, is dissected and released from the rostrum with an incision carried along the superior border of the choana extending to the area of the sphenopalatine artery. The anterior wall of the sphenoid sinus is taken down, the mucosa inside the sinus is removed and sent for histological analysis, separately from the primary lesion.

Usually, a Draf type IIA sinusotomy is combined with the procedure removing a pneumatized agger nasi or frontal cells that close the access to the frontal sinus. The concept consists in obtaining an accurate view of the frontal sinus mucosa intraoperatively and a wide sinusotomy for the endoscopic follow-up. As a final step, the bone beneath the lesion is widely drilled with a diamond burr and multiple biopsies of the margins of the resection are sent for immediate histological analysis (i.e., frozen sections).

When a supraorbital cell is present, the exposure is widened by coagulation and section of the anterior ethmoidal artery, drilling the upper part of the lamina papyracea and displacing the orbit. This maneuver permits the surgeon to reach the deep part of the cell with the instruments. Curved drills are currently used to facilitate the approach to the frontal infundibulum and large supraorbital cells. Despite these new curved drills, massive involvement of the supraorbital cell with a significant lateral extension requires an external osteoplastic frontal flap.

Type 2 Endoscopic Approach for Inverted Papilloma

Type 2 endoscopic resection (▶ Fig. 12.5**b**) corresponds to a medial endoscopic maxillectomy[8,23] and is indicated for those inverted papillomas that originate from the middle meatus, the ethmoid and/or the sphenoid sinuses, and the frontal infundibulum and involve the maxillary sinus, or when the lesion originates from the medial or posterior maxillary wall (▶ Fig. 12.3**b**). The nasolacrimal duct may or may not be included in the resection, depending on the anterior extension of the tumor. The basic limitation of this approach is the limited exposure of the anterior and lateral wall of the maxillary sinus.

This resection differs from a type 1 resection, as the vertical incision, performed with a diode laser along the maxillary line, is extended from the insertion of the middle turbinate on the lateral nasal wall caudally to section the inferior turbinate and reach the floor of the nasal fossa. From this point, a second mucosal incision with a corresponding osteotomy is continued posteriorly in the inferior meatus as far as the posterior wall of the maxillary sinus; therefore, including the whole medial wall of the maxillary sinus in the resection. During the osteotomy, it is important to pay attention to the junction of the palatine bone and the posterior maxillary wall to avoid damaging the descending palatine artery. The posterior and superior dissections are performed as described in the type 1 procedure. If there is a direct involvement of the nasolacrimal duct, or if a wider exposure of the sinus is required, the duct must be transected 2 to 3 mm below the Bèraud-Krause valve marsupializing the superior part to prevent postoperative stenosis. The nasolacrimal duct transection must be performed with a single cut. Multiple attempts with the scissors (i.e., crushing) increase the risk of postoperative stenosis. If the duct is

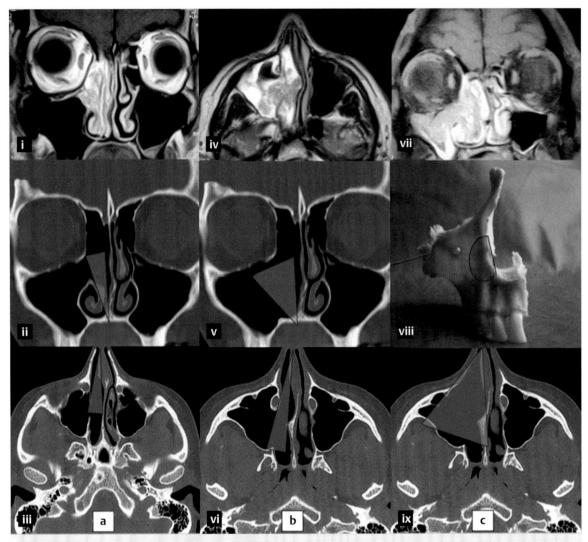

Fig. 12.5 a–c Schematic representation of the different surgical approaches for inverted papillomas with ethmoidal and maxillary involvement. See text for details. (a) Type 1 resection (i–iii). (b) Type 2 resection (iv–vi). (c) Type 3 resection (vii–ix).

accidentally damaged during surgery, a lacrimal stent must be placed for 1 month. A type 2 resection offers good exposure of the angle between the orbital floor and the nasolacrimal duct, which represents one of the common sites of persistence of disease; therefore, it must be drilled carefully avoiding periorbital or orbital injuries. Use of the new safe-tip microdrills is recommended to avoid harming vestibular and cutaneous areas.

Type 3 Endoscopic Approach for Inverted Papilloma

A type 3 endoscopic resection, also known as the modified Sturmann-Canfield operation or endonasal Denker operation[24] (▶ Fig. 12.5c and ▶ Fig. 12.6), is indicated for mucosal involvement of the anterior, lateral, and inferior walls of the maxillary sinus (where wide exposure of the

whole sinus is required), whether it is associated or not with involvement of the middle meatus, the ethmoid and/or sphenoid sinuses, and the frontal infundibulum. This procedure includes a medial maxillectomy and resection of the medial portion of the anterior wall of the maxillary sinus to obtain complete visualization of the antrum (▶ Fig. 12.3c).

The first surgical step is the mucosal incision just anterior to the inferior turbinate. Following a subperiosteal plane, the piriform crest and the anterior wall of maxillary sinus are dissected (depending on the case) until identification of the infraorbital nerve. Drilling of the anterior wall and the medial angle is tailored to expose the antrum. The nasolacrimal duct is isolated and cut below the sac. The dissection of the medial wall is then completed as described for type 1 and 2 resections. The second surgical step consists in detaching and removing

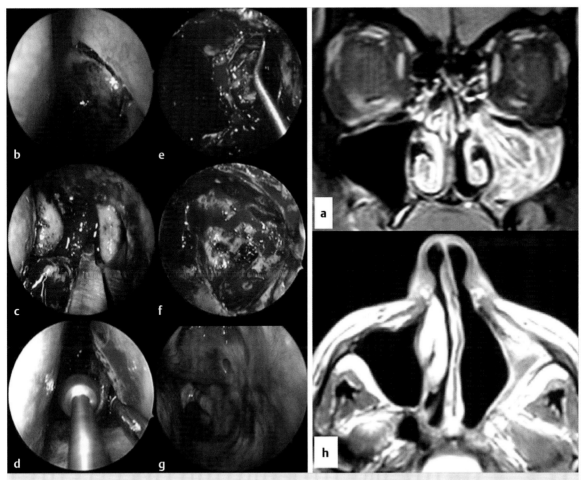

Fig. 12.6 a–h Type 3 resection of inverted papilloma. **(a)** Initial laser incision on the left maxillary line. **(b)** Identification and transection of the left nasolacrimal duct with microendoscopic scissors. **(c)** Drilling of the piriform crest and anterior wall of the left maxillary sinus with a microdrill. **(d)** Subperiosteal dissection of the mucosa of the left maxillary sinus with a curved microdissector. **(e)** Final result of the left maxillary cavity at the end of the surgery. **(f)** Postoperative endoscopic view of the left nasal fossa after 10 months. Complete re-epithelization of the maxillary cavity due to normal scar tissue formation can be observed. **(g)** Preoperative MRI scan: T1-weighted, fat-saturated, with gadolinium enhancement. Inverted papilloma involving the lateral wall of the left maxillary sinus. The typical cerebriform-columnar pattern is evident. **(h)** Postoperative MRI scan after 8 months showing no evidence of recurrence. Normal scar tissue fills the new maxillary cavity.

the lesion from the walls of the sinus following a subperiosteal plane. In patients with a very deep alveolar recess, exposure of the field can be obtained by drilling the bone at the junction between the floor of the nasal fossa and the alveolar recess. The mucosa can be easily removed using double-curved instruments and a 45° endoscope. Cotton wads can help in detaching mucosal remnants from the walls of the maxillary sinus. At this point, it is possible to drill the bone of the antrum to ensure that no mucosa is retained, paying attention not to harm the infraobital nerve. When the alveolar recess is very deep, curved drills are very helpful for drilling the bottom of the recess to achieve complete radicality. Hyperostosis in the site of origin of the inverted papilloma must be drilled out until the bony surface becomes smooth and macroscopically free from tumor.

Special Considerations–Frontal Sinus Involvement

The frontal sinus is a challenging site for endoscopic approaches because different conditions may be present, ranging from limited lesions growing from the ethmoid into the frontal recess to massive mucosal involvement by the disease (► Fig. 12.7). The surgical options are based on the possibility of dissecting the mucosa along the subperiosteal plane and drilling out the underlying bone. This may involve a Draf type IIB (for lesions growing from the ethmoid into the infundibulum of the frontal sinus) (► Fig. 12.8b) or a Draf type III (also known as the modified Lothrop procedure or median drainage) frontal sinusotomy (in the presence of a small frontal sinus and/ or tumor originating from the posterior wall of the

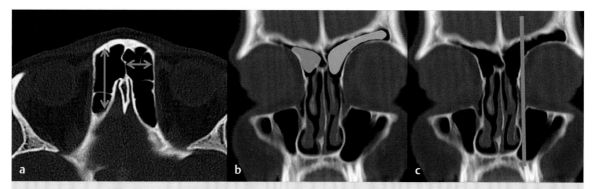

Fig. 12.7 a–c Factors influencing the choice of the surgical approach to the frontal sinus. **(a)** Configuration of the frontal recess. **(b)** Frontal sinus dimensions. Small right frontal sinus suitable for an endoscopic endonasal approach (light blue). Large left frontal sinus suitable for an external osteoplastic approach (light yellow). **(c)** Site and extension of the lesion. When the tumor arises or extends over an imaginary line passing through the lamina papyracea, the external approach is strongly recommended.

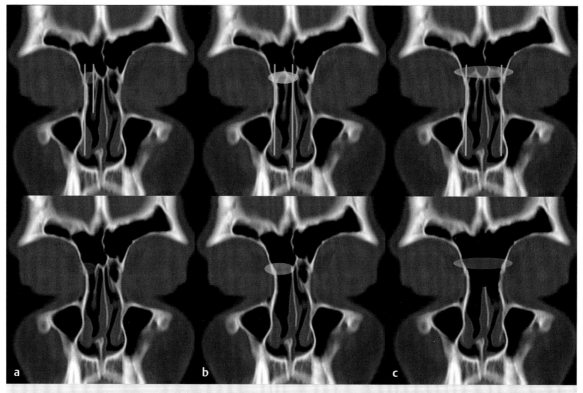

Fig. 12.8 a–c Frontal sinusotomies according to Draf. **(a)** Type IIA frontal sinusotomy. The extension of removal of the frontal floor is from the lamina papyracea to the middle turbinate. **(b)** Type IIB frontal sinusotomy. The extension is diverted medially from the lamina papyracea to the nasal septum. **(c)** Type III frontal sinusotomy. The frontal floor is removed from the ipsilateral lamina papyracea to the contralateral lamina papyracea.

frontal sinus) (▶ Fig. 12.8c) or a combined endoscopic approach with a frontal osteoplastic flap when there is massive mucosal involvement in a hyperpneumatized frontal sinus or within a largely pneumatized supra-orbital cell (type 4 approach) (▶ Fig. 12.9). Occasionally, the preoperative imaging cannot provide clear informa-tion about frontal mucosa involvement and this is defined

intraoperatively. The patients must be informed about the possibility of switching from a purely endoscopic endonasal technique to a combined one with an external osteoplastic approach. A Draf type IIB sinusotomy con-sists of removing the frontal sinus floor from the lamina papyracea to the septum. For this procedure, it is manda-tory to identify the first olfactory fiber that marks the

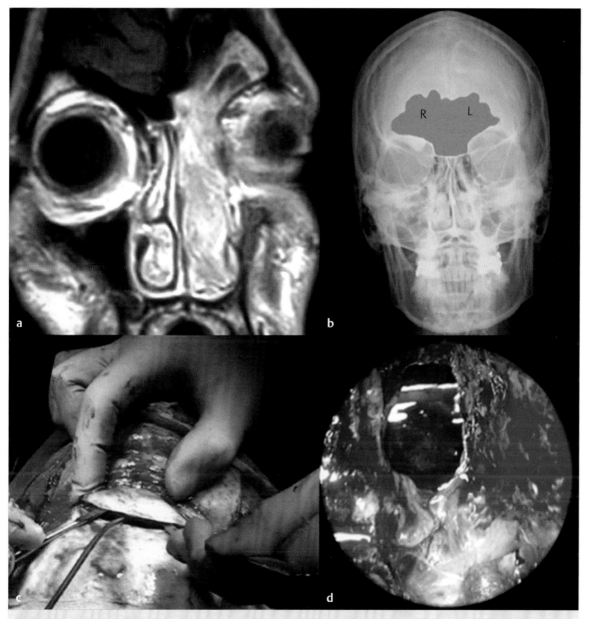

Fig. 12.9 a–d Combined endoscopic–osteoplastic approach for massive involvement of the left frontal sinus. **(a)** MRI scan: T1-weighted with gadolinium enhancement. Inverted papilloma involving the left frontal sinus and nasal cavity. **(b)** A 6-foot Caldwell view X-ray is necessary for drawing the frontal osteoplastic template. **(c)** Frontal bone osteoplasty. **(d)** Endoscopic view of the Draf IIB frontal sinusotomy. The external communication with the osteoplastic approach can be seen.

beginning of the anterior cranial fossa. The identification begins with a downward U-shaped incision starting about 1 cm behind and superiorly to the middle turbinate insertion on the lateral nasal wall, going up to the roof of the nasal fossa, anteriorly to the olfactory fissure (i.e., olfactory cleft), and then turning down on the septum. The mucosa is detached until the first olfactory fiber is identified. The bone lying anterior to that point can be safely drilled with a diamond burr, proceeding upwards until the frontal sinus floor is perforated. Then the natural

ostium can be connected to this perforation and the anterior portion of the middle turbinate is trimmed; thus, creating a large frontal access. The mucosa is pulled out and the underlying bone drilled.

In a Draf type III sinusotomy (modified Lothrop procedure or median drainage), the contralateral frontal sinus floor is removed to create wide exposure of the frontal sinuses, using the two-nostrils and four-hands technique to reach the lateral or superior regions of the sinus. Identification of the first olfactory fiber is now bilateral. The upper third of the anterior portion of the nasal septum is then removed using backbiting forceps and the frontal floor is drilled anteriorly and in between the two fibers. Intersinus septations are also removed. At the end of the operation, the "frontal T" formed by the septum and cribriform plate is created with the residual middle turbinates.[25,26]

If the tumor extends to a supraorbital cell with limited lateral extension, the exposure may be increased by laterally displacing the orbital soft-tissue contents after coagulating and sectioning the anterior ethmoidal artery (before drilling the upper part of the lamina papyracea).[27]

Type 4 Combined Endoscopic Resection with a Frontal Osteoplastic Approach for Inverted Papilloma

A type 4 approach consists of the combination of one of the previous types of endoscopic endonasal resection combined with a frontal osteoplastic flap (▶ Fig. 12.9). This procedure is indicated when there is massive frontal sinus involvement, especially in patients with a hyperpneumatized frontal sinus or within a large pneumatized supraorbital cell. A coronal incision is carried 1 cm behind the hairline from a point just anterior to the tragus to a mirror image point on the opposite one. Benefits in terms of contracture and cosmesis are achieved by shaping the incision with an anterior curve, the so-called "gull wing." Raney clips are applied to the wound edges for hemostasis. The

scalp flap is raised by blunt dissection in the subgaleal plane. In this step, it is important not to harm the supraorbital and supratrochlear nerves anteriorly or the temporal branch of the facial nerve laterally. Once the frontal region is adequately exposed, the periosteum is incised preserving wider margins than the bone window to provide a blood supply to the osseous flap. To determine the borders of the sinus, a template obtained from a 6-foot Caldwell view radiograph and preoperatively sterilized is applied to the frontal bone using the supraorbital rims for alignment, and its outline is marked. Using an oscillating saw, the frontal sinus is perforated trying to avoid accidental dural injuries. Once the lesion is removed, the attachment in the sinus bone is drilled to obtain greater radicality. The frontal sinus should not be obliterated after removal of inverted papillomas to facilitate postoperative endoscopic monitoring. The osteoplastic flap is then repositioned and fixed with titanium microplates. The procedure ends with suture of the periosteum/galea using 3–0 absorbable suture and stapling of the skin.

Special Considerations–Sphenoid Sinus Involvement

Inverted papillomas of the sphenoid sinus are rare and their direct contact with vital structures, such as optic nerve, internal carotid artery, or pituitary gland, requires accurate preoperative evaluation (▶ Fig. 12.10). The endoscopic technique is tailored to the extension of

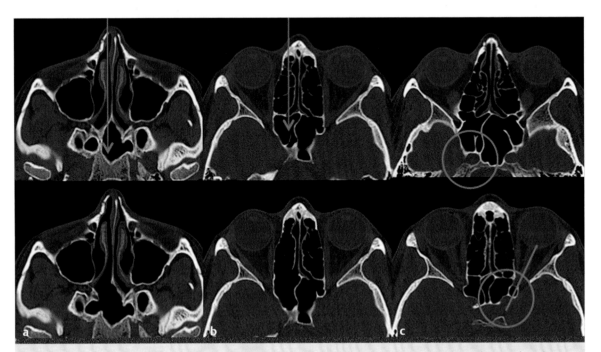

Fig. 12.10 a–c Endoscopic approaches for inverted papillomas of the sphenoid sinus. **(a)** Transnasal paraseptal approach to the sphenoid sinus. **(b)** Transethmoidal approach to the sphenoid sinus. **(c)** Vital structures adjacent to the sphenoid sinus. Internal carotid artery and optic nerve.

the tumor and the different anatomical variations of the sinus (sellar, presellar, or conchal-type pneumatization of the sphenoid sinus). The sphenoid sinus can be approached by a transethmoidal or a trans-ethmoidal-pterygoidal-sphenoidal (TEPS) route since the transnasal or direct paraseptal route does not allow adequate control of the lateral recess of the sphenoid sinus. When the tumor modifies the bony walls, it is necessary to remove the mucosa from critical areas such as the optic nerve, opticocarotid recess, sella turcica, internal carotid artery, and cavernous sinus area. Dissecting a tumor that can be associated with a high risk of damaging the optic nerve or internal carotid artery is not justified and should be tailored individually to every single patient. The only anatomical inconvenience in this site is a well-pneumatized pterygoid recess that can be reached only by a TEPS approach. A radical ethmoidectomy allows exposure of the anterior wall of the sphenoid sinus, the orbital apex, and the base of the pterygoid process. The anterior wall of the sphenoid sinus is then removed and the sphenopalatine artery is cauterized with bipolar forceps. Once the pterygopalatine fossa is opened, the vidian canal and foramen rotundum may be identified. The vidian artery is cauterized and the base of the pterygoid as well as the basisphenoid are drilled. A wide contralateral paraseptal approach, drilling of the rostrum to access the sphenoid sinus and removal of the intersphenoidal septum, are included in the procedure. The posterior third of the bony nasal septum is then removed. This contralateral access permits a wider angle of insertion of the surgical instruments, allowing access to the most lateral regions of the sphenoid sinus, while the wider space facilitates the use of a four-hands technique.[28]

Special Considerations–Intracranial or Intraorbital Involvement

Intracranial or orbital involvement is rare and involves two possible conditions: intracranial or orbital extension with or without intradural or periorbital invasion. In both situations, the mass has to be resected from the extranasal compartment and frozen biopsies of the dura or the periorbit must be performed to ascertain tissue invasion; in this case, the pathologic dura or periorbit must be resected. The skull base defect has to be enlarged to permit a resection that produces clear dural margins. Surgical experience in this field has increased in recent years and endoscopic skull base duraplasty of large defects can be performed using a multilayer technique using autologous free grafts such as fascia lata and septal cartilage, alone or combined with vascularized flaps like the nasoseptal flap, after drilling the bone around the defect to obtain a smooth and regular surface and undermining the dura from the intracranial skull base bone.[29,30]

12.1.4 Postoperative Care and Follow-up

The aim of the operation should be the complete removal of the lesion with tumor-free margins and the creation of a large sinonasal cavity that is easy to inspect endoscopically during the follow-up. At the end of the surgery, nasal packing is placed in the nasal fossa. On the second postoperative day, the packing is removed and endonasal endoscopic medication is performed. Hospitalization lasts approximately 4 days.

All patients receive antibiotic therapy with amoxicillin–clavulanate at a dose of 3 g/day for 10 days and steroid therapy with deflazacort 30 mg for 5 days reducing the dose to 7.5 mg (total 15 days), or prednisone 25 mg reducing the dose to 6.25 mg. After removal of the packing, irrigations with saline solution twice a day are recommended for at least 1 month. The first medication is performed 3 weeks after the discharge. Subsequently, the patients are followed by endoscopic examinations every 4 months during the first postoperative year then every 6 months for at least 4 years and once a year thereafter. Since recurrences have been reported several years after the primary surgery, a lengthy follow-up is recommended.[4,16]

Whenever sectioning of the nasolacrimal duct is performed, irrigation of the residual lacrimal pathway is performed at the end of surgery, after removal of the nasal packing, and 15 days later to preserve its patency. A lacrimal stent is not required during primary procedures. In the presence of postoperative epiphora, an endoscopic dacryocystorhinostomy may be performed.[16]

Postoperative MRI or CT scan is performed: (1) when a sinus previously involved by the lesion is not endoscopically accessible due to scar tissue (every 6 months for the first 2 years, and then once a year for the following 3 years); (2) in symptomatic patients; (3) when a residual or recurrent lesion has been histologically documented; or (4) when synchronous invasive SCC is detected histologically (every 4 months for the first year, then every 6 months for the following 4 years).[16,31]

12.1.5 Complications

Complications may be classified as early or late. In a recent manuscript reporting 212 patients treated with a purely endoscopic approach or endoscopic combined with frontal osteoplastic flap approach, we observed a total of 20 complications (9.4%) with 8 cases classified as early (3.7%) and 12 cases as late (5.7%). A review of the literature performed in the same paper revealed that the overall complication rate ranges between 0 to 20% (mean, 6.5%), with early and late complication rates ranging between 0 to 19.6% (mean, 4%) and 0 to 13.9% (mean, 2.5%), respectively.[16]

Immediate postoperative complications may include CSF leaks that have to be intraoperatively identified and treated by endoscopic duraplasty, and postoperative epistaxis that may require endoscopic surgical revision under general anesthesia. On the other hand, delayed complications include the presence of a mucocele usually in the frontal or the maxillary sinus and identified by an MRI performed in symptomatic patients or occasionally in asymptomatic patients who undergo MRI due to scar tissue formation obscuring the view of the previously involved sinus. The treatment of choice is endoscopic marsupialization.

Postsaccal lacrimal obstruction is another late complication due to scar-tissue formation. Endoscopic endonasal dacryocystorhinostomy must include a lacrimal stent that is kept for 1 month. Lastly, endoscopic revision surgery may be needed for rhinosinusitis (usually frontal or maxillary) that is unresponsive to medical therapy.[16]

12.1.6 Conclusions

Endoscopic endonasal resection can now be considered the gold standard in the treatment of the vast majority of inverted papillomas. The modern approach for the treatment of this tumor is outlined in the following guidelines: MRI is fundamental to establish a differential diagnosis; multiple biopsies are advocated for histopathological confirmation; subperiosteal removal of the lesion with frozen sections to obtain free margins of resection; endoscopic follow-up and, in selected cases, postoperative MRI. Thanks to this protocol, the rates of recurrence/persistence and complications have been significantly reduced.

Pearls and Pitfalls

- Three histologic subtypes of sinonasal papilloma can be identified: exophytic or fungiform papilloma, columnar cell papilloma, and inverted papilloma.
- Inverted papilloma displays a prevalent pattern of growth toward the underlying stroma, without any sign of transgression of the basement membrane.
- Endoscopically, a diagnosis of inverted papilloma is strongly suggested by the presence of a single or multiple unilateral polyps with multiple digitations and papillary surface.
- Endoscopic removal is the first line of treatment of inverted papilloma, except if the tumor originates or invades the most superior and lateral aspects of the frontal sinus.
- Radical extirpation of the inverted papilloma includes a subperiosteal dissection and subsequent drilling of the underlying bone; thus, effectively removing any remnant and preventing a recurrence.
- Strict follow-up guarantees early detection of residual/recurrent lesions, which may still be amenable to endoscopic resection.

12.2 Juvenile Angiofibroma

Piero Nicolai, Alberto Schreiber, Andrea Bolzoni Villaret, Davide Farina

12.2.1 Introduction

Juvenile angiofibroma (JA) is a benign, highly vascularized lesion that accounts for 0.05% of all head and neck tumors and typically affects young adolescent males. Its distribution worldwide appears to be quite variable, with a higher incidence in India and Egypt than in Europe. Data collected in Denmark indicate an incidence of 0.4 cases per million inhabitants per year.[32]

Upon microscopic examination, JA is composed of a fibrous stroma with scattered, variable-sized vessels without elastic fibers in their walls (► Fig. 12.11). Recent immunohistological and electron microscopic studies have suggested that JA could be considered more a vascular malformation (hamartoma) than a genuine tumor. Schick and colleagues[33] have studied this possibility in detail and postulated that JA may develop from incomplete regression of a branchial artery that arises in embryogenesis between days 22 and 24 and forms a temporary connection between the ventral and dorsal aorta. This artery commonly regresses and forms a vascular plexus that either involutes or may leave remnants, potentially leading to the development of JA at a pubertal age under hormonal stimulation of hormones to the development of JA.

This section reviews the recent advances in diagnosis and treatment of JA, with special reference to the introduction of endoscopic techniques and technological achievements that favored their application. The indications, limitations, and outcomes of an endoscopic approach are also discussed.

12.2.2 Site of Origin and Patterns of Spread

JA is considered to arise in the area of the sphenopalatine foramen, and subsequently spreads to adjacent anatomical sites with two different modalities: growth in areas that offer no (i.e., nasal cavity, nasopharynx) or minor (i.e., pterygopalatine and infratemporal fossa) resistance and erosion through the cortical of the basisphenoid into the cancellous bone. According to the former pattern, the lesion can grow laterally into the pterygopalatine and infratemporal fossa, typically displacing anteriorly the posterior wall of the maxillary sinus (► Fig. 12.12). Further lateral growth may place the lesion in close contact with the temporalis muscle, the masseter muscle, and the soft tissues of the cheek (► Fig. 12.13).

Posterior growth may follow several pathways from a medial to a lateral direction: along the vidian canal back

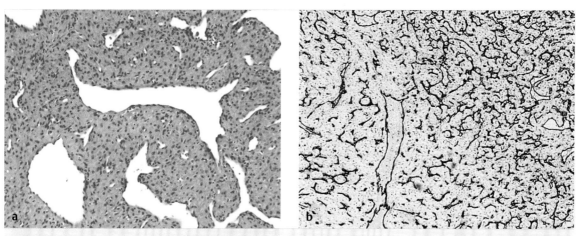

Fig. 12.11 a, b Microscopic appearance of juvenile angiofibroma. (**a**) H&E, and (**b**) immunohistochemistry for CD31. Vessel caliber is extremely variable, the muscular layer of vessels is often absent, and stromal cells usually have a spindle-shaped appearance.

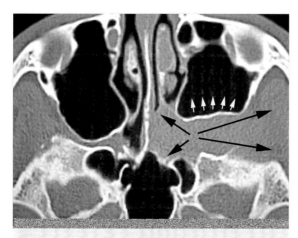

Fig. 12.12 CT scan (bone algorithm reconstruction) performed in an adolescent male for persistent nasal obstruction and facial pain on the left side. An expansile lesion with epicenter in the left sphenopalatine fossa extending medially to the nasal cavity and laterally to the infratemporal fossa (*black arrows*) is visible. The posterior wall of the maxillary sinus is anteriorly displaced (*white arrows*) but uninterrupted.

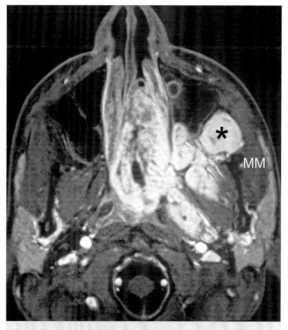

Fig. 12.13 Axial contrast-enhanced MRI: juvenile angiofibroma stage IIIb according to Andrews et al[42] for intracranial extradural extension (not shown) and massive involvement of the buccal (*star*) and masticatory space.
MM, masseter muscle.

to the foramen lacerum and to the genu of the internal carotid artery (ICA), medial to the maxillary nerve and subsequently lateral to the cavernous sinus, or more laterally along the inferior orbital fissure to the apex of the orbit and subsequently intracranially. Once JA has penetrated the medullary portion of the basisphenoid, it spreads inside the bone. The lesion can replace the entire greater wing of the sphenoid bone, with subsequent extension to the middle cranial fossa (▶ Fig. 12.14). Overall, intracranial extension of JA cannot be considered a rare event; however, the observation of intradural growth is exceedingly rare.[34]

12.2.3 Diagnostic Work-up

Physical Examination

Typical symptoms for JA are unilateral nasal obstruction and epistaxis; so these complaints in an adolescent boy should immediately arise suspicion. Progressive growth of the lesion may lead to obstruction of sinus drainage (▶ Fig. 12.15) with symptoms such as headache and facial

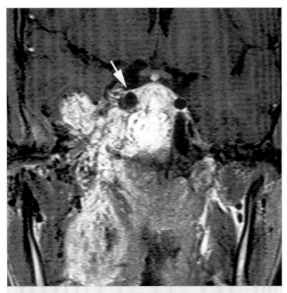

Fig. 12.14 Coronal contrast-enhanced MRI: a huge juvenile angiofibroma with encasement of the right cavernous tract of the internal carotid artery (*arrow*), massive infiltration of the great wing of the sphenoid, and subsequent extension into the middle cranial fossa.

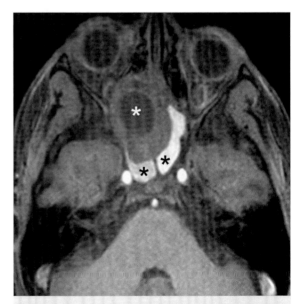

Fig. 12.15 Plain gadolinium-enhanced T1-weighted MRI: juvenile angiofibroma on the right side invading both sphenoid sinuses and the rostrum. The lesion displays a hypointense cystic component (*white star*); hyperintensity within both sphenoid sinuses (*black stars*) indicates retained blood products.

pain, and/or impairment of Eustachian tube function causing secretory otitis media with conductive hearing loss. Proptosis or swelling of the cheek clearly indicate that the lesion has extended into the orbit or the infratemporal fossa, respectively.

Endoscopy

Endoscopy usually shows a large, lobulated mass bulging behind the tail of the middle turbinate and filling the choana, with a smooth surface, clearly exhibiting signs of hypervascularization (▶ Fig. 12.16). Biopsy is not recommended, as it would expose the patient to an undue risk of massive hemorrhage.

Cross-sectional Imaging

Cross-sectional imaging classically depicts a markedly enhancing soft-tissue mass, centered at the level of the pterygopalatine fossa, which presents a characteristic dual pattern of bone involvement (remodeling and destruction); several newly formed vessels can be seen into the lesion and at its periphery. Both CT and MRI can equally demonstrate these findings. However, the latter is by far superior in showing cancellous bone invasion and, in lesions invading the middle cranial fossa, in assessing its relationships with the cavernous sinus and the dura.

Analyzing the imaging pattern, the differential diagnosis may include hemangiopericytoma, lobular capillary hemangioma, and paraganglioma. Nonetheless, all these

lesions are characterized by different patterns of growth and age distribution.

Identification of the pattern of vascularization is another important aspect that helps to select the most appropriate surgical strategy. Although some information may be obtained (or indirectly inferred) with angio-MRI, the complete map of all feeders (and their preoperative embolization) requires digital subtraction angiography. Generally, the internal maxillary and ascending pharyngeal arteries predominantly supply the lesion. When the lesion involves the skull base and comes in close contact with the ICA, the observation of vascular irrigation arising from branches of this vessel, such as the inferomedial trunk or the inferior hypophyseal artery, is common (▶ Fig. 12.17). Bilateral vascularization is seen in 36% of patients[35]; therefore, both carotid systems require angiographic assessment (▶ Fig. 12.18).

Preoperative Embolization

Preoperative embolization was introduced to decrease intraoperative bleeding, which in the most extensive lesions was previously associated with catastrophic hemorrhage, and has nowadays became a standard procedure when an interventional radiologist is available. In the early 1990s, McCombe et al[36] warned that the modifications induced by embolization at the interface between the lesion and adjacent tissues could contribute to incomplete excision. However, refinements in the technique and the availability of new embolization materials have minimized this hazard.

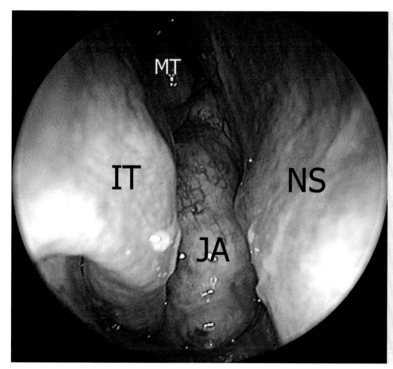

Fig. 12.16 Endoscopic appearance of juvenile angiofibroma (JA): lobulated hypervascularized mass with a smooth surface growing into the right nasal fossa, behind the tail of the middle turbinate and filling the choana.
IT, inferior turbinate; MT, middle turbinate; NS, nasal septum.

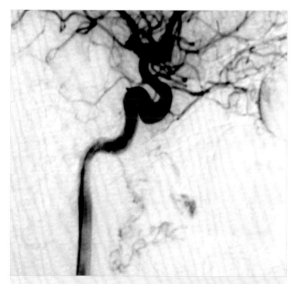

Fig. 12.17 Digital subtraction angiography shows small feeders arising from the internal carotid artery that supply the lesion.

Polyvinyl-alcohol particles are one of the most frequently used materials for embolization, which is usually planned no more than 24 to 48 hours before surgery to avoid the risk of revascularization. Traditionally, embolization is performed on collateral or terminal branches of the external carotid artery to avoid the unacceptable risk of neurologic sequelae arising from treatment of small feeders supplied by the ICA.

In the attempt to control intraoperative bleeding from these vessels in lesions with extensive skull base involvement, Tran Ba Huy et al[37] introduced a technique of direct embolization through a transnasal or lateral transcutaneous access with a mixture of cyanoacrylate, lipiodol, and tungsten powder. In view of the incidence of severe neurologic complications, described by the same team,[38] this technique has not gained much popularity. However, recent reports on a limited number of patients treated with a new embolic material, Onyx, with properties that seem to prevent its migration, have revived the interest in this procedure.[39,40] Occlusion of the ICA after balloon occlusion test is a another alternative available in the rare instances of lesions completely encircling the vessel (▶ Fig. 12.19).

Although in experienced hands it bears minimal risks of complications, preoperative embolization can be avoided in early-stage JA. In these cases, the sphenopalatine or internal maxillary artery is easily accessible through the posterior wall of the maxillary sinus and can be clipped and sectioned as the first step of the surgical procedure.

12.2.4 Staging Systems

Different staging systems have been proposed with the intent of easing comparison of different series and to stratify patients in relation to different surgical options. Among the proposals of classification made in the pre-endoscopic era, those from Radkowski et al[41] and Andrews

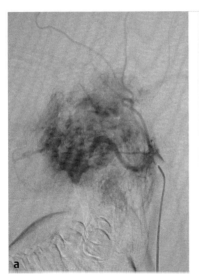
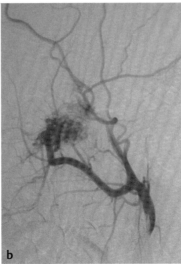

Fig. 12.18 a, b Digital subtraction angiography shows feeders from the homolateral (**a**) and contralateral (**b**) external carotid systems.

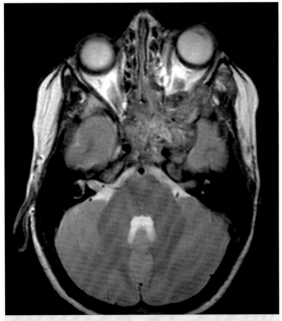

Fig. 12.19 Axial late contrast-enhanced MRI: the left ICA appears encased by the lesion that has also extensive contact with the contralateral ICA.

Table 12.1 Önerci et al staging system for juvenile angiofibroma[43]

Type I	Nose, nasopharyngeal vault, ethmoidal-sphenoidal sinuses, or minimal extension to pterygopalatine fossa
Type II	Maxillary sinus, full occupation of pterygopalatine fossa, extension to the anterior cranial fossa, and limited extension to the infratemporal fossa
Type III	Deep extension into the cancellous bone at the base of the pterygoid or the body and the greater wing of sphenoid, significant lateral extension to the infratemporal fossa or to the pterygoid plates posteriorly or orbital region, cavernous sinus obliteration
Type IV	Intracranial extension between the pituitary gland and internal carotid artery, tumor localization lateral to internal carotid artery, middle fossa extension, and extensive intracranial extension

Table 12.2 Snyderman et al staging system for juvenile angiofibroma[44]

Type I	No significant extension beyond the site of origin and remaining medial to the midpoint of the pterygopalatine space
Type II	Extension to the paranasal sinuses and lateral to the midpoint of the pterygopalatine space
Type III	Locally advanced with skull base erosion or extension to additional extracranial spaces, including orbit and infratemporal fossa, no residual vascularity following embolization
Type IV	Skull base erosion, orbit, infratemporal fossa Residual vascularity
Type V	Intracranial extension, residual vascularity M: medial extension L: lateral extension

et al[42] have been more extensively used. As expected, the staging systems recently suggested by Önerci et al[43] (▶ Table 12.1) and Snyderman et al[44] (▶ Table 12.2) provide more precise differentiation between lesions amenable to endoscopic surgery and those requiring an external or combined approach. Interestingly, the latter includes residual vascularity after embolization as a further classification parameter in addition to extent of the lesion.

12.2.5 Surgical Strategies and Perioperative Management

Surgery is unanimously considered the ideal treatment for JA. The advent of endoscopic surgery has revolutionized its treatment, which was traditionally based on anterior (transpalatal, transpharyngeal, transfacial through lateral rhinotomy, midfacial degloving, or Le Fort I osteotomy) and lateral (infratemporal and subtemporal) approaches. There is general agreement that lesions involving the nasal cavity, nasopharynx, sphenoid sinus, and pterygopalatine fossa can be appropriately resected through an endoscopic approach. Furthermore, recent experiences suggest that this technique can be successfully used even in JAs extending to the infratemporal fossa, orbit, and/or parasellar region by surgeons who have acquired the necessary expertise.[45,46] In cases with large infiltration of the skull base, extensive vascular contribution from the ICA, or encasement of the artery itself the need to associate an external approach, anterior or lateral basically according to the relationship of the lesion with the ICA and the surgeon's preference, should always be communicated and discussed with the patient. Well-known advantages of endoscopic approaches include the absence of scars, preservation of the anterior bony wall of the maxilla, the possibility with angled endoscopes to achieve excellent visualization of all sinus recesses, and finally a decreased morbidity and hospitalization time.

The key principle when approaching a JA endoscopically is to expose the lesion as extensively as possible without touching its surface so that bleeding is minimized. This is commonly achieved by resecting the middle turbinate and performing ethmoidectomy, sphenoidotomy, and a large middle antrostomy extended posteriorly to expose the sphenopalatine foramen. Resection of the posterior third of the nasal septum enhances the exposure of the nasopharyngeal portion of the lesion and enables easier use of the "two-handed" technique. The next step is removal of the posterior wall of the maxillary sinus, which is laterally widened in relation to the lateral extent of the lesion into the pterygopalatine/infratemporal fossa. Not infrequently in large-volume lesions, the posterior wall of the maxillary sinus is pushed forward and the JA extensively fills the sinus or the infratemporal fossa may be completely occupied. In these situations, the surgeon can improve lateral exposure of the lesion by resorting to the so-called Sturman-Canfield operation (or endonasal Denker), a procedure that allows endoscopic resection of the medial part of the anterior maxillary wall through the nostril, which is exposed through a vertical incision at the level of the piriform aperture, or, alternatively, by combining a second endoscopic approach through the anterior wall of the maxillary sinus.

Another important principle when dealing with large-volume lesions is that resection can rarely be achieved in a single bloc. In these situations, it is preferable to disassemble the lesion by first removing the nasal-nasopharyngeal portion, and subsequently addressing the projections deeply located in the infratemporal fossa and retropterygoid area. In our experience, the use of a diode laser is extremely helpful to minimize bleeding when sectioning the lesion. The cooperation of an assistant who helps the surgeon to release the JA from the adjacent soft tissues of the infratemporal fossa and retropterygoid area by gentle traction on the lesion itself is another key point to maintain a proper cleavage plain. Special attention must be paid to the identification of the maxillary nerve, which has to be dissected off the lesion and preserved. Whenever a portion of JA is in close contact with the ICA, it is addressed as a last step after achieving wide exposure of the critical area. The use of intraoperative navigation and Doppler is extremely beneficial to precisely identify the artery and avoid its injury. The procedure is completed by extensive drilling of the basisphenoid, which has been shown to markedly decrease the likelihood of leaving residual pathologic tissue behind.[47] In the resection of advanced lesions, substantial bleeding, either venous or arterial, may occur. Therefore, the cooperation of an anesthesiologist with special expertise in endoscopic skull base surgery is mandatory and the availability of a cell salvage machine and of any material (absorbable gelatin powder, sponge oxidized regenerated cellulose, microfibrillar collagen, or fibrin or synthetic sealants)[48] that helps the surgeon to control bleeding is urged. Until the intervention is completed, the presence of an interventional radiologist in the hospital who could take care of an uncontrolled ICA bleeding is another precautionary measure that should be considered. At the end of the procedure, light packing is placed in the nasal cavities, which is left in place for 24 to 48 hours.

Antibiotic therapy in the form of a wide-spectrum cephalosporin is perioperatively administered starting the day before surgery and is continued until the nasal packing is removed. Cleaning of the surgical cavity is performed under endoscopic control to remove clots and fibrin, and the patient is instructed to perform daily irrigations of the sinonasal cavity with saline solution to moisten secretions and minimize crust formation.

12.2.6 Postoperative Surveillance

Endoscopic examination has limited value in the identification of residual/recurrent JA in view of the submucosal pattern of growth of the lesion. MRI examination is therefore strongly recommended. Based on the experience reported by Kania et al,[49] who suggested obtaining a baseline CT in the immediate postoperative period for early identification of any suspicious residual disease, we have begun to scan patients with MRI the same day or the day after removal of nasal packing. With this timing, MRI does not reveal any of the inflammatory changes that, after 3 to 4 months, frequently challenge the differentiation between small residual lesions and active scar tissue. To date, none of our patients who had an early postoperative MRI have shown any residual lesion even at subsequent MRI examination, which is obtained every 6 months for at least 3 years. Persistent JA, either intentionally unresected due to unacceptable surgical hazard or detected by routine follow-up scans, needs close surveillance with contrasted MRI to assess its possible growth before establishing that treatment is actually required.

12.2.7 Outcome

Comparison of the results using external and endoscopic techniques is hindered by several biases related to stratification by staging and follow-up methodology. However, the recurrence rate of series with a consistent number of patients reported in the 1990s and treated with an external technique is around 36 to 40%.[50,51] More recently, Danesi et al[34] demonstrated that a transfacial approach (through lateral rhinotomy or midfacial degloving) can lead to excellent results, with only 13.5 and 18.2% of residual disease in lesions with extracranial and intracranial extent, respectively.

Endoscopic surgery is associated with a recurrence rate ranging from 0%[50,51] in series including only small/intermediate size lesions to 19.1%[45] when more advanced tumors are included. In our series of 46 patients, endoscopic resection achieved good results not only in stage I–II but also in stage IIIA–B lesions, according to Andrews et al,[42] with an overall rate of residual disease of 8.6%.[46] Interestingly, in spite of the fact that we extensively drilled the basisphenoid adjacent to the lesion, all four residual lesions, which were diagnosed by MRI within 24 months, were located at this site (▶ Fig. 12.20). This observation reinforces the recommendation to extend drilling well beyond the apparent margin of infiltration.

12.2.8 Is There Any Role for Nonsurgical Treatments?

Traditionally, the use of radiotherapy and even chemotherapy has been offered with the intent to provide an alternative treatment option in residual JAs for which surgery was considered to be associated with unacceptable morbidity.

Radiotherapy

The role of radiotherapy is still debated in view of the possible risk of development of sarcomatoid degeneration

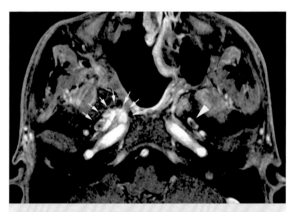

Fig. 12.20 Axial contrast-enhanced MRI with fat saturation performed 6 months after surgery: suspected persistent juvenile angiofibroma (*arrows*) at the level of the root of the pterygoid process in close proximity with the third branch of trigeminal nerve (detectable as a hypointense spot) and the anterior foramen lacerum. The *arrowhead* on the contralateral side indicates the position of the foramen ovale.

or radioinduced neoplasms in subsequent decades. However, it should be kept in mind that low dose (30–36 Gy) radiotherapy has been shown to be effective in cases of advanced or recurrent lesions deemed not amenable to complete resection with acceptable morbidity.[52] Furthermore, the availability of new techniques of stereotactic radiosurgery (i.e., Gamma Knife, Cyberknife) can optimize irradiation of the target volume by sparing uninvolved structures and may decrease potential morbidity. In our opinion, the indications for radiotherapy should be limited to residual lesions in critical areas, not amenable to a surgical resection and that have been clearly demonstrated to increase in size.

Chemotherapy

The first experience with chemotherapy dates to the 1980s, when successful results were obtained with two different drug schedules, including doxorubicin and dacarbazine, or vincristine, dactinomycin, and cyclophosphamide.[53] However, very few reports have appeared subsequently in the literature.[54]

In view of the well-known hormone dependence of JA, different forms of treatments based on estrogens or testosterone receptor blockers have been proposed. In a recent study, flutamide, a drug belonging to the latter class, was used as an adjuvant treatment to decrease the size of the lesion before surgery in advanced stage JAs. Volume reduction correlated with serum testosterone levels, and regression of the lesion was observed only in postpubertal patients.[55]

- Features of a JA include: (1) an epicenter at the level of the pterygopalatine fossa from where the lesion tends to spread along skull base foramina, fissures, and canals as well as the medullary portion of the basisphenoid; (2) high degree of vascularization arising from either the external or the ICA; (3) intimate and tight adherences to the posterosuperior wall of the nasopharynx.
- Endoscopy commonly shows a large, lobulated mass with a smooth and highly vascular surface bulging behind the tail of the middle turbinate and filling the posterior choana.
- Diagnostic work-up should usually include a contrasted CT or MRI. Angiography is only recommended as an interventional tool for preoperative, embolization of the tumor.
- The endoscopic approach is a safe and effective technique that allows removal of small and intermediate-sized JAs with low morbidity. Removal of large and invasive angiofibromas is possible but should only be entertained by experienced teams.
- Key principles to approach a JA endoscopically include:
  - To expose the lesion as extensively as possible without manipulating its surface so that bleeding is minimized
  - When dealing with large-volume lesions it is preferable to disassemble the lesion by first removing the nasal-nasopharyngeal portion, and subsequently addressing the projections located deep in the infratemporal fossa and retropterygoid area.
- Use of a diode laser is helpful to minimize bleeding when sectioning the lesion.
- Use of intraoperative navigation and Doppler is beneficial to precisely identify the ICA and avoid its injury.
- Recently suggested staging systems by Önerci et al[43] and Snyderman et al[44] provide the best differentiation between lesions amenable to endoscopic surgery and those requiring an external or combined approach.

represents about 3% of all malignant tumors involving the nasal cavity.[57] It can occur over a broad age range but shows a bimodal age distribution in the second and fifth decades.

Histologically, ENB consists of small round cell tumors of neuroendocrine origin, arising from precursor cells of the nasal neuroepithelium. Immunohistochemical staining is positive for synaptophysin, S-100, chromogranin, and neuron-specific enolase. It has a predilection for cervical lymph node metastasis, with an incidence that ranges from 5% at presentation to around 23% at long-term follow-up.[58] ENB also has the potential for distant metastasis, reported to be synchronous at presentation in about 6% of patients.[59]

Complete surgical resection (▶ Fig. 12.21) followed by adjuvant radiation therapy is considered standard treatment in most studies.[60] However, some institutions report success with alternative treatment paradigms, including surgery without radiation.[61] Chemotherapy has been introduced in the therapeutic armamentarium, although it is not recommended for routine treatment of ENB, but rather as part of a multimodality treatment in patients with advanced or metastatic disease or for palliation of terminal patients.[62]

Symptoms are related to the sites and invasion of the tumor, but initially are nonspecific. Presenting features may include unilateral nasal obstruction, epistaxis, rhinorrhea, sinus pain, or proptosis.

The Kadish staging system,[63] based on tumor extension, has been widely accepted and has proven to have a prognostic relevance. ENBs limited to the nasal cavity are classified as stage A, those involving the nasal cavity and extending into the paranasal sinuses are staged as B, and stage C includes those that spread beyond the nasal cavity and paranasal sinuses.

At our institution, the treatment policy for ENB has been a resection via either a traditional craniofacial approach or, increasingly more frequent, an endoscopic endonasal approach followed by adjuvant radiation

12.3 Esthesioneuroblastoma

Matteo de Notaris, Isam Alobid, Joaquim Enseñat, Manuel Bernal-Sprekelsen

12.3.1 Introduction

Esthesioneuroblastoma (ENB) is a rare malignant neoplasm that arises from the olfactory neuroepithelium situated at the roof of the nasal cavity, cribriform plate, upper portion of superior turbinate, and of the nasal septum.[56] Initially described by Berger and Luc in 1924, ENB

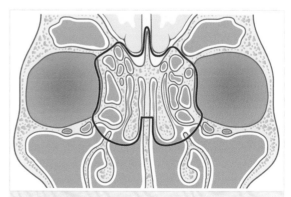

Fig. 12.21 Schematic drawing of the area to be resected endoscopically in extended esthesioneuroblastomas.

therapy (for high-grade and locally advanced tumors). The aim of this section is to analyze the natural history, diagnosis, surgical technique, multimodality treatment, and prognosis of ENB based on our experience and a review of the literature.

12.3.2 Imaging Features

ENBs are slow-growing masses that probably begin as relative small lesions in the superior olfactory recess, initially involving the anterior and middle ethmoid cells unilaterally. As they grow, ENBs tend to destroy surrounding bone, and can extend in any direction within the skull base. This invasion may extend superiorly into the ante-

rior cranial fossa, laterally into the orbit, and across midline into the contralateral nasal cavity. They can also obstruct the ostia of paranasal sinuses resulting in retention of secretions and opacification of the sinus in the imaging. Particular attention should be paid to the presence of cervical and retropharyngeal nodal metastases, which are present in 10 to 44% of cases at diagnosis.

A CT scan (▶ Fig. 12.22a) is particularly useful in assessing bone destruction, although it cannot distinguish olfactory neuroblastomas from other malignancies that arise in the same region. CT shows a homogeneous, soft-tissue attenuation mass with relatively homogeneous enhancement. Using this imaging technique, focal calcifications can occasionally be present and easily recognized.[64]

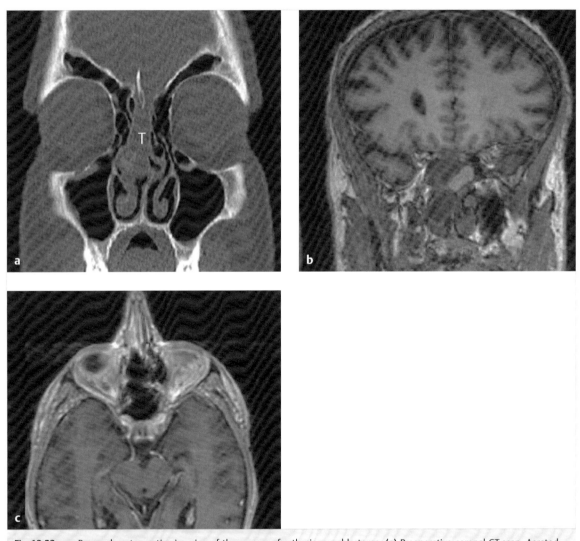

Fig. 12.22 a–c Pre- and postoperative imaging of three cases of esthesioneuroblastoma. **(a)** Preoperative coronal CT scan. Aerated maxillary and frontal sinuses. Kadish stage A tumor involving mainly the right nasal fossa at the olfactory cleft, reaching the skull base (cribriform plate) with no intracranial involvement (confirmed by MRI!). **(b)** Preoperative coronal MRI section (in T1) at the level of the planum sphenoidale showing invasion of the sphenoid sinus and partial erosion of the bony skull base with involvement of the dura in a Kadish stage C esthesioneuroblastoma. **(c)** Postoperative MRI showing complete removal.

MRI (▶ Fig. 12.22**b, c**) in T1 and T2 sequences displays ENB as a heterogeneous mass of intermediate signal. Gadolinium enhancement is variable, although usually is moderate to intense. When intracranial extension is present, cystic degeneration between the main tumor and the overlying brain is often present. This may be helpful in distinguishing ENB from other entities. The margins of these cysts sometimes enhance.[64]

12.3.3 Histologic Findings

ENB has a characteristic appearance, containing discrete nests, trabeculae and nodules of tumor cells, fibrous material, and prominent collections of stromal blood vessels. Uniform tumor cells have small, dark round, or oval nuclei, lack nucleoli, and show little cytoplasm. Its vascularity may be prominent. The eosinophilic fibrous material consists of fine, pale-pink fibrils resembling neural tissues, and may show immunohistochemical staining with antibody to S-100 protein. But the only histological feature of prognostic importance is the presence or absence of tumor necrosis. Cytological atypia and mitotic rate show little correlation to long-term outcome.

Histological differentiation is sometimes more difficult because these tumors exhibit little or no differentiation and can often be mistaken for other malignancies such as undifferentiated carcinoma, melanoma, lymphoma, or sarcoma. Its aggressive biologic behavior, which is usually reflected in its histologic grade, is characterized by cryptic submucosal spread, local recurrence, atypical distant metastases, and poor long-term prognosis.

12.3.4 Surgery

Combined transfacial and neurosurgical approaches have been the preferred techniques for a craniofacial resection because they allow an en bloc removal of the tumor and cribriform plates, protection of the brain, and assessment of intracranial tumor growth.

12.3.5 Principles

The oncologic principles of anterior craniofacial resection, as described by van Buren et al,[65] involve an en bloc resection of the tumor, including the ethmoid sinuses, superior nasal septum, and floor of the anterior cranial fossa, corresponding to the interorbital area (i.e., anterior craniofacial resection) or extended laterally to include part of the bony orbit or its soft-tissue contents (i.e., anterolateral craniofacial resection).

The external approach starts with a classic bicoronal scalp flap. Care is taken not to injure the frontotemporal branch of facial nerve. A large frontal based pericranial flap is then raised for the skull base reconstruction. A large bifrontal craniotomy with the base of the skull immediately above the superior orbital rim is performed and a free bone flap is then elevated. In the majority of cases, the tumor is found projecting from the cribriform plate of the ethmoid bone. If brain invasion is demonstrated, an intradural subfrontal approach is then performed. Two separate dural openings are realized on both sides, with the base of the opening being at the orbital roof. At midline, two ligatures are passed through the falx to safely cut the sinus on its anterior margin along with the falx to reach its inferior border. Finally, to get access to the anterior skull base region the frontal lobes are gently retracted; thus permitting the visualization of the floor of the anterior cranial fossa.

A bilateral subfrontal approach allows exposure of the entire surface of the anterior cranial base, offering the best view over the suprachiasmatic area. The optic nerves, the chiasm, the internal carotid artery and its bifurcation, and the anterior circle of Willis are under a symmetric and panoramic view.

Subsequently, a lateral rhinotomy incision is made, followed by a total ethmoidectomy and exposure of the whole skull base from below. This enables resection of the tumor en bloc.

12.3.6 Expanded Endoscopic Endonasal Approach to the Anterior Skull Base: Surgical Technique

Continuous technological and surgical development in functional endoscopic sinus surgery[63,66] led to a progressive reduction of the invasiveness associated with transcranial and craniofacial procedures to the anterior skull base during recent decades.

The endoscopic approach for endoscopic removal of ENB is the transcribriform module, which can be performed on one or on both sides (▶ Fig. 12.23 and ▶ Fig. 12.24). The limits of this approach are: anteriorly, the posterior wall of the frontal sinuses; laterally, the medial wall of the orbit; and posteriorly, the anterior part of the planum sphenoidale at the level of the posterior ethmoidal arteries.

As in all expanded endoscopic approaches, the first step to be planned and performed is to prepare the necessary flap for the skull base reconstruction. Thus, the procedure starts with the creation of a pedicled nasoseptal flap (Hadad-Bassagaisteguy flap),[67] which is used at the end of the procedure to reconstruct the anterior skull base. The flap can be stored in the maxillary sinus or in the nasopharynx during the subsequent tumor removal. We prefer to place this flap in the maxillary sinus to minimize possible visual interference of the target area. In cases of septal tumor infiltration a contralateral nasoseptal flap or one from the lateral nasal wall can be elevated[68] for the anterior skull base reconstruction.

Then, the first olfactory filament is identified at the top of the olfactory cleft, which delineates the posterior limit

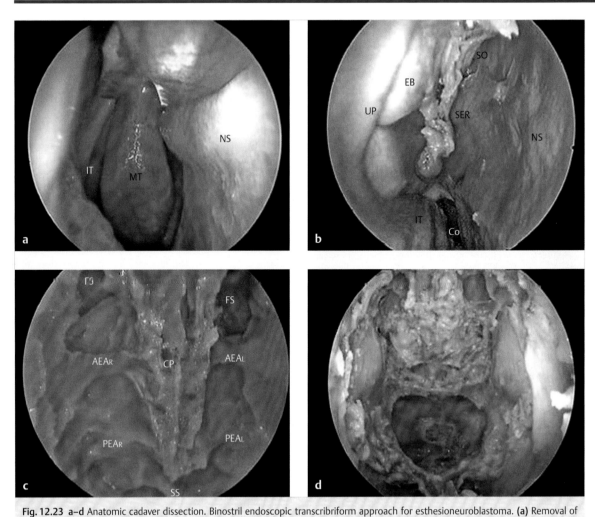

Fig. 12.23 a–d Anatomic cadaver dissection. Binostril endoscopic transcribriform approach for esthesioneuroblastoma. **(a)** Removal of the right middle turbinate. **(b)** Situation after removal of the right middle turbinate. **(c)** Full bilateral endoscopic exposure of the cribriform plate from the sphenoid sinus (posteriorly) to the recess of both frontal sinuses. **(d)** Situation of the anterior skull base at the cribriform plate after drilling of the planum sphenoidale (posteriorly) to the frontal sinus anteriorly.

AEA, anterior ethmoidal artery; AEAl, left anterior ethmoidal artery; AEAr, right anterior ethmoidal artery; Co, choana; CP, cribriform plate; EB, ethmoidal bulla; FS, frontal sinus; IT, inferior turbinate; MT, middle turbinate; NS, nasal septum; PEAl, left posterior ethmoidal artery; PEAr, right posterior ethmoidal artery; SER, sphenoethmoid recess; SO, sphenoid ostium; SS, sphenoid sinus; UP, uncinate process.

of the frontal sinus drilling. A Draf type IIB or a Draf type III is performed depending on whether the tumor has a unilateral or bilateral extension, respectively.

Tumor resection is performed piecemeal to allow a progressive centrifugal exposure of the margins, which are: septum superiorly and medially, the cribriform plate and ethmoidal roof superiorly, and the superior aspect of the lamina papyracea laterally. Necessarily, the entire anterior skull base needs to be skeletonized, which has to include a total anterior and posterior ethmoidectomy, removal of the middle and superior turbinate until the anterior aspect of the planum sphenoidale is reached, the superior aspects of affected septum (mucoperichondrium) are resected, the ethmoidal roof is completely exposed, and at least the superior aspect of the papyracea

needs to be resected. The cribriform plate subsequent resection is included after ligating or coagulating the ethmoidal arteries. In complete bilateral transcribriform resections the bone of the skull base needs to be drilled at the level of the first olfactory filament and the limit to the planum sphenoidale transversally and along the lateral aspect of the ethmoidal roof to achieve a quadrangular exposure of the dura of the anterior skull base.

When the dura is opened it is important to identify the falx cerebri anteriorly to coagulate bleeding from the sagittal sinus. Once the falx is detached from the crista galli the dura is resected together with the tumor and the olfactory bulb. Tumors involving the cribriform plate bilaterally need to have the mucosa from the anterior and posterior ethmoidal cells resected bilaterally for

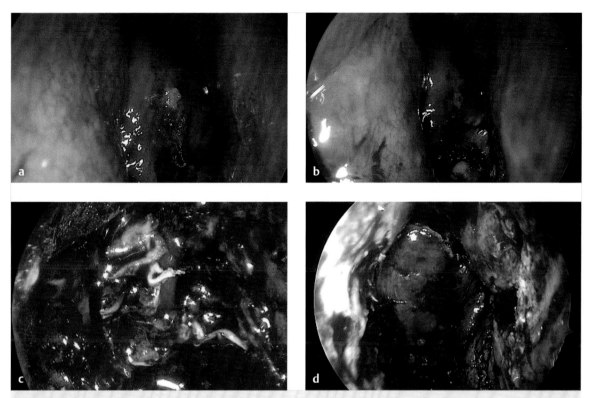

Fig. 12.24 a–d Intraoperative situation of a transcribriform approach for esthesioneuroblastoma. **(a)** Endoscopic view of a tumor in the right nasal fossa located between the nasal septum (to the right) and the middle turbinate (to the left) in the olfactory cleft. **(b)** Situation after a biopsy of the tumor for intraoperative confirmation. **(c)** Situation after tumor removal with opened anterior skull base and subsequent CSF leak (with fluorescein dye). Note the white fibers corresponding to olfactory filae. Frozen sections of the dura confirmed that it was not infiltrated. **(d)** Nasoseptal flap covering the anterior skull base defect.

histopathological analysis. Additional margins include the anterior septum and the mucosa from the inferior aspect of the posterior table of the frontal sinus.

While waiting for frozen sections of the soft-tissue margins, one can drill down the crista galli to facilitate the skull base reconstruction, which is performed at least with one or two layers of fascia lata (intra and extradural) covered by the nasoseptal flap.

12.3.7 Outcomes

The treatment of ENB includes surgery, primary radiation therapy, or combined surgery and radiation. Some authors also advocate chemotherapy.

In the following paragraphs, we will focus on the outcomes after endoscopic endonasal surgery. During recent decades, endoscopic endonasal surgery has increasingly become an accepted modality for the surgical treatment of sinonasal malignancies. Recently, a thorough review on the use of endoscopic techniques in the treatment of benign and malignant tumors in the paranasal sinuses and the anterior skull base has been published, including ENB[69]; however, the literature is sparse.[70,71]

Unger et al[72] described 14 patients who underwent endoscopic surgery and postoperative radiotherapy. Median follow-up was 58 months. Five patients had recurrence of disease (36%) at a mean of 36.6 months after combined endoscopic and radiotherapeutic treatment. At the time of publication, all patients were alive and at least 13 had no evidence of disease. In addition, one patient had a postoperative CSF leak requiring a second surgery and another patient developed chronic bilateral frontal sinusitis.

Castelnuovo et al[73] reported a series of 10 patients in whom a negative margin resection was achieved. Nine of the patients received postoperative radiotherapy and one received adjuvant chemotherapy. None of the patients showed local recurrence; however, one patient had neck metastasis 21 months after surgery and underwent subsequent neck surgery plus radiotherapy. With a median follow-up of 37 months, all patients were alive without disease.

In a study combining the experiences with endoscopic endonasal resection of ENB at the University of Pittsburgh and University of Miami,[71] 23 patients were retrospectively reviewed (19 patients had primary tumors and 4 were undergoing surgery for recurrent tumors). Complete removal with negative intraoperative margins was achieved in 17/19 of the patients undergoing surgery for primary tumors. Mean follow-up for the primary cases was 45.2 months, and all patients except one with cervical metastasis had no evidence of disease at their last follow-up.

12.3.8 Discussion

Staging

Most authors use the Kadish staging system,[63] as it reflects a prognosis. The main shortcoming of the Kadish classification is that the definition of stage C is too broad. Recognizing this inadequacy, other classifications have been proposed, such as that by Dulgerov and Calcaterra (based on the classical tumor size, node involvement, and metastasis status [TNM] system).[58]

Currently, there is no universally accepted epidemiologic, molecular, or pathological prognostic indicator; although it seems that the histopathologic grading described by Hyams et al[74] could offer some value in predicting survival.[75,76,77] Hirose et al describe a better survival linked to a high degree of S-100 immunopositivity and a low (< 10%) Ki-67 labeled index[78]; however, others have not corroborated this finding.

Controversies

Treatment of the Olfactory Bulb

It is said that the olfactory bulb and overlying dura should be removed with the specimen; however, there is no clear evidence to support the assertion that the whole bulb should be removed.[79] It is also a matter of discussion whether in unilateral tumors a bilateral (thus more radical) approach should be performed.

Purely Endoscopic Approach

Over the last several decades, the surgical management of ENB has undergone significant change. Cranial base surgery, developed in the 1950s, is a rapidly changing field. There has been a significant evolution over this time, leading to a continuing decrease in morbidity and mortality. ENBs that were previously treated via open craniotomy and facial incisions can now be treated endoscopically through the nose. Indications for these minimally invasive surgeries continue to grow parallel to our ability to repair the defects that separate the intracranial compartment from the sinonasal tract. Separation of the cranial cavity from the sinonasal tract after an open approach is accomplished through the use of pericranial flaps and free microvascular flaps. Novel procedures are also employed to close those defects that are created endoscopically, including pedicled nasoseptal flaps.[80,81,82,83] In addition, technologi-

cal advances such as intraoperative navigation allow surgeons to pinpoint and avoid critical structures, as well as confidently remove parts of the tumor that would otherwise be missed. A review of individual published series demonstrates that there is inconsistency and controversy of surgical techniques with surgeons performing resection of sinonasal tissues only (extracranial resection), removal of bone with preservation of dura (extradural resection), limited dural resections (preservation of olfactory bulb and tract), and complete transdural resection including the olfactory bulb and tract.[83] However, most rhinologists favor an endoscopic surgery supplemented by external beam radiation to the anterior fossa floor, primarily the olfactory bulb region, only if the tumor is early stage, confined to the nasal cavity, or with modest adjacent sinus involvement.

The European Position Paper on Endoscopic Management of Tumors of the Nose, Paranasal Sinuses, and Skull Base[69] has elaborated a list of absolute and relative indications for a pure endoscopic approach of malignant sinonasal tumors for surgeries with a curative intent (▶ Table 12.3).

Treatment of the Neck

Overall, metastases to the cervical lymph nodes develop in about 30% of patients. Because of the rarity of this malignancy, no definitive consensus regarding the optimal treatment has been reached and considerable controversy exists over its optimal management.

Approximately 5% of patients have metastasis to the cervical lymph nodes at presentation. This situation indicates the need for a neck dissection, radiotherapy, or a combination of the two modalities. In the clinical N0 neck, the "wait-and-see" option is a debated issue, as around 23% of patients may develop metastasis in the neck.[58]

However, as they may become clinically apparent at 2 years or more, or after initial treatment, delaying a neck dissection is an accepted option. An important drawback

Table 12.3 Relative and absolute contraindications for the use of endoscopic endonasal resection of malignant sinonasal tumors as a single approach

Relative contraindications	Absolute contraindications
Vascular invasion (internal carotid artery and cavernous sinus) Chiasm invasion Posterior fossa invasion Tumor below vertebra C2	When the following is necessary: • Orbital exenteration • Total or radical maxillectomy (medial maxillectomy is acceptable) Invasion of the skin Involvement of the frontal sinus anterior wall ± lateral recess Dura or brain involvement lateral to the midorbital roof or lateral to optic nerve Brain parenchyma invasion

is the fact that metastatic lymphadenopathy may be associated with the development of distant metastasis.

Long-term Follow-up

There are great variations in treatment for ENB. Some series advocate a protocol with surgery,[84,85] radiotherapy[86] alone, combined preoperative radiotherapy and surgery,[87] or combined surgery and postoperative radiotherapy.[88] Multimodal therapy has been shown to improve survival in these patients. Surgical treatment using craniofacial resection or the expanded endoscopic endonasal approach (particularly for locally contained low-grade tumor) is the treatment of choice. Neoadjuvant radiotherapy appears to be helpful.

When considering whether to proceed with an external or an endoscopic approach it may be helpful to know that a recent meta-analysis suggested that endoscopic surgery had better overall survival (OS) rates compared with open surgery with no significant difference between follow-up times in the endoscopic and open surgery groups.[89] Another important consideration is the absolute need for a long-term follow-up because of the extended interval for recurrent disease. While the 5-year interval is used for other malignant tumors of the head and neck, recurrence of ENB may show up at 10, 15, and even 20 years after treatment[90]; and, unlike most sinonasal malignancies, salvage surgery is possible. Local recurrence is possible in 33 to 50% of cases.[91]

Pearls and Pitfalls

- ENB is a small round cell tumor of neuroendocrine origin, arising from precursor cells of the nasal neuro-epithelium. It accounts for 6% of tumors arising in the nasal cavity and paranasal sinuses.
- ENB may present cervical lymphatics or distant metastasis, at the time of diagnosis (rare) or at long-term follow-up (more common).
- Both the modified Kadish staging system and the Hyams' histopathological classification predict survival.
- A complete surgical resection followed by adjuvant radiation therapy is considered standard treatment.
- Preoperative assessment usually includes both CT and contrasted MRI to respectively assess the tumor interface with the adjacent bones and soft tissues.
- A recent meta-analysis suggests that in selected patients endoscopic endonasal removal of ENB has similar or superior overall survival (OS) rates compared with open approaches.
- Endoscopic endonasal removal of ENB is advocated for Kadish stage A and B tumors as well as in selected cases of Kadish stage C.

12.4 Meningiomas

Nancy McLaughlin, Daniel M. Prevedello, Daniel Kelly, Juan Fernandez-Miranda, Ricardo L. Carrau, Amin B. Kassam

12.4.1 Introduction

Meningiomas account for about 30% of all primary brain tumors, constituting the largest subset of all intracranial tumors.[92] These generally benign lesions represent a heterogeneous group of neoplasms that can arise from various regions of the skull base. Although their natural history and clinical presentation might differ, the treatment goals remain the same regardless of their location: alleviate mass effect and maintain neurological function, while trying to achieve the most definitive resection as possible to prevent recurrence.[93] The management strategy must be individualized, weighing the benefits and risks of each option and considering the patient's preference in trying to achieve these goals.

Multiple skull base approaches have been developed over the years to reach these dural-based lesions. Transcranial skull base procedures may require extensive soft-tissue disruption, significant bone resection, brain retraction, and neurovascular manipulation to gain access to the pathology. Furthermore, traditional lateral transcranial approaches provide limited access to central areas such as the sella, subchiasmatic space, and the area ventral to the brainstem, particularly when the tumor is surrounded by cranial nerves along its perimeter.[94] Recently, many skull base surgery centers have adopted surgical approaches that are tailored to minimize surgical morbidity.[95] In general, the surgeon should perform the most complete tumor resection while maintaining the patient's quality of life by preserving neurologic function. Importantly, the degree of tumor resection should be tempered to minimize morbidity and should not occur at the expense of neurological function when possible; especially in patients with low-grade tumors where prolonged survival is expected.

In general there are four corridors to the reach the skull base: posterolateral, lateral, anterolateral, and anteromedial. During the past decade, numerous anatomical and clinical studies have documented the feasibility and safety of the expanded endonasal approaches (EEAs), which provide access to the ventral skull base via a central anteromedial corridor. As a result, the EEA allows for resection of skull base lesions within the anterior, middle, and posterior cranial fossae, located medial to the carotid in the sagittal plane and lateral to the carotid in the coronal plane[96,97,98,99]. Recent clinical studies have shown that transsphenoidal and expanded approaches can yield similar oncological results to those obtained with traditional open approaches for sinonasal, sellar, and skull base lesions.[21,94,100,101,102,103,104] These modular approaches are recognized as an important tool in the armamentarium of skull base surgeons. The overarching principle in selecting between the four skull base approaches is the relative position of the affected cranial nerves. In the case of meningiomas located centrally with the cranial nerves displaced laterally or superiorly along the perimeter, the direct ventral corridor of the EEA offers several advantages. It enables: (1) early tumor devascularization; (2) minimal pituitary gland, brain, and neurovascular manipulation; (3) direct access to the ventral osseous framework of the skull base such as the cribriform plate, clivus, and medial optic canal. Over the past decade there has been a shift in the underlying philosophy of skull base surgery to one that is predicated to achieve the most complete tumor removal through less invasive routes; therefore, optimizing both long-term survival as well as quality of life. This philosophy is particularly applicable to meningiomas, given that a significant proportion originate from the dura along median/central skull base and displace critical neurovascular structures along their perimeter.

In this section, we will provide an overview of skull base meningiomas treated via a fully expanded endoscopic endonasal route using the modular anatomical approaches. We will first discuss the surgical strategy in general and then specifically based on anatomic locations. These will include meningiomas of the olfactory groove, planum sphenoidale/tuberculum sellae, diaphragma sella, cavernous sinus, Meckel cave, posterior medial orbit, petroclival synchondrosis, clivus, and foramen magnum.

12.4.2 General Surgical Strategy

The ideal surgical strategy to resect meningiomas, whether they are of the convexity or of the ventral skull base, is to address the various compartments sequentially and systematically, in layers: bone, dura, and the capsule (with cytoreduction as needed). This starts with an initial wide osseous resection not only to reduce recurrence rates but also to provide critical circumferential exposure of the basal dura and the origin of the lesion. The next step is the systematic and circumferential devascularization and separation of the dural attachment of the tumor from its vascular supply. Finally, and only after circumferential devascularization, cytoreduction and extracapsular dissection is carried out. Consider the case of a large convexity meningioma: the procedure does not begin with a limited opening in the center of the tumor, but rather a wide circumferential bony exposure of the dura extending as much as possible to the margins of the tumor prior to cytoreduction and extracapsular dissection.

In the case of ventrally located meningiomas the perimeter position of the circumferentially displaced cranial nerves can create limitations in accessing the basal dural origin when approached via traditional lateral approaches. Over the first three decades of skull base surgery this resulted in the development of a series of well-described transcranial corridors to allow the surgeon to work between small windows at the depth of the corridor, between cranial nerves, or alternatively move and transpose the nerves. This experience demonstrated the ability to access otherwise previously inaccessible lesions; however, such approaches required various degrees of neurovascular manipulation and, therefore, consequent morbidity and impact on the quality of life. With the advancement of technology such as surgical image-guided navigation and high-definition optics, a more targeted approached using a similar strategy to that used for ventral skull base meningiomas as that for convexity, i.e., sequential layered resection of osseous, dural, and capsular dissection can be accomplished via an anterior medial corridor.

Meningiomas of the ventral skull base are ideal lesions for an EEA given they are in contact with the roof of the sinonasal tract and they are most often median lesions with critical neurovascular structures located on the perimeter. EEAs take advantage of these relationships to allow a resection without any brain retraction or neurovascular manipulation, and with minimal brain exposure. Removal of the involved bone and dura as part of the approach enables achieving a Simpson grade 1 resection. Once the approach is performed, these skull base tumors are virtually converted into convexity meningiomas, exposing the basal attachment of the tumor.[102] Direct access to the main vascular supply to the tumor allows for early devascularization (▶ Table 12.4 and ▶ Table 12.5). The dura-mater is broadly coagulated before opening. Early devascularization facilitates subsequent tumor cytoreduction using the same principles of microdissection.[105] During tumor removal, the extent of dissection and/or retraction is minimized thanks to the panoramic and dynamic view obtained with the zero degree endoscope and occasional visualization of paramedian areas with the angled endoscopes. The endoscope also has a magnification power that enables early and direct visualization of critical subchiasmatic perforators as well as superior hypophyseal arteries. Preserving these respective arteries has the potential to improve visual outcome and preserve pituitary function.[102]

In the ensuing discussion we will review key anatomical principles to approach the specific locations of ventral skull base meningiomas. Given that the endoscope takes physical space within the nasal passages, it should be remembered that in each of these regions a working corridor should provide space for bimanual dissection as well as for dynamic movement of the endoscope, which is critical for visualization.

Table 12.4 Series of purely endoscopic or endoscopic-assisted removal of ventral skull base meningiomas

Reference	Number of patients/ tumor location	Technique	Removal (% of GTR)	Outcome: visual or other cranial neuropathy	Endocrine outcome	Complication
Gardner et al (2008)[102]	35: 15 OG/PS, 13 TS, 5 PS with petrous involvement, 2 PC with significant secondary PS extension	Endoscopic EEA	OG/PS: 83% TS: 92%	100% resolution or improvement of preoperative visual symptoms	3% New pituitary permanent dysfunction	New neuro deficit: 3% CSF leak: 40% Meningitis: 0%
Dusick et al (2005)[101]	7: all TS	Endoscopic-assisted microsurgical TSS	57.1% (85.7% when NTR are included)	No worsening of vision Anosmia: 14.3% (1/7)	14.3% (1/7) loss of anterior axis	CSF leak: 42.3% (3/7) Meningitis: 0%
de Divitiis (2007)[105]	6: all TS	Extended endoscopic TSS	83%	Improvement of vision: 66.7% Temporary worsening of vision: 33.3%	16.7% new DI (1/6)	CSF leak: 16.7%
Kitano et al (2007)[120]	16: all TS	Sublabial extended TSS	GTR or NTR in 75% (12/16)	Improvement of visual acuity: 81% Worsening of vision at least in one eye: 38% (6/16) Anosmia: 12.5% (2/16)	NS	CSF leak: 12.5% (2/16) No meningitis
Dusick et al (2008)[117]	13: all TS	Endoscopic-assisted microsurgical TSS	54% (7/13) (87% when NTR are included)	NS	7.7% (1/13) loss of anterior axis (same patient as previous series)	NS
Wang et al (2009)[118]	7: all TS	Extended endoscopic endonasal TSS	85.7%	71.4% improvement No worsening	14.3% (1/7) transient DI	No CSF leak
Akutsu et al (2009)[112]	21: all CS	Endoscope-assisted micro-surgical TS decompression of the sellar floor	NS	88.2% improvement if ocular motility 33.3% resolution of trigeminal nerve disturbance	Normalization of hyperprolactinemia in 76.4% Recovery of GH deficiency (37.5%) and hypogonadism (33.35) New endocrine deficit: 4.8% (GH deficiency)	No CSF leak No meningitis

CS, cavernous sinus; CSF, cerebrospinal fluid; DI, diabetes insipidus; EEA, expanded endonasal approach; GH, growth hormone; GTR, gross total removal; NS, not specified; NTR, near-total removal; OG, olfactory groove; PS, planum sphenoidale; TS, tuberculum sella; TSS, transsphenoidal surgery.

Table 12.5 Summary of ventral skull base meningiomas treated via an EEA, with special emphasis on vascular supply and related cranial nerves

	Origin	Vascular supply	Related nerves	EEA approach
Olfactory groove	Cribriform plate; Frontosphenoid suture	AEA, PEA, anterior branch of the middle meningeal artery, superficial recurrent ophthalmic artery, meningeal branches of the ophthalmic artery; Branches of ACA, ACoA	Olfactory: superolateral; Optic nerve/chiasm: inferolateral	Transcribriform
Planum sphenoidale/ tuberculum sella	Planum sphenoidale, tuberculum sellae, chiasmatic sulcus, limbus sphenoidale	PEA, ACA, ACoA	Olfactory: inferolateral; Optic nerve/chiasm: superolateral	Transplanum/transtuberculum sella
Diaphragma sellae	Diaphragma sellae (suprasellar, intrasellar, both)	Suprasellar: branches of the internal carotid artery; Intrasellar: dural branches of ECA, branches of IMA and ICA	Optic apparatus: superolateral	Transtuberculum sella/ transsellar
Cavernous sinus (cavernous sinus proper)	Intradural or interdural	Medial clival and dorsal meningeal arteries (posterior roof); branches of the inferolateral trunk (lateral wall)	III, IV, V_1, V_2, VI	Transsellar (for sellar extension); Superior cavernous sinus
Meckel cave	Dural covering of Meckel cave	Inferolateral trunk, lateral branch of the dorsal meningeal artery	V_2, VI	Infrapetrous/quadrangular
Petrous apex	Petrous apex	Medial tentorial artery, dorsal meningeal artery	Displacement of cranial nerves depends on the location of the dural attachment in regards to the skull base foramina of cranial nerves V–XI	Medial petrous apex
Clival	Clival area	Medial clival and dorsal meningeal arteries, branches of the ICA, anterior meningeal branch of the VA, branches of the ascending pharyngeal arteries	Lateral displacement of cranial nerves; Upper clivus: II, II; Panclivus: V–X	Transclival; Panclivectomy (± pituitary transposition)
Petroclival	Petroclival area	Dorsal meningeal artery, subarcuate artery, branches of the middle meningeal, occipital, and ascending pharyngeal arteries	VI: medial; VII: caudal	Petroclival (builds on to the transclival and transpterygoid)
Foramen magnum	Anterior lip of foramen magnum	Predominantly from the ECA (branches of the ascending pharyngeal artery and occipital artery) and VA (anterior and posterior meningeal arteries)	Lateral displacement of cranial nerves IX–XII	Transodontoid and foramen magnum/ craniovertebral approach

ACA, anterior cerebral artery; ACoA, anterior communicating artery; AEA, anterior ethmoidal artery; ECA, external carotid artery; EEA, expanded endonasal approach; ICA, internal carotid artery; IMA, inferior mesenteric artery; PEA, posterior ethmoidal artery; VA, vertebral artery.

12.4.3 Anatomical Considerations and Limitations

Anterior Cranial Fossa: Olfactory Groove, Planum/Tuberculum, and Diaphragm Sella Meningiomas

For meningiomas located along the anterior cranial fossa, the rostral limit is the frontal sinus and the caudal limit is the sella turcica.[96] A guiding principle for EEAs is that the plane of the cranial nerves represents the lateral limit and when possible cranial nerves should not be crossed.[96,102] For olfactory groove meningiomas there is an additional concern, in that edematous frontal lobes are displaced circumferentially along the perimeter and may be vulnerable to the slightest manipulation, especially in the presence of subpial invasion and venous engorge-

ment.[106] The lateral limit of resection for olfactory groove meningiomas is the optic nerve and a useful surrogate marker is the meridian of the orbit or the position of the superior rectus muscle. The working corridor for olfactory groove meningiomas is a wide bilateral frontal sinusotomy (endoscopic Lothrop or Draf III) and anterior/posterior ethmoidectomies. Although the lateral boundaries of the transcribriform approach are the laminae papyracea, the superior-medial orbital roof at its attachment to the olfactory crest may be removed by displacing the periorbita and orbital contents, a maneuver that allows extension of the lateral access to the meridian of the orbit (▶ Fig. 12.25). Lesions located in the anterior fossa, presenting lateral to this point, are generally not accessed endonasally (at least not that specific lateral component).

Regarding the transplanum/transtuberculum approach the working corridor extends up to the posterior ethmoidal

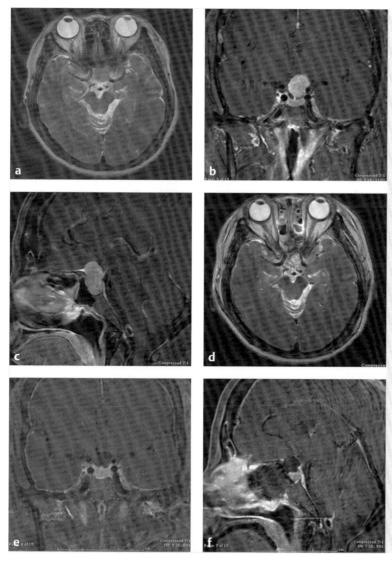

Fig. 12.25 a–f Tuberculum sella and diaphragma sella meningioma. A 57-year-old woman developed progressive left-sided vision loss. The brain MRI showed a sellar and suprasellar mass, which caused severe chiasmal compression and distortion of the left optic nerve. The lesion's epicenter was at the level of the tuberculum sella. It was distinct from the pituitary gland. The lesion enhanced homogeneously after gadolinium injection (a–c). Preoperative diagnosis was a tuberculum/diaphragm sella meningioma. On physical examination the patient had decreased visual acuity in the left eye with a left afferent papillary defect. The patient underwent a transsellar/transtuberculum/transplanum approach for removal of the mass. Intraoperative pathology confirmed the diagnosis of a benign meningioma. Postoperative examination showed complete resection of the meningioma (d–f). The patient's vision progressively improved and her pituitary function remained intact.

arteries and benefits of wide bilateral sphenoidotomies. The posterior ethmoidal artery represents the anterior boundary of the osseous exposure as the olfactory filaments are anterior to this landmark and olfaction can be jeopardized. Given that the principles of microsurgery must be maintained in endonasal surgery, extracapsular dissection of the lesion (following adequate debulking) requires early control of the critical neurovascular structure; in this case the paraclinoid ICA and optic nerve. In undertaking the sequential dissection, the critical lateral osseous boundaries are the medial opticocarotid recesses (mOCR) consisting of the lateral tubercular crest and middle clinoid. This bony exposure is mandatory and allows for the subsequent dural opening to extend laterally to the periosteal layer forming the internal ring of the paraclinoid ICA. In the process of detaching the meningioma from this region, the McConnell capsular artery is coagulated, which provides significant devascularization of the tumor. The dura along the interfalcine ligament and diaphragma is opened to the level of the internal ring providing for simultaneous access to the optic nerve at the falcine ligament and the ICA as it enters the subarachnoid space. This segment of the ICA gives off a critical branch, specifically the superior hypophyseal artery. The superior hypophyseal arteries from both sides meet under the chiasm creating a subchiasmatic plexus that represents the primary blood supply to the ventral optic apparatus. These very fine vessels are displaced along the perimeter of the tumor and must be preserved along with their respective descending infundibular branches.

Olfactory groove, planum sphenoidale/tuberculum sellae, and diaphragm sella meningiomas may chronically compress the optic apparatus producing secondary ischemia, rendering it sensitive to any degree of manipulation.[102] The posterior limit is the optic chiasm and anterior circulation.[102] Olfactory groove meningiomas displace the optic nerves inferolaterally and the chiasm posteriorly; whereas, the anterior cerebral and communicating arteries are dislocated superiorly and posteriorly.[106] Conversely, meningiomas of the planum sphenoidale/tuberculum sellae tend to displace the visual apparatus superolaterally along with the anterior cerebral arteries.[107] When these key structures remain on the perimeter of the lesion, the meningioma is accessible via an EEA. We generally divide these lesions into three categories according to their relationship to the cerebral vasculature: (1) cuff of cortex between the posterior aspect of the capsule and the vessels; (2) absence of a tissue cuff, with adherence of the vessels to the capsule; and (3) encasement of the vasculature within the tumor. While tumors that encase either the optic apparatus or the anterior cerebral arteries can be approached by an EEA, a lateral transcranial route should be given consideration as a standalone or a second-stage approach.[108]

Given that the optic nerve represents the lateral limit of the approach, the optic canal must therefore be identi-fied as it joins the orbital apex early in the exposure. An important consideration is extension of the tumor into the optic canal. Tumor extension into the canal is not a contraindication, as the ventral corridor enables easy access to the medial optic canal, allowing tumor resection along the inferior and medial portion of the nerve and consequently a very reliable means of optic nerve decompression.[102] The anteromedial corridor via EEA can access about 270° of the ventral and medial portion of the optic canal and this can be extended forward into the orbit into the retrobulbar space. This frequently represents the most difficult region to access via a traditional lateral approach, which conversely is better suited to address lateral portion of the optic canal.

With respect to rostral caudal extension, the height of anterior skull base meningiomas does not in itself limit the use of an EEA. Although vertical tumors can be difficult to access, strategic debulking of the tumors' base before removal of the inferior and anterior capsule prevents the frontal lobes from descending into the field and obscuring the view. Sometimes, very tall tumors need to be resected in stages, with a significant initial debulking; thus, allowing the descent of the tumor over time. The absence of a well-defined arachnoid plane between the tumor and the optic chiasm and ventral aspect of the brain due to subpial invasion may render a complete resection unsafe, independent of the approach. A trans-sellar approach may be required to access tumors that extend caudally, inside the sella turcica (the cavernous sinus and the cavernous ICA are the lateral limits).

Middle Cranial Fossa: Cavernous Sinus Meningiomas with and without Extension to the Meckel Cave

Given there are two leafs of dura (periosteal and meningeal), the cavernous sinus represents a diverticulum between these layers. Meningiomas within the cavernous sinus may have originated from either layer with subsequent lateral extension. In many situations the tumor may have originated lateral and be compressing the cavernous sinus, e.g., large sphenoid wing or anterior clinoid lesions.[109] Therefore cavernous sinus meningiomas represent a heterogeneous group and it is imperative to determine if they are truly located within the cavernous sinus or simply compressing it. During the resection of a cavernous sinus meningioma through an EEA, it is critical to avoid the superolateral compartment of the cavernous sinus to prevent injury to cranial nerves III, IV, V1, and VI. The cavernous sinus is actually a relatively small geographic space and often the Meckel cave is inadvertently mistaken as the inferior cavernous sinus. However, the Meckel cave represents a geographically distinct region that contains the gasserian ganglion and its branches. This region is very amenable to an anteromedial corridor (► Fig. 12.26) via the quadrangular space. The anatomical

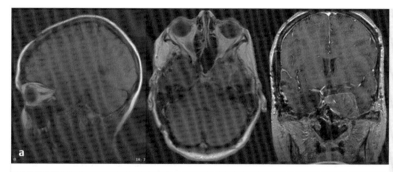

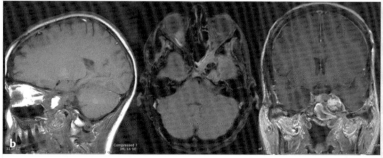

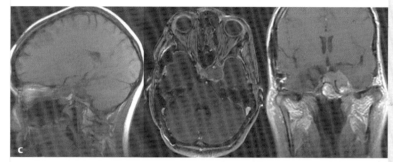

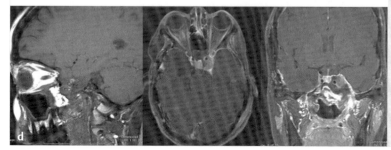

Fig. 12.26 a–d Cavernous sinus, sellar, and Meckel cave meningioma. A 35-year-old woman presented with a 1-week history of left ptosis, and decreased lateral and medial gaze in her left eye. Her symptoms improved with a bolus regimen of decadron. Known to have neurofibromatosis type 2, she had been diagnosed many years ago with a skull base meningioma involving the sella, cavernous sinus, Meckel cave, and middle fossa. She underwent eight resections including transcranial and endonasal procedures as well as stereotactic radiosurgery. Following her most recent surgery (**a, b**), the meningioma was characterized as atypical with a Ki-67 of 10%. To decompress her cranial nerves III–IV–V₁–VI, the patient underwent an expanded endonasal approach with removal of tumor within the sella and Meckel cave (**c, d**). This anteromedial approach enabled removal of the tumor median to the cavernous internal carotid artery, preventing transgression of the cranial nerves. The nasoseptal flap that had been elevated in a prior expanded endonasal approach was reused for closure of the skull base defect. Pathology demonstrated a meningioma with rhabdoid features and increased Ki-67 of 15%. Postoperatively, the patient had no new neurologic deficit, with moderate improvement of the left cranial nerve III neuropathy and mild improvement in disconjugate gaze. Adjuvant therapy was coordinated as subsequent steps.

boundaries of the quadrangular space are: the petrous ICA inferiorly, the paraclival ICA medially, cranial nerve VI superiorly (as it courses through the cavernous sinus representing a functional transition zone between the Meckel cave and cavernous sinus), and the maxillary division of the trigeminal nerve (V₂) laterally.[110]

A true superolateral cavernous sinus approach, lateral to the ICA siphon, is usually reserved for cases with already established cranial nerve deficits III, IV, VI or for meningiomas refractory to adjuvant therapy. Cavernous sinus meningiomas that extend and compress the optic nerves and/or chiasm may be considered for segmental resection to create a gap for subsequent radiosurgery;

thereby minimizing the risk of radiation optic neuropathy.[109,111] Similarly, cavernous sinus meningiomas that extend medially resulting in pituitary gland and stalk compression with consequent hypopituitarism may be debulked to recover function and create separation; thus minimizing postradiation pituitary dysfunction.[112,113]

Meningiomas involving the petrous apex can be reached through a medial petrous apex approach. The petrous (horizontal) and paraclival (vertical) segments of the ICA as well as cranial nerve VI at the Dorello canal are the lateral boundary of this approach. The petroclival approach is used to access lesions deeper along the midportion of the petrous bone as it adds on to the medial petrous apex exposure. This approach is limited laterally by the middle fossa and the ICA. A critical limitation is the distance between the petrous/paraclival ICA and the basilar artery. A quadrangular space with the basilar artery posterior-medially, cranial nerve VI superiorly, paraclival ICA anterior lateral, and vidian inferior is very helpful. The space is directly proportional to the distance between parallel lines of the posterior medial basilar artery and anterior lateral paraclival ICA.

Posterior Cranial Fossa: Petrous Apex, Petroclival, Clival, and Foramen Magnum Meningiomas

The infrapetrous approach builds on the infratemporal approach and is usually performed to access tumors below the petrous ICA into the petrous apex. This approach is limited laterally by cranial nerves VII and VIII. Meningiomas that involve the petrous apex, clivus, and the petroclival area may displace surrounding cranial nerves, rendering them susceptible to direct manipulation.[109,114,115] For these ventral posterior fossa lesions, the rostral limit is the dorsum sella and the caudal limit is the distal part of the clivus (anterior foramen magnum) and the craniocervical junction.[97] The anteromedial corridor to the posterior skull base is limited laterally by the cranial nerves. Cranial nerve III represents the lateral limit for exposure to the upper third of clivus and, together with cranial nerves V through X, limits the middle and lower third approaches.[97,99] Transodontoid and foramen magnum/craniovertebral approaches may extend the inferior exposure to the transclival approach (▶ Fig. 12.27) and allow access to the foramen magnum, ring of C1, odontoid, and upper body of C2.[115] The caudal margin of the craniocervical junction is the nasopalatine line drawn from the bony portion of the nasal septum to the hard palate and extended to the cervical spine. In general a lesion above this line can be accessed via an EEA; however, the lateral exposure and dissection must remain medial to the lower cranial nerves and in

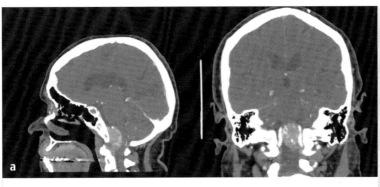

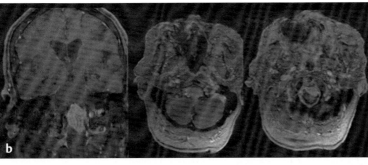

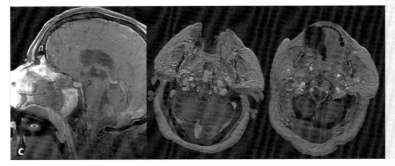

Fig. 12.27 a–c Foramen magnum meningioma. A 67-year-old woman presented with gait difficulties. Initial MRI showed an anterior lip foramen magnum lesion suggestive of a meningioma (**a, b**). She underwent a transclival approach with subtotal resection of the lesion. A small inferior residue was left to avoid spinal instability (**c**). Histopathological assessment documented a grade I meningioma. The patient was discharged without any neurological deficits.

particular hypoglossal canals bilaterally. The occipital bone can be drilled laterally expanding the clivectomy at the level of the inferior third of the clivus. It allows exposure of the jugular tubercle through a supracondylar approach. The medial condyle can also be drilled to allow proximal control of a vertebral artery in the subarachnoid space. However this is laterally limited at the 10 o'clock and 2 o'clock positions by the hypoglossal canal.

12.4.4 Preoperative Evaluation

Physical Examination

The preoperative physical examination includes a detailed neurological assessment with special focus on cranial nerve function. Olfaction is usually compromised by most of the olfactory groove meningiomas and it must be evaluated preoperatively. A complete neuro-ophthalmologic examination including visual acuity, assessment of anisocoria and ptosis, as well as visual fields using Goldman perimetry is mandatory for anterior fossa meningiomas.[106,107] Assessment of extraocular muscle function is important for meningiomas directly abutting cranial nerves III, IV, and VI anywhere along their course. Signs of intracranial hypertension detected by the presence of papilledema should be addressed preoperatively. For lesions in proximity or abutting the gasserian ganglion or branches of the trigeminal nerve, presence of facial numbness or facial pain should be noted preoperatively. Patients with petroclival meningiomas may present with palsies of cranial nerves V to XI.[115] Cranial nerves VII and VIII should be investigated with a detailed facial motor examination and an audiogram. Patients with large clival or foramen magnum lesions should have an evaluation of their lower cranial nerve function for any subclinical dysfunction.[100,114] In addition to evaluating the gag reflex, an endoscopic inspection of the pharynx may be indicated to assess for laryngeal function. Furthermore, consultation with a speech pathologist may help identify and/or quantify vocal cord and swallowing preoperative dysfunctions.

Cross-sectional Imaging

Routine CT scan assesses tumor location and its extent. On nonenhanced CT scans, most meningiomas appear as homogeneous masses hyperdense to the adjacent brain. Following contrast injection, meningiomas typically enhance homogeneously. CT scans determine the presence of associated calcifications, cysts, necrosis, and hemorrhage, which will contribute to inhomogeneous appearance. Adjacent brain edema and mass effect can be assessed preliminarily on CT imaging. Specific bony anatomy and associated pathological changes including hyperostosis or bony destruction are best evaluated with a CT scan with fine cuts through the skull base. A CT angiogram (CTA) is helpful, providing simultaneous information on the osseous, vascular, and ICA relationships; thus, identifying the safe corridors to be considered.

MRI, with and without gadolinium, is the preferred study for preoperative evaluation of meningiomas. They have a characteristic appearance on MRI regardless of their location. Meningiomas appear as isointense to the gray matter on T1-weighted sequences and iso- to hyperintense on T2-weighted sequences and enhance homogeneously following gadolinium injection. For each subtype of meningioma, the relationship with neurovascular structures in proximity with the tumor must be ascertained prior to treatment, as this will dictate the corridor. In addition, the extent of vasogenic white-matter edema in the surrounding brain must be noted in T2-weighted and FLAIR sequence. Ideally, preoperative CTA and MRI are fused and used for frameless stereotactic image guidance (Stryker, Kalamazoo, Michigan, United States). Extension of the tumor within the cavernous sinus, parasellar region, nasal cavity, and nasal sinuses must be addressed at the time of the first surgery[109]: 10 to 15% of skull base lesions have extension to the paranasal sinuses.[116]

In addition, a CTA or MR angiography should be obtained to detail the vessel anatomy and the effect of the tumor on important adjacent vessels. These investigations help evaluate the presence of vessel encasement and narrowing, which may suggest adventitial invasion.[114] If adventitial invasion is suspected on preoperative examination, a decision must be taken as to whether some tumor will potentially be left behind or if a vascular reconstruction is needed. A catheter angiogram may be warranted to evaluate the possibility of preoperative embolization. However, this is rarely recommended as the tumor frequently receives its blood supply from the ICA.

Endocrine Evaluation

Endocrine assessment of both anterior and posterior pituitary function should be performed preoperatively in patients undergoing surgery for meningiomas of the planum sphenoidale/tuberculum sella, diaphragma sella, and cavernous sinus with sellar extension. Although preoperative deficits are exceptional, they may arise transiently postoperatively.[117]

12.4.5 Surgical Technique: General Considerations Specific to Meningiomas Approached via an Expanded Endonasal Approach

Endoscopic and EEAs have been described in length in Chapters 8 and 9, respectively. In this section we will detail the general surgical techniques of osseus exposure, dural detachment/devascularization, and tumor capsule resection.[94,101,102,105,118]

For every modular approach, it is important to tailor the osseous resection to the extent of the disease. In general, the bone resection must be as wide as the entire area of the tumor attachment, appreciating that in some circumstances there maybe anatomic limitations such as the ICA or cavernous sinus. With respect to the actual tumor resection of a skull base meningioma via an EEA, we emphasize that the same principles of standard microsurgical approach be applied.[102,105,116] Namely, early tumor devascularization, serial internal debulking, and extracapsular dissection of neurovascular structures are sequentially performed in bimanually. Specifically, use of meticulous microsurgical techniques of gentle countertraction combined with sharp dissection, rather than grasping instruments, is the overriding principle that cannot be compromised under any circumstances.

The cytoreduction phase can be performed with mechanical instruments, such as two suctions or scissors; however, the advent of recent technology has allowed the development of powered instrumentation. We have avoided the use of thermal-based tools, such as ultrasonic aspirators, as the dispersion of heat can be potentially damaging to neurovascular structures. Mechanical automation such as the Myriad (NICO Corporation, Indianapolis, Indiana, United States) that is not associated to thermal energy seems the safest and most efficient tool for piecemeal removal.

Anterior Cranial Base Meningiomas

The osseous exposure is generally very similar for suprasellar meningiomas, specifically those located along the diaphragma sellae, tuberculum sellae, and planum sphenoidale. In each of these circumstances the initial step is drilling of the face of the sellae to allow for inferior displacement of the gland and early identification of the mOCR. Next, a V-shaped osteotomy using a high-speed drill with a hybrid burr is created using the posterior ethmoidal artery as the anterior limit, the optic canals as the lateral boundary, and the tuberculum as the posterior margin. The dissection separating the periosteal layer of the dura from the bone should be done in an anterior to posterior direction to avoid breaching the meningeal layer. Removal of the tuberculum sella is generally left as the last portion of the osseous stage, as there can be significant venous bleeding from the superior intercavernous sinus. Removal of the planum can be helpful and facilitate the anterior to posterior bony dissection that is required to avoid breaching the intercavernous sinus.

While dural detachment and devascularization have been discussed previously, there are a few key points worth reiterating. The lateral dural opening must be extended to the internal dural ring to gain control of the paraclinoid subarachnoid ICA. This facilitates the final extracapsular layer dissection, which follows a specific sequence extending from the ICA to the anterior communicating artery through to the contralateral ICA. It is imperative to assess the relationship of the vessels to the capsule on the preoperative imaging: cortical cuff, capsular adherence, or vascular encasement. The critical vessel to identify is the superior hypophyseal artery and its branches. Coagulation of the base of the tumor at the tuberculum/sellar junction should proceed only after identification of the stalk since it is most often adherent to the posterior margin of the capsule and can be easily damaged during this step.

For olfactory groove meningiomas, the posterior wall of the frontal sinus and the cribriform plate must be removed. However, for large olfactory groove meningiomas, it may also be necessary to remove the planum sphenoidale, tuberculum sellae, and face of the sphenoid to achieve appropriate rostrocaudal exposure, as well as removal of the medial roof of the orbits to achieve laterolateral adequate exposure.[96] In general both olfactory crests are removed first along with the laminae papyracea to provide the superior-medial orbitotomy, as described earlier. Next, the cribriform plate, which is often hyperostotic, is separated from the crista galli and again dissected in an anterior to posterior direction. The crista galli is the last portion of the osseous framework that is removed, as there may be significant venous bleeding from the inferior sagittal sinus.

The next layer of dural detachment and devascularization follows a specific sequence based on the primary sources of blood supply to these tumors. The first set, i.e., the anterior and posterior ethmoidal arteries, are easily access via this exposure and best identified as they emerge through their respective canals. Care should be taken to leave enough of a "stump" during sectioning to avoid retraction into the orbit and occurrence of a retrobulbar hematoma. The next set of vessels is the anterior falcine branches of the middle meningeal arteries. As their name suggests, these vessels are located along the anterior portion of the falx. Therefore the dural opening is made on either side of the falx and cytoreduction is undertaken as described previously. Once the free edge is identified, the falx is transected after the inferior sagittal sinus is coagulated.

Finally, extracapsular dissection is generally followed from a proximal to distal direction. The posterior proximal boundary is represented by the chiasm and the anterior communicating artery is identified and systematically followed through the interhemispheric fissure. Vascular branches are dissected with care: the preoperative pattern of cortical cuff, pial invasion, adherence, and vascular encasement guides the final dissection.

Middle Cranial Fossa Meningiomas

Clival meningiomas require drilling of the clivus between both paraclival segments of the ICA, whereas some foramen magnum meningiomas may also need resection of the odontoid process of the axis.[97] In these cases it is important to weigh the risk of craniocervical spinal instability and assess the need of fusion preoperatively.

The approaches used to access the middle coronal plane are grouped on the basis of their relationship to the petrous carotid artery and require different degrees of bony exposure of the paraclival and petrous ICA segments depending on whether the lesion is below the petrous ICA (medial petrous apex and the petroclival lesions) or above it (superior cavernous sinus and the Meckel cave).[98,110] In addition, opening of the clival dura at the level of the petrous ICA should be performed only under direct visualization as the abducens nerves travel in this space.

Large skull base meningiomas can be staged without associated morbidity. The nasoseptal flap can easily be elevated from the skull base during the second stage allowing for direct tumor access within a few minutes.

Skull Base Defect Reconstruction

Reconstruction of the skull base defect is essential to overall success of the EEA. It must be planned before approaching the tumor. This subject is covered in depth in Chapter 13. In our practice the preferred vascularized tissue used for reconstruction of the skull base defect is the Hadad-Bassagaisteguy nasoseptal flap.[67,81] The nasoseptal flap is raised at the beginning of the procedure in an anterior to posterior fashion, remaining pedicled on the posterior nasal artery. It is then stored in the nasopharynx until the end of the tumor dissection. The reconstruction starts with an inlay layer of collagen matrix membrane placed in the subdural space. Collagen matrix is easy to manipulate, which diminishes the risk of injuring the critical neurovascular structures as the graft is tucked around the dural defect. This first step significantly decreases egress of CSF through the defect.

Unlike the reconstruction following removal of sinonasal tumors, the septal mucosa is not invaded by meningiomas. Therefore, the full extent of the septal flap can be utilized for reconstruction. In cases where the entire anterior cranial fossa is exposed, there is often the need of supplementary tissue for reconstruction. Alternatives are the use of fat graft obliteration of the sphenoid sinus, followed by the nasoseptal flap touching the fat graft and covering the anterior fossa, the use of membrane grafts as fascia lata or alloderm (purified cadaveric dermis) to augment the area covered by the flap. The balloon of a 14-Fr Foley catheter is inflated under direct endoscopic visualization and keeps the reconstruction positioned against the defect for 3 to 6 days following surgery.

12.4.6 Complications

Major complications that occur with the EEA are similar in nature to those associated with traditional transcranial skull base approaches and include CSF leak, hemorrhage, pneumocephalus, cranial neuropathy, and cerebrovascular injuries specific to the location of the lesion, and infections.

We recently reviewed our experience with 100 patients who underwent an EEA for anterior fossa meningioma resection. Intraoperatively, vascular damage occurred in one patient with damage to an A2. Postoperatively the patient bled from a pseudoaneurysm with resultant neurological compromise. Worsening of vision occurred in 5% of the patients. New permanent pituitary dysfunction occurred in 6% of the initial series.[102] This later complication occurred early in our experience and was most probably secondary to thermal injury to the superior hypophyseal arteries during coagulation of the tuberculum. There was no 30-day mortality. Other complications encountered in this series of anterior fossa meningioma treated via an EEA included pulmonary embolus/deep venous thrombosis (< 5%), seizures (< 6%), pituitary dysfunction (< 4%), new cranial nerve deficit (< 2%), bacterial meningitis (< 2%), and myocardial infarction (< 1%).

A detailed assessment of complications following removal of ventral meningiomas of the middle and posterior cranial fossa is underway. As previously stated, cranial nerves V and VI, along with the ICA (horizontal and vertical segments), are at risk during EEAs to the middle fossa. For posterior fossa approaches, the brainstem, basilar artery, vertebral arteries and branches, as well as cranial nerves V to XII are at risk.

Whenever the dura is opened during a surgical procedure, there is unavoidably a risk of CSF leak. In the series of anterior fossa meningioma, the most frequent postoperative complication was CSF leak, which decreased significantly from levels around 30% initially in the series to levels below 6% once a vascularized nasoseptal flap became routine for reconstruction.[81] Lumbar drains are not routinely installed prior to transsellar or EEAs but may be considered for a high-flow CSF leak, intense arachnoid dissection, or obesity. Interestingly, the empiric use of a lumbar drain with the hope for CSF leak cessation proved to increase the risk for meningitis early in our series. In our practice, if a CSF leak is suspected during the postoperative period, there is a very low threshold to take patients back to the operating room for exploration and CSF leak identification and repair if necessary. With the association of the use of vascularized tissue for reconstruction and being aggressive with re-exploration and repair in cases of CSF leak, we have decreased cases of meningitis to below 1% among recent EEA cases.

12.4.7 Postoperative Care and Outcome

Skull base meningiomas removed via an EEA require close surveillance in an intensive care unit for the first 24 hours after surgery, with vital signs and neurologic assessment performed hourly. A CT scan without contrast should be obtained immediately after surgery to have a baseline imaging and document quantity of intracranial air. A postoperative MRI is obtained on postoperative day 1.

A detailed postoperative evaluation of cranial nerve function, motor, sensory, and cerebellar function is essential and must be compared with the preoperative evaluation. As such, in our series of anterior fossa meningiomas, 70% of patients with preoperative vision compromise had significant improvement in visual function, defined as improvement of two or more lines of Snellen visual acuity, or as improvement of visual field defect.[102] If required, detailed assessment of a specific component of the neurological examination may be complemented with an evaluation from a neuro-ophthalmologist, ear, nose, and throat (ENT) specialist, speech therapist, and physiotherapist.

Endocrine follow-up is indicated in the immediate postoperative period to assess the function of the anterior pituitary gland. Urinary output, specific urinary gravity, and serum sodium should be monitored closely as diabetes insipidus might occur transiently following procedures that might have altered the pituitary gland or pituitary stalk. In the setting of a new postoperative pituitary dysfunction, a consultation in endocrinology should be made to assure adequate postoperative follow-up.

Antibiotics are administered while the patient has endonasal packing, which might include a Foley catheter that abuts against a vascularized flap. Once the nasal packing is removed, patients are instructed to begin nasal irrigation two to three times per day to moisten the sinus mucosa, clean the nasal cavities and opened sinuses, decrease crusting, and overall decrease risk of infection. The patients are seen in clinic for postoperative follow-up 1 week after surgery for joint neurosurgical and ENT evaluation. At this time, patients are scoped with a rigid endoscope to assess the healing of the mucosa. If needed, patients are also debrided at that time.

Although results of EEAs for ventral skull base meningiomas are promising when performed in dedicated centers, the collective number of patients is still insufficient and postoperative follow-up is still too short to conclude on the superiority of the EEA surgical results versus those of the traditional transcranial.[101,102,105,112,116,118,119,120] Larger series and longer follow-up are required. More extensive drilling of the infiltrated bone and removal of the dural attachment may lead to a greater number of Simpson grade 1 resections, potentially reducing recurrence rates. Drilling of the bone and removal of the involved dura as performed through transcranial routes may be insufficient as compared with that achieved via the EEA.

12.4.8 Conclusion

The EEA is a safe and feasible procedure for the resection of ventral skull base meningiomas. In experienced hands, this approach yields favorable outcomes, enabling most complete tumor removal through a less invasive route.

It is important to acknowledge that specific issues such as vascular control, maintenance of microsurgical dissection, and reconstruction make these tumors some of the more challenging via an EEA. Therefore, the choice of a specific surgical route should be guided by tumor characteristics, patient comorbidities, and skill and experience of the operating team. Each patient should be evaluated with a 360° approach, considering the least destructive route with the least complications to achieve the most complete lesion resection.

Pearls and Pitfalls

- Meningiomas account for about 30% of all primary brain tumors constituting the largest subset of all intracranial tumors.
- EEAs can provide adequate access for anterior and central skull base meningiomas (from crista galli to the craniocervical junction).
- Access to anterior fossa meningiomas that present with lateral extension (up to the midorbital plane) require removal of the lamina papyracea to enable the displacement of the orbital soft tissues.
- Meningiomas of the planum sphenoidale/tuberculum sellae tend to displace the visual apparatus superolaterally along with the anterior cerebral arteries. This medial extension is accessed by an EEA better than with an anterolateral craniotomy, as the latter does require mobilization of the optic nerve.
- While tumors that encase either the optic apparatus or the anterior cerebral arteries can be approached by EEA, a lateral transcranial route should be considered as a standalone or a second-stage approach.
- Meningiomas that are separate from the vasculature by a cuff of cerebral cortex are the simplest and safest tumors to manage via an EEA.
- Meningiomas in direct dorsal contact with the vasculature are more complex, and safe dissection of their capsule requires a higher level of skill and experience of the endoscopic surgical team.
- Meningiomas with vascular encasement (e.g., anterior cerebral artery) are the most complicated and imply the highest risk requiring a very experienced EEA team to safely access, dissect, and control these critical vessels.
- The ideal surgical strategy to resect meningiomas is to address the various affected layers sequentially and systematically, removing bone, then dura, followed by circumferential devascularization, cytoreduction, collapse of the capsule, and extracapsular dissection.
- Specific issues such as vascular control, microsurgical dissection, and reconstruction make these tumors some of the most challenging via an EEA.

12.5 Chordoma

Eng H. Ooi, Ian J. Witterick, Fred Gentili

12.5.1 Introduction

Skull base chordomas are rare tumors that arise from embryonic notochordal tissue and comprise 6 to 8% of all central nervous system malignancies. Their most common location in the skull base is typically the clivus.[121] Their central location in the skull base and close proximity to critical neurovascular structures continues to pose significant challenges to skull base surgeons. Their propensity to infiltrate bone makes total removal very difficult resulting in a high incidence of recurrence. Surgical resection, which remains the initial management option, carries significant potential morbidity and reduced quality of life. Chordomas are generally slow-growing malignant tumors characterized by local infiltrative growth with invasion of surrounding structures, which if left untreated can result in severe disability or death. Distant metastases have been reported in 29% of cases.[121]

12.5.2 Clinical Features

Symptoms are variable and depend on the location and growth pattern of the tumor. Headache, neck pain, cranial nerve palsies, and visual changes are common presentations.[122,123] Patients with large tumors with brainstem compression may present with bulbar palsy, long tract signs, and ataxia. In many series an isolated abducens nerve palsy (i.e., diplopia) is the most common presenting feature reported.[124]

12.5.3 Pathology

Chordomas have traditionally been classified pathologically into chondroid and conventional types.[121] Conventional chordomas, the more common type, consists of multivacuolated cells with eosinophilia (physaliferous) arranged as nests and cords in a myxoid stroma. Chondroid chordomas were described as containing a significant chondroid component, which in the stroma resembles hyaline cartilage with neoplastic cells in the lacunae. The chondroid type was felt to have a better prognosis.[125] Other studies have not found significant differences in recurrence-free survival (RFS) rates between conventional and chondroid chordomas.[126,127] However, others feel the chondroid type may have been originally mistaken for low-grade chondrosarcomas that are known to have a better prognosis.[126,128,129] Immunohistochemistry has been helpful in the differentiation and diagnosis of chondrosarcomas and chordomas. While conventional and chondroid chordomas stain positive for vimentin, S-100, and cytokeratin, only conventional chordomas stain

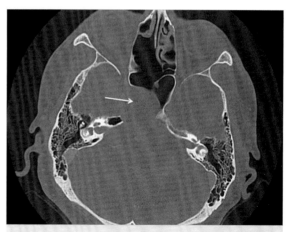

Fig. 12.28 CT axial view demonstrating a median clival tumor (*white arrow*) with bone erosion.

positive for cytokeratin, epithelial membrane antigen, and carcinoembryonic antigen.[130]

12.5.4 Imaging

Both CT and MRI are important and complementary in the diagnosis of chordomas. These diagnostic modalities are very helpful in delineating the extent of the tumor, its involvement and effects on surrounding neurovascular structures and brainstem, and in surgical planning.[131] CT scanning provides better bony delineation typically revealing a midline mass with destruction of clival bone (▶ Fig. 12.28). MRI delineates the soft-tissue boundaries of the tumor, usually showing a variable T1 signal and a hyperintense T2 signal.

Enhancement with gadolinium is usually moderate to high (▶ Fig. 12.29). While certain radiological features have been described as typical for chordomas, the differentiation between chordomas and chondrosarcomas cannot be definitively made on radiological features alone. Postoperative MRI is very useful in delineating the extent of resection and for follow-up. It is generally performed at 3 months after surgery and then at 6- to 12-monthly intervals (▶ Fig. 12.30).

12.5.5 Prognostic Factors

The mean survival for patients with a chordoma who do not receive treatment is less than a year.[121] It has been shown that the extent of resection is important and that more extensive resections are associated with better RFS rates than partial resection.[126,127] Female gender, tumor necrosis in a biopsy preradiation treatment, and tumor volume in excess of 70 mL were independent predictors of shortened OS.[132] Studies have shown that there appears to exist two subgroups of patients with biologically different tumor behavior. In one group,

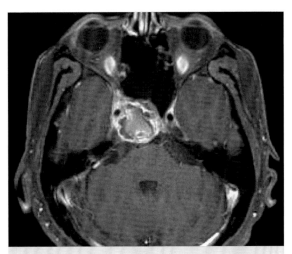

Fig. 12.29 MRI: T1-weighted axial view demonstrating the same lesion as shown in the CT scan in ▶ Fig. 12.28, enhanced with gadolinium.

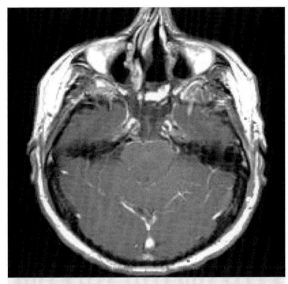

Fig. 12.30 Postoperative MRI: T1-weighted axial view demonstrating gross total resection of the tumor.

patients have a higher morbidity and mortality, with early recurrence and death usually within 4 years after initial diagnosis; in a second group, patients have more indolent tumors with longer survival.[123,133] In addition, expression of telomerase reverse transcriptase mRNA and p53 mutation is associated with an increased doubling time of residual tumor and a high probability of tumor recurrence.[133]

12.5.6 Anatomy of the Clivus

The clivus, the most common site for chordomas, slopes upward and forward from the foramen magnum to the dorsum sellae, with contributions from the basiocciput and basisphenoid bones. On each side of the clivus are the jugular tubercles with the hypoglossal canal and nerve passing between it and the occipital condyles. The lateral margins of the clivus inferiorly are the petro-occipital fissures grooved by the inferior petrosal sinus. Posterior to the clivus is the posterior cranial fossa with the vertebral arteries (VAs), vertebrobasilar junction (VBJ), basilar artery (BA), medulla, and pons. Lateral to the clivus is the foramen lacerum and the petroclival portion of the ICA. The abducens nerve runs superiorly and laterally just above the VBJ along the ventral face of the clivus prior to entering the Dorello canal and into the cavernous sinus. The clivus is divided into upper, middle, and lower thirds (▶ Fig. 12.31). The upper third relates to the dorsum sellae and sella. The middle third extends from the sella to the jugular tubercles. The lower third extends from jugular tubercles to the foramen magnum and occipital condyles.

12.5.7 Classification System

A classification system has been proposed based on the extent of skull base involvement and surgical approaches to remove the tumor[122] (▶ Table 12.6).

12.5.8 Management

Surgical resection plays an important role in the overall management of clival chordomas. Longer survival and disease-free recurrence rates are reported with more extensive tumor removal including recurrent cases.[100,123,128,134,135,136,137] Unfortunately there is no consensus on how the extent of surgical resection is reported in the literature. The terms radical,[122] gross total,[124,138] or total resection[128] have been used to describe the absence of residual tumor on intraoperative inspection and postoperative imaging. Other authors have used the terms radical excision[123] or subtotal resection[122,126,127] to describe a greater than 90% excision. Partial resection is generally defined as excision of less than 90% of the tumor.[122,123,126]

Selection of a surgical approach is based on the location, extent, and growth pattern of the tumor, its relation to vital neurovascular structures (ICA, VAs, BA, and cranial nerves), and whether one has to transgress these structures to access the tumor. Other considerations include the presence of intradural extension and whether an occipitocervical fusion is required. Radical resection is less likely if the tumor involves more than three anatomical sites and/or there is infiltration of vascular and/or neural structures.[139] Surgical approaches can be divided into open, endoscopic, or combined. The open approaches are anterior or laterally based, and are summarized in

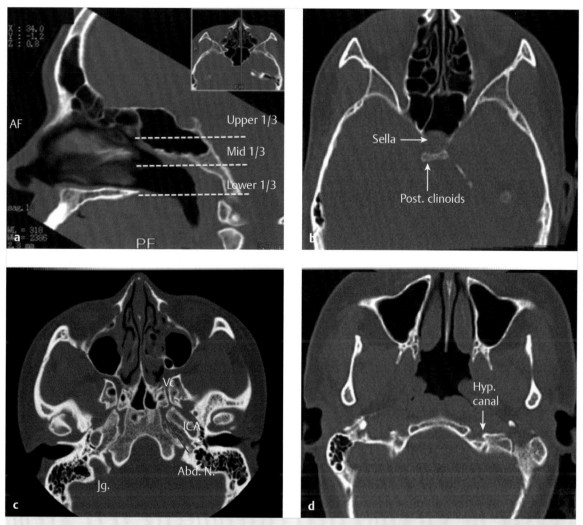

Fig. 12.31 a–d CT scans with sagittal (**a**) and axial views demonstrating division of the clivus into upper (**b**), middle (**c**), and lower (**d**) thirds.

Abd n., the *red arrow* demonstrates the course of the abducens nerve posterior and medial to the ICA; Hyp. canal, hypoglossal canal; ICA, internal carotid artery, petrous portion, demonstrating its relationship with the vidian canal; Jg., jugular fossa; Post. clinoids, posterior clinoids; Vc, vidian canal.

Table 12.6 Staging system for skull base chordomas[122]

Type	Description
I	Tumors restricted to one compartment or anatomical area of the skull base
II	Tumors that extent to two or more contiguous areas of the skull base and whose radical removal can be achieved using a single skull base approach
III	Tumors that extent to several contiguous compartments of the skull base and require two or more skull base approaches to achieve a radical removal

Table 12.7 Open approaches for clival chordomas

Anterior	Transbasal, cranio-orbitozygomatic, extended frontal, frontotemporal, transmaxillary, sublabial or transseptal extended transsphenoidal, transoral, pedicled rhinotomy, transmandibular-circumglossal, retropharyngeal approach
Lateral	Lateral transcondylar, transjugular, transpetrosal, infratemporal, retrosigmoid, pterional

Table 12.8 Results of open surgical approaches for skull base chordomas

Series	No. of patients	Extent of resection	Recurrence-free survival	Overall survival
Choi et al (2010)[123]	97	Not stated	25% recurrence rate	55% at 5 years; 36% at 10 years
Colli & Al-Mefty (2001)[126,127]	53	Radical 49.2% Subtotal 28.6% Partial 22.2%	50.7% at 5 years	85.9% at 5 years
Sen et al (2010)[139]	71	Radical 58%	49% recurrence rate	75% at 5 years
Gay et al (1995)[128]	46	Total 47%, near total 20%, subtotal 23%, partial 10%	76% at 5 years	Not stated
Tamaki et al (2001)[135]	17	Total 12%, near total 18%, subtotal 52%, partial 18%	51% at 5 years	Not stated

▶ Table 12.7. The extent of resection, recurrence free, and overall survival results of open surgery for skull base chordomas are summarized in ▶ Table 12.8.

The main operative complications are usually CSF leaks and neurological deficits. CSF leak rates range from 5.3 to 20.3%.[123,126,127,129,136,138,139] The rate of permanent postoperative neurological deficit ranges from 5.8 to 28.6%.[126,127,136] Operative mortality with open approaches is reported as ranging from 0 to 14.6%.[126,127] Other morbidity issues to consider with open approaches include facial scars, a need for temporary gastrostomy and/or tracheotomy in some patients, and ongoing speech and swallowing difficulties with some of the anterior open approaches.[123,140] Surgical seeding of chordomas has been reported along the operative route and even the abdomen where fat was harvested.[141] Care with harvesting surgical grafts and inclusion of the operative route for open approaches within the radiation therapy fields may reduce the risk of seeding.

12.5.9 Adjuvant Treatment

Proton beam radiotherapy is currently the most recommended adjuvant treatment for chordomas. This radiation modality allows delivery of high radiation doses with reported local tumor control rates of 87 and 81% at 3 and 5 years, respectively.[137] High-grade toxicity rates were reported as less than 10%. However, results have indicated a benefit only for tumors that were resected extensively. A better RFS at 4 years was reported for patients with chordomas treated with proton beam therapy compared with those treated without radiation (90.9 versus 38.5%, respectively).[126,127] Stereotactic radiosurgery has also been used for treatment of residual or recurrent chordomas.[142] Our protocol, however, has been to use intensity-modulated conformal radiotherapy postoperatively with comparable results.[124]

12.5.10 The Endoscopic Approach for Clival Chordoma Resection

An EEA for the resection of clival chordomas has been described and has gained rapid acceptance.[97,98,124,143,144,145]

Advantages and disadvantages of the endoscopic approach are summarized in ▶ Table 12.9. An EEA is indicated for median clival chordomas and can be combined with an open approach as a two-stage procedure. Relative contraindications for an EEA are extensive intradural invasion or significant lateral extension of the tumor.[124]

Surgical Preparation

Patients are positioned supine on the operating table and placed in Mayfield head-holders, with the head slightly flexed, and slightly rotated to the right to improve the view toward the clivus. We use computer-assisted surgical navigation (Stealth Station; Medtronic Inc., Jacksonville, Florida, United States) for anatomic guidance and a microvascular Doppler acoustic ultrasound to aid in confirming the position of the internal carotid and basilar arteries.[124]

Surgical Approach

We use a binarial, four-hands, two-surgeon technique with the endoscope usually placed in the right nostril by one surgeon who is responsible for maintaining the surgical field, while allowing the second surgeon to use instruments through both nostrils. The right middle turbinate is resected to create more room for the surgical corridor. Both middle turbinates can be resected if required

Table 12.9 Advantages and disadvantages of expanded endonasal approach

Advantages	Disadvantages
Most direct route to median tumor	Different anatomical perspective from that of open approaches
Minimal retraction of brain or cranial nerves	Different skills required, learning curve
Angled endoscope allows visualization around structures	Lack of binocular vision
Tumor invasion/extension has created a significant corridor that assists the dissection	

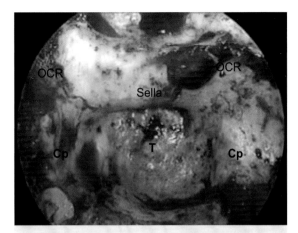

Fig. 12.32 Intraoperative image demonstrating the wide exposure of the sphenoid sinuses and clivus required for resection of the clival tumor.
Cp, carotid protuberance; OCR, medial opticocarotid recess; T, tumor.

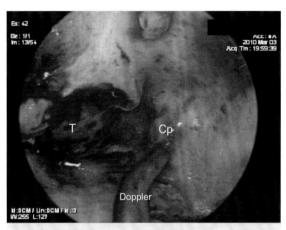

Fig. 12.33 Intraoperative image demonstrating use of the Doppler acoustic ultrasound probe in confirming the position of the petroclival carotid artery.
Cp, carotid protuberance; T, tumor.

depending on surgeon preference. We perform bilateral posterior ethmoidectomies and lateralize the left middle turbinate. Our preferred reconstruction option is to harvest a nasoseptal flap as described by Hadad et al.[67] We usually raise the flap contralateral to any lateral extension of the clival tumor that may require a transpterygoid approach. We recommend correcting any significant anterior septal deviations to improve the endoscopic corridor. A maxillary antrostomy is performed on the side of the flap pedicle so the flap can be tucked carefully out of the way into the maxillary sinus taking care not to twist the vascular pedicle.

Midline Exposure

A posterior septectomy is performed to widely expose the sphenoid rostrum. This step is critical to allow enough free space so the endoscope can be positioned out of the instrumentation field, allowing the instruments to pass bilaterally without impeding each other while still providing excellent illumination and magnification of the surgical target. Bilateral wide sphenoidotomies are performed, the posterior septal artery not used for the nasoseptal flap is cauterized, and the entire anterior face of the sphenoid is removed with a drill and/or Kerrison rongeurs with the dissection extended lateral toward the pterygoid process depending on the pneumatization of the lateral recess of the sphenoid.

This preparatory stage is critical to creating a single large box-shaped cavity with wide exposure of the sphenoid sinuses and clivus (▶ Fig. 12.32). The sella, opticocarotid recesses, petroclival carotid protuberances, and upper clivus should be easily visualized. The mucosa of the sphenoid sinus is stripped. Exposure of the middle and lower thirds of the clivus is achieved by removing the nasopharyngeal mucosa and stripping the pharyngo-

basilar fascia overlying it, as far inferiorly as the foramen magnum. The longus capitis muscles are identified and separated or removed as required. Drilling the maxillary crest and vomer flush with the nasal floor optimizes the inferior exposure as required.

The tumor often displaces the critical neurovascular structures dorsally or dorsolaterally due to its predominantly central component; thus, making an endoscopic endonasal approach ideal for this type of tumor. At this point the tumor is often visible, especially if the clivus is eroded anteriorly, thus reducing the amount of drilling required accessing it. On rare occasions where the tumor is not visible, then its location can be confirmed by intraoperative navigation. The intraoperative Doppler probe can be helpful in cases where the position of the paraclival internal carotid arteries is uncertain (▶ Fig. 12.33).

Lateral Exposure

Tumors that significantly extend lateral or posterolateral beyond the petroclival segment of the ICA may require a lateral craniotomy approach as the single procedure or combined with an endoscopic approach as a two-stage procedure. Two patients in our series of chordomas underwent a combined craniotomy approach for a significant lateral component (▶ Fig. 12.34) followed by an endoscopic approach.[124] Other authors have described endoscopic resection of tumors with lateral or posterolateral extension beyond the petroclival and petrous segments of the ICA.[145] This requires control of these segments through a transpterygoid approach with a wide maxillary antrostomy, resection of the posterior maxillary wall, and ligation of the sphenopalatine artery and other internal maxillary artery branches in the pterygopalatine and infratemporal fossae.[145]

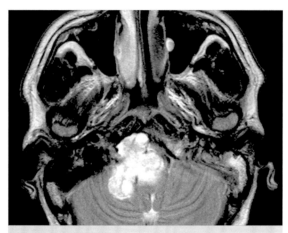

Fig. 12.34 MRI: T1-weighted axial view demonstrating a clival tumor with a significant lateral component. This was managed with a staged open lateral approach followed by an endoscopic endonasal approach for the midline anterior component.

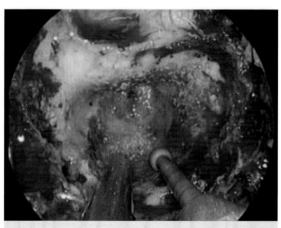

Fig. 12.35 Intraoperative image demonstrating drilling of the clivus. Usually the tumor has eroded the clival bone so the extent of drilling required is minimal and predominantly done to improve the exposure for resection of the tumor.

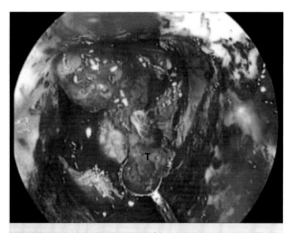

Fig. 12.36 Intraoperative image demonstrating intracapsular removal of the tumor (T) using a ring curette.

The vidian canal runs in a medial-to-lateral direction and is a key landmark as the anterior genu of the petrous ICA is found superior-medial to it (▶ Fig. 12.31c).[146] Drilling of the pterygoid wedge of bone proceeds in a caudal-to-rostral direction using the vidian canal as the superior limit thus protecting against inadvertent injury to the ICA. Drilling proceeds by skeletonizing the vidian nerve and artery along its inferior margin in a caudal-to-rostral direction.[98] The bone over the carotid protuberance is then removed using a high-speed drill until there is a thin eggshell layer of bone over the ICA that can be removed using fine Kerrison rongeurs. One has to remain aware of the course of the cranial nerves, especially the abducens nerve, as it runs posterior to the ICA heading toward the cavernous sinus.

Surgical Dissection

Drilling of the clivus is usually performed with a 3-mm coarse diamond burr (▶ Fig. 12.35). Bleeding from the cancellous bone during the drilling can be controlled with bone wax, Floseal (Baxter International Inc., Deerfield, Illinois, United States), gelatin foam (Gelfoam; Upjohn Co., Kalamazoo, Michigan, United States), microfibrillar collagen (Surgicel; Ethicon, Johnson & Johnson, Somerville, New Jersey, United States), Avitene (Ethicon, Johnson and Johnson, Somervillle, New Jersey, United States), or a combination of the above. The inner cortex is removed with a combination of drilling and Kerrison rongeurs. Gross total resection is performed whenever possible by creating as wide a corridor of exposure as possible and using microsurgical techniques and the endoscope for visualization.

Depending on the consistency of the tumor a variety of curette and suction techniques are used for removing the tumor (▶ Fig. 12.36). If the consistency is favorable (soft and "suckable") then a two-hand suction technique can be used to provide gentle countertraction in one hand while another suction is used in the other hand to perform internal debulking of the tumor. Dissection especially from brain stem should be performed under direct visualization avoiding blind traction, which can tear fine perforating vessels. Angled endoscopes may be useful in managing lateral extensions of tumor.

Intradural Dissection

In patients where the tumor has eroded dura and extended intracranially the dura mater is opened, being careful to coagulate the surface and underlying basilar venous plexus, which can bleed extensively. A midline incision in the dura is made initially to expose the

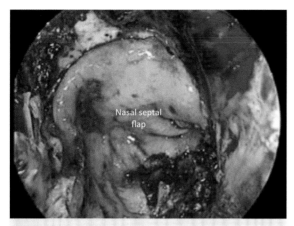

Nasal septal flap

Fig. 12.37 Intraoperative image demonstrating reconstruction of the clival defect with the nasoseptal flap.

the graft will "lift off" leading to CSF leakage. This is supplemented with fat and gelatin foam to pack the sphenoid sinus followed by fibrin glue (Tisseel; Baxter Canada Bioscience, Ontario, Canada). Our initial CSF leak rate was 33% with this method of reconstruction. This has been reduced to 13% with the recent use of a vascularized nasoseptal flap. Our current practice is to place the flap onto the fascia lata ensuring that it is in direct contact with the bone around the defect and (covering the entire defect) followed by tissue glue (► Fig. 12.37). We then place fat and gelatin foam over the flap followed by an inflated balloon of a Foley catheter (Foley no. 14) to bolster the reconstruction in position. The Foley balloon is deflated and removed 3 days after surgery. The inferior turbinate flap is an alternative if a nasal septal flap cannot be used due to previous surgery.[147] We do not use lumbar spinal drainage routinely.

intradural component of the tumor. Bleeding is controlled using the techniques described above. Bimanual microsurgical dissection above the petrous ICA should be done with care and under direct visualization because of the risk of injury to the abducens nerves located in this region. Intradural dissection is performed by internal debulking, capsular mobilization, and extracapsular dissection of vessels using endoscopic bipolar microcautery and sharp dissection.[97,98] The extent of resection is limited by adherence of the tumor to the brainstem perforators, vital neurovascular structures (e.g., BA and ICA) and the brainstem.

Reconstruction

Closure of the defect is performed using a multilayer reconstruction technique using fascia lata as an inlay graft, followed by a layer of fascia lata in an onlay fashion. Care is taken to avoid any folds in the fascia lata and to ensure that it is direct contact with a bony surface or else

Results of Endoscopic Clival Chordoma Resection

The reported results are summarized in ► Table 12.10. Recurrence rates appear equivalent with less postoperative morbidity when we compared our historical open resection results with our endoscopic group.[100] However, follow-up was shorter with smaller patient numbers compared with the open skull base resections.

12.5.11 Conclusion

The optimal management for clival chordomas is one that achieves as much as possible removal of the tumor, minimizing postoperative morbidity, and preserving function and quality of life, followed by adjuvant radiotherapy. The endoscopic approach has been shown to be safe and effective and seems ideal for median clival chordomas. Longer follow-up is required to confirm the advantages of this approach compared with open resections.

Table 12.10 Results of endoscopic clival chordoma resection

Series	No. of patients	Follow-up	Extent of resection	Results of surgery
Solares et al (2005)[144]	3	Follow-up 8–24 months	Not stated	1 died of other causes, 1 alive with no disease, 1 alive with residual disease
Jiang et al (2009)[143]	12	Follow-up 6–36 months	Not stated	8 alive no disease, 2 alive with residual disease, 1 patient with recurrence, 1 died from disease a year postoperative
Stippler et al (2009)[145]	20	Mean 13 months (1–45 months)	8 (66.7%) total resections, 2 (16.7%) near total, and 2 (16.7%) subtotal resections	10% recurrence rate 5 patients (25%) had progression of residual disease during follow-up
Dehdashti et al (2008)[124]	12	Median 16 months (4–26 months)	7 (58%) gross total resection, 5 (42%) subtotal resections	No recurrence and no mortalities
Frank et al (2006)[148]	9	Mean 27 months (15–69 months)	3 radical, 5 subtotal, 1 partial	1 recurrence, 3 (33%) died of disease progression

Pearls and Pitfalls

- Clivalchordomas are rare tumors that arise from embryonic notochordal tissue and comprise 6 to 8% of all central nervous system malignancies.
- Chordomas can be classified pathologically into conventional and chondroid types. The latter have been associated to have a more favorable prognosis.
- Common symptoms of clivalchordomas include headache, neck pain, cranial nerve palsies, and visual changes.
- CT and MR imaging are complementary in the diagnosis of chordomas.
- The optimal management for clivalchordomas is surgical removal of the tumor followed by adjuvant radiotherapy. Some evidence suggests that proton beam radiotherapy is the best option.
- EEA is indicated for median and paramedianclivalchordomas. Extensive intradural invasion or significant lateral extensions are relative contraindications. However, an EEA can be combined with an open approach as a two-stage procedure to cover extensive lateral and inferior extensions.
- Use of intraoperative navigation and acoustic Doppler sonography is extremely beneficial to identify and preserve the ICA.
- The extent of tumor resection is an important prognostic marker. However, in consideration of the prognosis of this tumor, the degree of resection should be weighed against potential complications and sequelae. Surgical morbidity should be minimized, and function and quality of life preserved.

References

[1] Busquets JM, Hwang PH. Endoscopic resection of sinonasal inverted papilloma: a meta-analysis. Otolaryngol Head Neck Surg 2006; 134: 476–482

[2] Calcaterra TC, Thompson JW, Paglia DE. Inverting papillomas of the nose and paranasal sinuses. Laryngoscope 1980; 90: 53–60

[3] Weissler MC, Montgomery WW, Turner PA, Montgomery SK, Joseph MP. Inverted papilloma. Ann Otol Rhinol Laryngol 1986; 95: 215–221

[4] Tomenzoli D, Castelnuovo P, Pagella F et al. Different endoscopic surgical strategies in the management of inverted papilloma of the sinonasal tract: experience with 47 patients. Laryngoscope 2004; 114: 193–200

[5] Waitz G, Wigand ME. Results of endoscopic sinus surgery for the treatment of inverted papillomas. Laryngoscope 1992; 102: 917–922

[6] Lund VJ. Optimum management of inverted papilloma. J Laryngol Otol 2000; 114: 194–197

[7] Sham CL, Woo JKS, van Hasselt CA. Endoscopic resection of inverted papilloma of the nose and paranasal sinuses. J Laryngol Otol 1998; 112: 758–764

[8] Kamel RH. Transnasal endoscopic medial maxillectomy in inverted papilloma. Laryngoscope 1995; 105: 847–853

[9] Yamaguchi KT, Shapshay SM, Incze JS, Vaughan CW, Strong MS. Inverted papilloma and squamous cell carcinoma. J Otolaryngol 1979; 8: 171–178

[10] Hyams VJ. Papillomas of the nasal cavity and paranasal sinuses. A clinicopathological study of 315 cases. Ann Otol Rhinol Laryngol 1971; 80: 192–206

[11] Pelausa EO, Fortier MAG. Schneiderian papilloma of the nose and paranasal sinuses: the University of Ottawa experience. J Otolaryngol 1992; 21: 9–15

[12] Kapadia SB, Barnes L, Pelzman K, Mirani N, Heffner DK, Bedetti C. Carcinoma ex oncocytic Schneiderian (cylindrical cell) papilloma. Am J Otolaryngol 1993; 14: 332–338

[13] Mansell NJ, Bates GJ. The inverted Schneiderian papilloma: a review and literature report of 43 new cases. Rhinology 2000; 38: 97–101

[14] Krouse JH. Endoscopic treatment of inverted papilloma: safety and efficacy. Am J Otolaryngol 2001; 22: 87–99

[15] Mirza S, Bradley PJ, Acharya A, Stacey M, Jones NS. Sinonasal inverted papillomas: recurrence, and synchronous and metachronous malignancy. J Laryngol Otol 2007; 121: 857–864

[16] Lombardi D, Tomenzoli D, Buttà L et al. Limitations and complications of endoscopic surgery for treatment for sinonasal inverted papilloma: a reassessment after 212 cases. Head Neck 2011; 33: 1154–1161

[17] Myers EN, Fernau JL, Johnson JT, Tabet JC, Barnes EL. Management of inverted papilloma. Laryngoscope 1990; 100: 481–490

[18] Maroldi R, Farina D, Palvarini L, Lombardi D, Tomenzoli D, Nicolai P. Magnetic resonance imaging findings of inverted papilloma: differential diagnosis with malignant sinonasal tumors. Am J Rhinol 2004; 18: 305–310

[19] Lee DK, Chung SK, Dhong HJ, Kim HY, Kim HJ, Bok KH. Focal hyperostosis on CT of sinonasal inverted papilloma as a predictor of tumor origin. AJNR Am J Neuroradiol 2007; 28: 618–621

[20] Yousuf K, Wright ED. Site of attachment of inverted papilloma predicted by CT findings of osteitis. Am J Rhinol 2007; 21: 32–36

[21] Snyderman CH, Carrau RL, Kassam AB et al. Endoscopic skull base surgery: principles of endonasal oncological surgery. J Surg Oncol 2008; 97: 658–664

[22] Landsberg R. Attachment-oriented endoscopic surgical approach for sinonasal inverted papilloma. Oper Tech Otolaryngol Head Neck Surg 2006; 17: 87–96

[23] Sukenik MA, Casiano R. Endoscopic medial maxillectomy for inverted papillomas of the paranasal sinuses: value of the intraoperative endoscopic examination. Laryngoscope 2000; 110: 39–42

[24] Brors D, Draf W. The treatment of inverted papilloma. Curr Opin Otolaryngol Head Neck Surg 1999; 7: 33–38

[25] Draf W. Endonasal micro-endoscopic frontal sinus surgery: the Fulda concept. Oper Tech Otolaryngol Head Neck Surg 1991; 2: 234–240

[26] Kountakis S, Brent A, Draf W. The Frontal Sinus. Berlin, Germany: Springer-Verlag; 2005

[27] Nicolai P, Tomenzoli D, Lombardi D, Maroldi R. Different endoscopic options in the treatment of inverted papilloma. Oper Tech Otolaryngol Head Neck Surg 2006; 17: 80–86

[28] Castelnuovo P, Locatelli D. The Endoscopic Surgical Technique "Two Nostrils–Four Hands". Tuttlingen, Germany: Endo-Press; 2006

[29] Bignami M, Pistochini A, Meloni F, Delehaye E, Castelnuovo P. A rare case of oncocytic Schneiderian papilloma with intradural and intraorbital extension with notes of operative techniques. Rhinology 2009; 47: 316–319

[30] Locatelli D, Rampa F, Acchiardi I, Bignami M, De Bernardi F, Castelnuovo P. Endoscopic endonasal approach for repair of cerebrospinal fluid leaks: Nine-year experience. Neurosurgery 2006; 58 Suppl 2: 246–256

[31] Nicolai P, Castelnuovo P. Benign tumors of the sinonasal tract. In: Flint P, Haughey B, Lund V, et al, eds. Cummings Otolaryngology: Head and Neck Surgery. 5th ed. Philadelphia: Mosby Elsevier; 2010:717–727.1

[32] Glad H, Vainer B, Buchwald C et al. Juvenile nasopharyngeal angiofibromas in Denmark 1981–2003: diagnosis, incidence, and treatment. Acta Otolaryngol 2007; 127: 292–299

[33] Schick B, Plinkert PK, Prescher A. Aetiology of angiofibromas: reflection on their specific vascular component [in German]. Laryngorhinootologie 2002; 81: 280–284

[34] Danesi G, Panciera DT, Harvey RJ, Agostinis C. Juvenile naso-pharyngeal angiofibroma: evaluation and surgical management of advanced disease. Otolaryngol Head Neck Surg 2008; 138: 581–586

[35] Wu AW, Mowry SE, Vinuela F, Abemayor E, Wang MB. Bilateral vascular supply in juvenile nasopharyngeal angiofibromas. Laryngoscope 2011; 121: 639–643

[36] McCombe A, Lund VJ, Howard DJ. Recurrence in juvenile angiofibroma. Rhinology 1990; 28: 97–102

[37] Tranbahuy P, Borsik M, Herman P, Wassef M, Casasco A. Direct intratumoral embolization of juvenile angiofibroma. Am J Otolaryngol 1994; 15: 429–435

[38] Casasco A, Houdart E, Biondi A et al. Major complications of percutaneous embolization of skull-base tumors. AJNR Am J Neuroradiol 1999; 20: 179–181

[39] Lehmann M, Ulrich S, Reineke U, Hamberger U, Dietrich U, Sudhoff H. Intratumoral Onyx embolisation in the management of juvenile nasopharyngeal angiofibroma [in German] HNO 2010; 58: 853–857

[40] Herman B, Bublik M, Ruiz J, Younis R. Endoscopic embolization with onyx prior to resection of JNA: a new approach. Int J Pediatr Otorhinolaryngol 2011; 75: 53–56

[41] Radkowski D, McGill T, Healy GB, Ohlms L, Jones DT. Angiofibroma. Changes in staging and treatment. Arch Otolaryngol Head Neck Surg 1996; 122: 122–129

[42] Andrews JC, Fisch U, Valavanis A, Aeppli U, Makek MS. The surgical management of extensive nasopharyngeal angiofibromas with the infratemporal fossa approach. Laryngoscope 1989; 99: 429–437

[43] Önerci M, Oğretmenoğlu O, Yücel T. Juvenile nasopharyngeal angiofibroma: a revised staging system. Rhinology 2006; 44: 39–45

[44] Snyderman CH, Pant H, Carrau RL, Gardner P. A new endoscopic staging system for angiofibromas. Arch Otolaryngol Head Neck Surg 2010; 136: 588–594

[45] Ardehali MM, Samimi Ardestani SH, Yazdani N, Goodarzi H, Bastaninejad S. Endoscopic approach for excision of juvenile nasopharyngeal angiofibroma: complications and outcomes. Am J Otolaryngol 2010; 31: 343–349

[46] Nicolai P, Villaret AB, Farina D et al. Endoscopic surgery for juvenile angiofibroma: a critical review of indications after 46 cases. Am J Rhinol Allergy 2010; 24: 67–72

[47] Howard DJ, Lloyd G, Lund V. Recurrence and its avoidance in juvenile angiofibroma. Laryngoscope 2001; 111: 1509–1511

[48] Ong YK, Solares CA, Carrau RL, Snyderman CH. New developments in transnasal endoscopic surgery for malignancies of the sinonasal tract and adjacent skull base. Curr Opin Otolaryngol Head Neck Surg 2010; 18: 107–113

[49] Kania RE, Sauvaget E, Guichard JP, Chapot R, Huy PT, Herman P. Early postoperative CT scanning for juvenile nasopharyngeal angiofibroma: detection of residual disease. AJNR Am J Neuroradiol 2005; 26: 82–88

[50] Lloyd G, Howard D, Phelps P, Cheesman A. Juvenile angiofibroma: the lessons of 20 years of modern imaging. J Laryngol Otol 1999; 113: 127–134

[51] Gullane PJ, Davidson J, O'Dwyer T, Forte V. Juvenile angiofibroma: a review of the literature and a case series report. Laryngoscope 1992; 102: 928–933

[52] McAfee WJ, Morris CG, Amdur RJ, Werning JW, Mendenhall WM. Definitive radiotherapy for juvenile nasopharyngeal angiofibroma. Am J Clin Oncol 2006; 29: 168–170

[53] Goepfert H, Cangir A, Lee YY. Chemotherapy for aggressive juvenile nasopharyngeal angiofibroma. Arch Otolaryngol 1985; 111: 285–289

[54] Schick B, Kahle G, Hässler R, Draf W. Chemotherapy of juvenile angiofibroma—an alternative? [in German] HNO 1996; 44: 148–152

[55] Thakar A, Gupta G, Bhalla AS et al. Adjuvant therapy with flutamide for presurgical volume reduction in juvenile nasopharyngeal angiofibroma. Head Neck 2011; 33: 1747–1753

[56] Neuronal origin of human esthesioneuroblastoma. N Engl J Med 1982; 307: 1457–1458

[57] Berger LLR. Esthesioneuroepithelioma olfactif. Bull Assoc Franç Etude Cancer 1924; 13: 410–421

[58] Rinaldo A, Ferlito A, Shaha AR, Wei WI, Lund VJ. Esthesioneuroblastoma and cervical lymph node metastases: clinical and therapeutic implications. Acta Otolaryngol 2002; 122: 215–221

[59] Koka VN, Julieron M, Bourhis J et al. Aesthesioneuroblastoma. J Laryngol Otol 1998; 112: 628–633

[60] Dulguerov P, Allal AS, Calcaterra TC. Esthesioneuroblastoma: a meta-analysis and review. Lancet Oncol 2001; 2: 683–690

[61] Demiroz C, Gutfeld O, Aboziada M, Brown D, Marentette LJ, Eisbruch A. Esthesioneuroblastoma: is there a need for elective neck treatment? Int J Radiat Oncol Biol Phys 2011; 81: e255–e261

[62] Fitzek MM, Thornton AF, Varvares M et al. Neuroendocrine tumors of the sinonasal tract. Results of a prospective study incorporating chemotherapy, surgery, and combined proton-photon radiotherapy. Cancer 2002; 94: 2623–2634

[63] Kadish S, Goodman M, Wang CC. Olfactory neuroblastoma. A clinical analysis of 17 cases. Cancer 1976; 37: 1571–1576

[64] Yu T, Xu YK, Li L et al. Esthesioneuroblastoma methods of intracranial extension: CT and MR imaging findings. Neuroradiology 2009; 51: 841–850

[65] Van Buren JM, Ommaya AK, Ketcham AS. Ten years' experience with radical combined craniofacial resection of malignant tumors of the paranasal sinuses. J Neurosurg 1968; 28: 341–350

[66] Kennedy DW. Functional endoscopic sinus surgery. Technique. Arch Otolaryngol 1985; 111: 643–649

[67] Hadad G, Bassagasteguy L, Carrau RL et al. A novel reconstructive technique after endoscopic expanded endonasal approaches: vascular pedicle nasoseptal flap. Laryngoscope 2006; 116: 1882–1886

[68] Zanation AM, Carrau RL, Snyderman CH et al. Nasoseptal flap takedown and reuse in revision endoscopic skull base reconstruction. Laryngoscope 2011; 121: 42–46

[69] Lund VJ, Stammberger H, Nicolai P et al. European Rhinologic Society Advisory Board on Endoscopic Techniques in the Management of Nose, Paranasal Sinus and Skull Base Tumours. European position paper on endoscopic management of tumours of the nose, paranasal sinuses and skull base. Rhinol Suppl 2010: 1–143

[70] Gallia GL, Reh DD, Salmasi V, Blitz AM, Koch W, Ishii M. Endonasal endoscopic resection of esthesioneuroblastoma: the Johns Hopkins Hospital experience and review of the literature. Neurosurg Rev 2011; 34: 465–475

[71] Folbe A, Herzallah I, Duvvuri U et al. Endoscopic endonasal resection of esthesioneuroblastoma: a multicenter study. Am J Rhinol Allergy 2009; 23: 91–94

[72] Unger F, Haselsberger K, Walch C, Stammberger H, Papaefthymiou G. Combined endoscopic surgery and radiosurgery as treatment modality for olfactory neuroblastoma (esthesioneuroblastoma). Acta Neurochir (Wien) 2005; 147: 595–601, discussion 601–602

[73] Castelnuovo P, Bignami M, Delù G, Battaglia P, Bignardi M, Dallan I. Endonasal endoscopic resection and radiotherapy in olfactory neuroblastoma: our experience. Head Neck 2007; 29: 845–850

[74] Hyams VJ. Olfactory neuroblastoma. In: Hyams V, Batsakis J, Michaels L, eds. Tumours of the Upper Respiratory Tract and Ear. Washington DC: Armed Forces Institute of Pathology; 1988:240–248

[75] Foote RL, Morita A, Ebersold MJ et al. Esthesioneuroblastoma: the role of adjuvant radiation therapy. Int J Radiat Oncol Biol Phys 1993; 27: 835–842

[76] Miyamoto RC, Gleich LL, Biddinger PW, Gluckman JL. Esthesioneuroblastoma and sinonasal undifferentiated carcinoma: impact of histological grading and clinical staging on survival and prognosis. Laryngoscope 2000; 110: 1262–1265

[77] Koch M, Constantinidis J, Dimmler A, Strauss C, Iro H. Long-term experiences in the therapy of esthesioneuroblastoma [in German] Laryngorhinootologie 2006; 85: 723–730

[78] Hirose T, Scheithauer BW, Lopes MB et al. Olfactory neuroblastoma. An immunohistochemical, ultrastructural, and flow cytometric study. Cancer 1995; 76: 4–19

[79] Carta F, Kania R, Sauvaget E, Bresson D, George B, Herman P. Endoscopy skull-base resection for ethmoid adenocarcinoma and olfactory neuroblastoma. Rhinology 2011; 49: 74–79

[80] Rivera-Serrano CM, Bassagaisteguy LH, Hadad G et al. Posterior pedicle lateral nasal wall flap: new reconstructive technique for large defects of the skull base. Am J Rhinol Allergy 2011; 25: e212–e216

[81] Kassam AB, Thomas A, Carrau RL et al. Endoscopic reconstruction of the cranial base using a pedicled nasoseptal flap. Neurosurgery 2008; 63 Suppl 1: ONS44–ONS52, discussion ONS52–ONS53

[82] Hadad G, Rivera-Serrano CM, Bassagaisteguy LH et al. Anterior pedicle lateral nasal wall flap: a novel technique for the reconstruction of anterior skull base defects. Laryngoscope 2011; 121: 1606–1610

[83] Snyderman CH, Gardner PA. "How much is enough?" endonasal surgery for olfactory neuroblastoma. Skull Base 2010; 20: 309–310

[84] Biller HF, Lawson W, Sachdev VP, Som P. Esthesioneuroblastoma: surgical treatment without radiation. Laryngoscope 1990; 100: 1199–1201

[85] Beitler JJ, Fass DE, Brenner HA et al. Esthesioneuroblastoma: is there a role for elective neck treatment? Head Neck 1991; 13: 321–326

[86] Parsons JT, Mendenhall WM, Mancuso AA, Cassisi NJ, Million RR. Malignant tumors of the nasal cavity and ethmoid and sphenoid sinuses. Int J Radiat Oncol Biol Phys 1988; 14: 11–22

[87] Simon JH, Zhen W, McCulloch TM et al. Esthesioneuroblastoma: the University of Iowa experience 1978–1998. Laryngoscope 2001; 111: 488–493

[88] Oberman HA, Rice DH. Olfactory neuroblastomas: a clinicopathologic study. Cancer 1976; 38: 2494–2502

[89] Devaiah AK, Andreoli MT. Treatment of esthesioneuroblastoma: a 16-year meta-analysis of 361 patients. Laryngoscope 2009; 119: 1412–1416

[90] Levine PA. Would Dr. Ogura approve of endoscopic resection of esthesioneuroblastomas? An analysis of endoscopic resection data versus that of craniofacial resection. Laryngoscope 2009; 119: 3–7

[91] Bradley PJ, Jones NS, Robertson I. Diagnosis and management of esthesioneuroblastoma. Curr Opin Otolaryngol Head Neck Surg 2003; 11: 112–118

[92] Claus EB, Bondy ML, Schildkraut JM, Wiemels JL, Wrensch M, Black PM. Epidemiology of intracranial meningioma. Neurosurgery 2005; 57: 1088–1095, discussion 1088–1095

[93] Drummond KJ, Zhu JJ, Black PM. Meningiomas: updating basic science, management, and outcome. Neurologist 2004; 10: 113–130

[94] Dehdashti AR, Ganna A, Witterick I, Gentili F. Expanded endonasal approach for anterior cranial base and suprasellar lesions: indications and limitations. Neurosurgery 2009; 64: 677–687, discussion 687–689

[95] Bambakidis NC, Kakarla UK, Kim LJ et al. Evolution of surgical approaches in the treatment of petroclival meningiomas: a retrospective review. Neurosurgery 2007; 61 Suppl 2: 202–209, discussion 209–211

[96] Kassam A, Snyderman CH, Mintz A, Gardner P, Carrau RL. Expanded endonasal approach: the rostrocaudal axis. Part I. Crista galli to the sella turcica. Neurosurg Focus 2005; 19: E3

[97] Kassam A, Snyderman CH, Mintz A, Gardner P, Carrau RL. Expanded endonasal approach: the rostrocaudal axis. Part II. Posterior clinoids to the foramen magnum. Neurosurg Focus 2005; 19: E4

[98] Kassam AB, Gardner P, Snyderman C, Mintz A, Carrau R. Expanded endonasal approach: fully endoscopic, completely transnasal approach to the middle third of the clivus, petrous bone, middle cranial fossa, and infratemporal fossa. Neurosurg Focus 2005; 19: E6

[99] Kassam AB, Prevedello DM, Thomas A et al. Endoscopic endonasal pituitary transposition for a transdorsum sellae approach to the interpeduncular cistern. Neurosurgery 2008; 62 Suppl 1: 57–72, discussion 72–74

[100] Carrabba G, Dehdashti AR, Gentili F. Surgery for clival lesions: open resection versus the expanded endoscopic endonasal approach. Neurosurg Focus 2008; 25: E7

[101] Dusick JR, Esposito F, Kelly DF et al. The extended direct endonasal transsphenoidal approach for nonadenomatous suprasellar tumors. J Neurosurg 2005; 102: 832–841

[102] Gardner PA, Kassam AB, Thomas A et al. Endoscopic endonasal resection of anterior cranial base meningiomas. Neurosurgery 2008; 63: 36–52, discussion 52–54

[103] Tabaee A, Anand VK, Barrón Y et al. Endoscopic pituitary surgery: a systematic review and meta-analysis. J Neurosurg 2009; 111: 545–554

[104] Zada G, Kelly DF, Cohan P, Wang C, Swerdloff R. Endonasal transsphenoidal approach for pituitary adenomas and other sellar lesions: an assessment of efficacy, safety, and patient impressions. J Clin Neurosurg 2003; 98: 350–358

[105] de Divitiis E, Cavallo LM, Esposito F, Stella L, Messina A. Extended endoscopic transsphenoidal approach for tuberculum sellae meningiomas. Neurosurgery 2007; 61 Suppl 2: 229–237, discussion 237–238

[106] Hentschel SJ, DeMonte F. Olfactory groove meningiomas. Neurosurg Focus 2003; 14: e4

[107] Chi JH, McDermott MW. Tuberculum sellae meningiomas. Neurosurg Focus 2003; 14: e6

[108] de Divitiis E, Esposito F, Cappabianca P, Cavallo LM, de Divitiis O. Tuberculum sellae meningiomas: high route or low route? A series of 51 consecutive cases. Neurosurgery 2008; 62: 556–563, discussion 556–563

[109] Heth JA, Al-Mefty O. Cavernous sinus meningiomas. Neurosurg Focus 2003; 14: e3

[110] Kassam AB, Prevedello DM, Carrau RL et al. The front door to Meckel's cave: an anteromedial corridor via expanded endoscopic endonasal approach- technical considerations and clinical series. Neurosurgery 2009; 64 Suppl: ons71–ons82, discussion ons82–ons83

[111] Pendl G, Schröttner O, Eustacchio S, Ganz JC, Feichtinger K. Cavernous sinus meningiomas—what is the strategy: upfront or adjuvant gamma knife surgery? Stereotact Funct Neurosurg 1998; 70 Suppl 1: 33–40

[112] Akutsu H, Kreutzer J, Fahlbusch R, Buchfelder M. Transsphenoidal decompression of the sellar floor for cavernous sinus meningiomas: experience with 21 patients. Neurosurgery 2009; 65: 54–62, discussion 62

[113] Couldwell WT, Kan P, Liu JK, Apfelbaum RI. Decompression of cavernous sinus meningioma for preservation and improvement of cranial nerve function. Technical note. J Neurosurg 2006; 105: 148–152

[114] Boulton MR, Cusimano MD. Foramen magnum meningiomas: concepts, classifications, and nuances. Neurosurg Focus 2003; 14: e10

[115] Liu JK, Gottfried ON, Couldwell WT. Surgical management of posterior petrous meningiomas. Neurosurg Focus 2003; 14: e7

[116] Derome PJ, Guiot G. Bone problems in meningiomas invading the base of the skull. Clin Neurosurg 1978; 25: 435–451

[117] Dusick JR, Fatemi N, Mattozo C et al. Pituitary function after endonasal surgery for nonadenomatous parasellar tumors: Rathke's cleft cysts, craniopharyngiomas, and meningiomas. Surg Neurol 2008; 70: 482–490, discussion 490–491

[118] Wang Q, Lu XJ, Li B, Ji WY, Chen KL. Extended endoscopic endonasal transsphenoidal removal of tuberculum sellae meningiomas: a preliminary report. J Clin Neurosci 2009; 16: 889–893

[119] Fatemi N, Dusick JR, de Paiva Neto MA, Malkasian D, Kelly DF. Endonasal versus supraorbital keyhole removal of craniopharyngiomas and tuberculum sellae meningiomas. Neurosurgery 2009; 64 Suppl 2: 269–284, discussion 284–286

[120] Kitano M, Taneda M, Nakao Y. Postoperative improvement in visual function in patients with tuberculum sellae meningiomas: results of the extended transsphenoidal and transcranial approaches. J Neurosurg 2007; 107: 337–346

[121] Eriksson B, Gunterberg B, Kindblom LG. Chordoma. A clinicopathologic and prognostic study of a Swedish national series. Acta Orthop Scand 1981; 52: 49–58

[122] Al-Mefty O, Borba LA. Skull base chordomas: a management challenge. J Neurosurg 1997; 86: 182–189

[123] Choi D, Melcher R, Harms J, Crockard A. Outcome of 132 operations in 97 patients with chordomas of the craniocervical junction and upper cervical spine. Neurosurgery 2010; 66: 59–65, discussion 65

[124] Dehdashti AR, Karabatsou K, Ganna A, Witterick I, Gentili F. Expanded endoscopic endonasal approach for treatment of clival chordomas: early results in 12 patients. Neurosurgery 2008; 63: 299–307, discussion 307–309

[125] Heffelfinger MJ, Dahlin DC, MacCarty CS, Beabout JW. Chordomas and cartilaginous tumors at the skull base. Cancer 1973; 32: 410–420

[126] Colli B, Al-Mefty O. Chordomas of the craniocervical junction: follow-up review and prognostic factors. J Neurosurg 2001; 95: 933–943

[127] Colli BO, Al-Mefty O. Chordomas of the skull base: follow-up review and prognostic factors. Neurosurg Focus 2001; 10: E1

[128] Gay E, Sekhar LN, Rubinstein E et al. Chordomas and chondrosarcomas of the cranial base: results and follow-up of 60 patients. Neurosurgery 1995; 36: 887–896, discussion 896–897

[129] Sekhar LN, Pranatartiharan R, Chanda A, Wright DC. Chordomas and chondrosarcomas of the skull base: results and complications of surgical management. Neurosurg Focus 2001; 10: E2

[130] Ishida T, Dorfman HD. Chondroid chordoma versus low-grade chondrosarcoma of the base of the skull: can immunohistochemistry resolve the controversy? J Neurooncol 1994; 18: 199–206

[131] St Martin M, Levine SC. Chordomas of the skull base: manifestations and management. Curr Opin Otolaryngol Head Neck Surg 2003; 11: 324–327

[132] O'Connell JX, Renard LG, Liebsch NJ, Efird JT, Munzenrider JE, Rosenberg AE. Base of skull chordoma. A correlative study of histologic and clinical features of 62 cases. Cancer 1994; 74: 2261–2267

[133] Pallini R, Maira G, Pierconti F et al. Chordoma of the skull base: predictors of tumor recurrence. J Neurosurg 2003; 98: 812–822

[134] Sen C, Triana A. Cranial chordomas: results of radical excision. Neurosurg Focus 2001; 10: E3

[135] Tamaki N, Nagashima T, Ehara K, Motooka Y, Barua KK. Surgical approaches and strategies for skull base chordomas. Neurosurg Focus 2001; 10: E9

[136] Samii A, Gerganov VM, Herold C et al. Chordomas of the skull base: surgical management and outcome. J Neurosurg 2007; 107: 319–324

[137] Ares C, Hug EB, Lomax AJ et al. Effectiveness and safety of spot scanning proton radiation therapy for chordomas and chondrosarcomas of the skull base: first long-term report. Int J Radiat Oncol Biol Phys 2009; 75: 1111–1118

[138] Al-Mefty O, Kadri PA, Hasan DM, Isolan GR, Pravdenkova S. Anterior clivectomy: surgical technique and clinical applications. J Neurosurg 2008; 109: 783–793

[139] Sen C, Triana AI, Berglind N, Godbold J, Shrivastava RK. Clival chordomas: clinical management, results, and complications in 71 patients. J Neurosurg 2010; 113: 1059–1071

[140] DeMonte F, Diaz E, Jr, Callender D, Suk I. Transmandibular, circumglossal, retropharyngeal approach for chordomas of the clivus and upper cervical spine. Technical note. Neurosurg Focus 2001; 10: E10

[141] Arnautović KI, Al-Mefty O. Surgical seeding of chordomas. Neurosurg Focus 2001; 10: E7

[142] Martin JJ, Niranjan A, Kondziolka D, Flickinger JC, Lozanne KA, Lunsford LD. Radiosurgery for chordomas and chondrosarcomas of the skull base. J Neurosurg 2007; 107: 758–764

[143] Hong Jiang W, Ping Zhao S, Hai Xie Z, Zhang H, Zhang J, Yun Xiao J. Endoscopic resection of chordomas in different clival regions. Acta Otolaryngol 2009; 129: 71–83

[144] Solares CA, Fakhri S, Batra PS, Lee J, Lanza DC. Transnasal endoscopic resection of lesions of the clivus: a preliminary report. Laryngoscope 2005; 115: 1917–1922

[145] Stippler M, Gardner PA, Snyderman CH, Carrau RL, Prevedello DM, Kassam AB. Endoscopic endonasal approach for clival chordomas. Neurosurgery 2009; 64: 268–277, discussion 277–278

[146] Vescan AD, Snyderman CH, Carrau RL et al. Vidian canal: analysis and relationship to the internal carotid artery. Laryngoscope 2007; 117: 1338–1342

[147] Fortes FS, Carrau RL, Snyderman CH et al. The posterior pedicle inferior turbinate flap: a new vascularized flap for skull base reconstruction. Laryngoscope 2007; 117: 1329–1332

[148] Frank G, Sciarretta V, Calbucci F, Farneti G, Mazzatenta D, Pasquini E. The endoscopic transnasal transsphenoidal approach for the treatment of cranial base chordomas and chondrosarcomas. Neurosurgery 2006; 59 Suppl 1: ONS50–ONS57, discussion ONS50–ONS57

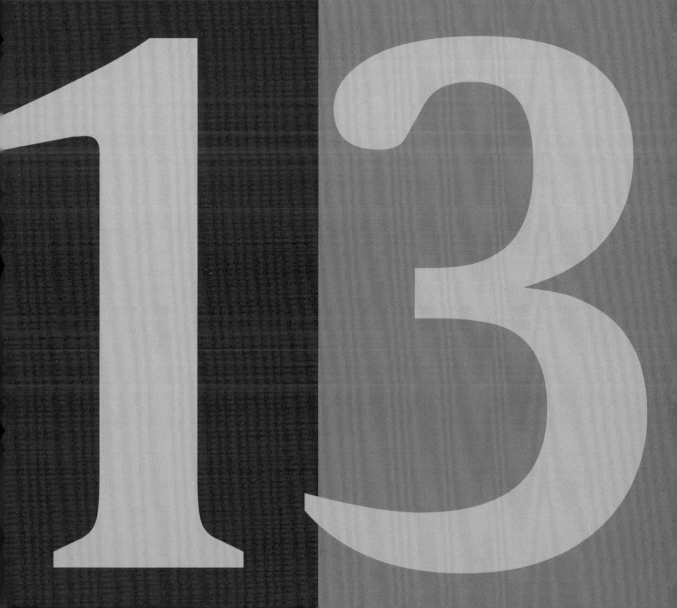

Chapter 13

Dural Reconstruction

13

13 Dural Reconstruction

Paolo Castelnuovo, Andrea Pistochini, Stefania Gallo

13.1 Introduction

13.1.1 The "Pre-endoscopic" Era

Paranasal sinus tumors are rare, accounting for 3% of all head and neck malignancies. Local extension of these tumors can result in invasion of the skull base and surgery remains the cornerstone in the treatment of extended diseases.[1] In 1954, Smith reported a case in which the craniofacial concept was applied for the first time; a neurosurgeon and a head and neck surgeon working in conjunction resected an ethmoidal-orbital tumor en bloc with the cribriform plate and the anterior wall of the sphenoid sinus in the specimen.[2] However, Smith's work was not readily appreciated. It was not until 1963, when Ketcham published a series of 17 anterior craniofacial resections, that this surgical procedure became the touchstone for the treatment of malignancies approaching or involving the anterior skull base, and became widely recognized as the gold standard.[3]

Since then, advances in surgical techniques and reconstruction have refined the indications and scope of craniofacial resection. In addition, improved radiologic imaging techniques have allowed surgeons to better assess the extent of tumors, thus permitting better staging and more precise surgery through safer approaches.[4] However, despite this, craniofacial resection is not without complications. The operative mortality has been reported to be less than 5%, but overall complication rates range from 25 to 65%.[5]

13.1.2 The "Endoscopic" Era

Since its introduction and first applications by Messerklinger in the 1970s, transnasal endoscopic surgery has spread all over the world, thanks to the contribution of Stammberger, Wigand, Kennedy, Draf, Lund, Castelnuovo, and others, and represents the gold standard in the treatment of inflammatory diseases of the sinonasal tract. Its indications rapidly expanded during the second half of the 1980s to include a wide spectrum of other pathologic conditions, such as lacrimal pathway stenoses, choanal atresia, cerebrospinal fluid (CSF) leaks, ophthalmic orbitopathy, and pituitary tumors.[6,7] More recently, due to refinement in surgical instrumentation and endoscopes and to increasing surgical experience and confidence, endoscopic surgery has been demonstrated to be an effective and reliable treatment for most benign sinonasal and nasopharyngeal tumors also extended to the skull base. In the late 1990s, some isolated reports addressed the possibility of applying the endoscopic technique to manage carefully selected cases of malignant tumors of the sinonasal tract as well.[8,9,10,11]

Detailed anatomical studies have improved knowledge of the skull base anatomy from the endoscopic perspective. This progress, together with the use of intraoperative image guidance and customized instruments, has enabled skull base surgeons to approach deeply seated lesions using minimal-access techniques. The feasibility and the safety of these extended approaches have been well established and reported in numerous studies.[12] As a result, current expanded endonasal approaches can provide access to the anterior, middle, and posterior cranial fossa.[13]

One of the main requisites for performing expanded endonasal approaches is the ability to work according to a four-hands surgical technique. The first author to promote the endoscopic technique using more than two hands was Mark May in 1990. He suggested technical modifications that allow the use of more surgical instruments in a single nasal cavity and require the collaboration of two surgeons.[14] In addition, a wider exposure of the surgical field is guaranteed by a subtotal resection of the nasal septum. Briner and Simmen have recently emphasized the positive aspects of this technique, in particular regarding a reduction in the duration of surgery, improved vision of the surgical field, and optimization of the resources.[15] In recent years, the experience of other authors in the neurosurgical field has demonstrated how this technique can be extended to the treatment of advanced pathologies in the anterior, middle, and, in selected cases, posterior skull base.[16,17,18,19,20]

13.1.3 Skull Base Reconstruction

The efficacy of any surgical procedure for skull base tumor resection also is determined by the ability to repair the resulting defect, which has been a major challenge over the past decade.

Reconstruction procedures after craniofacial resection include simple and more sophisticated options, among which pericranial flaps and galeal-pericranial flaps have received the widest approval.[21,22]

The overall goals of reconstruction after endoscopic expanded approaches are similar to those of traditional open skull base surgery and include separation of the cranial cavity from the sinonasal tract, protection of neurovascular structures, preservation or restoration of cosmesis, preservation or rehabilitation of function, and avoidance of dead spaces.[23] Separation of the cranial cavity from the sinonasal tract prevents postoperative CSF leaks, pneumocephalus, and intracranial infections, such as ascending bacterial meningitis and abscesses, and protects cranial nerves and major vessels against desiccation and infection.

Early endoscopic reconstructive techniques were based on experience with the repair of defects following spontaneous CSF leaks and accidental or iatrogenic trauma. Multiple reports have validated that small cranial base defects can be reconstructed with a wide variety of free grafting techniques, achieving success in more than 95% of patients.[24]

However, when applied to the larger and more complex defects produced by expanded endonasal approaches, these techniques proved to be inadequate. In these cases, reconstruction is challenging not only because of the size of the defects but also because of the lack of supporting structures. High flow of CSF at the middle and posterior skull base and the presence of adjacent delicate neurovascular structures (such as optic chiasm, internal carotid artery, cranial nerve VI), are other factors that further limit this technique.

Subsequent refinements of free grafting techniques, such as multilayer repair, reduced the CSF leak rate at anterior skull base,[25] but its incidence remained high for large defects located at the middle and posterior skull base.[13,26]

A rapid and reproducible drop in postoperative complications after traditional open approaches followed the adoption of vascularized flaps (generally galeal-pericranial flap overturned through the craniotomy)[27] and a similar development was needed for an endoscopic technique. Emulating this evolution, many pedicled vascularized flaps have been developed (i.e., the Hadad-Bassagaisteguy flap) for use in the reconstruction of skull base defects resulting from endoscopic expanded approaches, resulting in a decrease of CSF leak incidence to < 5%.[28]

13.2 Skull Base Reconstruction

13.2.1 Available Materials (Grafts and Flaps)

In 1926, Walter Dandy published one of the of the first successful surgical closures of a CSF leak, using a frontal craniotomy and employing fascia lata.[29] In 1948, Dohlman reported an extracranial approach (naso-orbital incision) to close an ethmoidal roof defect, using a nasoseptal mucosal flap.[30] In 1952, Oskar Hirsch was the first to use an exclusive endonasal approach (transseptal-transsphenoidal) for skull base reconstruction at sphenoid sinus level, employing a mucosal perichondrial flap harvested from the nasal septum.[31]

Since then, many different materials have been proposed to aid the closure of dural defects. In general, autologous grafts, allogenic transplants, and various synthetic biomaterials have been evaluated as substitutes for dura closure. Experimental testing of new materials has been performed in only a few animal studies and limited information is provided in the literature on the healing mechanism that takes place after duraplasty.[32]

Histologically, the dura mater is composed of a rich network of collagen fibers with intermingled fibroblasts and is covered by subdural neuroepithelium. The process of wound healing after dura repair using a degradable transplant is believed to occur by endogenous tissue (fibroblast migration from dura borders) replacing the graft, resulting ultimately in a thick scar. Collagen grafts are extremely effective in this context. Nondegradable materials, on the other hand, cannot be replaced by endogenous tissue due to their resistance against enzymatic and cellular processes; when they are biocompatible, they become covered with a thin layer of tissue during the healing process. These synthetic biomaterials enveloped in connective tissue layers without causing foreign-body reactions were found acceptable for duraplasty since they showed no adherence to the cortex and only moderate extradural fibrosis.[33] Anyway, although rare, synthetic graft-related complications have been reported in the literature, in terms of local inflammation and infections.[34,35]

It is stated that the ideal material for duraplasty should be: (1) autologous, to avoid all potential risks of heterogeneous grafts; (2) free of biological hazards to avoid HIV infection, hepatitis, and other communicable diseases[36]; (3) able to facilitate fibroblastic migration and connective tissue deposition; and (4) associated with a good cost–effectiveness ratio.

Skull base reconstruction is generally described according to reconstructive procedures with free grafts or with vascularized flaps:

Free Grafts

The grafting techniques employ tissues that are totally detached from the donor site, and transferred and implanted into the receiver site. They lack their own vascularization; therefore, they need a well-vascularized bed that can provide nourishment to the graft itself guaranteeing the success of the grafting. The reconstruction can be performed with a single layer (overlay technique) or multiple layers (multilayer technique) of tissue. The latter is defined "simple" if using only one kind of material or "combined" if materials with different histologic nature are employed.

The most employed tissues are:
- Fascia lata is a favored autologous grafting material that is easy to harvest and large grafts can be obtained. It can be used in association with other grafts, whether free or pedicled. Its consistency is very similar to the dura and its healing properties are good.
  (In the authors' experience, the iliotibial tract [ITT] has the best characteristics in terms of thickness, pliability, and strength. ITT is a continuation of the fascia lata in the lateral thigh extending from the iliac crest to the infracondylar tubercle of the tibia [Gerdy tubercle], with a mean length of 400 mm and mean width of 90 mm[37] [▶ Fig. 13.1]. Its mean thickness at the femoral

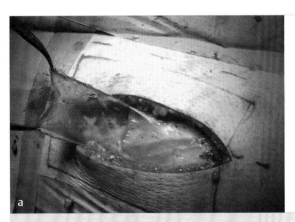
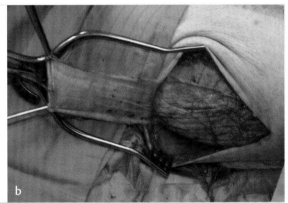

Fig. 13.1 **a, b** Harvesting of the graft of fascia lata (**a**) compared with the one made at the iliotibial tract (**b**). The better consistency of this second graft is evident.

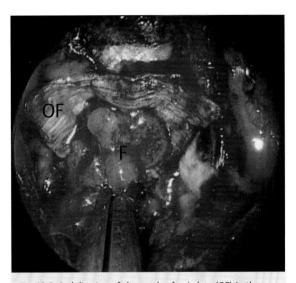

Fig. 13.2 Stabilization of the overlay fascia lata (OF) in the repair of a skull base defect made by using a small piece of fat (F), both fixed with fibrin glue.

condyle varies from 2.2 to 1.6 mm and varies in inverse proportion to the patient's age.[38] The ITT is harvested in the middle third of the thigh together with subcutaneous fat, if required. The wound is closed with double subcutaneous sutures to avoid muscle prolapse.)

- Fascia temporalis is easier to harvest but is thinner and weaker than the fascia lata, and only smaller grafts can be obtained.
- Mucoperiosteum/mucoperichondrium harvested from septum or turbinates.
- Cartilage can be harvested from the nasal septum, the ear concha, or tragus.
- Bone can be harvested from the nasal septum or turbinates and shows rapid reabsorption.

- Fat can be used as an obliteration material, possibly in combination with fascia, in cases of poorly pneumatized sinuses. Some further applications are to stabilize the overlay graft or, taken in small pieces, a "cushionlike device" between grafts in the multilayer duraplasty (▶ Fig. 13.2).
- Heterologous materials such as bovine or human lyophilized dura have been used widely; however, since there has been evidence of transmission of prion-associated diseases, they should no longer be used routinely.[39]
- Synthetic material such as Gore-Tex patches, porous polyethylene implants, or bone-substitute material such as hydroxyapatite are episodically mentioned in literature. Contact of the latter with brain surface or other neurologically sensitive structures should be strictly avoided.[40]

Vascularized Flaps

Surgical advances made over the past decade allowed large lesions affecting the dura, as well as intradural tumors, to be reached with the transnasal endoscopic approach. This necessitated the development of additional techniques to provide a predictable, reliable, and safe closure.

Vascularized flaps provide the best means to achieve this goal. In this case, tissues maintain a connection with the donor site (pedicle) and are transferred to the receiver site, which has to be adjacent, through sliding and rotation movements. They have their own vascularization.

An ideal flap should be simple to design, resist trauma, produce little or no morbidity, provide an adequate surface area, and have an arc of rotation that permits its transposition without the tendency to return to its original position. In general, local flaps obtained from areas that are adjacent to the defect are preferable to regional flaps and these latter are preferable to flaps that are obtained from distant areas or that require a microvascular transfer.

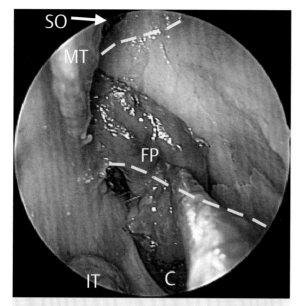

Fig. 13.3 Endoscopic view of right nasal fossa with a 0°, 4 mm scope, during cadaver dissection. The yellow dashed line indicates the section of the flap at level of the sphenoethmoidal recess upon and below the tails of middle turbinate (MT) and superior turbinate, between the sphenoidal ostium (SO) and the choana (C). The flap pedicle (FP) can be better mobilized if undermined also at level of the pterygoid and sphenopalatine region drilling the bone beneath.

Below is a brief summary of the different vascularized flaps described in the literature and employed for skull base reconstruction:

Hadad-Bassagaisteguy Flap

The Hadad-Bassagaisteguy flap (HBF) is a vascular pedicle flap supplied by the posterior nasoseptal arteries.[41] These arteries arise from the posterior nasal artery, which is one of the terminal branches of the maxillary artery. The posterior nasoseptal arteries supply the entire length of the nasal septum and anastomose with the ethmoidal arteries, the greater palatine artery, and the anterior facial artery. The flap is designed according to the size and shape of the anticipated defect, although it is best to overestimate the size and then trim the flap if needed.

The HBF had a profound impact on the advancement and acceptance of expanded endonasal approaches because the incidence of postsurgical CSF leaks dramatically decreased to < 5%[42]; thus, allowing the expansion of endoscopic skull base procedures.[26] The HBF has become a mainstay reconstructive option after expanded endonasal approaches due to its versatility, wide arc of rotation, generous size, and relative ease of harvesting. Loss of the flap occurred in patients who had undergone extensive radiation therapy to the area of the posterior choana.[28]

Harvesting of the HBF includes the use of two parallel incisions along the axis of the nasal septum. An inferior incision is made over the maxillary crest and a superior incision is made 1 to 2 cm below the most superior aspect of the septum to preserve the olfactory epithelium. A vertical incision at the mucocutaneous junction joins these two horizontal incisions anteriorly.

Posteriorly, the superior incision extends laterally over the rostrum of the sphenoid sinus at the inferior aspect of the sphenoid ostium, while the inferior incision extends along the posterior free border of the nasal septum, and then laterally along the arch of the posterior choana. A strip of the mucosa between the sphenoid rostrum incisions contains the posterior septal arteries and forms a relatively long and narrow pedicle that facilitates a long reach and wide arc of rotation[41] (▶ Fig. 13.3).

It is also important to raise the pedicle to a level that is as close as possible to the sphenopalatine foramen to gain maximum length. To make the pedicle free at this level, drilling the base of the pterygoid is needed.

Maximal length of the flap is obtained by placing the anterior vertical incision at the mucocutaneous junction. A wider flap can be harvested by placing the inferior incision at the lateral nasal floor in the inferior meatus. All incisions can be modified according to reconstructive or oncologic requirements. Subperichondrial elevation of the HBF frees its paddle and pedicle so it can be then stored in the nasopharynx or inside the antrum.[43]

This flap, when applied directly or placed over traditional fascia grafts, should provide very strong support and rapid epithelialization, especially in critical areas. A double elevation from both sides of the septum is described also.[44]

Posterior Pedicle Inferior Turbinate Flap

The use of vascularized flaps from the inferior turbinate is not a new concept. Anteriorly based flaps have been described for the closure of septal perforations and for the internal lining of nasal defects. The posterior pedicle inferior turbinate flap (PPITF) is based on the inferior turbinate artery, a terminal branch from the posterolateral nasal artery, which is a terminal branch from the sphenopalatine artery.[45] It is best to identify first the sphenopalatine artery as it exits the sphenopalatine foramen and follow it distally to identify the posterolateral nasal artery. Two parallel incisions are performed following the sagittal plane of the inferior turbinate; the superior one just above the inferior turbinate, at the maxillary fontanelle level, and the inferior one following the caudal margin of the turbinate. A vertical cut made along the anterior head of the turbinate connects the two previous incisions. The mucoperiosteum is elevated, providing about 4.97 cm^2 surface area.[46]

Posterior Pedicle Middle Turbinate Flap

The posterior pedicle middle turbinate flap (PPMTF) is suitable for the reconstruction of defects at the cribriform plate, fovea ethmoidalis, planum sphenoidale, or sella turcica.[47] Its blood supply comes from the middle turbinate branch of the sphenopalatine artery that runs through the posterior attachment and constitutes its pedicle.

Its harvesting entails the elevation of its mucoperiosteum in a superior-to-inferior direction, exposing the turbinate bone medially and laterally. After removal of the turbinate bone, further elevation of the flap posteriorly exposes the pedicle that can be mobilized and released from all surrounding attachments. A complete release allows a wider arc of rotation and greater length.

A significant limitation of the PPMTF is the technical difficulty involved with its dissection due to the anatomical variability. As is the case with the PPITF, the surface area of the PPMTF is somewhat limited at 5.6 cm².

Transpterygoid Transposition of the Temporoparietal Fascia Flap

The temporoparietal fascia flap (TPFF) is a pedicled flap based on the anterior branch of the superficial temporal artery, which is one of the terminal branches of the external carotid artery. It has been used as a reconstructive option in a variety of defects in the head and neck, including intraoral defects, and oronasal and nasocutaneous fistulas, as well as skull base defects after traditional craniofacial resections.[48]

To perform this technique, a wide exposure of the pterygopalatine fossa and the infratemporal fossa is needed; a transpterygoid corridor is tailored exposing the anterior aspect of the pterygoid plates and the bone is reduced with a high-speed drill to enlarge the tunnel and allow transposition of the TPFF into the nasal cavity.

Harvesting of the TPFF follows a conventional coronal incision. Transposition of the TPFF into the infratemporal fossa follows a tunnel created by separating the temporalis muscle from the lateral orbital wall and from the pterygomaxillary fissure. The TPFF is then tied to a guide wire, inserted under endonasal endoscopic visualization, and pulled into the nasal cavity.

The TPFF has a predictable vascular anatomy, good arch of rotation, long vascular pedicle length and a rich vascularity that allows it to survive and heal even under unfavorable conditions. It can cover a surface area of 17 × 14 cm.[49]

Transfrontal Pericranial Flap

The pericranial and galeopericranial flaps are the most commonly used reconstructive options for traditional anterior cranial base procedures. These are pedicled axial flaps based on the supraorbital and supratrochlear arteries, which yield a very large surface area.[50] Their use after endoscopic skull base techniques requires introduction of the externally harvested flap into the nasal cavity through a bony window at the upper aspect of the nasion.

The pericranial flap can be harvested via a standard coronal incision or using an endoscopic assisted technique.[51] A Draf III frontal sinusotomy is needed as part of the corridor and to secure the drainage of the frontal sinuses.

Oliver Pedicled Palatal Flap

The Oliver modification of the palatal flap (OPPF) transposes the vascularized mucoperiosteal tissue of the hard palate into the nasal cavity through the greater palatine foramen.[52]

It yields a large surface area that ranges between 12 and 18.5 cm and its long pedicle allows a large arc of rotation that can reach multiple areas of the skull base.[53]

The OPPF is an excellent alternative when previous expanded endonasal approaches and/or open skull base surgical procedures have eliminated all other reconstructive options. One potential complication of the flap is the persistence of an oronasal fistula. To avoid this complication, the nasal floor mucosa is elevated and preserved with a differential flap. Another potential problem is that the OPPF introduces oral bacterial flora into the surgical field.

Microvascular Free Flaps

A further evolution of these flaps is a microvascular free flap. Once the flap's pedicle is isolated and transected, it can be transferred at a distance and revascularized with microvascular anastomosis of the pedicle with vessels of the receiver site. Typically, branches of the external carotid arterial system, and the facial artery in particular, are readily accessible for the artery from the flap. The external jugular vein and its venous tributaries, such as the posterior facial vein, are extremely reliable recipient vessels for the venous anastomosis. The superficial temporal vessels are potential recipient vessels because of their proximity to the lateral skull base. However, the artery, and particularly the vein, may be of moderate caliber or poor quality; thus, unreliable. Because most of the commonly used free flaps in skull base reconstruction have long pedicles, the superficial temporal vessels can usually be avoided in preference to large-caliber neck vessels without the need for vein jump graft.[54]

Their use is reserved for cases of surgical revision of large duraplasty for persistent CSF leak. They can be fascia-muscle-cutaneous, and generally employed for soft-tissue reconstruction, such as the radial forearm flap, the anterolateral thigh flap, the latissimus dorsi flap, the rectus abdominis flap, and the trapezius flap. Otherwise, they can be osteo-muscle-cutaneous, generally for combined bone reconstruction, such as the fibular flap, the scapular flap, and the iliac crest flap.

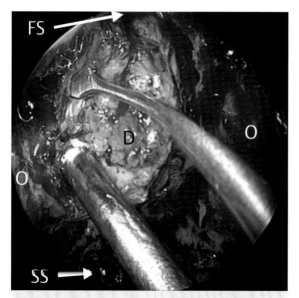

Fig. 13.4 Endoscopic view with a 45°, 4 mm scope during endoscopic transnasal craniectomy. The nasal septum is removed, the ethmoidal roof from the frontal sinus (FS) to the sphenoidal sinus (SS), from orbit (O) to orbit is removed together with the crista galli. At this step of surgery, before resecting the dura (D), it is important to undermine the epidural space also coagulating and cutting the ethmoidal arteries to provide an adequate space for positioning the intracranial extradural layer of the duraplasty.

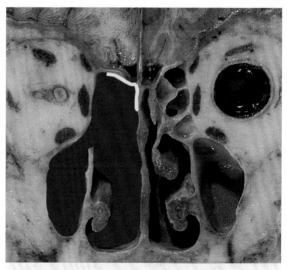

Fig. 13.5 Scheme showing the position of the overlay extracranial layer (yellow) positioned to cover small skull base defects at level of the olfactory fissure. The red line indicates dura.

13.2.2 Indications and Duraplasty Techniques

The aim of this surgery is the closure of the defect avoiding seepage of CSF. The criterion that guides the repair is "integration of the borders." No matter what type of technique is used, the preparatory stage of duraplasty must include appropriate exposure of the defect, undermining of the dural margins (when possible), and smoothing of the defect edges to get an adhesion effect for the graft/flap (▶ Fig. 13.4). As general rule, meticulous management of the tissues is required for the best integration and a dedicated surgical team for performing the reconstruction is recommended.

The main surgical reconstructive procedures can be divided into: (1) free graft techniques (including the "multilayer technique"); and (2) pedicled flaps, which can be otherwise combined together in selected cases.

Free Graft Techniques

Overlay Technique

The most simple reconstruction technique is the overlay technique, indicated in cases of small defects in the olfactory fissure (▶ Fig. 13.5). In this area, preparation of the tissues in the site of the defect does not include dissection of the dural margin away from the bony border, since the dura in this area is extremely fragile because of the olfactory pores and any consequent dural tear would mean a useless enlargement of the defect. The graft, which is usually either mucoperichondrial or mucoperiosteal and removed from the homolateral or contralateral nasal cavity, is put in place with the mucosa side facing the nasal cavity and is firmly secured, applying pressure from the center outwards, to avoid air remaining trapped between the graft and the defect. Hence, for any overlay technique the receptor site must be stripped of its mucosal layer in the area to be covered by the graft/flap. If used, fibrin glue is placed along the graft margins but not under it; this avoids a gap between graft and the receiving site.

The removal of benign fibro-osseous tumors or inverted papillomas that involve the skull base can occasionally require just a reinforcement of a seemingly intact dura, which can be performed with a free graft of overlaid mucoperichondrium or mucoperiosteum.[55] This procedure is most commonly used when the olfactory fissure has been drilled for removal of the tumor but no intradural dissection has been performed. The minimum amount of liquorrhea secreted from the olfactory filaments is kept under control with an overlay graft.

Underlay Technique

In the underlay technique the (free) graft is placed between the dura and the bone of the skull base (epidural) or between the dura and the brain (subdural). It is recommended to create the underlay graft larger in diameter than the dural defect, to overlap the defect and to compensate for shrinking of the graft during healing.

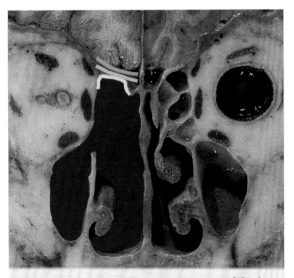

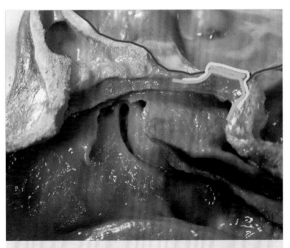

Fig. 13.7 Using the gasket-seal technique the margins of the fascia layers are kept outside of the defect to avoid dural undermining at the level of risky anatomical areas. The first layer (yellow) is maintained in position using a fragment of cartilage whose margins are inserted into the defect (green). The third layer (light blue) is used to stabilize the duraplasty. The red line indicates the dura.

Fig. 13.6 Scheme showing the correct positioning of the three layers in the multilayer technique. The first intracranial intradural layer is green, the second intracranial extradural underlay layer is light blue, and the extradural, extracranial, overlay layer is yellow. The red line indicates dura. The intracranial layers have to be at least 30% larger than the defect.

Multilayer Technique

The combination of underlay and overlay grafts, or flaps in association with intracranial intradural grafts, is termed multilayer technique. Free tissue grafting yields adequate and reproducible results not only in patients who present small defects, such as those following transsellar surgery, but is still an option for the repair of larger defects, such as those after endonasal endoscopic craniectomy at anterior skull base level, using large fascial grafts.

The underlying principle of multilayered reconstruction is to re-establish the tissue barriers. The technique usually involves the application of three layers:

- The first layer is usually made up of fascia (lata or temporal) or dural substitutes placed intracranially and intradurally to serve as a guide for fibroblast migration. This first layer must be one-third larger than the dural defect.
- The second intracranial and extradural layer (underlay) guarantees the plasty with greater stability. Any difficulty encountered when inserting the margins of the fascia in the epidural gap can be overcome by using fragments of bone or autologous cartilage removed from the nasal cavities or from the ear concha. In these cases, the appropriately shaped fragments are used to push in the fascia in a suitable manner. However, patients undergoing reconstruction in this fashion should not be submitted to radiotherapy since there is a risk of developing a sequestrum and possible necrosis.
- The third layer, extracranial and intranasal (overlay), facilitates the sealing capacity of the plasty by guiding the repair mechanisms of the nasal mucosa. This layer

can be made of fascia or free grafts of septal mucoperichondrium or of septal or turbinal mucoperiosteum (▶ Fig. 13.6). It is worth noting that healing and re-epithelialization is much more rapid when mucoperiosteum is used as a third layer, rather than fascia lata, which can sometimes become necrotic even after 1 to 2 months.

The **"fat-plug" technique** is a variant of the multilayer technique in which a fat lobule is used as intracranial intradural graft.[56,57]

The **"gasket-seal closure"** technique is another kind of multilayer reconstruction, used mostly at the sphenoethmoidal-planum level and clivus level (middle and posterior cranial fossae) where dural undermining is more risky due to the proximity of neurovascular structures (optic nerve and chiasm, superior hypophyseal artery, cranial nerve VI) (▶ Fig. 13.7).

This technique allows fixing the graft margins intradurally without risking damage to these neurovascular structures. To accomplish this, the graft is placed on the dural defect and its central portion is pushed inside the defect with the aid of a shaped fragment of septal or conchal cartilage, which is fixed beyond the dural border to seal the closure while still keeping the margins of the fascia outside the skull base[58] (▶ Fig. 13.8). As with the other closure techniques, it is recommended that no nasal or sinus mucosa be "buried" under any graft or flap to avoid the formation of mucocele.

The **obliterative technique,** largely used in the past to fill sinus cavities where a CSF leak was present, has a high

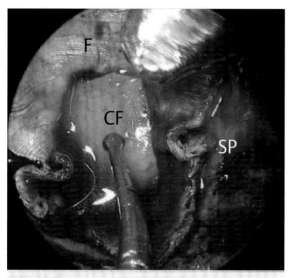

Fig. 13.8 The endoscopic view (45°, 4 mm scope) of the repair of a dural defect located at the sphenoethmoidal plane (SP) shows the positioning of the cartilage fragment (CF) over the first fascial layer (F) whose margins are kept outside of the defect. The insertion of the cartilage borders inside the margins of the defect helps to stabilize the duraplasty.

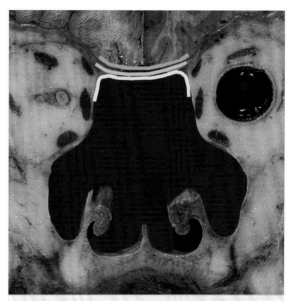

Fig. 13.9 Endoscopic duraplasty after endoscopic transnasal craniectomy is performed with a three-layer technique. The first is the intradural layer of duraplasty (green), 30% larger than the dural defect. The second layer (light blue) is intracranial and extradural, tacked between the previously undermined dura and the residual anterior skull base. The third (yellow) is the extracranial layer covering all the exposed anterior skull base. The red line indicates the dura.

risk of reabsorption of the fat lobule with recurrence of rhinoliquorrea and/or inflammatory complications. In our experience, two cases of arachnoidal cyst at level of middle cranial fossa were observed when bone defect at the Sternberg canal was untreated. In these cases, the multilayer duraplasty technique foresees direct closure of the bone defect. This is the reason why we prefer the multilayer technique instead of simply filling the sinus cavity with fat.

Skull Base Reconstruction After Endonasal Endoscopic Anterior Skull Base Craniectomy

This skull base reconstruction is a multilayer technique used for large defects extending from orbit to orbit laterally, and from the frontal recess to the sphenoethmoidal-planum anteroposteriorly (▶ Fig. 13.9). The key point to perform an optimal skull base reconstruction following endoscopic transnasal craniectomy is to properly dissect the dura over the orbital roof(s) laterally, the planum sphenoidale posteriorly, and the posterior wall of the frontal sinus anteriorly before starting the resection of the dura itself. The dura is subsequently cauterized with bipolar cautery, incised, and circumferentially removed with angled scissors as far away possible from the suspected area of tumor spread (wide free margin).

The material employed is usually fascia lata or ITT for all the three layers; bone and cartilage are avoided because of the frequent need for postoperative adjuvant radiotherapy.

- For the first intradural layer of duraplasty, the graft must be 30% larger than the dural defect and split anteriorly on the midline to adjust to the falx cerebri in case of bilateral resection, in order to compensate its shrinking during healing.[59] It is sometimes necessary to section the falx to facilitate the insertion of the first intradural layer.
- The second layer, intracranial and extradural, needs to be sized precisely and tacked between the previously undermined dura and the residual bony anterior skull base. Pieces of fatty tissue are adopted to eliminate the dead space between the second and third layers and to flatten the residual bared anterior skull base.
- The third layer, extracranial, has to cover all the exposed anterior skull base, but without overlapping the frontal and/or sphenoidal sinusotomy(ies).

Each layer is properly fixed with fibrin glue along the borders and the last layer is stabilized with oxidized cellulose and smoothed from its center toward the margins to guarantee better adhesion due to the its capillary adhesion effect. This is why the employment of other stabilizing devices, such as balloons, are debatable in our setting, even if they are routinely used by other schools of surgery.[60]

At the end of the procedure, the frontal sinusotomy (Draf III) can be stented with a rolled Silastic (Dow Corning, Midland, Michigan, United States) sheath to allow subsequent frontal sinus débridement, with no risks for the duraplasty and avoiding scarring in patients who are submitted to radiotherapy.

Attempts have been made to suture dural grafts endonasally in the vicinity of the defects and/or the remaining dura, to prevent intraoperative and postoperative displacement. Special U-clip anastomotic suture devices, originally developed for cardiovascular anastomosis, have been used.[61]

Vascularized Flap Technique

The HBF is the preferred flap, though not the only option, for the reconstruction of anterior, middle, and posterior large skull base defects. Middle and inferior turbinate flaps are best suited for limited defects, usually confined to a single area of the skull base. Use of the inferior turbinate pedicled flap is limited by its size and configuration. It is better used for the reconstruction of limited posterior and inferior defects, such as those in the clivus. To increase its coverage, it is feasible to raise bilateral PPITFs, or alternatively another pedicled flap can be used in conjunction with an inferior turbinate flap to address larger defects. The superior position of the middle turbinate pedicle flap allows it to reach defects of the cribriform plate, planum sphenoidale, sella, and fovea ethmoidalis areas better than the PPITF.

In patients with more extensive defects, the pericranial flap and the TPFF are more suitable options. Anterior defects, such as those resulting from a transcribriform skull base resection, are ideally suited for a reconstruction with the transfrontal pericranial flap. Given its pedicle location, the transfrontal pericranial flap is best suited for the reconstruction of cribriform and planar defects; however, it can be extended to cover defects of the sella and clivus. Posterior defects of the clivus or defects of the middle cranial fossa are best addressed with a TPFF; thus, making it an option for large planum, sella, clivus and craniovertebral junction defects. If these flaps are not available, the Oliver palatal flap provides coverage for planum, sella, and clivus defects down to the level of the foramen magnum.

Despite the fact that the widespread use of pedicled flaps has improved the outcome of duraplasty procedures, a reconstruction technique must be chosen according to the following criteria.

Anatomical and Mechanical Factors

These are linked with the site of the defect and its borders, since alignment of the borders is very important. The three cranial fossae differ because of their adjacent structures. To achieve success, it is essential to control the margins, particularly when dealing with intracranial grafts:

- In the anterior cranial fossa, epidural detachment is not very difficult and is necessary for receiving the extradural intracranial layer of the plasty, which should normally be spread out within the epidural space

to guarantee sealing of the duraplasty. The olfactory fissure is an exception in this case because it is impossible to detach the epidural plane (olfactory foramen) without tearing the dura itself (for this reason, the overlay technique is applied here). On the other hand, the ethmoidal roof offers the possibility of both lateral and posterior detachment; dissection of the anterior plane is possible with an extensive median frontal sinusotomy and simultaneous removal of the crista galli.

- In the middle fossa, the problematic issues are the optic nerve, the chiasm that is vascularized by the small arterial branches of the superior hypophyseal artery structure (in fact, the vision can be harmed through even the slightest damage to these vessels), the hypophyseal stalk (functional damage can result from minor trauma or maneuvers), and the internal carotid artery. In this area, epidural detachment must be handled very gently or even avoided, using the "gasket-seal" closure technique.

- In the posterior cranial fossa, the critical points encountered include the position of cranial nerve VI as it passes through the Dorello canal, the presence of the basilar artery, the greater CSF pressure, and the different spatial arrangement of the grafts because of the force of gravity.

If these aspects are considered, it is evident that the multilayer technique with free grafts is much easier to carry out in the anterior cranial fossa.

A subject of some controversy is the use of autologous bone/cartilage grafts or rigid allografts to support the reconstruction or to prevent brain herniation.[62] Currently, the concern for delayed brain herniation seems more theoretical than practical, as the phenomenon is extremely rare and not found in large series.[63]

Biological Factors

A distinction must be made between dural reconstruction following the removal of benign or malignant tumors. In case of malignancy, possible spread due to proximity, or through the lymphatic or perineuronal systems, or because of the presence of multiple focal sites (adenoid cystic carcinoma) advises against the use of material harvested from the nasal fossae for reconstruction purposes (since the nasal tissue might contain neoplastic components). From a statistical point of view, malignant tumors most frequently affect the anterior cranial fossa, while benign tumors or ones of low malignancy, such as meningiomas, hypophyseal adenomas, and gliomas, affect the middle and posterior fossae. The removal of a hypophyseal adenoma when no presurgical or intrasurgical rhinoliquorrea is manifest does not even require duraplasty. Grafts are usually autologous; fascia in particular allows tissue integration, with dural repair occurring through "cell migration."

When radiotherapy is expected, free grafts of bone or cartilage should not be used since they are at high risk of postradiotherapy necrosis. On the contrary, the fascia very rarely shows late phenomena of postradiotherapy necrosis. For instance, in the middle or posterior fossa it is possible to use the "gasket-seal" closure technique only when no radiotherapy is foreseen. It is important to remember that certain types of uncommon borderline aggressive behaving lesions (i.e., hemangiopericytoma) could require postsurgical radiotherapy.[64]

13.3 Postoperative Care and Follow-up

Recommendations in the literature concerning nasal packing, bed rest, and need for lumbar drainage are variable.[65] At the Varese/Brescia ear, nose, and throat departments, except for cases with impaired general conditions or those treated with more extensive cranioendoscopic approaches, patients are transferred directly to the general ward after surgery, with no need for intensive care. Nondegradable nasal packs are generally removed 1 to 2 days after surgery and bed rest is maintained for 2 days with trunk and head raised 25°. The importance of postoperative bed rest was apparently overrated in the past and no clear recommendations can be found in the literature.

Antibiotic prophylaxis is administered for 24 to 48 hours, starting at the time of induction of general anesthesia, and discontinuing following the removal of the nasal packing. A single agent antibiotic covering grampositive organisms (broad-spectrum cephalosporin, such as cefazolin, if no history of penicillin allergy is referred) may be adequate to prevent serious central nervous system infectious complications. In addition to intravenous antibiotics given during hospitalization, following discharge a topical aminoglycoside nasal spray or ointment (generally gentamicin) with gram-negative coverage is used in all patients until the wound cavity is considered well healed (2–3 months postoperatively).[66]

The patient is regularly monitored with complete blood tests 1, 5, and 10 days after surgery and a daily check of vital parameters (temperature). A brain computed tomography (CT) scan is performed within 24 hours after surgery for early detection of any signs of postoperative pneumoencephalus and is repeated if necessary. If a contrast-enhanced radiologic examination is performed after the application of a nasoseptal flap, any lack of contrast enhancement suggests ischemia of the flap itself and may warrant re-exploration or removal of the nasal packing to relieve the pressure.[67]

Endoscopic endonasal examinations are performed every day during hospitalization and then scheduled at progressive intervals (7, 14, 21 days; 1, 3, 6, and 12 months) at the outpatient department, with the aim to clean the nasal cavities of crusts and remove scarring tissue. Further endoscopic examinations may be reasonable according to the individual requirements of each patient. Occasionally, additional support to the skull base plasty may be performed placing degradable sponges over the intranasal layer.

Indications for a lumbar spinal drain remain unclear and no consensus can be found in the literature. In comparable indications, those authors who routinely use lumbar drainage do not appear to achieve (statistically) better outcomes than those using this measure less frequently or even not at all.[68,69] In our experience, lumbar spinal drain is not used in the absence of intracranial hypertension.

If an early CSF leak is suspected in the first postoperative days, a lumbar drainage can be inserted to decrease intracranial pressure and facilitate healing, but if a CSF leak is a certainty then a revision of the duraplasty should be performed immediately.

After discharge, patients are usually advised against blowing their nose, bending forward, and involving in physical efforts for at least 1 month. Patients are then closely followed by a multidisciplinary oncologic team (otorhinolaryngologist, neurosurgeon, maxillofacial surgeon, medical oncologist, radiotherapist, and endocrinologist). Radiological evaluations with gadolinium-enhanced magnetic resonance imaging (T1, T2, FLAIR, CISS, fat-saturated sequences) are usually planned every 6 months for the first 5 years and then once a year up to 10 to 15 years, according to the histology of the tumor. Obviously, each patient will require a personal follow-up program.

13.4 Results

A comprehensive review of the literature on skull base reconstruction is offered by the European Position Paper on Endoscopic Management of Tumours of the Nose, Paranasal Sinuses and Skull Base, published in 2010.[65] A total of 1,123 cases treated from 1991 to 2009 in different care units were revised in reference to diagnostic evaluations, surgical procedures, type of skull base reconstruction, and complications.

Use of a wide spectrum of isolated use and combinations of grafting materials appear to have no significant impact on outcome. Twenty-four authors reported primary closure rates equal to or greater than 90%, seven authors reported 87.5 to 89.6%, one author 67%, and another 50%. Secondary closure rate was 100% in 19 papers and between 93.4 and 97% in 6 papers.

Our experience shows a primary closure mean rate of 90.4% on 219 cases of skull base reconstruction performed after tumor removal (91.1% success after pure endoscopic approaches, and 88.7% success after combined external-endoscopic approaches). Secondary closure rate was 100%, reached in 15 cases with a surgical revision of the skull base plasty and in 6 cases setting a lumbar spinal drain (for details about postoperative complications, see Chapter 14).

13.5 Conclusions

The best choice of technique and material relates to experiences reported in the literature and to the expertise of the individual surgeon. Almost all autologous grafting materials work well while reports on allogenic material are episodic. The literature demonstrates a clear trend favoring the use of autologous material, especially fascia lata, which is easy to harvest and provides large grafts. It is very similar to dura in texture and consistency and its autologous nature avoids all potential risks of heterogeneous grafts.

An "ideal" duraplasty has to consider multiple factors that might influence the choice of the surgical technique. Defect dimension is only one aspect to be considered. Site of the defect and histologic type and biological behavior of the tumor are important as well, especially in relation to the need for postoperative radiotherapy.

In our experience, the safest procedure for anterior skull base reconstruction is the multilayer technique using the ITT, which can be used even when postoperative radiotherapy is required.

Gentle handling is mandatory when duraplasty has to be performed near important and/or vital neurovascular structures of the middle and posterior cranial fossae and dedicated minimally traumatic surgical techniques (i.e., "gasket-seal" closure technique, fat "bath-plug") are available to avoid damage.

Multilayer techniques must be conveniently combined with a nasoseptal flap in the treatment of middle and posterior cranial fossae defects. The introduction of the HDF changed the outcome of tumor resection with a dramatic decrease in the rate of postoperative CSF leaks. Bone and cartilage grafts must be avoided when postoperative radiotherapy is anticipated (▶ Table 13.1).

In revision surgery of a large defect, the use of free microvascular free flaps must be considered. They are best indicated in cases of: (1) revision surgery in which the galeal-pericranial flap was previously harvested; (2) secondary reconstruction with loss of the frontal bone and serious intracranial infections; (3) reconstruction of adjacent facial structures such as the orbit, nose, and maxilla; and (4) in previously irradiated patients with extensive defects.[70] Adequate experience in endoscopic CSF leak repair is considered mandatory before surgeons should attempt larger dural resections and/or transdural surgery.

Table 13.1 Recommended modalities of skull base reconstruction

Site of lesion	Histology	Recommended skull base reconstruction
Olfactory fissure	Benign	Overlay free graft Overlay pedicled graft
Ethmoidal roof	Benign	Multilayer free grafts ± pedicled flap
	Malignant	Multilayer fascia
Anterior skull base	Benign	Multilayer free grafts ± pedicled flap
	Malignant	Multilayer fascia
Middle skull base/posterior skull base	Benign	Multilayer free grafts (GS) ± pedicled flap (HBF)
	Malignant	Multilayer fascia ± pedicled flap (HBF)

GS, gasket-seal technique; HBF, Hadad-Bassagaisteguy flap.

Pearls and Pitfalls

- Ideal material for duraplasty should be: (1) autologous, (2) free of biological hazards, (3) able to facilitate fibroblastic migration and connective tissue deposition, and (4) associated with a good cost–effectiveness ratio.
- Adequate autologous free graft materials include: fascia lata, temporalis fascia, mucoperiosteum or mucoperichondrium, mucosa, fat, cartilage, bone.
- Heterologous materials such as bovine or human lyophilized dura or fascia lata, or synthetic material such as Gore-Tex patches and porous polyethylene implants, or bone-substitute material such as hydroxyapatite can be used but are not preferred due to possible lack of integration or infections.
- Pedicled mucosal or fascial flaps are preferred for reconstruction of larger skull base defects, as they represent the most reliable option.
- The following vascularized flaps are available: the HBF, the posterior pedicle inferior turbinate flap, the posterior pedicle middle turbinate flap, the transpterygoid transposition of temporoparietal fascia flap, the transfrontal pericranial flap, and the Oliver pedicled palatal flap.
- A microvascular free flap must be considered in patients with previous radiotherapy, who failed customary techniques for a large duraplasty or for persistent CSF leak.
- When indicated, dural reconstruction should be performed in a multilayer fashion involving the application of three layers.
- In this case the first layer, fascia (i.e., fascia lata or temporal fascia) or a dural substitute has to be placed intracranially and intradurally. Importantly, this first layer must be one-third larger than the dural defect.
- In the second layer, fascia (i.e., fascia lata or temporal fascia) is placed underlay intracranial extradurally.
- In the third layer, fascia or free grafts of septal mucoperichondrium, or of septal or turbinate mucoperiosteum, are placed onlay extracranial intranasally.

References

[1] Shah JP, Kraus DH, Bilsky MH, Gutin PH, Harrison LH, Strong EW. Craniofacial resection for malignant tumors involving the anterior skull base. Arch Otolaryngol Head Neck Surg 1997; 123: 1312–1317

[2] Smith RR, Klopp CT, Williams JM. Surgical treatment of cancer of the frontal sinus and adjacent areas. Cancer 1954; 7: 991–994

[3] Cantù G, Riccio S, Bimbi G et al. Craniofacial resection for malignant tumours involving the anterior skull base. Eur Arch Otorhinolaryngol 2006; 263: 647–652

[4] Ganly I, Patel SG, Singh B et al. Craniofacial resection for malignant paranasal sinus tumors: Report of an International Collaborative Study. Head Neck 2005; 27: 575–584

[5] Ganly I, Patel SG, Singh B et al. Complications of craniofacial resection for malignant tumors of the skull base: report of an International Collaborative Study. Head Neck 2005; 27: 445–451

[6] Lund VJ. Extended applications of endoscopic sinus surgery—the territorial imperative. J Laryngol Otol 1997; 111: 313–315

[7] Castelnuovo P, Dallan I, Battaglia P, Bignami M. Endoscopic endonasal skull base surgery: past, present and future. Eur Arch Otorhinolaryngol 2010; 267: 649–663

[8] Jorissen M. The role of endoscopy in the management of paranasal sinus tumours. Acta Otorhinolaryngol Belg 1995; 49: 225–228

[9] Stammberger H, Anderhuber W, Walch C, Papaefthymiou G. Possibilities and limitations of endoscopic management of nasal and paranasal sinus malignancies. Acta Otorhinolaryngol Belg 1999; 53: 199–205

[10] Castelnuovo P, Battaglia P, Locatelli D, Delù G, Sberze F, Bignami M. Endonasal micro-endoscopic treatment of malignant tumors of the paranasal sinuses and anterior skull base. Oper Tech Otolaryngol Head Neck Surg 2006; 17: 152–167

[11] Nicolai P, Castelnuovo P, Lombardi D et al. Role of endoscopic surgery in the management of selected malignant epithelial neoplasms of the naso-ethmoidal complex. Head Neck 2007; 29: 1075–1082

[12] Zada G, Kelly DF, Cohan P, Wang C, Swerdloff R. Endonasal transsphenoidal approach for pituitary adenomas and other sellar lesions: an assessment of efficacy, safety, and patient impressions. J Neurosurg 2003; 98: 350–358

[13] Kassam A, Carrau RL, Snyderman CH, Gardner P, Mintz A. Evolution of reconstructive techniques following endoscopic expanded endonasal approaches. Neurosurg Focus 2005; 19: E8

[14] May M, Hoffmann DF, Sobol SM. Video endoscopic sinus surgery: a two-handed technique. Laryngoscope 1990; 100: 430–432

[15] Briner HR, Simmen D, Jones N. Endoscopic sinus surgery: advantages of the bimanual technique. Am J Rhinol 2005; 19: 269–273

[16] Kassam AB, Gardner P, Snyderman C, Mintz A, Carrau R. Expanded endonasal approach: fully endoscopic, completely transnasal approach to the middle third of the clivus, petrous bone, middle cranial fossa, and infratemporal fossa. Neurosurg Focus 2005; 19: E6

[17] Frank G, Sciarretta V, Mazzatenta D, Farneti G, Modugno GC. Pasquini E. Transsphenoidal endoscopic approach in the treatment of Rathke's cleft cyst. Neurosurgery 2005; 56: 124–128; discussion 129

[18] de Divitiis E, Cappabianca P, Cavallo LM. Endoscopic transsphenoidal approach: adaptability of the procedure to different sellar lesions. Neurosurgery 2002; 51: 699–705; discussion 705–707

[19] Castelnuovo P, Pistochini A, Locatelli D. Different surgical approaches to the sellar region: focusing on the "two nostrils four hands technique". Rhinology 2006; 44: 2–7

[20] Locatelli D, Canevari FR, Acchiardi I, Castelnuovo P. The endoscopic diving technique in pituitary and cranial base surgery: technical note. Neurosurgery 2010; 66: E400–E401, discussion E401

[21] Cantù G, Solero CL, Pizzi N, Nardo L, Mattavelli F. Skull base reconstruction after anterior craniofacial resection. J Craniomaxillofac Surg 1999; 27: 228–234

[22] Patel SG, Singh B, Polluri A et al. Craniofacial surgery for malignant skull base tumors: report of an international collaborative study. Cancer 2003; 98: 1179–1187

[23] Neligan PC, Mulholland S, Irish J et al. Flap selection in cranial base reconstruction. Plast Reconstr Surg 1996; 98: 1159–1166; discussion 1167–1168

[24] Hegazy HM, Carrau RL, Snyderman CH, Kassam A, Zweig J. Transnasal endoscopic repair of cerebrospinal fluid rhinorrhea: a meta-analysis. Laryngoscope 2000; 110: 1166–1172

[25] Castelnuovo PG, Delù G, Locatelli D et al. Endonasal endoscopic duraplasty: our experience. Skull Base 2006; 16: 19–24

[26] Harvey RJ, Nogueira JF, Schlosser RJ, Patel SJ, Vellutini E, Stamm AC. Closure of large skull base defects after endoscopic transnasal craniotomy. Clinical article. J Neurosurg 2009; 111: 371–379

[27] Freije JE, Gluckman JL, Vanloveren H, McDonough JJ, Shumrick KA. Reconstruction of the anterior skull base after craniofacial resection. Skull Base Surg 1992; 2: 17–21

[28] El-Sayed IH, Roediger FC, Goldberg AN, Parsa AT, McDermott MW. Endoscopic reconstruction of skull base defects with the nasal septal flap. Skull Base 2008; 18: 385–394

[29] Dandy W. Pneumocephalus (intracranial pneumatocele or aerocele). Arch Surg 1926; 12: 949–982

[30] Dohlman G. Spontaneous cerebrospinal rhinorrhoea; case operated by rhinologic methods. Acta Otolaryngol Suppl 1948; 67: 20–23

[31] Hirsch O. Successful closure of cerebrospinal fluid rhinorrhea by endonasal surgery. Arch Otolaryngol 1952; 56: 1–12

[32] Barbolt TA, Odin M, Léger M, Kangas L, Holste J, Liu SH. Biocompatibility evaluation of dura mater substitutes in an animal model. Neurol Res 2001; 23: 813–820

[33] Schick B, Wolf G, Romeike BF, Mestres P, Praetorius M, Plinkert PK. Dural cell culture. A new approach to study duraplasty. Cells Tissues Organs 2003; 173: 129–137

[34] Sade B, Oya S, Lee JH. Non-watertight dural reconstruction in meningioma surgery: results in 439 consecutive patients and a review of the literature. Clinical article. J Neurosurg 2011; 114: 714–718

[35] El Majdoub F, Löhr M, Maarouf M, Brunn A, Stenzel W, Ernestus RI. Transmigration of fibrino-purulent inflammation and malignant cells into an artificial dura substitute (Neuro-Patch): report of two cases. Acta Neurochir (Wien) 2009; 151: 833–835

[36] Anand VK, Murali RK, Glasgold MJ. Surgical decisions in the management of cerebrospinal fluid rhinorrhoea. Rhinology 1995; 33: 212–218

[37] Birnbaum K, Siebert CH, Pandorf T, Schopphoff E, Prescher A, Niethard FU. Anatomical and biomechanical investigations of the iliotibial tract. Surg Radiol Anat 2004; 26: 433–446

[38] Goh LA, Chhem RK, Wang SC, Chee T. Iliotibial band thickness: sonographic measurements in asymptomatic volunteers. J Clin Ultrasound 2003; 31: 239–244

[39] Cappabianca P, Esposito F, Cavallo LM et al. Use of equine collagen foil as dura mater substitute in endoscopic endonasal transsphenoidal surgery. Surg Neurol 2006; 65: 144–148; discussion 149

[40] Ismail AS, Costantino PD, Sen C. Transnasal Transsphenoidal Endoscopic Repair of CSF Leakage Using Multilayer Acellular Dermis. Skull Base 2007; 17: 125–132

[41] Hadad G, Bassagasteguy L, Carrau RL et al. A novel reconstructive technique after endoscopic expanded endonasal approaches: vascular pedicle nasoseptal flap. Laryngoscope 2006; 116: 1882–1886

[42] Shah RN, Surowitz JB, Patel MR et al. Endoscopic pedicled nasoseptal flap reconstruction for pediatric skull base defects. Laryngoscope 2009; 119: 1067–1075

[43] Kassam AB, Thomas A, Carrau RL et al. Endoscopic reconstruction of the cranial base using a pedicled nasoseptal flap. Neurosurgery 2008; 63 Suppl 1: ONS44–ONS52; discussion ONS52–ONS53

[44] Nyquist GG, Anand VK, Singh A, Schwartz TH. Janus flap: bilateral nasoseptal flaps for anterior skull base reconstruction. Otolaryngol Head Neck Surg 2010; 142: 327–331

[45] Murakami CS, Kriet JD, Ierokomos AP. Nasal reconstruction using the inferior turbinate mucosal flap. Arch Facial Plast Surg 1999; 1: 97–100

[46] Fortes FSG, Carrau RL, Snyderman CH et al. The posterior pedicle inferior turbinate flap: a new vascularized flap for skull base reconstruction. Laryngoscope 2007; 117: 1329–1332

[47] Prevedello DM, Barges-Coll J, Fernandez-Miranda JC et al. Middle turbinate flap for skull base reconstruction: cadaveric feasibility study. Laryngoscope 2009; 119: 2094–2098

[48] Fallah DM, Baur DA, Ferguson HW, Helman JI. Clinical application of the temporoparietal-galeal flap in closure of a chronic oronasal fistula: review of the anatomy, surgical technique, and report of a case. J Oral Maxillofac Surg 2003; 61: 1228–1230

[49] Fortes FS, Carrau RL, Snyderman CH et al. Transpterygoid transposition of a temporoparietal fascia flap: a new method for skull base reconstruction after endoscopic expanded endonasal approaches. Laryngoscope 2007; 117: 970–976

[50] Yoshioka N, Rhoton AL. Vascular anatomy of the anteriorly based pericranial flap. Neurosurgery 2005; 57 Suppl: 11–16, discussion 11–16

[51] Zanation AM, Snyderman CH, Carrau RL, Kassam AB, Gardner PA, Prevedello DM. Minimally invasive endoscopic pericranial flap: a new method for endonasal skull base reconstruction. Laryngoscope 2009; 119: 13–18

[52] Oliver CL, Hackman TG, Carrau RL et al. Palatal flap modifications allow pedicled reconstruction of the skull base. Laryngoscope 2008; 118: 2102–2106

[53] Hackman T, Chicoine MR, Uppaluri R. Novel application of the palatal island flap for endoscopic skull base reconstruction. Laryngoscope 2009; 119: 1463–1466

[54] Aviv JE, Sultan MR. Free flaps in skull base surgery. In: Donald PJ, ed. Surgery of the Skull Base. Philadelphia: Lippincott-Raven; 1998:607–621

[55] Bignami M, Pistochini A, Meloni F, Delehaye E, Castelnuovo P. A rare case of oncocytic Schneiderian papilloma with intradural and intraorbital extension with notes of operative techniques. Rhinology 2009; 47: 316–319

[56] Wormald PJ, McDonogh M. 'Bath-plug' technique for the endoscopic management of cerebrospinal fluid leaks. J Laryngol Otol 1997; 111: 1042–1046

[57] Wormald PJ, McDonogh M. The bath-plug closure of anterior skull base cerebrospinal fluid leaks. Am J Rhinol 2003; 17: 299–305

[58] Leng LZ, Brown S, Anand VK, Schwartz TH. 'Gasket-seal' watertight closure in minimal-access endoscopic cranial base surgery. Neurosurgery 2008; 62: 342–343

[59] Villaret AB, Yakirevitch A, Bizzoni A et al. Endoscopic transnasal craniectomy in the management of selected sinonasal malignancies. Am J Rhinol Allergy 2010; 24: 60–65

[60] Snyderman CH, Kassam AB, Carrau R, Mintz A. Endoscopic reconstruction of cranial base defects following endonasal skull base surgery. Skull Base 2007; 17: 73–78

[61] Gardner P, Kassam A, Snyderman C, Mintz A, Carrau R, Moossy JJ. Endoscopic endonasal suturing of dural reconstruction grafts: a novel application of the U-Clip technology. Technical note. J Neurosurg 2008; 108: 395–400

[62] Neovius E, Engstrand T. Craniofacial reconstruction with bone and biomaterials: review over the last 11 years. J Plast Reconstr Aesthet Surg 2010; 63: 1615–1623

[63] Nicolai P, Battaglia P, Bignami M et al. Endoscopic surgery for malignant tumors of the sinonasal tract and adjacent skull base: a 10-year experience. Am J Rhinol 2008; 22: 308–316

[64] Schiariti M, Goetz P, El-Maghraby H, Tailor J, Kitchen N. Hemangiopericytoma: long-term outcome revisited. Clinical article. J Neurosurg 2011; 114: 747–755

[65] Lund VJ, Stammberger H, Nicolai P et al. European Position Paper on Endoscopic Management of Tumors of the Nose, Paranasal Sinuses and Skull Base. Rhinol Suppl 2010; 1: 1–143

[66] Brown SM, Anand VK, Tabaee A, Schwartz TH. Role of perioperative antibiotics in endoscopic skull base surgery. Laryngoscope 2007; 117: 1528–1532

[67] Kang MD, Escott E, Thomas AJ et al. The MR imaging appearance of the vascular pedicle nasoseptal flap. AJNR Am J Neuroradiol 2009; 30: 781–786

[68] Gendeh BS, Mazita A, Selladurai BM, Jegan T, Jeevanan J, Misiran K. Endonasal endoscopic repair of anterior skull-base fistulas: the Kuala Lumpur experience. J Laryngol Otol 2005; 119: 866–874

[69] Muscatello L, Lenzi R, Dallan I, Seccia V, Marchetti M, Sellari-Franceschini S. Endoscopic transnasal management of cerebrospinal fluid leaks of the sphenoid sinus. J Craniomaxillofac Surg 2010; 38: 396–402

[70] Califano J, Cordeiro PG, Disa JJ et al. Anterior cranial base reconstruction using free tissue transfer: changing trends. Head Neck 2003; 25: 89–96

Chapter 14

Prevention and Management of Complications

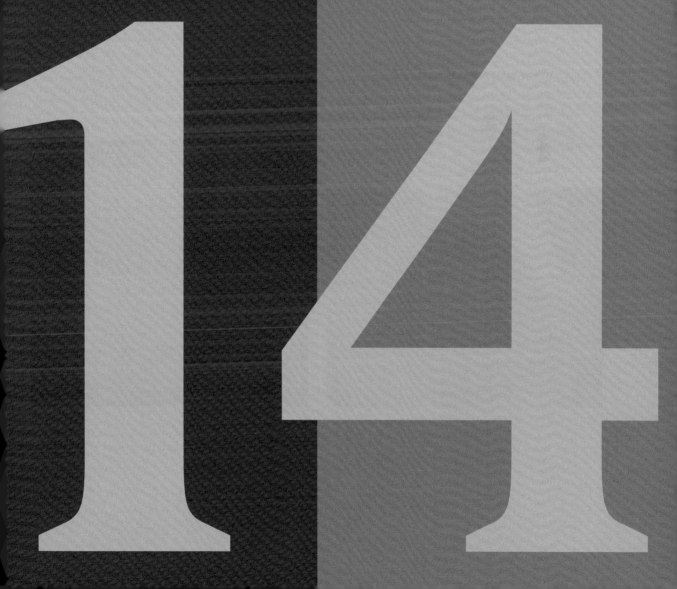

14 Prevention and Management of Complications

Ernesto Pasquini, Giorgio Frank

14.1 Introduction

Over the last decade, the advent of extended endoscopic approaches has promoted endoscopic endonasal surgery from a sellar pathology to skull base surgery.[1] To take advantage of this new technique, training is required to become familiar with two-dimensional vision, endoscopic anatomy, the surgical approaches in general, and the new instrumentation.[2]

In the following chapter the most frequent complications occurring during endoscopic skull base surgery are described, with suggestions as to how to prevent them and how to treat them using the endoscopic technique. The first step in avoiding complications is to perform only operations for which the surgeon is highly trained. A training program, such as that suggested by Snyderman et al (2007),[2] may be a useful instrument for assisting the surgeon in handling incremental and modular surgical difficulties.

Complications may be classified as vascular, neurological, endocrinological, cerebrospinal fluid (CSF) leak and infective.

14.2 Vascular Complications

Vascular complications may be related to the approach phase and/or to vascular dissection during tumor resection; these may be categorized into arterial or venous hemorrhages.

14.2.1 Vascular Complications in the Approach Phase

Arterial Hemorrhages

The most frequent arterial hemorrhages are represented by bleeding from the branches of the external carotid artery; only rarely is there bleeding from the internal carotid artery (1% of procedures).[3,4] The maxillary artery and its branch the sphenopalatine artery are part of the external carotid artery system and are more frequently involved during endoscopic skull base surgery.

The main trunk of the sphenopalatine artery (▶ Fig. 14.1) or its branches (the septal branch and the posterior nasal or external branch) may be the sources of the bleeding (▶ Fig. 14.2). When using a midline transsphenoidal approach, the septal branch may be lacerated accidentally during the enlargement of the ostium sphenoidalis and the external nasal branch may be interrupted at the tail of the middle turbinate when performing a middle turbinectomy.[5] Conversely, interruption of the main trunk of the sphenopalatine artery is planned when performing an ethmoidopterygo-sphenoidal approach.[6] The sphenopalatine artery reaches the nasal cavity through the sphenopalatine foramen, which is located medially to the attachment of the middle turbinate at the posterosuperior corner of the maxillary sinus. To expose the main trunk of the sphenopalatine

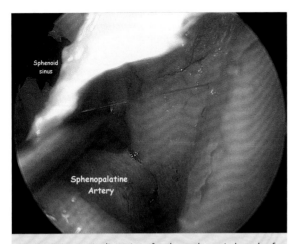

Fig. 14.1 Anatomic dissection of cadaver: the main branch of sphenopalatine artery is easily recognizable because of displacement of mucoperiosteum covering the vertical process of palatine bone and pterygoid process.

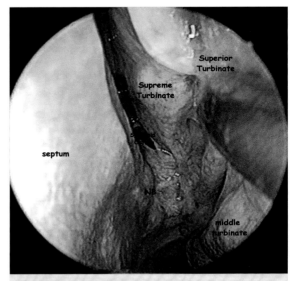

Fig. 14.2 Anatomic dissection of cadaver: between the tail of the superior turbinate and the supreme turbinate, the nasal branch (NB) of the sphenopalatine artery is clearly visible, along with its relationship with the choana, septum, and sphenoid ostium.

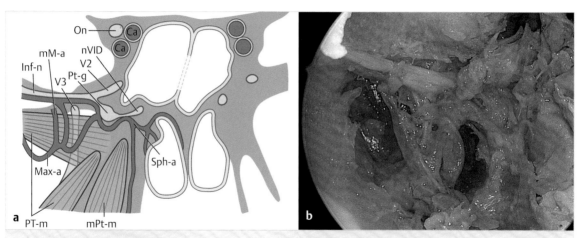

Fig. 14.3 a, b Scheme (**a**) and anatomic dissection (**b**) of the pterygopalatine and infratemporal fossae. Ca, carotid artery; Inf-n, infrorbital nerve; Max-a, maxillary artery; mM-a, middle meningeal artery; mPt-m, medial pterigoid muscle; nVID, vidian nerve; ON, optic nerve; Pt-g, pterygopalatine ganglion; PT-m, pterigoid muscle; Sph-a, sphenopalatine artery.

artery, the foramen should be opened using rongeurs, after which it should be cauterized or clipped before its transection. In all cases, bleeding of the main trunk or of the branches of the sphenopalatine artery requires meticulous coagulation of the vessel, not only to stop the blood loss but also to prevent possible delayed epistaxis.

The main trunk or branches of the maxillary artery are involved during endoscopic approaches to the pterygopalatine or infratemporal fossae (▶ Fig. 14.3), such as during the removal of a juvenile angiofibroma. In fact, during this procedure, the identification, coagulation, and interruption of the maxillary artery should anticipate the tumor removal either to prevent hemorrhage from its laceration or to reduce the blood supply to the tumor. To control the maxillary artery, simple coagulation may not be sufficient and a clipping of the vessel trunk may be preferred.

Hemorrhage from the Internal Carotid Artery

Hemorrhage from the internal carotid artery (ICA) is a rare complication of transsphenoidal surgery.[3,4] The incidence of arterial lesions during transsphenoidal surgery varies between 0.4% for expert surgeons and 1.4% for surgeons who are less expert.[3] Raymond[7] pointed out an incidence of 1% bleeding during or after transsphenoidal pituitary surgery, with a morbidity of 24% and a mortality of 14%.

Some anatomical variations may lead to this serious complication. The most important anatomical variants are[8]:

- Bulging of the ICA within the sphenoidal sinus at the level of the parasellar tract where, in 4% of cases, the bony wall may be lacking
- Sphenoidal septa inserting on the prominence of the internal carotid

- Reduced intercarotid space
- The persistence of the trigeminal artery, consisting of a connection between the carotid–vertebral system (▶ Fig. 14.4 and ▶ Fig. 14.5)
- The presence of vascular malformations, such as an aneurysm (▶ Fig. 14.6 and ▶ Fig. 14.7).

Other factors that may favor these arterial hemorrhages are: carcinomas encroaching on the wall of the arteries, and the presence of scar tissue derived from previous surgical procedures or from radiotherapy.

Although the possibility of injuring the carotid artery through a transsphenoidal route is remote, the same thing cannot be said for cases of extended surgical approaches requiring an anatomical dissection in the proximity and along the pathway of the ICA. The surgical routes or corridors used to gain access to the ventral skull base have been described and identified by Kassam et al[9,10,11] according to their relationship to the four main segments of the ICA (ascending parapharyngeal segment, horizontal petrous segment, vertical paraclival/parasellar segment, paraclinoid segment).

In carrying out these approaches, knowledge of the course of the ICA and its landmarks is of paramount importance to avoid vascular complications. The main landmarks are the medial clinoid process for the identification of the paraclinoid segment of the artery, the vidian canal for the junction between the horizontal petrous portion of the carotid and its ascending paraclival portion, and the Eustachian tube for the parapharyngeal artery (▶ Fig. 14.6).

Some devices, such as a neuronavigator[12] (▶ Fig. 14.8) and Doppler[13] are useful supports for the early identification of the vessel. When the anatomy is normal, they simply confirm previous anatomical identification but, in the presence of anatomical variants, such as an anomalous

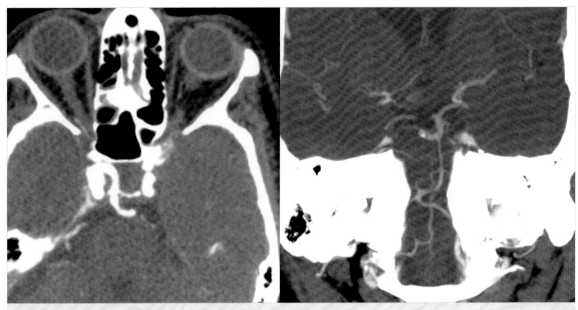

Fig. 14.4 Angio-CT of the persistent trigeminal artery. It is clear how the artery crosses the sella cavity ending at the basilar artery. The middle and the inferior parts of the basilar artery are hypoplastic after this junction.

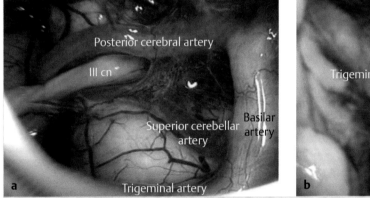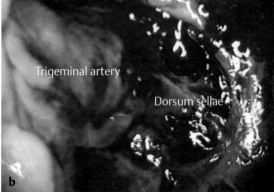

Fig. 14.5 a, b Endoscopic endosellar view after tumor removal (a). The suprasellar view clearly shows the persistent trigeminal artery connecting to the upper part of the basilar artery and running behind the medial wall of the cavernous sinus (b). cn, Cranial nerve.

course of the vessel, they are of paramount importance in selecting the safest approach and identifying the vessel in an unexpected location.

However, if a carotid injury occurs, the surgeon should be able to control the bleeding. In such dramatic circumstances, teamwork with the second surgeon is of great importance. In fact, the second surgeon has to hold the endoscope at a specific distance from the source of the bleeding while trying to maintain clear vision and using a suction device to eliminate the blood from the field. On the other hand, the first surgeon should control the bleeding by compressing the vessel with pledgets. Then, moving the pledget aside, the edges of the bleeding site are cauterized using bipolar coagulation.[14] If cauterization fails and/or when the bleeding source is extradural and the dura is intact, packing should be considered. Conversely, packing in a surgical field with an opened dura should be avoided because the bleeding could become intradural. The contribution of the anesthesiologist during these maneuvers is crucial. In fact, the anesthesiologist should maintain the blood pressure and vascular volume assuring adequate cerebral perfusion. With the same aim, if the patient is in a semisitting position and/or with the head elevated, the surgeon should restore the supine position with the head at heart level.

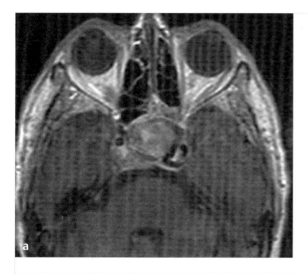
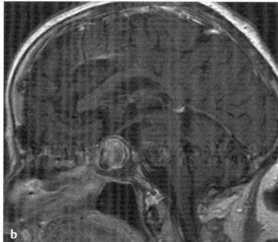
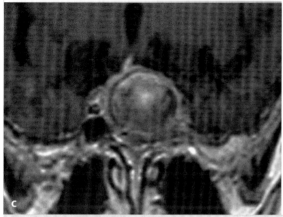

Fig. 14.6 a–c MRI scans showing an adenoma in 70-year-old woman with mild hyperprolactinemia. (a) Axial view; (b) sagittal view; (c) coronal view.

After the bleeding is controlled, an angiography should be performed to confirm the presence of either a pseudoaneurysm at the site of the vascular injury or the effectiveness of the collateral circulation.[7] The first therapeutic choice could be to repair the vessel through the endovascular placement of a stent, thus occluding the tear in the vessel wall and maintaining the blood flow. The second therapeutic choice is an endovascular permanent occlusion of the ICA, including the site of bleeding.[7,15] This option can be considered only if adequate collateral circulation exists. Otherwise, a bypass should be performed before there is occlusion of the vessel.

There is still disagreement regarding the value of routinely performing a preoperative balloon occlusion test.[16] Due to the invasiveness of the procedure, its use is advisable in only selected cases where the risk of carotid injury is greater than that of the test.

Venous Hemorrhage

During skull base surgery, although foreseeable, some venous hemorrhage is unavoidable due to the presence of venous structures in the approach pathway.[8]

This condition may occur during a midline transsphenoidal approach in the presence of a wide intercavernous connection that may be unavoidable during the opening of the sellar meningeal layer. Similarly, there are venous sinuses that are to be transected during some extended transsphenoidal approaches: in the supradiaphragmatic approach, to gain access to the diaphragma and expose the pituitary stalk, transection of the superior intercavernous sinus is planned[17]; in the transclival approach, to open the dura and gain access to the intradural space, the basilar venous plexus has to be transected. Bipolar coagulation is generally effective, particularly after the dura has been opened. Otherwise, several hemostatic materials may contribute to controlling venous bleeding (Floseal, Avitene, Gelfoam).

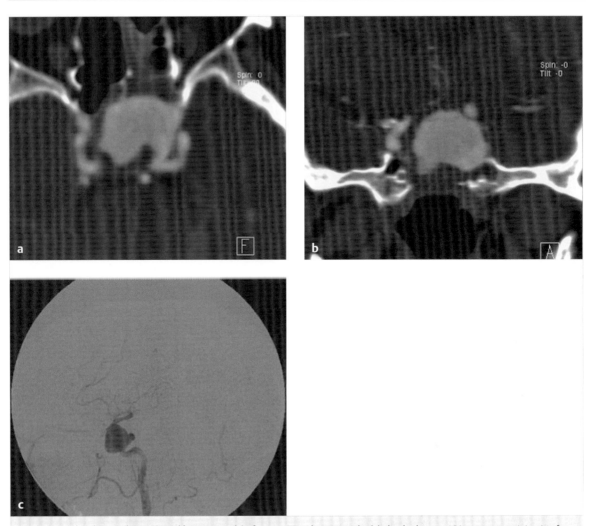

Fig. 14.7 Axial and coronal views (**a** and **b**, respectively) of angio-CT and angiography (**c**) clearly show an ICA aneurysm originating from the right ICA.

Some venous hemorrhages are not foreseeable and avoidable. A similar situation occurs when the cavernous sinus is opened erroneously, due to a wrong surgical trajectory. To prevent such a complication, it is necessary to open the dura in the midline, bearing in mind the anatomical landmarks (sphenoidal septa, parasellar carotid protuberances, and opticocarotid recesses) and/or using devices such as a neuronavigator. To control the bleeding from the cavernous sinus, bipolar coagulation may be harmful, increasing the diameter of the tear due to the retraction of the cauterized margins. In such a situation, the use of hemostatic agents (Avitene, Floseal, Gelfoam) is preferable. Some of these agents (Avitene and Floseal) have the advantage of being removable by washing, without interfering with the visual control of the surgical field.

14.2.2 Vascular Complications in the Dissecting Phase

The rules of microsurgery are the same for endoneurosurgery.[14,18] The surgeon operates using both hands, one for suction and the other for dissection; tumor debulking requires sharp extracapsular dissection and only after this step can the tumor be removed. Unfortunately, even respecting such rules, bleeding may occur and great attention should be applied to hemostasis. Management of extradural arterial or venous bleeding is identical to that in the approach phase. However, the management of intradural bleeding is more intuitive, being a compromise between what can be done and what is more convenient. The hemostatic techniques used are simple packing and irrigation with warm water (effective for venous oozing),

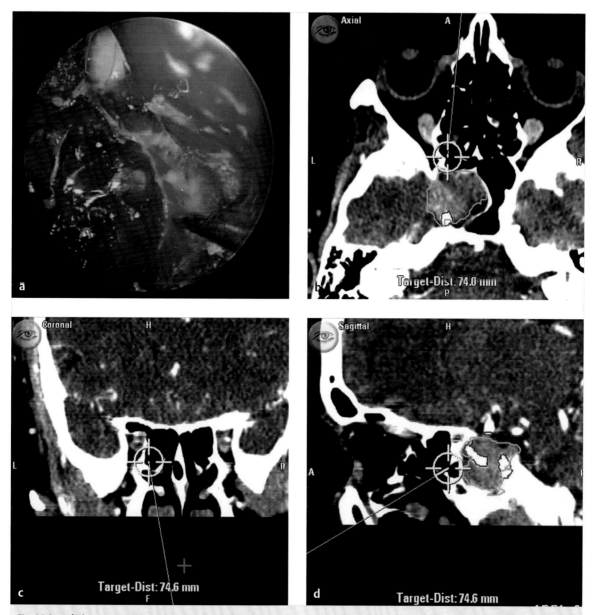

Fig. 14.8 a–d The neuronavigation system shows the position of the ICA before the cavernous sinus opening into a nonfunctioning adenoma invading the left cavernous sinus.

the use of hemostatic agents (effective for venous bleeding and also for mild arterial bleeding), and the use of bipolar cauterization (especially necessary for arterial bleeding). The experience of the surgeon guides the choice of the technique because each technique has advantages and disadvantages. The packing-waiting-washing technique is time consuming and is mainly effective in stopping minor oozing of blood. On the other hand, the use of hemostatic agents is effective for venous bleeding, but some nonremovable agents may hide the presence of retrograde bleeding toward the brain. Focal bipolar cauterization is the technique of choice for arterial

bleeding, but its use is limited by the functional role of the bleeding vessel.

Despite a meticulous hemostatic technique, the absolute avoidance of postoperative hematoma seems to be impossible.[4] Asymptomatic hematomas in the surgical field discovered incidentally in routine postoperative neuroradiological controls (computed tomography [CT] scan or magnetic resonance imaging [MRI]) are not infrequent and do not require treatment, but should be monitored until their disappearance. Conversely, symptomatic hematomas should be promptly treated: an endonasal reintervention may be sufficient, but sometimes a craniotomic procedure is necessary, particularly when the surgeon suspects that the bleeding source is a major arterial vessel.

14.3 Other Complications

14.3.1 Neurological Complications

Neurological complications may be the consequence of vascular damage or may be due to direct injury of the nervous tissue (for example, the curettes that pierce the diaphragma sellae and penetrate the nervous tissue) and nerves. It is assumed that that endoscopic skull base surgery is more conservative with respect to craniotomic microsurgery. In fact, craniotomic approaches to the ventral skull base require brain manipulation even if incremental demolition of the bone of the skull base minimizes it. Furthermore, craniotomic approaches follow a lateromedial direction, and access to midline lesions requires dissection of the vasculonervous structures displaced at the periphery of the expanding mass. Conversely, endoscopic skull base approaches allow extracerebral direct access to the ventral skull base, avoiding brain manipulation and vasculonervous dissection. These are the reasons why endoscopic approaches are well tolerated and why they are called minimally invasive.

In the following text we describe the cranial nerves that are most frequently involved in endoscopic approaches, specifying the most frequent points of risk.

Olfactory Nerve

Anosmia is the clinical consequence of bilateral damage to the olfactory nerves and/or of the resection of the neurosensorial olfactory mucosa. Bilateral olfactory nerve damage is rarely due to the approach, and is more frequently due to the involvement of the olfactory pathways by the tumor itself which frequently has anosmia as a presenting symptom. The unilateral sacrifice of the olfactory nerve is generally without functional consequences, but the olfactory mucosa, located in the cribriform plate and medial wall of superior turbinate, should be maintained to preserve the olfaction.

Optic Nerve and Chiasm Injury

The sellar and suprasellar regions are limited superolaterally and posteriorly by the optic nerve and the chiasm. When using an endoscopic approach, the zone at maximum risk for the optic nerve is the optic canal. The optic nerve may be damaged by direct and indirect trauma and its recovery ability is very low. Therefore, utmost care should be taken not only to avoid direct injury to the nerve, but also to avoid indirect damage, such as that which can be induced by excessive heating during the drilling of the optic canal. When using a transethmoidal approach to the sella, the surgeon should be aware of

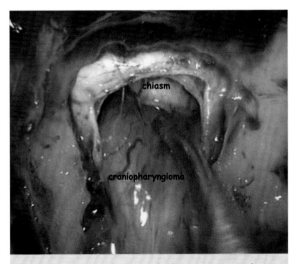

Fig. 14.9 Transtuberculum supradiaphragmatic approach: dissection of craniopharyngioma from the chiasm.

the presence of the Onodi variants of the posterior ethmoidal cells since this anatomical variant increases the risk of direct optic nerve injury. In an extended transtuberculum sellae approach, the optic canals represent the lateral limit of the opening and, being well visible, they are to be preserved.[17] Furthermore, in a transtuberculum approach intended to open the dura of the suprasellar area, the surgeon should be aware of the displacement of the chiasm, which may be pushed immediately behind the dura and is at risk of damage during this phase[17] (▶ Fig. 14.9). Finally it is of paramount importance during the dissection phase to preserve the superior meningohypophysial artery, which is the main vascular supply to the chiasm. The easiest way to avoid damage to this artery is to keep intact the arachnoidal plane, where the artery and its terminal thin branches are located.

Oculomotor, Trochlear, and Abducens Nerve Injuries

Lesions to these nerves induce ophthalmoplegia. The zone at risk for damage is mainly the cavernous sinus.[13] Cranial nerves III and IV course the lateral wall of the cavernous sinus, where they are embedded and protected between the endosteal and meningeal layers that make up the lateral wall. Cranial nerve VI runs free in the cavernous sinus, with a mediolateral ascending course to the superior orbital fissure. The abducens nerve is also at risk of damage during the opening of the clival dura; in this circumstance, the opening should be in the midline and, if possible, it should start in the lower part of the clival dura where the nerve can more easily be identified, at the level of vertebrobasilar junction where it emerges a few millimeters above the latter junction.

Trigeminal Nerve Injury

Lesions to the branches of the trigeminal nerve induce neuralgia, anesthesia, or both (painful anesthesia). There are different zones at risk regarding damage to the branches of the trigeminal nerve.

The first branch of the trigeminal nerve, the ophthalmic branch, may be injured in the parasellar area where it courses the lateral wall of the cavernous sinus; by avoiding transection of the lateral wall, the nerve is preserved. The second and the third branches of the trigeminal nerve, the maxillary branch and the mandibular branch respectively, are at risk of damage mainly during the transmaxillary approach to the pterygopalatine and infratemporal fossae.[19] In this approach, the course of the infraorbital nerve indicates the lateral limit of the resection of the posterior wall of the maxillary sinus. The infraorbital nerve is a branch of the maxillary branch of the trigeminal nerve. The maxillary nerve is reached by following the infraorbital nerve backward. It emerges from the cranium through the foramen rotundum and courses the lateral wall of the sphenoid sinus where it is covered by a bony prominence called the trigeminal prominence. The mandibular branch of the trigeminal nerve emerges from the cranium through the foramen ovale and it courses the infratemporal fossa, running from above to below anteriorly to the bone canal of the horizontal petrous segment of the ICA.

Vidian Nerve Injury

The vidian nerve derives from the union of the greater petrosal nerve, which arises from the facial nerve at the geniculate ganglion, and the deep petrosal nerve, which originates from the carotid sympathetic plexus (▶ Fig. 14.2). The vidian nerve plays an important role in maintaining normal lacrimation and nasopharyngeal physiology. Damage to the vidian nerve may lead to a loss of lacrimation with desiccation of the cornea and dry nose due to damage to the parasympathetic fibers. The vidian nerve runs in the vidian or pterygoid canal together with the vidian artery. The vidian canal is located in the floor of the sphenoid sinus where, in well-pneumatized sinuses, it is visible as a prominence. However, in the presellar and conchal variants of the sphenoid sinus, this prominence is not visible and, therefore, its exposure should start at the level of the pterygoid process. In a subperiosteal approach performed along the face of the pterygoid process, the vidian canal is located 5 to 6 mm posteromedially to the sphenopalatine foramen. The posterior end of the vidian canal delimits the genu between the petrous carotid artery and the paraclival artery. This is an important landmark for the carotid artery and, indirectly, for the trigeminal Meckel ganglion, which is located in a space bounded by the horizontal

and paraclival carotid arteries medially and inferiorly, by the maxillary branch laterally, and the abducens nerve superiorly. Kassam recommended drilling the vidian canal in its ventral surface, between 3 and 9 o'clock, to avoid injuring the carotid artery with the drill.[20]

Facial and Vestibulocochlear Nerves

The facial nerve and the vestibulocochlear nerves are positioned too laterally to be involved when using endoscopic endonasal approaches, even if, in exceptional circumstances, the internal auditory canal can be reached following the tumor along its direction of growth.

Glossopharyngeal, Vagus, and Hypoglossal Nerves

The glossopharyngeal, vagus, and hypoglossal nerves are also distant from the surgical corridors normally used in the endoscopic endonasal approach. The surgeon should keep them in mind when carrying out an approach to the jugular foramen or to the foramen magnum. In the latter circumstance (i.e., during an approach to the foramen magnum) the posterior half of the occipital condyle should be preserved to avoid hypoglossal nerve injury.[10]

14.3.2 Endocrine Complications

Endocrine complications, caused by the manipulation of the pituitary gland, the pituitary stalk, and the hypothalamus, may worsen the postoperative course of endoscopic skull base procedures aimed at the sellar/suprasellar regions. Their occurrence is not strictly dependent on the surgical technique (i.e., endoscopic or microscopic, transsphenoidal, or craniotomic), but also on the experience of the surgeon[3] and the type of lesion (nonpituitary pathologies are more likely be accompanied by hypopituitarism and/or diabetes insipidus). Therefore, patients should undergo a strict follow-up by a multidisciplinary team, which should include an endocrinologist.[21,22] In the early postoperative course, the priority is the assessment of the pituitary adrenal axis; other axes, pituitary thyroid, pituitary gonadal, and pituitary growth hormone, may be evaluated later, since their impairment is not life threatening. Most centers use a routine postoperative glucocorticoid coverage. However, even in this case it is advisable, beginning on the second or third postoperative day, to reduce the replacement therapy and to monitor the morning cortisol plasma levels to assess the need for substitutive therapy.[21] If the levels of morning plasma cortisol are borderline, we prefer to continue the replacement therapy, planning the definitive provocative test of the pituitary–adrenal axis after 1 month.[23]

Any damage to the posterior pituitary and/or the pituitary stalk and/or the hypothalamus may produce disorders of water balance.[21] Water balance is controlled by antidiuretic hormone (ADH), which is synthetized in the supraoptic and paraventricular nuclei of the hypothalamus that terminate in the posterior pituitary, where ADH is stored and released into the circulation. A decrease in ADH production induces diabetes insipidus (DI), which is manifested clinically with a large volume of dilute urine due to inability to concentrate the urine. As a result, plasma osmolarity rises and patients experience a marked increase in thirst. If fluid intake is unable to compensate for urine output, serum osmolarity and sodium increase. Most commonly DI begins within 48 hours of surgery. DI may resolve itself and then may recur and remain permanently (triphasic pattern). Sometimes, during the period between the remission and the recurrence, a transitory phase of inappropriate secretion of ADH may develop due to the release of the stored hormone.

An excess of ADH, due to damage of the posterior pituitary or of the secreting hypothalamic neurons, induces the syndrome of inappropriate ADH secretion (SIADH), which clinically manifests as a fall of urine output (which is concentrated) and preservation of fluid intake; therefore, hyponatremia and hypo-osmolarity increase. It occurs mostly on the 7th postoperative day[21] and it is transitory.

The incidence of these two water disorders varies according to the pathology, and is more frequent in non-adenomatous disease.[24] After transsphenoidal surgery for adenoma, transient DI requiring desmopressin therapy at some time during hospitalization was reported in 12.4%[24] of patients, and long-term treatment was noted in 2% of all patients.

SIADH occurs frequently in a subclinical transient form; the incidence of symptomatic SIADH is estimated to be around 2.1%.[25] Early diagnosis and treatment of these water disorders is mandatory to obviate severe disturbances that may be lethal. Therefore, the continuous 24-hour monitoring of fluid intake and urine output, the assessment of urinary specific gravity, and serum electrolyte monitoring are necessary in all patients who have undergone surgery of the sellar suprasellar region. In case of DI, the increasing value of hypernatremia may require correction with desmopressin therapy; conversely in SIADH, treatment of hyponatremia requires fluid restriction.

14.3.3 Cerebrospinal Fluid Leak

The leakage of CSF from the subarachnoid space into the paranasal sinuses and, finally, into the nasal cavities may produce disastrous intracranial complications such as meningitis and pneumocephalus. This is the reason why CSF leak repair is mandatory. Generally, the incidence of a CSF leak after pituitary surgery is about 2.3%,[26] but a higher incidence is reported after extended transsphenoidal approaches.[27]

A CSF leak may occur intraoperatively or postoperatively. An intraoperative CSF leak appears as the flow of clear fluid from the suprasellar cisterns. Sometimes a tear in the cisterns is not evident and the CSF oozes through a macroscopically intact arachnoid membrane; a Valsalva maneuver is always suggested to confirm the presence of a leak. A postoperative CSF leak normally occurs within a few days of surgery. The main reasons for a delayed CSF leak are laceration of previously intact suprasellar membranes or displacement of the graft. The features leading to such a complication are mostly uncontrollable expiratory reflexes, such as sneezing, coughing, or vomiting. Smooth arousal from anesthesia and preoperative instructions to carry out sneezing with an open mouth are useful expedients in preventing such events.

In postoperative CSF leaks, different algorithms have been proposed to confirm the diagnosis. Suspicion that clear fluid leaking from the nose is CSF may be confirmed using the tilt test (head flexed). However, the certainty that the fluid is CSF may be reached only by the beta-2 transferrin test or the beta-trace protein test.[28] Unfortunately, these two highly sensitive tests, based on a specific marker of CSF, are not widely available. The intrathecal fluorescein test may be used to confirm the CSF leak. Furthermore this test is strongly suggested as a guide during surgery to indicate the sites of the leak and to confirm the effectiveness of the repair.[29] Regarding intraoperative or early postoperative CSF leaks, radiological evaluation (high-resolution CT and/or magnetic resonance cisternography[30,31]) is not necessary.

Management of a Skull Base Defect

According to the Esposito-Dusik classification,[32] we believe that the repair should be tailored to the grade of the CSF leak: grade 0, no leak (no repair); grade 1, small leak without an obvious diaphragmatic defect (simple reinforcement with fat and/or mucoperiosteum from the middle turbinate or septum may be sufficient); grade 2, a moderate leak with a definite diaphragmatic defect (a multilayer repair is suggested: fat + fascia lata + mucoperiosteum); grade 3, a large diaphragmatic/dural defect (multilayer repair or a pedicled flap is required[27]; ▶ Fig. 14.10). The material available for a plastic repair may be heterologous or autologous. At present, we prefer to use only autologous material because it allows stable healing with viable material. A debate still exists on the use of lumbar drainage.

This conservative management is used by us in only two circumstances: (1) recurrent small leakage after a previous plastic repair; and (2) the presence of CSF hypertension

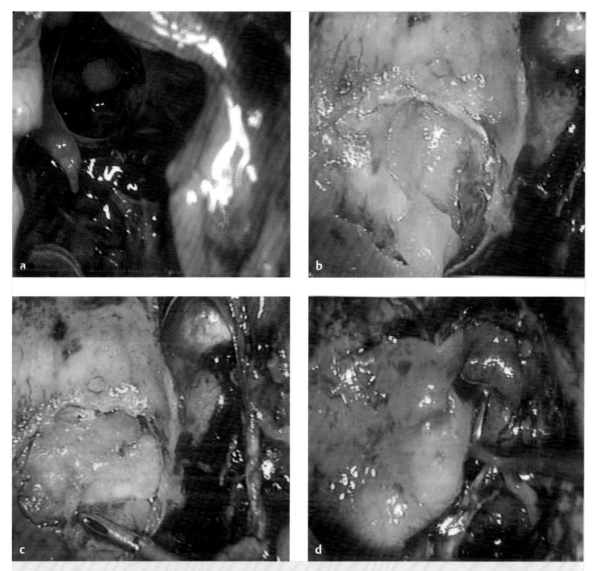

Fig. 14.10 a–d Multilayer plastic reconstruction after adenoma removal. **(a)** Diaphragm defect. **(b)** Abdominal fat inserted in the sellar cavity. **(c)** Bone lamina inserted between the dura and the sellar bone. **(d)** Mucoperiosteum flap from middle turbinate overlaying the bone defect.

suggesting the use of lumbar drainage to support the plastic repair, since it reduces the pressure on the graft.

It should be kept in mind that lumbar drainage may precipitate a rare and severe complication of CSF leak: tension pneumocephalus. Pneumocephalus normally occurs concomitantly with a CSF leak and may be considered an indirect sign of this complication due to the fact that there is a CSF outflow from the intracranial spaces and an air inflow at the same time. It is normally asymptomatic. There are few reports stating that lumbar drainage may increase the volume of the penetrating air, inducing intracranial hypertension and clinical deteriora-

tion of the patient. In this rare condition, it is mandatory to remove the lumbar drainage and to repair the fistula directly at the site of origin.[33]

14.3.4 Infections

Two main types of infection may occur: systemic infections (urogenital, pulmonary, and cardiac infections) and local infections. The former depend on the length of time for the operation, the recovery time, and bed rest, and on factors related to the general health conditions of the patient; they are not affected by antibiotic prophylaxis.[34] Management of systemic infections is part of general health care and is not addressed in this chapter.

Conversely, local infection at the surgical site (rhinosinusitis, meningitis) is related to the surgical procedure. Endonasal skull base surgery is clean-contaminated surgery.[35] A direct connection between the nasal cavity and the intracranial cavity and multiple passages with the use of surgical instruments through a contaminated field occurs systematically during endonasal surgery. Despite the theoretical high risk of intracranial contamination with sinus nasal flora, the experience gained up to now shows a reduction in the incidence of rhinosinusitis and central nervous system infections.

Four factors influence the reduction of infections of the surgical field: antibiotic prophylaxis, sealed closure of the dural defect, prompt management of the postoperative CSF leak, and operative and postoperative management of the sinonasal cavity.

Antibiotic Prophylaxis

Antibiotics[35] should prevent infection, reducing the "infectious load," and, since endoscopic skull base surgery is clean-contaminated surgery, antibiotic prophylaxis is highly recommended. A standardized regimen of antibiotic prophylaxis maintains a low incidence of postoperative infection, decreasing the risk of infection resulting from resistant organisms, allergic reactions and side-effects, antibiotic-related complications such as *Clostridium difficile* enterocolitis, and thrombophlebitis from intravenous lines. Multiple factors influence the choice of antibiotic prophylaxis; these are mainly patient demographics and the nature of the surgical procedure.

Our antibiotic prophylaxis scheme is short-term prophylaxis with cephazolin (an initial dose of 2 g and then 1 g 6 hours postoperatively). In patients allergic to penicillin, clindamycin is used. In the case of infection, antibiotic therapy is mandatory.

Sealed Closure of the Dural Defect and Management of Postoperative Cerebrospinal Fluid Leak

Whenever there is suspected or evidence of a CSF leak, meticulous waterproof closure of the exposed dural defect is mandatory. When there is an evident or persistent leak, we recommend carrying out revision plastic surgery as soon as possible to reduce the time of exposure involving the sinus flora and the intracranial

cavity. In our experience, all cases of postoperative meningitis have occurred in patients with a postoperative CSF leak.[5,13]

Operative and Postoperative Management of the Sinonasal Tract

All surgical injury of the mucosa reduces mucociliary transport in the nose and sinus cavities. Moreover, if the sinus mucosa is removed, the new epithelium is not ciliated and secretions do not flow easily. If the natural ostium patency of the sinus is not respected, it may possibly lead to acute or, more frequently, chronic sinusitis and, over the long term, a postsurgical mucocele. Therefore, to prevent acute or chronic alterations of the sinuses and nasal cavity functioning and/or infection and/or postsurgical mucocele, the avoidance of unnecessary stripping of the mucosa, the preservation of sinus patency, and the correction of the operative lateralization of the middle turbinate, which would compress the ethmoidal cells, is of utmost importance.

In the postoperative period we suggest frequent nasal cleaning with hypotonic solution and a transnasal endoscopic examination 3 to 4 weeks after the surgical procedure. An earlier examination should be performed in patients who have undergone an extended approach or who have disturbing sinus symptoms, such as rhinorrhea, a foul smell, and/or nasal obstruction.

14.4 Final Remarks

Endoscopic skull base surgery is the most recent development of endoscopic transsphenoidal surgery and is based on the use of expanded endonasal approaches. The key to its good acceptance lies in the direct extracerebral access to the ventral skull base, avoiding brain manipulation and vasculonervous dissection. Otherwise, the endoscopic technique follows the same rules of microsurgery. It is a technique that can give great results, but it may pose many pitfalls for the surgeon. Safety can be maintained by following some golden rules: (1) perform only those operations for which the surgeon is highly trained; (2) prevent complications by strictly following the technical rules; (3) be prepared to treat complications, which unfortunately occur even in the best hands, using careful and cautious management. The latter statement implies that such procedures have to be performed by surgeons only, or in centers where all competencies are present; providing the possibility of switching to open surgery, having rapid access to endovascular treatment, and having an intensive care unit.

Pearls and Pitfalls

- Prevention of serious complications requires correct selection of patients, and a surgical team who has mastered the skull base anatomy from the endoscopic perspective, can perform meticulous dissection, and deliver perioperative care with utmost attention to detail.
- Bimanual dissection and minimal traction of intracranial tumors are advocated to avoid inadvertent avulsion of the surrounding vessels.
- Sacrificing or injuring small perforating vessels to the brainstem and optic chiasm often lead to ischemic deficits as they contribute important blood supply.
- Control of small-vessel bleeding is best achieved using bipolar electrocauterization or by irrigating with warm water (40–42°) for several minutes.
- Various hemostatic materials may help to control venous sinus bleeding (Floseal, Tachosil, Avitene, Gelfoam, Tabotamp).
- Hypotensive anesthesia as an attempt to control bleeding is contraindicated as it results in cerebral hypoperfusion!
- Options for the acute management of large-vessel injuries include bipolar electrocauterization of the vessel, direct compression or compressive packing of the vessel, suture repair, reconstruction using aneurysm clips, and circumferential ligation or clipping of the vessel. However, there is clinical and experimental evidence to suggest that focal pressure with crushed muscle is the best way to stop the ensuing catastrophic arterial hemorrhage and enable stabilization of the patient and subsequent transfer to the angiography suite.
- After intraoperative major vascular injury, an immediate angiography is essential. In most patients neuroradiological intervention is possibly indicated (i.e., balloon occlusion or embolization). A repeat angiography excludes a delayed pseudoaneurysm.
- Neurological complications may be due to direct injury of neural tissue or the consequence of vascular damage (i.e., ischemia or hemorrhage).
- Endocrine complications are most commonly due to the manipulation of the pituitary gland, the pituitary stalk, and the hypothalamus.
- Four factors influence the reduction of infections of the surgical field: antibiotic prophylaxis, sealing of the dural defect, prompt management of a postoperative CSF leak, and operative and postoperative management of the sinonasal cavity.

References

[1] Cappabianca P, Cavallo LM, Esposito F, De Divitiis O, Messina A, De Divitiis E. Extended endoscopic endonasal approach to the midline skull base: the evolving role of transsphenoidal surgery. Adv Tech Stand Neurosurg 2008; 33: 151–199

[2] Snyderman C, Kassam A, Carrau R, Mintz A, Gardner P, Prevedello DM. Acquisition of surgical skills for endonasal skull base surgery: a training program. Laryngoscope 2007; 117: 699–705

[3] Ciric I, Ragin A, Baumgartner C, Pierce D. Complications of transsphenoidal surgery: results of a national survey, review of the literature, and personal experience. Neurosurgery 1997; 40: 225–236; discussion 236–237

[4] Laws ER, Jr. Vascular complications of transsphenoidal surgery. Pituitary 1999; 2: 163–170

[5] Frank G, Pasquini E, Farneti G et al. The endoscopic versus the traditional approach in pituitary surgery. Neuroendocrinology 2006; 83: 240–248

[6] Pasquini E, Sciarretta V, Farneti G, Mazzatenta D, Modugno GC. Frank G. Endoscopic treatment of encephaloceles of the lateral wall of the sphenoid sinus. Minim Invasive Neurosurg 2004; 47: 209–213

[7] Raymond J, Hardy J, Czepko R, Roy D. Arterial injuries in transsphenoidal surgery for pituitary adenoma; the role of angiography and endovascular treatment. AJNR Am J Neuroradiol 1997; 18: 655–665

[8] Renn WH, Rhoton AL, Jr. Microsurgical anatomy of the sellar region. J Neurosurg 1975; 43: 288–298

[9] Kassam A, Snyderman CH, Mintz A, Gardner P, Carrau RL. Expanded endonasal approach: the rostrocaudal axis. Part I. Crista galli to the sella turcica. Neurosurg Focus 2005; 19: E3

[10] Kassam A, Snyderman CH, Mintz A, Gardner P, Carrau RL. Expanded endonasal approach: the rostrocaudal axis. Part II. Posterior clinoids to the foramen magnum. Neurosurg Focus 2005; 19: E4

[11] Kassam AB, Gardner P, Snyderman C, Mintz A, Carrau R. Expanded endonasal approach: fully endoscopic, completely transnasal approach to the middle third of the clivus, petrous bone, middle cranial fossa, and infratemporal fossa. Neurosurg Focus 2005; 19: E6

[12] Lasio G, Ferroli P, Felisati G, Broggi G. Image-guided endoscopic transnasal removal of recurrent pituitary adenomas. Neurosurgery 2002; 51: 132–136; discussion 136–137

[13] Frank G, Pasquini E. Endoscopic endonasal cavernous sinus surgery, with special reference to pituitary adenomas. Front Horm Res 2006; 34: 64–82

[14] Kassam A, Snyderman CH, Carrau RL, Gardner P, Mintz A. Endoneurosurgical hemostasis techniques: lessons learned from 400 cases. Neurosurg Focus 2005; 19: E7

[15] Archondakis E, Pero G, Valvassori L, Boccardi E, Scialfa G. Angiographic follow-up of traumatic carotid cavernous fistulas treated with endovascular stent graft placement. Am J Neuroradiol 2007; 28: 342–347

[16] Sorteberg A, Bakke SJ, Boysen M, Sorteberg W. Angiographic balloon test occlusion and therapeutic sacrifice of major arteries to the brain. Neurosurgery 2008; 63: 651–660, 660–661

[17] Frank G, Pasquini E, Doglietto F et al. The endoscopic extended transsphenoidal approach for craniopharyngiomas. Neurosurgery 2006; 59 Suppl 1: ONS75–ONS83; discussion ONS75–ONS83

[18] Snyderman CH, Carrau RL, Kassam AB et al. Endoscopic skull base surgery: principles of endonasal oncological surgery. J Surg Oncol 2008; 97: 658–664

[19] Pasquini E, Sciarretta V, Farneti G, Ippolito A, Mazzatenta D, Frank G. Endoscopic endonasal approach for the treatment of benign schwannoma of the sinonasal tract and pterygopalatine fossa. Am J Rhinol 2002; 16: 113–118

[20] Kassam AB, Vescan AD, Carrau RL et al. Expanded endonasal approach: vidian canal as a landmark to the petrous internal carotid artery. J Neurosurg 2008; 108: 177–183

[21] Ausiello JC, Bruce JN, Freda PU. Postoperative assessment of the patient after transsphenoidal pituitary surgery. Pituitary 2008; 11: 391–401

[22] Vance ML. Perioperative management of patients undergoing pituitary surgery. Endocrinol Metab Clin North Am 2003; 32: 355–365

[23] Agha A, Tomlinson JW, Clark PM, Holder G, Stewart PM. The long-term predictive accuracy of the short synacthen (corticotropin) stimulation test for assessment of the hypothalamic-pituitary-adrenal axis. J Clin Endocrinol Metab 2006; 91: 43–47

[24] Nemergut EC, Zuo Z, Jane JA, Jr, Laws ER, Jr. Predictors of diabetes insipidus after transsphenoidal surgery: a review of 881 patients. J Neurosurg 2005; 103: 448–454

[25] Hensen J, Henig A, Fahlbusch R, Meyer M, Boehnert M, Buchfelder M. Prevalence, predictors and patterns of postoperative polyuria and hyponatraemia in the immediate course after transsphenoidal surgery for pituitary adenomas. Clin Endocrinol (Oxf) 1999; 50: 431–439

[26] Cappabianca P, Cavallo LM, Esposito F, Valente V, De Divitiis E. Sellar repair in endoscopic endonasal transsphenoidal surgery: results of 170 cases. Neurosurgery 2002; 51: 1365–1371; discussion 1371–1372

[27] Kassam AB, Thomas A, Carrau RL et al. Endoscopic reconstruction of the cranial base using a pedicled nasoseptal flap. Neurosurgery 2008; 63 Suppl 1: ONS44–ONS52; discussion ONS52–ONS53

[28] Bachmann-Harildstad G. Diagnostic values of beta-2 transferrin and beta-trace protein as markers for cerebrospinal fluid fistula. Rhinology 2008; 46: 82–85

[29] Stammberger H, Greistorfer K, Wolf G, Luxenberger W. Surgical occlusion of cerebrospinal fistulas of the anterior skull base using intrathecal sodium fluorescein [in German] Laryngorhinootologie 1997; 76: 595–607

[30] El Gammal T, Sobol W, Wadlington VR et al. Cerebrospinal fluid fistula: detection with MR cisternography. AJNR Am J Neuroradiol 1998; 19: 627–631

[31] Lloyd KM, DelGaudio JM, Hudgins PA. Imaging of skull base cerebrospinal fluid leaks in adults. Radiology 2008; 248: 725–736

[32] Esposito F, Dusick JR, Fatemi N, Kelly DF. Graded repair of cranial base defects and cerebrospinal fluid leaks in transsphenoidal surgery. Neurosurgery 2007; 60 Suppl 2: 295–303; discussion 303–304

[33] Candrina R, Galli G, Bollati AJ. Subdural and intraventricular tension pneumocephalus after transsphenoidal operation. J Neurol Neurosurg Psychiatry 1988; 51: 1005–1006

[34] Carrau RL, Snyderman C, Janecka IP, Sekhar L, Sen C, D'Amico F. Antibiotic prophylaxis in cranial base surgery. Head Neck 1991; 13: 311–317

[35] Brown SM, Anand VK, Tabaee A, Schwartz TH. Role of perioperative antibiotics in endoscopic skull base surgery. Laryngoscope 2007; 117: 1528–1532

Chapter 15
Surgical Results

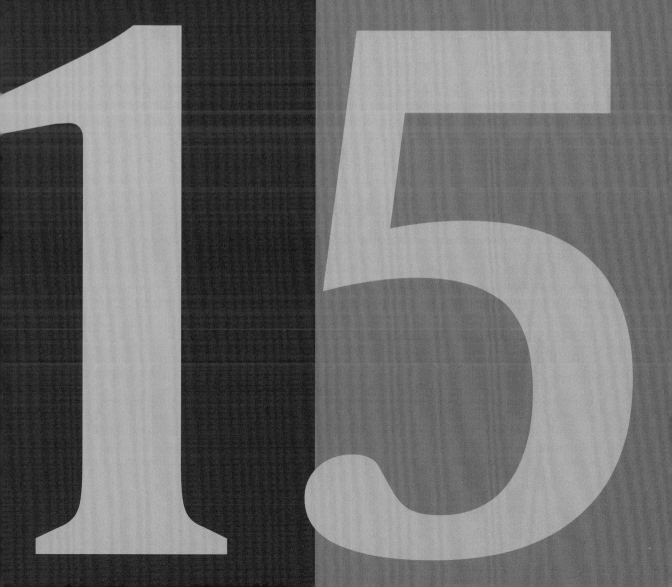

15 Surgical Results

15.1 Long-term Outcome of Endonasal Resection of Sinonasal and Skull Base Malignancies (Fulda, Kassel School)

Ulrike Bockmühl, Wolfgang Draf[†]

15.1.1 Introduction

One of the most dramatic changes in the practice of skull base surgery has been the adoption of endonasal endoscopic techniques for the treatment of pathologies within the sinonasal complex and at the anterior and central skull base. In the late 1980s, Wolfgang Draf pioneered the endonasal resection of sinonasal and anterior skull base lesions using the microscope and/or endoscope. For more than 30 years he focused on the development, refinement, and progression of endonasal surgical techniques placing special emphasis on the frontal sinus and promoting the concept of minimal invasive functional surgery. His progressive application of endonasal surgery to the management of benign tumors and malignant sinonasal tumors contributed to a revolution in their surgical treatment. Based on his experience, surgical skills, anatomical knowledge, and use of dedicated instrumentation and neuronavigation systems, Wolfgang Draf taught many scholars from all over the world, especially in frontal sinus and anterior skull base tumor surgery; thereby, establishing the "Fulda School." His department was the leading center for endonasal surgery in Germany. As one of his senior surgeons who has worked with him for several years I carry on his concepts in Kassel (Germany).

In this chapter we present the review of a series of 151 patients treated during a 10-year period in Fulda, Germany. We offer special emphasis on the comparison between the outcomes of endonasal endoscopic surgery and those of external approaches.

15.1.2 Surgical and Oncological Principles of Endonasal Tumor Surgery

As described in Chapter 8 a key concept of endonasal tumor surgery is the adequacy of the surgical corridor. Its access can be adapted and enlarged as necessary while still obviating some of the morbidity associated with an open procedure. In our series, endonasal surgery was performed with 4-mm rigid endoscopes (0 and 45°) alone or in combination with the microscope using video equipment (camera, monitors and recording system), appropriate straight, angled, and double-angled instruments, microdebrider, long stem and curved drills, intranasal acoustic Doppler sonography, and a surgical navigation system.

The goal of endonasal tumor surgery was the complete removal of the lesion with negative margins. Therefore, we followed two main surgical strategies:

- "En bloc" resection, which was achieved in only small neoplasms and in those malignancies limited to the nasoethmoidal complex filling the nasal cavity. It means dissection around the tumor from all sides (lateral, caudal, and cranial) along normal anatomical structures resulting in an "in toto" tumor removal. ▶ Fig. 15.1 demonstrates one example.
- Debulking of the tumor. This means a piecemeal, layered tumor removal clearly identifying the limits between normal and diseased mucosa so that the tumor can be resected with adequate safety margins. One example is shown in ▶ Fig. 15.2.

Basically, our endonasal tumor resections start anteriorly and consist of the following steps:

- Tumor debulking to clearly identify the site of origin and the anterior skull base.
- Cauterization of the nasal branches of the sphenopalatine artery(ies) by bipolar instrumentation.
- Drilling out of the frontal sinus (drainage type III according to Draf[1]). In cases of unilateral pathology a type II drainage is adequate.
- Removal of the posterior two-thirds of the nasal septum, detachment of the vomer from the sphenoidal rostrum, and drilling out of a large sphenoidotomy.
- Subperiosteal dissection of the nasoethmoidosphenoidal complex (performed one-sided in unilateral pathologies as shown in ▶ Fig. 15.3).
- If required, enlargement of the dissection including medial maxillectomy and resection of the nasolacrimal duct.
- Removal of the surgical specimen either transnasally or transorally.
- Routine use of intraoperative histological analysis (frozen sections).
- Removal of the lamina papyracea, cribriform plate, crista galli, or olfactory bulb was only performed if invaded by tumor.
- Duraplasty with a "three-layer" technique using autologous fascia lata as an intradural layer, intracranial extradural layer (underlay), and extradural layer (onlay), stabilized with fibrin glue. We do not utilize vascularized septal flaps routinely, as the septum is frequently involved by tumor.

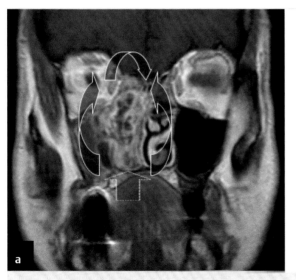
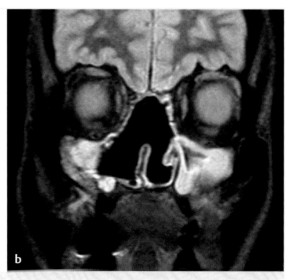

Fig. 15.1 **a, b** "En bloc" tumor resection of an adenocarcinoma of the right ethmoid sinuses with infiltration of the anterior skull base. **(a)** Coronal MRI. *Blue arrows* indicate preparation of surrounding area along normal anatomical structures. **(b)** Coronal MRI scan 4 years postoperatively showing no signs of recurrence.

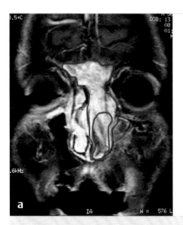
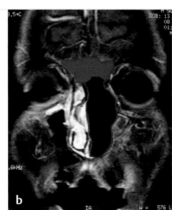
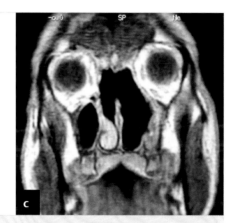

Fig. 15.2 **a–c** Example of piecemeal, multilayer tumor removal of a squamous cell carcinoma associated with an inverted papilloma. **(a)** Coronal MRI with outlined tumor extension (red). **(b)** Coronal MRI indicating sequential tumor debulking (black and blue areas). **(c)** Coronal MRI 3 years postoperatively showing no signs of recurrence.

15.1.3 Results of Endonasal Surgery for Malignancies

Patient and Tumor Characteristics

Between January 1995 and December 2004, 151 patients with malignant tumors of the paranasal sinuses and the anterior skull base were treated primarily with surgery at the Department of Otorhinolaryngology, Klinikum Fulda gAG, Teaching Hospital of the Philipps-University Marburg, Fulda, Germany. Of these, 61 patients were operated exclusively endonasally using endoscopes and/or microscopes.

The mean age at presentation was 56.8 years (median 55 years, range 22–90 years) in the group of patients who underwent endonasal tumor resection, and 54.7 years (median 56 years, range 16–78 years) in the group of patients whose tumors were removed via external approaches. The male to female ratio was 35:26 in the endonasal approach group and 60:30 in the external approach group. Follow-up of the patients was performed on an outpatient basis after therapy was completed. Follow-up ranged from 29 to 215 months (mean 60 and 70 months, median 62 and 66 months, respectively). In the first year, the patients were seen at 3, 6, and 12 months, and subsequently yearly. They were examined with nasal

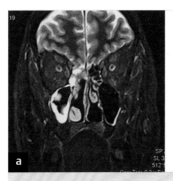
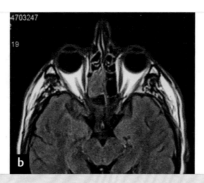
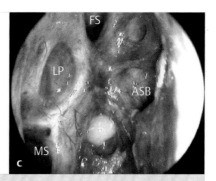

Fig. 15.3 a–c Circumscribed unilateral adenocarcinoma at the right anterior skull base. **(a)** Preoperative coronal MRI. **(b)** Preoperative axial MRI. **(c)** Endoscopic view 3 years postoperatively showing a unilateral anterior skull base (ASB) resection with a small type II frontal sinus (FS) opening.
ASB, anterior skull base; FS, frontal sinus; LP, lamina papyracea; MS, maxillary sinus opening.

endoscopy and yearly magnetic resonance imaging (MRI) scans. Biopsies were taken from any area suspicious for recurrent tumor. The cause of death was determined at autopsy or by clinical examination at the Fulda Hospital.

Tumors were classified according to the Union Internationale Contre le Cancer (UICC) staging system[1] except chordomas and metastases. Tumor localization, extent of sinus involvement, especially involvement of the sphenoid sinus, and infiltration of orbit and brain were assessed from radiological findings based on computed tomography (CT) and MRI, from findings at surgery, and from histological evaluation. The clinicopathological data of the tumors are summarized in ▶ Table 15.1. Tumor infiltration of the brain and the orbit was present in 20 and 22 patients, respectively. Those lesions were removed via external approaches, which mainly comprised the midfacial degloving, subcranial approach according to Raveh,[2] lateral rhinotomy in combination with an orbital exenteration, or other combined approaches. In 55 patients the sphenoid sinus was involved. Of these, 15 malignancies were resected endonasally and 40 via external approaches. Only 15 patients showed local or distant metastases at the time of presentation. Forty-one tumor resections were incomplete, i.e., with positive margins (15 after endonasal and 26 after external operation).

Survival Results

Survival analysis was applied to all 151 patients comprising all clinicopathological parameters and surgical approaches. Statistical analysis of data was performed using SPSS 10.0 (Chicago, Illinois, United States). Survival curves were calculated using the Kaplan–Meier product limit estimate[2] performed between each single parameter and the disease-specific survival and the disease-free survival (recurrence free and metastases free), respectively (▶ Fig. 15.4 and ▶ Fig. 15.5). The differences of the survival curves were tested for statistical significance with the log-rank test. Values of $p < 0.05$ were considered to be

Table 15.1 Clinicopathological tumor characteristics

Characteristic	Surgical approach		Total (n = 151)
	Endonasal (n = 61)	External (n = 90)	
Histology			
Adenocarcinoma	12	21	33
Squamous cell carcinoma	10	22	32
Esthesioneuroblastoma	10	14	24
Adenoid cystic carcinoma	2	9	11
Chordoma	3	10	13
Sarcoma	4	6	10
Melanoma	3	3	6
Other	17	5	22
Stage			
pT1	–	–	–
pT2	16	12	28
pT3	21	14	35
pT4a	15	37	52
pT4b	–	14	14
Chordoma/metastases	9	13	22
Type of disease at presentation			
Primary tumor	35	58	93
Residual	8	8	16
Recurrent	10	23	33
Metastases	8	1	9
Tumor origin			
Nasal cavity	14	10	24
Maxillary sinus	1	15	16
Ethmoid cells	28	40	68
Sphenoid sinus	5	1	6
Olfactory bulb/ epithelium	10	14	24
Clivus	3	10	13

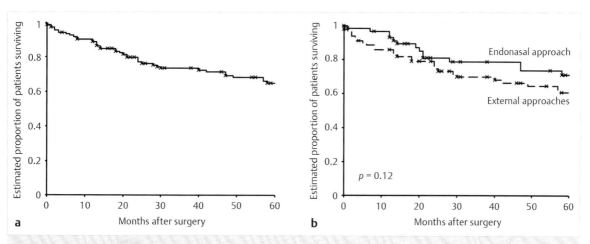

Fig. 15.4 a, b Kaplan–Meier plots presenting disease-specific survival for the entire study cohort of paranasal sinus malignancies (a), and results following the specific surgical approach (b).

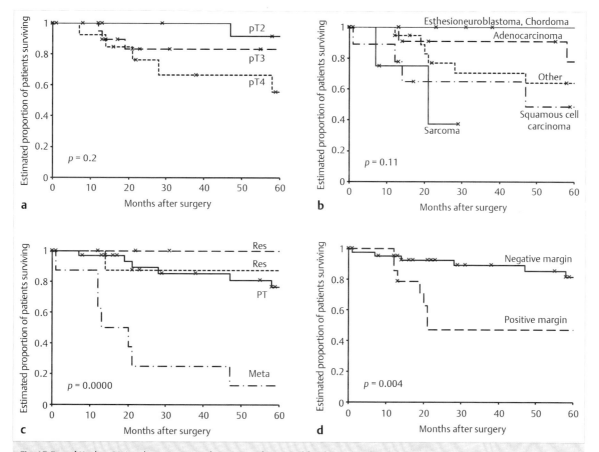

Fig. 15.5 a–d Kaplan–Meier plots presenting disease-specific survival for the group of patients whose tumors were resected endonasally according to pT stage (a), histological tumor type (b), type of disease (c), and status of surgical margins (d).
Meta, metastasis; PT, primary tumor; Rec, recurrent tumor; Res, residual tumor.

statistically significant. Deaths from causes other than the index tumor or recurrence/metastases were not considered treatment failures, and these patients were censored in each analysis involving the length of survival.

Cox proportional hazards regression models[3] were used to examine the relative impact of variables demonstrated to be statistically significant in univariate analysis or those likely to have an effect on outcome. The stepwise backward/forward procedures provided by the SPSS software were employed to further reduce the number of variables in the Cox models. For assessing and comparing the Cox models a Wald test with significance level 0.05 was used for both inclusion and exclusion of variables.

At the closeout date, 51 of the 151 patients had died due to their tumor: 36 from local recurrences, and 15 of metastatic spread. Sixteen patients died after endonasal resection and 35 died following external procedures. Of these, 12 and 24 patients developed local recurrences, and 4 and 11 patients showed metastases, respectively. A total of 16 patients were salvaged with additional surgery. Five patients died of unrelated causes. Hence it follows, 87 patients were alive and free of disease, and 8 patients were alive with disease. The 5-year disease-specific survival rate of the entire study cohort was 67% (▶ Fig. 15.4a). In the group of patients whose lesions were removed endonasally the 5-year disease-specific survival rate was 72% compared with 60% in the group of external tumor resection (▶ Fig. 15.4b). However, the log-rank test indicated no statistical significant difference.

The results of a univariate Kaplan–Meier analysis indicated statistically significant differences for pT stage, histology, and status of surgical margins, as well as infiltration of the orbit, brain and/or sphenoid sinus according to the disease-specific survival within the entire group. In the external approach group the log-rank test revealed significant correlations with disease-specific survival for histological tumor type, type of disease (primary or recurrent/persistent tumor), and infiltration of the brain and/or sphenoid sinus. In the endonasal group only the type of disease and the status of surgical margins were of statistical significance (▶ Fig. 15.5c, d). For the status of sphenoid sinus infiltration and the pT stage there was a tendency for significance regarding the disease-specific survival only (▶ Fig. 15.5a). Regarding histology, our analysis indicated that, among the main tumor types, esthesioneuroblastoma had the most favorable prognosis followed by adenocarcinoma. In contrast, squamous cell carcinoma showed a 5-year survival rate of only 50% in (▶ Fig. 15.5b).

Multivariate Cox regression analysis identified factors that significantly affected the outcome. For disease-specific recurrence, and metastases-free survival, the backward and the forward procedure for variable inclusion/exclusion determined the set of remaining variables, which are listed in ▶ Table 15.2. Of these, independent predictors of survival were pT stage, status of surgical margins, and infiltration of the brain.

Table 15.2 Results of the multivariate Cox regression analysis*

	Whole tumor group (*p* value; *n* = 151)	Approach used for tumor removal (*p* value)	
		Endonasal (*n* = 61)	External (*n* = 90)
Disease-specific survival			
pT stage (UICC)	0.004	–	–
Type of disease	0.0003	–	0.003
Status of surgical margins	–	0.031	–
Infiltration of the brain	–	–	0.011
Recurrence-free survival			
pT stage (UICC)	–	–	0.036
Type of disease	0.025	–	0.006
Status of surgical margins	0.035	–	0.046
Infiltration of the brain	0.022	–	–
Metastasis-free survival			
pT stage (UICC)	0.038	–	0.006
Type of disease	0.002	–	0.002
Infiltration of the brain	0.033	–	–

*Only significant *p* values are shown.
UICC, Union Internationale Contre le Cancer.

Summary

Malignant sinonasal neoplasms are rare pathologies, accounting for 3 to 5% of all head and neck cancers.[4] Moreover, due to the fact that early symptoms mimic those of rhinosinusitis, they are usually diagnosed at an advanced stage. Other features of sinonasal malignancies are their histologic heterogeneity and the variable geographical distribution of histologies.[4,5,6,7,8]

A craniofacial resection combined with adjuvant radiation therapy or chemoradiotherapy is still considered the gold standard for therapy of sinonasal and anterior skull base malignancies.[5,9,10,11,12,13,14,15,16,17,18,19] During the past 15 years endonasal endoscopic surgery has been extensively used to manage malignancies and the evolution of this technique has been demonstrated clearly to be associated with decreased morbidity, complication, and hospitalization time, and, when compared with external approaches, the endoscopic procedure has shown similar success rates.[5,7,20,21,22]

Selection of a surgical approach depends on patient comorbidities, tumor characteristics, and the level of skill and experience of the surgical team. The need for an external or combined procedure may be suggested by preoperative imaging but in few instances a definite decision can be taken only during the surgical procedure. Consequently, the possibility of converting from an endoscopic to an external procedure must be always discussed with the patient prior to operation.

As in external procedures, the target of endonasal tumor surgery is the complete removal of the lesion with negative margins. However, the goals of surgery depend on the histology and extent of the neoplasm. Whereas in many squamous cell carcinomas, adenocarcinomas, or esthesioneuroblastomas a radical removal can be achieved by the endonasal endoscopic resection, a complete resection of adenoid cystic carcinomas that involve the cranial base is usually not possible due to perineural extension. In those cases the goal of surgery is to resect as much as possible without compromising function of the orbit or cranial nerves. Then, adjunctive radiation therapy is an important part of treatment. Primary curative chemoradiotherapy may be considered the first choice therapy in high-grade malignancies that involve critical structures such as brain, optic nerves, carotid artery, or cavernous sinus, precluding complete resection. Surgical salvage may be considered for residual tumors following treatment, such as for nasopharyngeal carcinoma. Furthermore, endoscopic debulking of tumors may be indicated for palliation of symptoms: pain, epistaxis, nasal obstruction, and visual loss and cranial neuropathies secondary to compression.

Reported survival rates for traditional craniofacial resection of sinonasal and anterior skull base malignancies ranged from 44 to 61% at 5 years.[5,8,9,12,13,14] Since prospective studies comparing results of endoscopic surgery and traditional craniofacial resection are not feasible due to the rarity of these pathologies as well as for ethical reasons, we and others attempted to retrospectively compare the two techniques.[23] The "Fulda School" 5-year disease-specific survival rate of the 61 patients whose tumors were removed exclusively endonasally was 72% compared with 60% after external tumor resection (mean follow-up time > 60 months). Eloy et al[15] also analyzed two groups of patients treated at the same institution with either transnasal endoscopic ($n = 18$) or craniofacial resection ($n = 48$) for tumors involving the anterior skull base and found an overall survival after 3 years of 94.4% compared with 83.3%, which was not statistically significant between the two groups. Two other large series reported on 184[7] and 120[21] patients, respectively, undergoing either endoscopic surgery alone or in combination with frontal or subfrontal craniotomy to resect a sinonasal and anterior skull base cancer. At mean follow-up times of 34.1 and 37 months, the 5-year disease-specific survival for the entire patient cohorts in the two series was quite similar: 81.9 versus 87%. However, when estimating 5-year disease-specific survival in relation to histology, there were statistically significant differences as shown in ▶ Table 15.3. As in external approaches, in endonasal surgery it is also of vital importance to achieve a complete tumor removal, and additionally survival depends on stage and infiltration of surrounding structures.[7,21,23]

In our experience, contraindications of endonasal tumor surgery include deep invasion of brain, orbit, or hard palate as well as erosion of the nasal bones, and involvement of the anterior wall or upper lateral portion of the frontal sinus.

Conclusion

In conclusion, despite some limitations (i.e., histological heterogeneity and limited cohort of cases due to the rarity of these lesions), our 5-year disease-specific survival rates indicate that endonasal surgery is an effective alternative to standard external approaches and has to be considered as one of the first line therapeutic options in the management of sinonasal and anterior skull base malignancies.[18] However, the extent of surgery should not be compromised by the endoscopic technique. Treatment decisions should be made on a case-by-case basis. One must pay careful consideration to a multimodality therapy capable of achieving radical and complete treatment of the pathology, while minimizing the morbidity and preserving quality of life for the patient.

Open questions remain regarding long-term outcomes and stratification of survival by histology and stage. The role of other treatment options including radiotherapy,

Table 15.3 Reported 5-year disease-specific survival rates of sinonasal and anterior skull base malignancies according to the surgical approach

Histologic tumor type	5-year disease-specific survival (%)				
	Traditional craniofacial resection			Endonasal resection	
	Shah et al[16]	Ganly et al[18]	Patel et al[15]	Nicolai et al[7]	Fulda school
Adenocarcinoma	57	52	57.5	80.4	75
Squamous cell carcinoma	51	43.6	53	60.7	50
Esthesioneuroblastoma	100	–	82.6	100	100
All tumors	58	53.3	60	91.4	72
Mean follow-up (months)	55	19	25	34.1	65
Number of patients	115	334	1,307	134	61

chemotherapy, combined chemoradiotherapy, or biological modifiers has to be explored. Quality of life should be assessed preoperatively and postoperatively. Therefore, the current levels of evidence for the effectiveness of endonasal tumor surgery are mainly level 3 (case series) and level 4 (expert option).[22] To reach higher levels of evidence it is necessary to perform randomized, collaborative, international, multicenter trials; and, this will be the challenge for the next decade.

Pearls and Pitfalls

- Malignant sinonasal neoplasms account for 3 to 5% of all head and neck cancers.
- Most sinonasal malignancies present with unilateral nasal obstruction, nasal discharge, loss of smell, epistaxis, and headache.
- The UICC classification is used for most sinonasal malignant tumors. The modified Kadish staging system is most commonly used for esthesioneuroblastoma.
- Squamous cell carcinoma is the most common malignant tumor of the paranasal sinuses, although in parts of central and south Europe, adenocarcinoma predominates.
- Five-year disease-specific survival rate of endonasal resected malignancies ranged between 70 and 90% compared with 50 to 70% after traditional craniofacial resection. This difference, however, is in great part due to a strong selection bias.
- These 5-year disease-specific survival rates indicate that for properly selected patients endonasal endoscopic surgery should be considered a first choice therapeutic option in the management of sinonasal and anterior skull base malignancies.
- With regard to the endonasal approach, the status of the surgical margins was found to be the only independent predictor of survival in our analysis.
- Irrespective of the surgical approach our analysis revealed that the pT stage and type of disease (primary tumor, residual tumor, etc.) are independent predictors of disease-specific survival. Type of disease, status of surgical margins, and infiltration of the brain were independent predictors for recurrence-free survival and for metastases-free survival.
- Among the different tumor histologies we found that esthesioneuroblastomas have the most favorable prognosis.
- The goals of surgery depend on the histopathology and extent of the neoplasm.
- Contraindications for endonasal tumor surgery with curative intent are extensive invasion of brain, soft tissues of the orbit, skin, erosion of hard palate or the nasal bones, and involvement of the anterior wall or upper lateral portion of the frontal sinus.

15.2 Endoscopic Resection of Sinonasal and Skull Base Tumors (Varese, Brescia School)

Paolo Castelnuovo, Mario Turri-Zanoni, Paolo Battaglia, Piero Nicolai

15.2.1 Introduction

Advances in imaging techniques and increased experience with endoscopic surgery have led to a revived interest in the management of benign and malignant tumors of the sinonasal tract and adjacent skull base. The indications for endoscopic resection of sinonasal neoplasms have been expanded during recent years, owing to the multiangle, magnified view of the surgical field, the availability of powered instrumentation, and the attachment-oriented surgical strategy. When compared with external approaches, this evolution has been shown to decrease morbidity, complication, and hospitalization time, and has shown similar success rates.

A review of the outcomes reported in the literature in the last 15 years shows that endoscopic resection of benign and malignant tumors of the sinonasal tract and adjacent skull base is a feasible and safe surgical option.[22] We validate this statement by reporting our extensive endoscopic experience in the management of sinonasal and skull base lesions at the departments of otorhinolaryngology of the universities of Varese, Pavia, and Brescia, from the early 1990s until December 2010.

Currently, most benign and malignant sinonasal tumors can be managed through an exclusively endoscopic endonasal approach, achieving results that are comparable with those of external traditional approaches. However, there are still situations that require an external or a combined procedure.

Overall, the golden point for the skull base procedures is to choose the best surgical corridor toward the pathology.[24] In fact, it is of paramount importance that the chosen route to the target allows safe and adequate management of the pathology without crossing cranial nerves or other vital structures. The endoscopic endonasal corridor is preferred when it provides the most direct access to the tumor with the least manipulation of neural and vascular structures; thus, if nerves or vessels need to be mobilized to reach the tumor an alternative approach should be considered.[25] Based on this statement, we believe that every surgical option should be available to the management team and that the surgical choice should be tailored on a given patient.

The choice of a surgical approach depends on patient comorbidities, tumor characteristics, and the level of skill and confidence of the surgeons. The need for an external or combined procedure may be suggested by preoperative imaging studies but in a few cases a definitive decision can be taken only during the surgical procedure. Consequently, the possibility of switching from an endoscopic to an external procedure must be always discussed with the patient prior to surgery.

Hence, the surgical team, which for tumors involving the anterior skull base necessarily includes both an otolaryngologist and a neurosurgeon, should be experienced in all these techniques to be able to perform "multiportal" surgical approaches. Moreover, to optimize outcomes, endoscopic resections of sinonasal and skull base tumors should be performed only by teams of surgeons with long-standing experience in the endoscopic management of inflammatory diseases and cerebrospinal fluid (CSF) leaks together with a thorough knowledge of surgical oncologic principles (for the management of malignancies).

15.2.2 Fibro-osseous Lesions

Benign fibro-osseous lesions are slow-growing diseases, comprising distinct entities with significant clinical and histological overlap. In this group, the most frequent histotype is the osteoma, followed by fibrous dysplasia and ossifying fibroma.

Surgical Techniques

While it is generally agreed that the "wait and scan" policy is the therapeutic standard for small and asymptomatic fibro-osseous lesions, surgery is indicated for those with symptoms.[22] Traditionally, the surgical removal of sinonasal fibro-osseous lesions was performed by an extranasal approach with acceptable esthetic results and very low recurrence rate.[26,27] Moreover, for removing

frontal sinus fibro-osseous lesions, the gold standard is still considered the external osteoplastic approach.[28] The advantage of the extranasal surgical technique is that it offers a better overview of the lesion and a potentially shorter operation time. The disadvantages are the lower patient acceptance, the cicatrization, and higher morbidity due to longer hospitalization.

In recent years, endoscopic transnasal removal has been increasingly performed, depending on the localization and size of the lesion (▶ Fig. 15.6). The endoscopic approach can be used not only for the fibro-osseous lesions of the ethmoidal and maxillary sinuses, but can be also extensively applied to the region of the frontal recess and sinus. Endoscopic resection of a frontal sinus osteoma was first reported in 1992.[29] Subsequently, the development of dedicated instruments together with the refinement of surgical techniques have continuously expanded the indications for an endoscopic endonasal resection of a fibro-osseous lesion. Lesions involving the ethmoid and sphenoid sinuses, the medial wall of the maxillary sinus, and even the inferior and medial wall of the orbit can be resected transnasally. Frontal lesions are always suitable for a purely endoscopic endonasal resection if they are located medially to a virtual sagittal plane passing through the lamina papyracea, if they originate from the inferior portion of the posterior frontal sinus wall, and if the anteroposterior diameter of the frontal sinus is at least 10 mm.[30] In 2001, Schick and Draf reported a significant series of 34 frontoethmoidal osteomas, 68% of which were approached endoscopically, with incomplete endonasal resection of only three.[31] To define the indication of endoscopic endonasal approach, Chiu et al developed a classification system for frontal sinus osteomas in 2005, recommending endoscopic resection

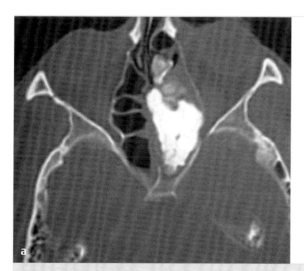
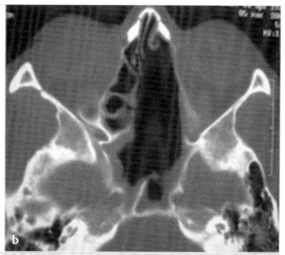

Fig. 15.6 a, b Preoperative and postoperative radiological images demonstrate the results obtained in the resection of a large osteoma filling the left anteroposterior ethmoidal compartment using the endoscopic endonasal approach. **(a)** Preoperative CT scan in axial view. **(b)** Result after the endoscopic endonasal cavitation of the lesion shown in **(a)**.

of grade I and II lesions and extranasal removal of grade III and IV lesions.[32] In 2007, we reported our experience in the management of 26 patients with frontal sinus osteomas, approached with a purely endoscopic technique in 11 patients, with no recurrence observed after a mean 40 months follow-up.[30]

Recently, the introduction of multiangled scope and angled drills, together with the Draf type III median drainage procedure and four-hands/two-nostrils technique, has allowed the resection of lesions localized more and more laterally, extending over the limits previously described. In this respect, the study by Seiberling and Wormald in 2009 has shown that the removal of large osteomas localized far laterally or filling the entire frontal sinus is possible and successful transnasally, with no recurrence of the lesion after 3 years mean follow-up.[33] Furthermore, the experience with 24 osteomas in the frontal recess and sinus described by Ledderose and Leunig in 2010 confirms the possibility of resecting laterally located lesions by means of a purely endoscopic endonasal approach.[34]

Results of Endonasal Surgery

Over the years, we have increased our experience in the management of sinonasal fibro-osseous lesions and we treated 129 such patients between June 1996 and December 2010 in the departments of otorhinolaryngology of the Universities of Varese, Pavia, and Brescia. Our cohort included 61 women and 68 men and their age at surgery ranged from 11 to 85 years (mean 44.2 years). The majority of these patients (63%) complained of facial pain and headache. The frontal sinus was the most frequent location (64/129, 49.6%), followed by the ethmoid complex in 37/129 (28.6%), and by simultaneous frontoethmoidal involvement in 20/129 (15.5%) cases, while the maxillary (3/129, 2.4%) and sphenoid (1/129, 0.8%) sinuses were seldom involved. In 6/129 (4.6%) cases, the lesions also involved the orbital region.

A purely endoscopic approach was performed in 87/129 (67.5%) patients. In 33 (25.6%) patients a combined procedure was used, while in 9 patients (6.9%) a purely external approach was performed (osteoplastic flap with coronal incision in 8 cases and Howard-Lynch frontoethmoidectomy in one of our first cases). For the endoscopic group, the mean hospital stay was 3.9 days (range 3–7 days) while in the combined and external groups the mean stay was 5.3 days (range 4–13 days). No serious immediate or delayed complications were observed after surgery. In the purely endoscopic group, preoperative assessment showed involvement of the skull base in five patients who were previously informed and scheduled for a skull base duraplasty during the osteoma resection. Moreover, two patients (1.6%) had a persistence of osteoma after the surgical resection. In both cases, the residual disease (1 and 1.4 mm) was localized on the frontal

sinus floor. Currently, the two persisting lesions are stable in size and are under CT surveillance. At the time of writing, we have observed no recurrence in the radically treated patients, at a mean follow-up of 67.5 months (range 4–184 months).

In our series, the tumors ranged in size from 6 to 60 mm at their maximum diameter, with a median size of 19 mm. There were no statistical differences between the median sizes of osteomas in the endoscopic group compared with those in the external or combined group when using the independent sample t-test ($p = 0.14$), confirming that the dimensional parameter was not the first criterion in planning the surgical approach.

An attempt to evaluate the toughness of osteomas can be performed preoperatively by CT densitometry but, unfortunately, it can be precisely defined only during the surgical procedure. Actually, in our experience, the toughness of the lesion required switching from an endoscopic endonasal to a combined external procedure in 2/129 (1.6%) far lateral frontal osteomas, due to the low speed of the angled drill. This limitation will be overcome in the next few years with the introduction of high-speed multiangled drills.

The localization of the lesion certainly represents a critical feature in the choice of the most appropriate surgical technique for obtaining the best exposure of the bony lesion and its boundaries.[35] Remarkably, if we stratify our data according to the year of surgery, we observe that from 2008 onwards we were able to manage transnasally most of the lesions localized lateral to the virtual sagittal plane through the lamina papyracea, taking advantage of the four-hands/two-nostrils technique, the Draf type III median drainage, and the angled instrumental and scope evolutions. Now, even intraorbital invasion is no longer an absolute contraindication for the endoscopic approach, which can be employed in selected cases, thus avoiding external access.

However, radical removal cannot be achieved with a purely endoscopic endonasal approach in cases of: small anteroposterior diameter of the frontal sinus in relation to a large frontal sinus volume (in this case, intrasinus maneuverability of angled instruments is reduced); erosion of the posterior wall of the frontal sinus with large intracranial multilobulated osteoma; extension of the tumor through the anterior frontal plate; relevant posttraumatic anatomical changes in frontal bone structure; lateral or superolateral orbital wall attachment of the lesion. In these latter cases, the lesion can be better exposed and drilled out through an osteoplastic flap sinusotomy, whether combined or not with the endoscopic endonasal approach, to achieve a radical resection. A large base of insertion on the posterior or anterior wall of the frontal sinus is a condition that makes a purely endoscopic endonasal resection of the osteoma more difficult, but it should not be considered an absolute contraindication. In these cases, we try to remove the lesion transnasally, according to the cavitation technique, with a surgical team ready to perform a combined external approach, if required. However, in the case of a lesion massively eroding the anterior or posterior frontal wall, an external approach is usually recommended and reconstruction is also required to maintain a regular frontal outline anteriorly and to close the intracranial space posteriorly.

Conclusion

At the present time, we conclude that endoscopic resection even of large and adversely located sinonasal and skull base osteomas is feasible, safe, and efficacious, obtaining the radical removal in most of the cases, with a success rate similar to that of extranasal approaches. Moreover, the endoscopic technique enables shorter hospitalization time, preserves the natural endonasal drainage pathways, or creates new ones, but requires longer surgical training and greater experience.[34] Finally, it should be noted that even when an osteoma is removed through an extranasal approach, endonasal surgery might be helpful to preserve or rehabilitate the natural drainage pathways, especially in the frontal sinus region.[36]

15.2.3 Inverted Papilloma

Surgical Techniques

Historically, the gold standard for the management of sinonasal inverted papillomas was an external approach (i.e., lateral rhinotomy, Caldwell-Luc procedure, or midfacial degloving) and medial maxillectomy.[37] Vrabec reported a recurrence rate of only 2% (in a mean follow-up of 8.9 years) using a lateral rhinotomy with a modified Weber-Ferguson incision.[38] Of late, an endoscopic resection has been given increasing consideration because it obviates the morbidity of an external approach (▶ Fig. 15.7). The advantage of the endoscopic technique is the absence of a facial incision, negligible

facial swelling, shorter in-patient time, and a reduction in postoperative pain and dysesthesia.[22] In addition, the endoscope offers improved visualization with enhanced discrimination of tumor from normal tissue.

In the first endoscopic experiences, the anterior wall and floor of the maxillary sinus were difficult to access and the Caldwell-Luc approach was still required to remove diseased mucosa in these areas. More recently, however, the endoscopic medial maxillectomy technique has meant that the whole lining of the maxillary sinus can be removed endoscopically and this has superseded the Caldwell-Luc approach in the vast majority of cases.[39] Similarly, the difficult removal of all diseased mucosa in the frontal sinus by endoscopic means was overcome by the introduction of the median drainage approach, according to the Draf type III[31,40] or the modified endoscopic Lothrop procedure.[41]

Nevertheless, whenever extensive mucosal involvement inside a supraorbital cell extending far laterally over the orbit or a massive involvement of the frontal sinus mucosa was identified, an osteoplastic flap using a coronal approach was required to remove all diseased mucosa.

Results of Endonasal Surgery

In our experience, a total of 348 patients affected by sinonasal inverted papilloma were treated at the departments of otorhinolaryngology of the universities of Varese, Pavia, and Brescia from November 1991 to December 2010. Only patients treated by a purely endoscopic or combined (endoscopic associated with external) approach and with at least 3 years of follow-up were considered eligible for inclusion in the analysis. The patients who fulfilled the inclusion criteria were 212 (167 men, 45 women), with a mean age at surgery of 56.5 years (range 20–86 years). To the best of our knowledge, this is the largest case series presented to date in English publications focusing on the role of endoscopic surgery in the management of inverted papilloma. Fifty-six patients (26.4%) had been

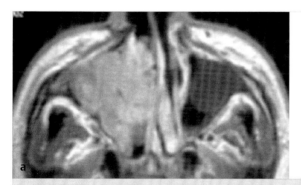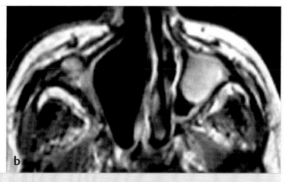

Fig. 15.7 a, b Preoperative and postoperative radiological images demonstrate the results obtained in the resection of a tight maxillary inverted papilloma staged T3, according to the Krouse classification system, using the endoscopic endonasal approach. (a) The typical "cerebriform-columnar pattern is evident in the MRI scan. (b) MRI scan after a type 2 endoscopic resection of the lesion shown in (a).

treated previously at other institutions with endoscopic (21.4%) or external (5%) approaches. Unilateral nasal obstruction was the presenting symptom in 89.9% of patients; other complaints included hyposmia-anosmia (18.7%), rhinorrhea (18.2%), headache (17.3%), epistaxis (11.8%), and epiphora (6%). The diagnosis was serendipitous in seven asymptomatic patients (3%). In 100 patients (47.2%), the lesion originated from the nasoethmoidal complex, in 92 patients (43.4%) from the maxillary sinus, in 11 patients (5.2%) from the frontal sinus, and in 9 patients (4.2%) from the sphenoid sinus. Bilateral involvement was present in seven patients (3.3%). Lesions were staged according to Krouse[42] as follows: 16 (7.5%) T1, 78 (36.8%) T2, 104 (49.1%) T3, and 14 (6.6%) T4. An exclusively endoscopic approach was used in 198 patients (93.4%): 88 patients (44.4%) received a type 1 resection, 62 patients (31.3%) received a type 2 (with resection of the nasolacrimal duct in 38 cases), and 48 patients (24.3%) received a type 3. The different types of endoscopic procedures have been extensively described in a previous publication.[43] Fourteen patients (6.6%) underwent an endoscopic approach combined with an osteoplastic flap. The main observed complication was CSF leak in 2.8% of the patients that was identified and treated by endoscopic duraplasty intraoperatively.

A complete endoscopic excision was achieved by disassembling the lesion in oriented blocks, starting at the endonasal portion and progressively reaching the area of attachment, where the dissection was performed along the subperiosteal plane followed by drilling of the underlying bone.[44] This modular resection implies that all the involved subsites with possible foci of microinvasive or invasive squamous cell carcinoma can be located at definitive histological analysis. Numerous publications on inverted papilloma differ widely in the reported incidence of associated squamous cell carcinoma, ranging from 0[45] to 53%.[46] A review of 63 case series[47] shows that the incidence of pathological changes in inverted papilloma was 1.1% of cases with atypia, 1.9% with dysplasia, 7.1% with synchronous carcinoma, and 3.6% with development of metachronous carcinoma in a mean time interval of 52 months (range 6–180 months).

In our series, definitive histology assessment found areas of mild dysplasia in three patients (1.4%) and moderate dysplasia in two patients (0.9%). Carcinoma in situ was detected in three patients (1.4%) and squamous cell carcinoma in eight patients (3.8%). In five-eighths of patients with squamous cell carcinoma, adjuvant postoperative radiation therapy (60–65 Gy) on the primary site was planned.

Remarkably, we have to consider that the estimated malignancy potential increased up to 11% for recurrent disease.[22] Recently, several authors have emphasized the need to modulate the surgical technique according to the site of attachment and extension of the inverted papilloma to minimize recurrence.[48] It is worth remembering that the term "recurrence" merely indicates residual disease in the majority of cases and is directly related to the surgical approach and the "care" with which the inverted papilloma is removed.[49] Therefore, a recurrence might be attributed primarily to the inability of the surgeon to achieve complete resection rather than to the intrinsic characteristics of the tumor itself. Consistently with this statement, a recent "position article" confirms that the outcome of treatment relates to how thoroughly the diseased mucosa is removed.[22] In fact, Bielamowicz et al found a statistically significant difference between the recurrence rates in patients treated with a medial maxillectomy (20%) versus those treated with a limited conservative resection (47%).[50]

Moreover, Mirza et al[47] reviewed 63 case series (2,109 patients) of inverted papilloma resection and found that recurrence rates were 12.8% for endoscopic procedures (484 patients), 17.0% for lateral rhinotomy with medial maxillectomy (1,025 patients), and 34.2% for limited resections such as nasal polypectomy (600 patients). In our series, 199 patients (93.9%) were free of disease in December 2010, after a mean follow-up of 65.8 months (ranging from 36 to 204 months). Recurrence was observed in the remaining 13 cases (6.1%). The mean interval between surgical treatment and diagnosis of recurrence was 29 months (range 6–70 months). All the recurrences were observed at the same site of the primary lesion and after endoscopic removal. The recurrences were treated by a purely endoscopic approach in 11 cases and by a combined approach in the remaining two cases. The recurrence rate of 6.1% observed in our series of 212 patients is comparable with data for both endoscopic and external approaches present in the literature (4–22%).[51,52]

When comparing the results of external and endoscopic techniques it should be noted that the postoperative follow-up period was shorter in the endoscopic group (3 years, mean) than in the external one (5 years, mean). However, similarly to Buchwald's report,[53] we underline that the most recurrent disease occurs in the first 9 to 12 months. This statement was confirmed in our series as well, in which most of the recurrences (8/13, 61.5%) were diagnosed within 36 months. Nevertheless, we maintain that at least 5 years of follow-up are to be recommended. Finally, the meta-analysis performed by Busquets[54] also supports the long-term efficacy of the endoscopic technique for the resection of inverted papilloma, with a recurrence rate of 12%, lower than the 20% encountered in the nonendoscopic group.

Conclusion

In conclusion, a review of the literature shows that endoscopic removal of inverted papillomas, when properly planned and in expert hands, yields similar, if not better, results than those of external approaches.[22]

15.2.4 Juvenile Nasopharyngeal Angiofibroma

Surgical Techniques

There is general agreement that surgery plays a key role in the management of juvenile nasopharyngeal angiofibroma (JNA). The fact that many approaches (suprahyoid, transpalatal, transmaxillary through a lateral rhinotomy or a midfacial degloving, facial translocation, Le Fort I, infratemporal approach, craniofacial resection) have been described, clearly indicates that there is no "ideal" technique but, rather, that the surgeon should have several different techniques available that can be used according to the extent of disease.

During recent years, the transnasal endoscopic approach has emerged as a viable alternative to external techniques for the management of small to intermediate size JNAs, in view of the excellent visualization of the surgical field through multiangled exposure, the low morbidity without any external scar or osteotomy, and short hospitalization times. The first reports about endoscopic resections were published during the 1990s and included low-staged JNA (Andrews stages I and II). They showed the feasibility of the procedure, with recurrence rates similar to external approaches but with reduced risks and morbidity.[55]

Our selection policy for an endoscopic approach has evolved over the years together with our increasing expertise, with a progressive shift from stages I and II toward selected Andrews stages IIIA and IIIB. Basically, all patients with lesions involving the nasopharynx, pterygopalatine fossa, nasal fossa, sphenoid sinus, maxillary sinus, ethmoid, infratemporal fossa, basisphenoid, and parasellar regions were considered eligible for endoscopic surgery.[56]

Contraindications for an endoscopic approach are still a matter of debate but, in our opinion, lesions associated with an extensive vascular supply from the internal carotid artery (ICA), its encasement, or with intracranial extension lateral to the paraclival segment of ICA are better treated with midfacial degloving or subtemporal craniotomy to fully expose the horizontal portion of the ICA.[57] Moreover, endoscopic surgery is deemed contraindicated in residual lesions involving critical areas (ICA, optic nerve, cavernous sinus, dura), where adhesions increase the risk of severe uncontrolled complications during dissection of the lesion.

Radiotherapy

With regard to therapeutic strategies in alternative to surgery, it is still a matter of debate whether radiotherapy can be considered a safe therapeutic option in young patients who have the likelihood of developing sarcomatoid degeneration of residual JNA or radioinduced neoplasms in the following decades. Kuppersmith et al[57] proposed the use of intensity-modulated radiotherapy for treatment of extensive and persistent JNA to limit irradiation of noble structures. They reported no acute toxicity and only two limited cases of late toxicity with epistaxis and persistent rhinitis. No patient developed recurrence (defined as growth). Reddy et al[58] treated 15 patients affected by advanced JNA (Andrews types IIIb and IV) with radiotherapy. Local control obtained was 85%, with two patients with local persistence. Five (33%) patients developed late complications, including cataracts, transient central nervous system syndrome, and basal cell carcinoma of the skin. In our opinion, radiotherapy might be recommended as an adjuvant therapy for unresectable tumors, failure of complete tumor removal, or for extensive intracranial extension.

Results of Endonasal Surgery

From January 1994 to December 2010, 93 patients affected by JNA were treated by a purely endoscopic resection at the departments of otorhinolaryngology of the universities of Varese, Pavia, and Brescia. All patients were Caucasian males, ranging in age from 10 to 49 years (mean 17.6 years). In our series, involvement of the pterygopalatine fossa was detected in 81 (87%) cases, of the sphenoid sinus in 58 (62.4%), infratemporal fossa in 35 (37.6%), maxillary sinus in 9 (9.7%), and ethmoid sinus in only 5 (5.4%). In 14 (15%) patients, there was an intracranial extradural extension. Intraorbital involvement was detected in four cases (4.3%). Lesions were classified according to the Andrews[59] staging system as follows: stage I, 7 (7.5%) patients; stage II, 44 (47.5%) patients; stage IIIA, 28 (30%) patients (▶ Fig. 15.8); stage IIIB, 14 (15%) patients. All patients underwent a purely endoscopic resection of angiofibroma with mean hospitalization time of 6.8 days (range 2–36 days). No minor or major postoperative complications were observed. At the moment, all patients are still undergoing regular follow-up (mean 74.5 months, range 1–197 months).

The amount of blood loss during JNA excision is intimately linked to the tumor vascular supply and to the quality of the embolization.[56] In the pre-embolization era, intraoperative bleeding was so dramatic that the procedure was a true challenge for the surgeon and was associated with high rates of persistent disease and considerable morbidity. In early 1970s, the introduction of this technique,[60] which is commonly performed 48 hours before surgery, has revolutionized the treatment of JNA by dramatically decreasing intraoperative bleeding (60–70%)[61] and therefore making the assessment of tumor borders more accurate at dissection. Glad et al[61] showed that the embolization procedure decreased intraoperative blood loss to 650 ml in the embolized group as compared with an average of 1,200 ml in the nonembolized group (p < 0.05). Similarly, the need for preoperative

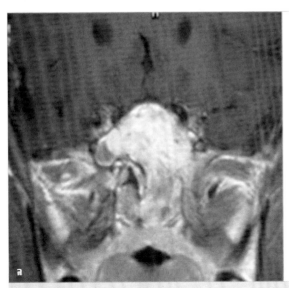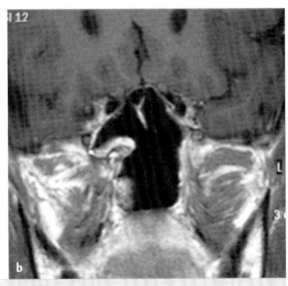

Fig. 15.8 a, b Preoperative and postoperative radiological images demonstrate the results obtained in the resection of a JNA, stage III A according to Andrews, using the endoscopic endonasal approach. **(a)** Preoperative coronal MRI. **(b)** Postoperative MRI after the endoscopic removal of the JNA shown in **(a)**.

blood transfusion was reduced ($p < 0.005$).[61] The methods of embolization currently available provide excellent devascularization of feeders coming from the internal maxillary artery and its branches as well as from the ascending pharyngeal artery, but are associated with an unacceptable risk of major neurologic complications[62] for the ICA feeders. In the event of encasement of the ICA, which nowadays is a very rare event, the balloon occlusion test and sacrifice of the ICA or, as a less invasive procedure, stenting of the intratemporal carotid artery, may be considered.[63] Another source of criticism against embolization is the experience of Lloyd et al, who considered this procedure to be a risk factor for persistence because of the increased difficulty in identifying tumor margins particularly at the interface with the basisphenoid.[64]

With regard to vascularization, 19 (20.4%) patients in our cohort presented an adjunctive blood supply from the contralateral external carotid artery system through the maxillary, sphenopalatine, and/or pharyngeal arteries. Moreover, 28 (30.1%) patients also had a vascular supply from the ICA, through siphon vessels, the mandibular artery, and/or the ophthalmic artery. Embolization was performed uneventfully in 86 (92.5%) patients, while in 7 (7.5%), in view of the limited size of the lesion with no major lateral extension, the procedure was not applied and surgery therefore included the exposure of the pterygopalatine fossa as a first step and bipolar cauterization or clipping of the maxillary artery. In our series, intraoperative or postoperative blood transfusion was required in 25 patients (26.9%).

Nowadays, the efficacy and safety of endoscopic excision of JNA is supported by excellent results from several operative series published in recent years. The rate of recurrent disease after endoscopic removal of JNA has ranged between the 0% reported by Schick,[65] Wormald,[66] and Gupta[67] in series of 5, 7, and 28 patients, respectively, and the 36.3% reported by Munoz del Castillo.[68]

During the endoscopic resection of a large volume JNA, disassembling of the lesion step by step can prove extremely helpful, thus providing a greater area for moving the instruments around the lesion and adequate exposure of the interface with the adjacent tissues.

Notably, in all series reported in the literature, the residual disease and the recurrence rate were rather low for smaller staged lesions, increasing in the higher staged tumors. However, the recurrence rate seems to be more related to the involvement of specific sites such as basisphenoid, pterygopalatine fossa, anterior skull base, cavernous sinus, and infratemporal fossa. In a review of preoperative CT and MRI scans on 72 patients, Lloyd et al demonstrated that 93% of the recurrences occurred in patients with imaging evidence of invasion of the sphenoid diploe through the pterygoid canal.[64] What seems to be important for preventing recurrences is the drilling out of the cancellous bone of the basisphenoid, particularly around the vidian canal, to remove any residual disease that may not be immediately evident.[69]

Until 2006, we followed all patients according to a schedule including endoscopic and MRI examination 4 months after surgery and then every 6 months to detect residual disease or recurrence. In the recent years, we changed this policy with reference to the experience reported by Kania et al,[70] and we now perform a MRI scan the same day the patient has the nasal packing removed or the day after, for early identification of any suspicious residual disease. The early postoperative MRI does not show any of the inflammatory changes that, after 3 to 4 months, frequently make the differentiation between small residual lesions and active scar tissue challenging. To date none of the patients who had an early postoperative MRI has shown any residual lesion, even at a subsequent MRI examination.

In our cohort, the postoperative MRI scan detected a residual disease localized in critical areas such as the basisphenoid, pterygoid root, cavernous sinus, or anterior skull base in nine patients (9.7%). The best treatment option for patients with residual disease and what should be the most appropriate follow-up protocol are still debated. At the time of writing, only two of our patients with persistent disease have required endoscopic surgical revision due to progressive growth. The other seven persistent lesions are nearly stable in size and are currently under MRI surveillance. In fact, Önerci[71] suggested that a "wait-and-see" policy for intracranial residual disease might be preferable to infratemporal craniofacial resection. In addition, one recent interesting case report reintroduced the concept of spontaneous involution of JNA. The patient described was never treated and was followed for 8 years, during which time the lesion constantly decreased in size.[72] In this regard, Reddy et al have noted that regression of a residual lesion may take up to 3 years.[58]

Comparison of the results between external and endoscopic techniques in terms of recurrence rate, amount of bleeding, and hospitalization time is hindered by several biases related mainly to stratification by staging and follow-up methodology. However, the recurrence rate of series with a consistent number of patients reported in the 1990s and treated with an external technique is around 36 to 40%.[64,73] More recently, Danesi et al demonstrated that a transfacial approach (through lateral rhinotomy or midfacial degloving) can lead to excellent results, with only 13.5 and 18.2% of residual disease in lesions with extracranial and intracranial extent, respectively.[74]

Conclusion

In conclusion, as shown by our results and in accordance with the reports of other authors, endoscopic resection achieved good results not only in stages I to II but also in Andrews stage IIIa and b lesions, without any major complication and with an acceptable overall rate of residual disease (9.7% in our series). Moreover, endoscopic surgery allows better exposure and visualization of JNA projections due to angled telescopes, avoids unsightly scars, doe not interfere with craniofacial bone growth, and it decreases postoperative pain and hospitalization time. Refinement in surgical techniques and dedicated instrumentation could make it possible to expand the indications further to lesions with intracranial extradural extension.

15.2.5 Malignant Tumors of the Sinonasal Tract and Adjacent Skull Base

Surgical Techniques

A major advance in the management of sinonasal malignancies was the introduction of craniofacial resection by Ketcham et al in the 1960s.[75] By including the anterior skull base in the surgical specimen, this intervention has dramatically improved the local control of tumors encroaching upon the roof of the ethmoid. However, this approach has been associated with a morbidity and perioperative mortality that is not negligible.

Nowadays, craniofacial resection with or without adjuvant postoperative radiotherapy, according to the extent and the biological aggressiveness of the single tumor, still remains as the "gold standard" for malignant lesions in contact with or transgressing the anterior skull base. An international collaborative study reported by Patel et al[15] based on 1,307 patients who underwent a standard anterior craniofacial resection, associated with adjuvant treatment in 39% of cases, showed a 5-year overall survival of 54% and a 5-year disease-specific survival of 60%.

The growing expertise of surgeons in endoscopic procedures, improvements in imaging studies to increase the accuracy of preoperative diagnosis, together with technological refinement of endoscopic equipment[76] have all contributed to gradually expand the indications for an endoscopic approach to resect selected cases of malignant tumors. The first endoscopic experiences in sinonasal malignancy treatment emerged in the late 1990s[77,78] and were limited to lesions involving the nasoethmoidal box, but not encroaching upon the anterior skull base.

Over the past decade, data from several centers worldwide have demonstrated that endoscopic resection of malignant sinonasal tumors can be extended to include the dura of the anterior skull base (endoscopic resection with transnasal craniectomy), from the posterior wall of the frontal sinus back to the planum sphenoidale and between the orbits.[79] In addition, endoscopic resection has been shown to allow precise localization of the tumor origin, which surprisingly is often limited despite a bulky mass filling the nasal cavity. Hence, the extent of the endoscopic resection can be tailored to specific tumor characteristics (histotype, site of origin, and proximity to critical areas) preserving uninvolved structures, with subsequent reduced functional sequelae.

In several reports, the endoscopic approach has shown acceptable morbidity and outcomes, suggesting that this technique can be included among the surgical options available for the management of this kind of cancer. However, all patients scheduled for endoscopic resection with transnasal craniectomy have to be informed about the possibility of switching to a combined cranioendoscopic approach in the presence of unexpected extensive dural involvement. In fact, the involvement of the dura in close proximity to the lamina papyracea or over the orbital roof detected in either the preoperative or the intraoperative setting required combining an endoscopic approach with an external one (cranioendoscopic resection).[15]

At that time, extension into the frontal sinus, involvement of the lacrimal pathway or of the bony walls of the maxillary sinus (with the exception of the medial one), erosion of the nasal fossa floor, extension into the pterygopalatine or infratemporal fossa, involvement of the orbit, and erosion of the skull base were all considered contraindications for an exclusively endoscopic approach.[80] On the other hand, simple contact of the tumor with "high-risk" areas, such as the lamina papyracea, the cribriform plate, or the roof of the ethmoid, without radiologic signs of bone erosion and knowledge of the volume of the lesion were not considered contraindications.

Results of Endonasal Surgery

Most publications analyzing the efficacy of endoscopic surgery in the management of sinonasal cancers have concentrated on a homogeneous cohort of patients with a specific histology. In olfactory neuroblastoma histotypes, the well-known propensity of the lesion to be associated with late recurrences, and therefore with a need for long-term follow-up, contributed to mitigate the enthusiasm toward the excellent results achieved by endoscopic surgery, which is commonly used in combination with postoperative radiotherapy. Folbe et al[81] recently reported the results of a study performed at two US centers on 23 patients (10.5% were modified Kadish stage A, 58.9% stage B, 26.3% stage C, and 5.3% stage D). All but one patient, who required the association with a transcranial approach to clear a positive margin along the supraorbital dura, had the tumor resected endoscopically. Postoperative radiotherapy was administered in 16 patients. After a mean follow-up time of 45.2 months, all patients were free of disease at the primary site.

The outcome of endoscopic surgery followed by radiotherapy in adenocarcinoma has been reported by Bogaerts et al[8] in a series of 44 patients, including 1 patient who was T1, 26 who were T2, 5 who were T3, and 9 who were T4a for sphenoid sinus involvement, and 3 who were T4b for limited dural involvement. Median follow-up, as well as follow-up of patients alive at the end of follow-up, was 36 months. Of note, no contralateral dissection was undertaken if the tumor was unilateral and the resection was rarely extended to include the dural plane. Twelve (27%) patients experienced local recurrence, which was diagnosed within 24 months of primary treatment in eight cases. Retreatment included a second endoscopic procedure in nine patients and craniofacial resection in three patients. The 5-year disease-specific survival was 83%, and was not influenced by the occurrence of local recurrence or T stage. In view of the

observation of local recurrences in areas that were quite different from the initial presentation, we have suggested the opportunity to include the entire bilateral ethmoid labyrinth in the resection. This would be justified by the fact that exposure to leather or wood dust, which is often associated with adenocarcinoma, renders all the mucosa of the nasoethmoidal complex vulnerable to developing adenocarcinoma foci. Another experience of a small number ($n = 12$) of patients with adenocarcinoma (6 T2, 5 T3, and 1 T4) was associated with a 91.6% 5-year disease-free survival after a median follow-up of 30 months.[82]

The two largest series reporting on 184[7] and 120[21] patients, who underwent an endoscopic approach to resect a sinonasal and anterior skull base cancer, were almost concomitantly published. The first was our 10-year experience in two tertiary care Italian centers, while the second summarized the oncologic results on a cohort of patients treated at the MD Anderson Cancer Center in Houston over a 16-year period. Both series included patients in whom endoscopic surgery was used either alone (72.8 versus 77.5%) or in combination with frontal or subfrontal craniotomy (27.2 versus 22.5%). The distribution of patients in relation to histology reflected the variable prevalence of histologies found in various geographical areas. In the Italian series, adenocarcinoma was the most frequent lesion (37%), while olfactory neuroblastoma was prevalent (17%) in the US experience. With no major differences in the mean follow-up time (34.1 versus 37 months), the 5-year disease-specific survival in the two series for the entire patient cohort was also quite similar: 81.9 versus 87%.

Throughout the years, we have increased our experience in the endoscopic management of sinonasal and skull base malignancies, totaling 320 patients (220 male and 100 female) by December 2010. In this cohort, an endoscopic resection was performed in 260 (81.3%) patients and a cranioendoscopic resection in the remaining 60 (18.7%). Among the 260 treated patients endoscopically, 137 underwent an exclusively endoscopic resection without endonasal craniectomy and 123 underwent endoscopic resection in association with transnasal craniectomy. The distribution of tumors in relation to T category was as follows: 77 (24.1%) T1 (73 and 4 in the endoscopic resection and cranioendoscopic resection group, respectively); 70 (21.9%) T2 (69 endoscopic resection without endonasal craniectomy and 1 cranioendoscopic resection); 58 (18.1%) T3 (45 endoscopic resection and 13 cranioendoscopic resection); 38 (11.8%) T4a (28 endoscopic resection and 10 cranioendoscopic resection); and 77 (24.1%) T4b (45 endoscopic resection and 32 cranioendoscopic resection). The most frequent histotypes encountered in our series remained adenocarcinoma (43.4%), followed by squamous cell carcinoma (11.9%), olfactory neuroblastoma (10.6%, ▶ Fig. 15.9), mucosal melanoma (7.8%), and adenoid cystic carcinoma (5%). Mean hospitalization time was 3.4 days (range 1–10 days)

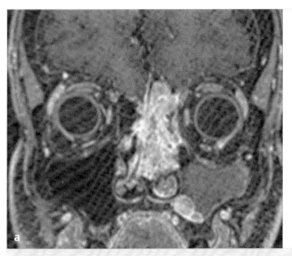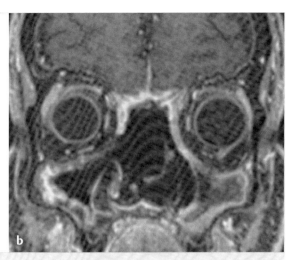

Fig. 15.9 a, b Preoperative and postoperative radiological images demonstrate the results obtained in the resection of a left olfactory neuroblastoma, staged T4bN0M0, Kadish C, using the endoscopic endonasal approach. (a) Preoperative coronal MRI using dynamic 3D VIBE sequence. (b) Postoperative MRI performed 6 months after the endoscopic resection with transnasal craniectomy (ERTC) associated with adjuvant radiotherapy (66 Gy).

in the endoscopic resection group and increased to 13.4 days (range 10–35 days) in the cranioendoscopic resection group.

Overall, 158 (49.3%) patients received some form of adjuvant treatment. Postoperative radiotherapy was planned in the case of significant skull base involvement (pT3), intracranial extension and dural infiltration (pT4a–b), close margins to the orbital content or the frontal sinus, and in cases of unresectable residual disease. All cases of olfactory neuroblastoma, except those not extending up to the skull base, received adjuvant radiotherapy. All patients who underwent a cranioendoscopic resection as a primary treatment underwent postoperative radiotherapy, except those with melanoma. In both endoscopic resection and cranioendoscopic resection groups, chemotherapy was added to radiotherapy in cases of high risk of systemic dissemination of the disease. Chemotherapy alone was administered in the case of osteosarcoma, Ewing sarcoma, recurrent non-Hodgkin lymphoma, and recurrent undifferentiated carcinoma.

All patients were prospectively followed according to a protocol that included monthly endoscopic examinations and MRI every 4 months during the first year; endoscopic examination and MRI every 2 and 6 months during the 2nd year; thereafter, both examinations at 6-month intervals. Follow-up ranged from 1 to 157 months (mean 43.8 months) for the entire patient population. Five-year overall survival was 72.5% for the entire population of the study, varying from 79 to 48.3% ($p = 0.036$) in the endoscopic and cranioendoscopic group, respectively (▶ Fig. 15.10a). Moreover, we found no statistically significant difference in 5-year disease-specific survival between patients treated with endoscopic surgery alone and those who received cranioendoscopic resection (87.2

versus 63%; $p = 0.5$), according to that observed by Hanna et al21 (▶ Fig. 15.10b). When 5-year disease-specific survival was estimated in relation to histology, by stratifying patients into four groups with comparable biological aggressiveness (epithelial and nonepithelial, such as adenocarcinoma, squamous cell carcinoma, and adenoid cystic carcinoma; olfactory neuroblastoma; melanoma; miscellaneous), we found a statistically significant difference (values of 88.8, 100, 41.3, and 82.3% respectively; $p < 0.0001$) (▶ Fig. 15.10c).

In our cohort, recurrence of the disease was observed in 22.9% of the patients (73/320) during a postoperative period ranging from 2 to 83 months (mean 22.7 months). Five-year recurrence-free survival was 78.6, 72.7, and 48.8% for the endoscopic transnasal craniectomy, endoscopic resection without craniectomy, and cranioendoscopic resection groups, respectively (▶ Fig. 15.10d). The overall complication rate in our series was 13.1% (8.8% in the endoscopic resection group and 31.6% in the cranioendoscopic resection group), comparable with the 11% of complications reported by Hanna et al.[21] Two cases of fatalities in patients with T4b lesions and extensive dural infiltration treated by cranioendoscopic resection occurred in our series, while no deaths were reported in the MD Anderson experience. Not unexpectedly, the most frequent major complication in both series was CSF leak, with a prevalence of 4.6% in our series and 3% in Hanna's cohort.[21] A recent analysis performed by our group on a subset of 62 patients who underwent endoscopic removal of tumor with dural resection (endoscopic transnasal craniectomy) showed that the occurrence of CSF leak is clearly related to the learning curve of the surgical team and to the refinement of surgical techniques.[79]

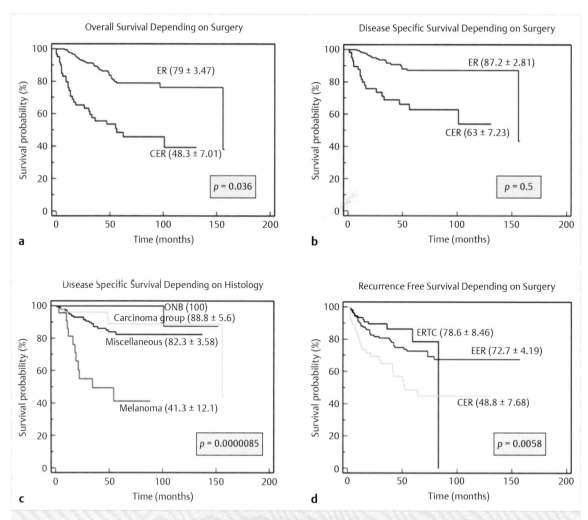

Fig. 15.10 a–d Survival rates in our series of 320 sinonasal and skull base malignancies. (a) Five-year overall survival in relation to the surgical approach. (b) Five-year disease-specific survival in relation to the surgical approach. (c) Five-year disease-specific survival depending on histology. (d) Five-year recurrence-free survival in relation to the surgical approach. A value of $p \leq 0.05$ was considered statistically significant.

CER, cranioendoscopic resection; EER, endoscopic resection without endonasal craniectomy, exclusively endoscopic resection; ER, endoscopic resection (without or with transnasal craniectomy); ERTC, endoscopic resection with transnasal craniectomy; ONB, olfactory neuroblastoma.

Since a prospective study comparing the results of endoscopic surgery and craniofacial resection is unfeasible, due to the rarity of sinonasal tumors as well as for ethical reasons, some authors have attempted to retrospectively compare the two techniques. Eloy et al[20] analyzed two groups of patients treated at the same institution with either transnasal endoscopic ($n = 18$) or craniofacial resection ($n = 48$) for tumors involving the anterior skull base. A statistically significant difference in terms of median hospital stay (3.5 versus 7.0 days) and median operative time (261.5 versus 625.5 minutes) in favor of endoscopic resections was observed, while the prevalence of perioperative complications was very similar in the two groups (27.8 versus 25.0%). Since there was no statistically significant difference

in overall survival between the two groups, the authors concluded that early and intermediate stage anterior skull base malignancies can be safely and successfully treated with transnasal endoscopic resection. However, there was a quite striking difference in the distribution of tumor local extent and histology, with olfactory neuroblastoma and squamous cell carcinoma being the most frequent histotype in the endoscopic and craniofacial resection groups, respectively. Devaiah and Andreoli[83] performed a meta-analysis on 361 patients treated from 1992 to 2008 for olfactory neuroblastoma. Although endoscopic surgery yielded statistically significant better survival rates than open surgery, the results must be interpreted with caution due to the differences in follow-up times and Kadish stage distribution between the two groups. Finally, we maintain that a precise comparison between the results obtained with endoscopic surgery and craniofacial resection is unreliable because of the heterogeneous composition of patient series in terms of histology, stage, and follow-up time.

However, when evaluating long-term outcomes on the whole, endoscopic approaches should be comparable, on one hand, with traditional external techniques such as midfacial degloving or lateral rhinotomy for tumors not reaching the anterior skull base and, on the other, with craniofacial resection for tumors in contact with or transpassing the anterior skull base.[9]

The absence of facial incisions and osteotomies, less postoperative pain, decreased hospitalization time, improved visualization of tumor borders, and reduced morbidity and mortality rate are commonly cited as the major advantages of endoscopic surgery compared with the external approach. Furthermore, when resection of the skull base is performed transnasally, retraction on the frontal lobes with the ensuing possible complications is avoided. On the other hand, as shown in our series as well, resection of the dura and the consequent duraplasty increase the likelihood of CSF leak.

Conclusion

In conclusion, although our series, as well the other experiences reported in the literature, suffers from some limitations (i.e., histological heterogeneity and limited cohort of cases due to the rarity of these lesions), the 5-year overall and disease-specific survival rates seem to indicate that endoscopic surgery (alone or combined with adjuvant treatment), when properly planned and performed by experienced surgeons, may be an effective alternative to standard approaches in the management of selected malignancies of the sinonasal tract.[9] Therefore, the endoscopic approach has nowadays acquired an accepted role with precise indications in the whole armamentarium available for the treatment of sinonasal and skull base malignancies, and has to be considered one of the therapeutic options, together with the other surgical approaches and radiochemotherapy, in a perspective of an oncologic multimodal therapy capable of achieving radical and complete treatment of the pathology, while minimizing the morbidity for the patient.

However, changes in clinical practice should be rooted in methodologically sound evidence. At the moment, the levels of evidence in endoscopic tumor surgery are mainly level 3 (case series) and level 4 (expert opinion). In the next decade, we need to reach higher levels of evidence. For this purpose, the first step has been the setting up of a large database of cases with benign and malignant sinonasal and skull base tumors, to collect the clinical history of the patient, the imaging data, the pathological findings, and the kind of surgical management and postoperative treatment.[22] The website permits the collection of large series of patients, particularly of rare neoplasms, which will increase our knowledge of their biological behavior. The final step will be to perform collaborative, multicenter, randomized, controlled trials to compare the endoscopic approach with the conventional one in the management of benign and malignant sinonasal and skull base tumors.[22] This is a unique opportunity for an international and interdisciplinary collaboration that will result in benefits for a wide range of patients affected by sinonasal and skull base tumors.

In fact, there are still open issues and questions, which could and should be answered. Longer follow-ups are needed to provide meaningful information on the outcome of those tumors that can relapse well beyond the usual 5-year period. Stratification of survival data by histology and stage is required to have a better understanding of the impact that these variables have on outcome. The role of adjuvant therapies (radiotherapy, chemotherapy, biological modifiers) also needs to be explored with the intent of identifying patients that can benefit from these therapies, thus avoiding overtreatment in those with a less aggressive disease. Tailoring target-treatment can be aided by expanding the study of specific biological markers. Prospective quality-of-life evaluation should also be included in the pre- and posttreatment assessment of patients.

Pearls and Pitfalls

- Unilateral nasal obstruction is the most common presentation of both benign and malignant sinonasal tumors. This complaint should never be neglected and the presence of a tumor should be ruled out.
- In patients with suspected sinonasal tumors the use of contrast-enhanced CT and MRI is standard.
- Inverted papillomas, osteomas, and JNAs are the most frequent benign tumors.
- Adenocarcinoma, esthesioneuroblastoma, squamous cell carcinoma, adenoid cystic carcinoma, and malignant melanoma are the most frequent malignancies for which an endoscopic surgery is indicated.
- The overall complication rate in our series was 13.1% (8.8% in the endoscopic approach group and 31.6% in the combined cranioendoscopic approach group).
- The most frequent major complication in our series was CSF leak, with a prevalence of 4.6%. A recent analysis, performed by our group on a subset of patients who underwent endoscopic removal of tumor with dural resection, showed that the occurrence of CSF leak is clearly related to the learning curve of the surgical team and to the refinement of surgical techniques.
- The 5-year disease-specific survival rates in patients treated with endoscopic surgery alone and those who received cranioendoscopic resection were 87.2 versus 63%.

- The 5-year recurrence-free survival rates were 72.7 and 48.8% for the endoscopic surgery and cranioendoscopic resection groups, respectively.
- There are some general contraindications for endoscopic approaches in both benign and malignant tumors: massive involvement of the lacrimal pathways, extension of the lesion to the maxillary sinus walls (except the medial one), to the orbital soft tissues, to the superior and lateral part of the frontal sinus, and to the floor of the nasal cavity (i.e., hard palate), and involvement of the brain.
- Similar to external approaches, advanced malignant pathologies following endoscopic surgery require adjuvant treatment (radiotherapy with or without chemotherapy).

References

[1] Draf W. Endonasal frontal sinus drainage type I–III according to Draf. In: Kountakis S, Senior B, Draf W, eds. The Frontal Sinus. Berlin Heidelberg New York: Springer; 2005:219–232

[2] Kaplan E, Meier P. Nonparametric estimation from incomplete observations. Journal of the American Statistical Association 1958; 53: 457–481

[3] Cox D. Regression models and life tables (with discussion). J R Stat Soc, B 1972; 34: 187–220

[4] Barnes L, Eveson JW, Reichart P, Sidransky D. World Health Organization Classification of Tumours: Pathology and Genetics Head and Neck Tumours. Lyon, France: IARC; 2005

[5] Nicolai P, Villaret AB, Bottazzoli M, Rossi E, Valsecchi MG. Ethmoid adenocarcinoma—from craniofacial to endoscopic resections: a single-institution experience over 25 years. Otolaryngol Head Neck Surg 2011; 145: 330–337

[6] Cantu G, Solero CL, Mariani L et al. Intestinal type adenocarcinoma of the ethmoid sinus in wood and leather workers: a retrospective study of 153 cases. Head Neck 2011; 33: 535–542

[7] Nicolai P, Battaglia P, Bignami M et al. Endoscopic surgery for malignant tumors of the sinonasal tract and adjacent skull base: a 10-year experience. Am J Rhinol 2008; 22: 308–316

[8] Bogaerts S, Vander Poorten V, Nuyts S, Van den Bogaert W, Jorissen M. Results of endoscopic resection followed by radiotherapy for primarily diagnosed adenocarcinomas of the paranasal sinuses. Head Neck 2008; 30: 728–736

[9] Nicolai P, Castelnuovo P, Bolzoni Villaret A. Endoscopic resection of sinonasal malignancies. Curr Oncol Rep 2011; 13: 138–144

[10] Ganly I, Patel SG, Singh B et al. Craniofacial resection for malignant tumors involving the skull base in the elderly: an international collaborative study. Cancer 2011; 117: 563–571

[11] Shah JP, Sundaresan N, Galicich J, Strong EW. Craniofacial resections for tumors involving the base of the skull. Am J Surg 1987; 154: 352–358

[12] Harvey RJ, Dalgorf DM. Chapter 10: Sinonasal malignancies. Am J Rhinol Allergy 2013; 27 Suppl 1: S35–S38

[13] van der Laan TP, Bij HP, van Hemel BM et al. The importance of multimodality therapy in the treatment of sinonasal neuroendocrine carcinoma. Eur Arch Otorhinolaryngol 2013; 270: 2565–2568

[14] Chi A, Nguyen NP, Tse W, Sobremonte G, Concannon P, Zhu A. Intensity modulated radiotherapy for sinonasal malignancies with a focus on optic pathway preservation. J Hematol Oncol 2013; 6: 4–8

[15] Patel SG, Singh B, Polluri A et al. Craniofacial surgery for malignant skull base tumors: report of an international collaborative study. Cancer 2003; 98: 1179–1187

[16] Shah JP, Kraus DH, Bilsky MH, Gutin PH, Harrison LH, Strong EW. Craniofacial resection for malignant tumors involving the anterior skull base. Arch Otolaryngol Head Neck Surg 1997; 123: 1312–1317

[17] Suarez C, Llorente JL, Fernandez De Leon R, Maseda E, Lopez A. Prognostic factors in sinonasal tumors involving the anterior skull base. Head Neck 2004; 26: 136–144

[18] Ganly I, Patel SG, Singh B et al. Craniofacial resection for malignant paranasal sinus tumors: Report of an International Collaborative Study. Head Neck 2005; 27: 575–584

[19] Bockmühl U. Malignant tumors of the paranasal sinuses and the anterior skull base. In: Anniko M, Bernal-Sprekelsen M, Bonkowsky V, Bradley P, Iurato S, eds. Otorhinolaryngology, Head and Neck Surgery. Berlin Heidelberg New York: Springer; 2010:297–305

[20] Eloy JA, Vivero RJ, Hoang K et al. Comparison of transnasal endoscopic and open craniofacial resection for malignant tumors of the anterior skull base. Laryngoscope 2009; 119: 834–840

[21] Hanna E, DeMonte F, Ibrahim S, Roberts D, Levine N, Kupferman M. Endoscopic resection of sinonasal cancers with and without craniotomy: oncologic results. Arch Otolaryngol Head Neck Surg 2009; 135: 1219–1224

[22] Lund VJ, Stammberger H, Nicolai P et al. European Rhinologic Society Advisory Board on Endoscopic Techniques in the Management of Nose, Paranasal Sinus and Skull Base Tumours. European Position Paper on Endoscopic Management of Tumours of the Nose, Paranasal Sinuses and Skull Base. Rhinol Suppl 2010: 1–143

[23] Bockmühl U, Minovi A, Kratzsch B, Hendus J, Draf W. Stellenwert der Endonasalen micro-endoscopic tumor surgery: state of the art [in German]. Laryngorhinootologie 2005; 84: 884–891

[24] Castelnuovo P, Dallan I, Battaglia P, Bignami M. Endoscopic endonasal skull base surgery: past, present and future. Eur Arch Otorhinolaryngol 2010; 267: 649–663

[25] Snyderman CH, Pant H, Carrau RL, Prevedello D, Gardner P, Kassam AB. What are the limits of endoscopic sinus surgery?: the expanded endonasal approach to the skull base. Keio J Med 2009; 58: 152–160Review

[26] Strek P, Zagólski O, Składzień J, Kurzyński M, Dyduch G. Osteomas of the paranasal sinuses: surgical treatment options. Med Sci Monit 2007; 13: CR244–CR250

[27] Mugliston TA, Stafford NJ. A cranio-facial approach to large osteomas of the fronto-ethmoidal region. J Laryngol Otol 1985; 99: 979–983

[28] Dubin MG, Kuhn FA. Preservation of natural frontal sinus outflow in the management of frontal sinus osteomas. Otolaryngol Head Neck Surg 2006; 134: 18–24

[29] Busch RF. Frontal sinus osteoma: complete removal via endoscopic sinus surgery and frontal sinus trephination. Am J Rhinol 1992; 4: 139–143

[30] Bignami M, Dallan I, Terranova P, Battaglia P, Miceli S, Castelnuovo P. Frontal sinus osteomas: the window of endonasal endoscopic approach. Rhinology 2007; 45: 315–320

[31] Schick B, Steigerwald C, el Rahman el Tahan A, Draf W. The role of endonasal surgery in the management of frontoethmoidal osteomas. Rhinology 2001; 39: 66–70

[32] Chiu AG, Schipor I, Cohen NA, Kennedy DW, Palmer JN. Surgical decisions in the management of frontal sinus osteomas. Am J Rhinol 2005; 19: 191–197

[33] Seiberling K, Floreani S, Robinson S, Wormald PJ. Endoscopic management of frontal sinus osteomas revisited. Am J Rhinol Allergy 2009; 23: 331–336

[34] Ledderose GJ, Betz CS, Stelter K, Leunig A. Surgical management of osteomas of the frontal recess and sinus: extending the limits of the endoscopic approach. Eur Arch Otorhinolaryngol 2011; 268: 525–532

[35] Georgalas C, Goudakos J, Fokkens WJ. Osteoma of the skull base and sinuses. Otolaryngol Clin North Am 2011; 44: 875–890, vii

[36] Castelnuovo P, Giovannetti F, Bignami M, Ungari C, Iannetti G. Open surgery versus endoscopic surgery in benign neoplasm involving the frontal sinus. J Craniofac Surg 2009; 20: 180–183

[37] Calcaterra TC, Thompson JW, Paglia DE. Inverting papillomas of the nose and paranasal sinuses. Laryngoscope 1980; 90: 53–60

[38] Vrabec DP. The inverted Schneiderian papilloma: a 25-year study. Laryngoscope 1994; 104: 582–605

[39] Tanna N, Edwards JD, Aghdam H, Sadeghi N. Transnasal endoscopic medial maxillectomy as the initial oncologic approach to sinonasal neoplasms: the anatomic basis. Arch Otolaryngol Head Neck Surg 2007; 133: 1139–1142

[40] Yoon BN, Batra PS, Citardi MJ, Roh HJ. Frontal sinus inverted papilloma: surgical strategy based on the site of attachment. Am J Rhinol Allergy 2009; 23: 337–341

[41] Chen C, Selva D, Wormald PJ. Endoscopic modified lothrop procedure: an alternative for frontal osteoma excision. Rhinology 2004; 42: 239–243

[42] Krouse JH. Development of a staging system for inverted papilloma. Laryngoscope 2000; 110: 965–968

[43] Tomenzoli D, Castelnuovo P, Pagella F et al. Different endoscopic surgical strategies in the management of inverted papilloma of the sinonasal tract: experience with 47 patients. Laryngoscope 2004; 114: 193–200

[44] Lombardi D, Tomenzoli D, Buttà L et al. Limitations and complications of endoscopic surgery for treatment for sinonasal inverted papilloma: A reassessment after 212 cases. Head Neck 2011; 33: 1154–1161

[45] Mansell NJ, Bates GJ. The inverted Schneiderian papilloma: a review and literature report of 43 new cases. Rhinology 2000; 38: 97–101

[46] Yamaguchi KT, Shapshay SM, Incze JS, Vaughan CW, Strong MS. Inverted papilloma and squamous cell carcinoma. J Otolaryngol 1979; 8: 171–178

[47] Mirza S, Bradley PJ, Acharya A, Stacey M, Jones NS. Sinonasal inverted papillomas: recurrence, and synchronous and metachronous malignancy. J Laryngol Otol 2007; 121: 857–864

[48] Landsberg R. Attachment-oriented endoscopic surgical approach for sinonasal inverted papilloma. Oper Tech Otolaryngol Head Neck Surg 2006; 17: 87–96

[49] Lund VJ. Optimum management of inverted papilloma. J Laryngol Otol 2000; 114: 194–197

[50] Bielamowicz S, Calcaterra TC, Watson D. Inverting papilloma of the head and neck: the UCLA update. Otolaryngol Head Neck Surg 1993; 109: 71–76

[51] Lawson W, Patel ZM. The evolution of management for inverted papilloma: an analysis of 200 cases. Otolaryngol Head Neck Surg 2009; 140: 330–335

[52] Minovi A, Kollert M, Draf W, Bockmühl U. Inverted papilloma: feasibility of endonasal surgery and long-term results of 87 cases. Rhinology 2006; 44: 205–210

[53] Von Buchwald C, Larsen AS. Endoscopic surgery of inverted papillomas under image guidance—a prospective study of 42 consecutive cases at a Danish university clinic. Otolaryngol Head Neck Surg 2005; 132: 602–607

[54] Busquets JM, Hwang PH. Endoscopic resection of sinonasal inverted papilloma: a meta-analysis. Otolaryngol Head Neck Surg 2006; 134: 476–482

[55] Kamel RH. Transnasal endoscopic surgery in juvenile nasopharyngeal angiofibroma. J Laryngol Otol 1996; 110: 962–968

[56] Nicolai P, Villaret AB, Farina D et al. Endoscopic surgery for juvenile angiofibroma: a critical review of indications after 46 cases. Am J Rhinol Allergy 2010; 24: e67–e72

[57] Kuppersmith RB, Teh BS, Donovan DT et al. The use of intensity modulated radiotherapy for the treatment of extensive and recurrent juvenile angiofibroma. Int J Pediatr Otorhinolaryngol 2000; 52: 261–268

[58] Reddy KA, Mendenhall WM, Amdur RJ, Stringer SP, Cassisi NJ. Long-term results of radiation therapy for juvenile nasopharyngeal angiofibroma. Am J Otolaryngol 2001; 22: 172–175

[59] Andrews JC, Fisch U, Valavanis A, Aeppli U, Makek MS. The surgical management of extensive nasopharyngeal angiofibromas with the infratemporal fossa approach. Laryngoscope 1989; 99: 429–437

[60] Roberson GH, Biller H, Sessions DG, Ogura JH. Presurgical internal maxillary artery embolization in juvenile angiofibroma. Laryngoscope 1972; 82: 1524–1532

[61] Glad H, Vainer B, Buchwald C et al. Juvenile nasopharyngeal angiofibromas in Denmark 1981–2003: diagnosis, incidence, and treatment. Acta Otolaryngol 2007; 127: 292–299

[62] Casasco A, Houdart E, Biondi A et al. Major complications of percutaneous embolization of skull-base tumors. AJNR Am J Neuroradiol 1999; 20: 179–181

[63] Sanna M, Khrais T, Menozi R, Piaza P. Surgical removal of jugular paragangliomas after stenting of the intratemporal internal carotid artery: a preliminary report. Laryngoscope 2006; 116: 742–746

[64] Lloyd G, Howard D, Phelps P, Cheesman A. Juvenile angiofibroma: the lessons of 20 years of modern imaging. J Laryngol Otol 1999; 113: 127–134

[65] Schick B, el Rahman el Tahan A, Brors D, Kahle G, Draf W. Experiences with endonasal surgery in angiofibroma. Rhinology 1999; 37: 80–85

[66] Wormald PJ, Van Hasselt A. Endoscopic removal of juvenile angiofibromas. Otolaryngol Head Neck Surg 2003; 129: 684–691

[67] Gupta AK, Rajiniganth MG, Gupta AK. Endoscopic approach to juvenile nasopharyngeal angiofibroma: our experience at a tertiary care centre. J Laryngol Otol 2008; 122: 1185–1189

[68] Muñoz del Castillo F, Jurado Ramos A, Bravo-Rodríguez F, Delgado Acosta F, López Villarejo P. [Endoscopic surgery of nasopharyngeal angiofibroma] Acta Otorrinolaringol Esp 2004; 55: 369–375

[69] Howard DJ, Lloyd G, Lund V. Recurrence and its avoidance in juvenile angiofibroma. Laryngoscope 2001; 111: 1509–1511

[70] Kania RE, Sauvaget E, Guichard JP, Chapot R, Huy PT, Herman P. Early postoperative CT scanning for juvenile nasopharyngeal angiofibroma: detection of residual disease. AJNR Am J Neuroradiol 2005; 26: 82–88

[71] Onerci M, Oğretmenoğlu O, Yücel T. Juvenile nasopharyngeal angiofibroma: a revised staging system. Rhinology 2006; 44: 39–45

[72] Spielmann PM, Adamson R, Cheng K, Sanderson RJ. Juvenile nasopharyngeal angiofibroma: spontaneous resolution. Ear Nose Throat J 2008; 87: 521–523

[73] Gullane PJ, Davidson J, O'Dwyer T, Forte V. Juvenile angiofibroma: a review of the literature and a case series report. Laryngoscope 1992; 102: 928–933

[74] Danesi G, Panciera DT, Harvey RJ, Agostinis C. Juvenile nasopharyngeal angiofibroma: evaluation and surgical management of advanced disease. Otolaryngol Head Neck Surg 2008; 138: 581–586

[75] Ketcham AS, Wilkins RH, Vanburen JM, Smith RR. A combined intracranial facial approach to the paranasal sinuses. Am J Surg 1963; 106: 698–703

[76] Ong YK, Solares CA, Carrau RL, Snyderman CH. New developments in transnasal endoscopic surgery for malignancies of the sinonasal tract and adjacent skull base. Curr Opin Otolaryngol Head Neck Surg 2010; 18: 107–113

[77] Thaler ER, Kotapka M, Lanza DC, Kennedy DW. Endoscopically assisted anterior cranial skull base resection of sinonasal tumors. Am J Rhinol 1999; 13: 303–310

[78] Stammberger H, Anderhuber W, Walch C, Papaefthymiou G. Possibilities and limitations of endoscopic management of nasal and paranasal sinus malignancies. Acta Otorhinolaryngol Belg 1999; 53: 199–205

[79] Villaret AB, Yakirevitch A, Bizzoni A et al. Endoscopic transnasal craniectomy in the management of selected sinonasal malignancies. Am J Rhinol Allergy 2010; 24: 60–65

[80] Nicolai P, Castelnuovo P, Lombardi D et al. Role of endoscopic surgery in the management of selected malignant epithelial neoplasms of the naso-ethmoidal complex. Head Neck 2007; 29: 1075–1082

[81] Folbe A, Herzallah I, Duvvuri U et al. Endoscopic endonasal resection of esthesioneuroblastoma: a multicenter study. Am J Rhinol Allergy 2009; 23: 91–94

[82] Jardeleza C, Seiberling K, Floreani S, Wormald PJ. Surgical outcomes of endoscopic management of adenocarcinoma of the sinonasal cavity. Rhinology 2009; 47: 354–361

[83] Devaiah AK, Andreoli MT. Treatment of esthesioneuroblastoma: a 16-year meta-analysis of 361 patients. Laryngoscope 2009; 119: 1412–1416

Index

Note: Page numbers set **bold** or *italic* indicate headings or figures, respectively.